	DSA	Digital subtraction angiography
	DST	Dexamethasone suppression test
E	EBV	Epstein-Barr virus
	ECG, EKG	Electrocardiogram
	ECHO	Echocardiography
	EEG	Electroencephalogram
	EGD	Esophagogastroduodenoscopy
	ELISA	Enzyme-linked immunosorbent assay
	EMG	Electromyography
	ENG	Electroneurography
	EP	Evoked potential
	EPS	Electrophysiologic study
	ER	Estrogen receptor
	ERCP	Endoscopic retrograde cholangiopancreatography
	ESR	Erythrocyte sedimentation rate
	EUG	Excretory urography
F	FBS	Fasting blood sugar
	FDPs	Fibrin degradation products
	Fe	Iron
	FSH	Follicle-stimulating hormone
	FSPs	Fibrin split products
	FTA-ABS	Fluorescent treponemal antibody absorption test
	FTI	Free thyroxine index
G	G-6-PD	Glucose-6-phosphate dehydrogenase
	GB series	Gallbladder series
	GE reflux	Gastroesophageal reflux scan
	GGT	Gamma-glutamyl transferase
	GGTP	Gamma-glutamyl transpeptidase
	GH	Growth hormone
	GHb, GHB	Glycosylated hemoglobin
	GI series	Gastrointestinal series
	GTT	Glucose tolerance test
H	HAA	Hepatitis-associated antigen
	HAI	Hemagglutination inhibition
	HAV	Hepatitis A virus
	Hb, Hgb	Hemoglobin
	HB_cAb	Hepatitis B core antibody
	HB_cAg	Hepatitis B core antigen
	HBV	Hepatitis B virus
	HCG	Human chorionic gonadotropin
	HCO_3^-	Bicarbonate
	Hct	Hematocrit
	HDL	High-density lipoprotein

5
F
H   virus
F   B27

ued on inside back cover

Mosby's
Diagnostic
and Laboratory
Test Reference

Mosby's
Diagnostic
and Laboratory
Test Reference

Fourth Edition

Kathleen Deska Pagana, PhD, RN

Professor
Department of Nursing
Lycoming College
Williamsport, Pennsylvania

Timothy James Pagana, MD, FACS

Surgical Oncologist
Williamsport, Pennsylvania

Illustrated

 Mosby

St. Louis Baltimore Boston Carlsbad
Chicago Minneapolis New York Philadelphia Portland
London Milan Sydney Tokyo Toronto

Mosby

Dedicated to Publishing Excellence

**A Times Mirror
Company**

Publisher: Nancy L. Coon
Editor: Loren S. Wilson
Editor: Brian Dennison
Project Manager: Deborah Vogel
Project Specialist: Mary E. Drone
Designer: Bill Drone
Manufacturing Supervisor: Don Carlisle
Cover Art: Teresa Breckwoldt

FOURTH EDITION

Copyright © 1999 by Mosby, Inc.

Previous editions copyrighted 1992, 1995, 1997

Composition by Graphic World, Inc.
Lithography/color film by Graphic World, Inc.
Printing/binding by R. R. Donnelley & Sons Company

Mosby, Inc.
11830 Westline Industrial Drive
St. Louis, Missouri 63146

Library of Congress Cataloging in Publication Data

Pagana, Kathleen Deska, 1952-
    Mosby's diagnostic and laboratory test reference / Kathleen Deska Pagana, Timothy James Pagana. — 1999-2000 ed.
      p.   cm.
    Includes bibliographical references and index.
    ISBN 0-323-00288-9
    1. Diagnosis, Laboratory—Handbooks, manuals, etc.   2. Nursing—Handbooks, manuals, etc.   I. Pagana, Timothy James, 1949-   .   II. Title.
    [DNLM: 1. Laboratory Techniques and Procedures handbooks.
2. Nursing Care handbooks.   QY 39P128m 1998]
    RB38.2.P337   1998
    616.07'5—dc21
    DNLM/DLC
    for Library of Congress   98-27246
                                             CIP

98 99 00 01 02 / 9 8 7 6 5 4 3 2 1

We lovingly dedicate this book to our daughters

Jocelyn Marie Pagana

Denise Kathleen Pagana

Theresa Noel Pagana

Mosby's Diagnostic and Laboratory Test Reference provides the user with an up-to-date, essential reference that allows easy access to clinically relevant laboratory and diagnostic tests. A unique feature of this handbook is its consistent format, which allows for quick reference without sacrificing the depth of detail necessary for a thorough understanding of diagnostic and laboratory testing. All tests begin on a new page and are listed in alphabetical order by their complete name. The alphabetical format is a strong feature of the book; it allows the user to locate tests quickly without having to place them in an appropriate category or body system. The User's Guide to Test Preparation and Procedures delineates the responsibilities for health care providers to ensure that the tests are accurately and safely performed. This guide should eliminate test repetition because of problems in patient preparation, test procedures, and/or collection techniques. Every feature of this book is geared to provide pertinent information in a sequence that best simulates priorities in the clinical setting.

The following information is provided, whenever possible, for effective diagnostic and laboratory testing.

Name of test. Tests are listed by their complete name. A complete list of abbreviations and alternate test names follows each main entry.

Type of test. This section identifies whether the test is, for example, an x-ray procedure, ultrasound, nuclear scan, blood test, urine test, sputum test, or microscopic examination of tissue. This section helps the reader identify the source of the laboratory specimen or location of the diagnostic procedure.

Normal findings. When applicable, normal values are listed for the infant, child, adult, and elderly person. Also, when appropriate, values are separated into male and female. It is important to realize that normal ranges of laboratory tests vary from institution to institution. This variability is even more obvious among the various laboratory textbooks. For this reason, we have deliberately chosen *not* to add a table of normal values as an appendix, and we encourage the user to check the normal values at the institution where the test is performed. This should be relatively easy, since most laboratory reports include normal values.

Possible critical values. These values give an indication of results that are well outside the usual range of normal. These results generally require immediate intervention.

Test explanation and related physiology. This section provides a concise, yet comprehensive description of each test. It includes fundamental information about the test itself, specific indications for the test, how the test is performed, what disease or disorder the various results may show, how it will affect the patient or client, and relevant pathophysiology that will enhance understanding of the test.

Contraindications. These data are crucial because they alert the user to patients who should not have the test. Patients frequently highlighted in this section include those who are pregnant, are allergic to iodinated or contrast dyes, or have bleeding disorders.

Potential complications. This section alerts the user to potential problems that will necessitate astute assessments and interventions. For example, if a potential complication is renal failure, the implication may be to hydrate the patient before the test and force fluids after the test. A typical potential complication for many x-ray procedures is allergy to iodinated dye. Patient symptoms and appropriate interventions are described in detail.

Interfering factors. This section contains pertinent information because many factors can invalidate the test or make the test results unreliable. An important feature of this section is the inclusion of drugs that can interfere with test results. Drugs that increase or decrease test values are always listed at the end of this section for consistency and quick access. A drug symbol (𝕩) is used to emphasize these drug interferences.

Procedure and patient care. This section emphasizes the role of nurses and other health care providers in diagnostic and laboratory testing by addressing psychosocial and physiologic interventions. Patient education and rationales are included. For quick access to essential information, this section is divided into *before, during,* and *after* time sequences.

Before. This section addresses the need to explain the procedure and to allay patient concerns or anxieties. If a consent is usually required, this is listed as a bulleted item in this section. Other important features of this section include requirements such as fasting, obtaining baseline values, and performing bowel preparations.

During. This section gives specific directions for clinical specimen studies (e.g., urine and blood studies). An estimate of approximate amount of a specimen is sometimes given; wever, this amount may vary from institution to institution. gnostic procedures and their variations are described in a nbered, usually step-by-step format. Important information h as who performs the test, where the study is performed, ient sensation, and duration of the procedure is bulleted for phasis. The duration of the procedure is very helpful for ient teaching because it indicates the time generally allotted each study.

After. This section includes vital information that the nurse or er health care provider should heed or convey following the . Examples include factors such as maintaining bed rest, nparing pulses with baseline values, encouraging fluids, and erving for signs and symptoms of sepsis.

Home care responsibilities. These boxes are new to this tion. They were added in response to the increasing emphasis early discharge and outpatient testing. As a result, patients l their families have the responsibility for detecting potential -related problems in the home setting. The boxes emphasize areas for assessment and provide instructions for what to do en problems are detected.

Abnormal findings. As the name implies, this section lists the normal findings for each study. Increased or decreased values listed when appropriate.

Notes. This blank space at the end of the tests facilitates ividualizing the studies according to the institution per- ming the test. Variations in any area of the test (e.g., patient paration, test procedure, normal values, or postprocedural e) can be noted.

This logical format emphasizes clinically relevant information; clarity of this format will facilitate a quick understanding of ntent essential to both students and health care providers. lor has been used to help locate tests and highlight critical ormation (e.g., possible critical values). Color is also used in numerous illustrations that are included to enhance the der's understanding of many diagnostic procedures (e.g., nchoscopy, fetoscopy, ERCP, pericardiocentesis, TEE). Many les are used to simplify complex material on topics such as oimmune diseases, hepatitis testing, and protein electro- resis. Extensive cross-referencing exists throughout the book t permits full understanding and helps the user tie together or ate related studies such as those on the cardiac enzymes PK, LDH, AST).

For easy access, a listing of abbreviations for test name included on the book's endpapers. Appendix A includes a lis studies according to *body systems*. This listing may familia the user with other related studies the patient or client may n or the user may want to review. This should be especially use for students and health care providers working in speciali areas. Appendix B provides a listing of studies according to type. This listing may help the user read and learn about simil performed tests and procedures (e.g., x-rays of the skull, ch and abdomen). Appendix C provides a list of typical abbre tions and units of measurement. Finally, a comprehensive in includes the names of all tests and their synonyms and any ot relevant terms found within the tests.

Many new studies such as bone densitometry, genetic testi octreotide nuclear scanning and sleep apnea studies have b added. All other studies have been revised and upda Outdated studies have been eliminated.

We sincerely thank our editors for their enthusiasm continual support. We are most grateful to the many stude nurses, and other health care providers who made the first th editions of this book so successful. This success validated need for a user-friendly and quick reference approach laboratory and diagnostic testing.

We invite additional comments from users of this book so t we may continue to provide useful, relevant diagnostic laboratory test information to users of future editions.

Kathleen D. Pagara

T.J. Pagana

Contents

Health care economics demand that laboratory and diagnostic testing be performed accurately and in the least amount of time possible. Tests should not have to be repeated because of problems in patient preparation, test procedure, and/or specimen collection technique. The following guidelines delineate the responsibilities for health care providers to ensure safety for test procedures and accuracy in test results. Guidelines are described for the following major types of tests: blood, urine, stool, x-ray, nuclear scanning, ultrasound, and endoscopy.

Blood tests

Overview

Blood studies are used to assess a multitude of body processes and disorders. Common studies include enzymes, serum lipids, electrolyte levels, red and white blood cell counts, clotting factors, hormone levels, and levels of breakdown products such as blood urea nitrogen.

Multiphasic screening machines can perform many blood tests quickly and simultaneously using a very small blood sample. An example of this is the *sequential multiple analyzer* (SMA), which is the name of one instrument used for automatically testing a specific group of tests. For example, an SMA-12 performs twelve tests. Another example is the Chem-7, which performs seven chemistry studies. The advantage of these machines is that results are available quickly and the cost is cheaper when compared to individually performing each test.

Guidelines

- Observe universal precautions in collecting a blood specimen.
- Check whether fasting is required. Many studies, such as fasting blood sugar and cholesterol levels, require fasting for a designated time.
- If ordered, withhold medications until the blood is drawn.
- Note the time of day that the blood test is drawn. Some blood test results (such as those for cortisol) vary according to a diurnal pattern, and this must be considered when blood levels are interpreted.
- Note the patient's position for certain tests. For example, renin levels are affected by body position.

- Collect the blood in the proper color-coded test tube. Blood collection tubes have color-coded stoppers to indicate the presence or absence of different types of additives (preservatives and anticoagulants). A preservative prevents change in the specimen, and an anticoagulant inhibits clot formation or coagulation. Charts are available from the laboratory indicating the type of tube needed for each particular blood test.
- Follow the recommended "order of draw" when collecting tubes. Draw specimens into nonadditive tubes (e.g., red-top) before drawing them into tubes with additives. Fill the tubes in the following order:
  1. Blood culture tubes (to maintain sterility)
  2. Nonadditive tubes (e.g., red-top)
  3. Coagulation tubes (e.g., blue-top)
  4. Heparin tubes (e.g., green-top)
  5. Ethylenediaminetetraacetic acid–K3 (EDTA-K3) tubes (e.g., lavender-top)
  6. Oxalate/fluoride tubes (e.g., gray-top)
- To obtain valid results, do not fasten the tourniquet for longer than 1 minute. Prolonged tourniquet application can cause stasis and hemoconcentration.
- Collect the blood specimen from the arm without an intravenous (IV) device, if possible. IV infusion can influence test results.
- Do not use the arm bearing a dialysis arteriovenous fistula for venipuncture unless the physician specifically authorizes it.
- Because of the risk of cellulitis, do not take specimens from the side on which a mastectomy or axillary lymph node dissection was performed.
- Follow the unit guidelines for drawing blood from an indwelling venous catheter such as a triple-lumen catheter. Guidelines will specify the amount of blood to be drawn from the catheter and discarded before blood is collected for laboratory studies. The guidelines will also indicate the amount and type of solution needed to flush the catheter after drawing the blood to prevent it from being clogged by blood.
- Do not shake the blood specimen. Hemolysis may result from vigorous shaking and invalidate test results.
- Collect blood cultures before the initiation of antibiotic therapy. Blood cultures are often drawn when the patient

manifests a fever. Often two or three cultures are taken at 30-minute intervals from different venipuncture sites.

- Skin punctures can be used for blood tests on capillary blood. Common puncture sites include the fingertips, earlobes, and heel surfaces. Fingertips are often used for small children, and the heel is the most commonly used site for infants.
- Record the exact time when the specimen was collected. Indicate any drugs that the patient is taking.
- Ensure that the blood tubes are correctly labeled and delivered to the laboratory.
- After the specimen is drawn, apply pressure or a pressure dressing to the venipuncture site. Assess the site for bleeding.
- If the patient fasted before the blood test, reinstitute appropriate diet.

Urine tests

Overview

Urine tests are easy to obtain and provide valuable information about many body system functions such as kidney function, glucose metabolism, and various hormone levels. The ability of the patient to obtain specimens appropriately should be assessed to determine the need for assistance.

Guidelines

- Observe universal precautions in collecting a urine specimen.
- Use the first morning specimen for routine urinalysis because it is more concentrated. To collect a first morning specimen, have the patient void before going to bed and collect the first urine specimen immediately on rising.
- *Random* urine specimens can be collected at any time. They are usually obtained during daytime hours and without any prior patient preparation.
- If a *culture and sensitivity (C&S)* study is required or if the specimen is likely to be contaminated by vaginal discharge or bleeding, collect a *clean-catch* or *midstream* specimen. This requires meticulous cleansing of the urinary meatus with an iodine preparation to reduce contamination of the specimen by external organisms. Then the cleansing agent must be completely removed, since it may contaminate the specimen. Obtain the *midstream* collection by:
  1. Having the patient begin to urinate in a bedpan, urinal, or toilet and then stop urinating (This washes the urine out of the distal urethra.)

2. Correctly positioning a sterile urine container, into which the patient voids 3 to 4 ounces of urine

3. Capping the container

4. Allowing the patient to finish voiding

- One-time *composite* urine specimens are collected over a period that may range anywhere from 2 to 24 hours. To collect a timed specimen, instruct the patient to void and discard the first specimen. This is noted as the "start time" of the test. Instruct the patient to save all subsequent urine in a special container for the designated period of time. Remind the patient to void before defecating so that urine is not contaminated by feces. Also, instruct the patient not to put toilet paper in the collection container. A preservative is usually used in the collection container. At the end of the specified time period, have the patient void and then add this urine to the specimen container, thus completing the collection process.

- Collection containers for 24-hour urine specimens should hold 3 to 4 L of urine and have tight-fitting lids. They should be labeled with the patient's name, the starting collection date and time, the ending collection date and time, the name of the test, the preservative, and storage requirements during collection.

- Many urine collections require preservatives to maintain their stability during the collection period. Some specimens are best preserved by being kept on ice or under refrigeration.

- *Urinary catheterization* may be needed for patients unable to void. This procedure is not preferred because of the risk of introducing organisms and because of patient discomfort.

- For patients with an *indwelling urinary catheter*, obtain a specimen by attaching a small-gauge (e.g., 25-gauge) needle to a syringe and aseptically inserting the needle into the catheter at a point distal to the sleeve leading to the balloon. Aspirate urine and then place it in a sterile urine container. The urine that accumulates in the plastic reservoir bag should never be used for a urine test.

- Urine specimens from infants and young children are usually collected in a disposable pouch called a *U bag*. This bag has an adhesive backing around the opening to attach to the child. Once the bag is in place, check the child every 15 minutes to see if an adequate specimen has been collected. Remove the specimen as soon as possible after the collection, and then label it and transport it to the laboratory.

- Indicate on the laboratory slip any medications that may affect test results.

Stool tests

Overview

The examination of feces provides important information that aids in the differential diagnosis of various gastrointestinal disorders. Fecal studies may also be used for microbiologic studies, chemical determinations, and parasitic examinations.

Guidelines

- Observe universal precautions in collecting a stool specimen.
- Collect stool specimens in a clean container that has a fitted cover.
- Do not mix urine and toilet paper with the stool specimen. Both can contaminate the specimen and alter the results.
- Fecal analysis for occult blood, white blood cells, or qualitative fecal fat requires only a small amount of a randomly collected specimen.
- Quantitative tests for daily fecal excretion of a particular substance require a minimum of a 3-day fecal collection. This collection is necessary because the daily excretion of feces does not correlate well with the amount of food ingested by the patient in the same 24-hour period. Refrigerate specimens or keep them on ice during the collection period. Collect stool in a 1-gallon container.
- Some fecal collections require dietary restrictions before the collection (e.g., tests for occult blood).
- A small amount of fecal blood that is not visually apparent is termed *occult blood*. Chemical tests using commercially prepared slides are routinely used to detect fecal blood. Numerous commercial slide tests use guaiac as the indicator. These guaiac tests are routinely done on nursing units in the hospital.
- Consider various factors (such as other diagnostic tests and medications) in planning the stool collection. For example, if the patient is scheduled for x-ray studies using barium sulfate, collect the stool specimen first. Various medications (e.g., tetracyclines and antidiarrheal preparations) affect the detection of intestinal parasites.
- Correctly label and deliver stool specimens to the laboratory within 30 minutes after collection. If you are unable to deliver the specimen within 30 minutes, it may be refrigerated for up to 2 hours.

X-ray studies

Overview

Because of the ability of x-rays to penetrate tissues, x-ray studies provide a valuable picture of body structures. X-ray studies can be as simple as a routine chest x-ray film or as complex as dye-enhanced cardiac catheterization. With the increasing concern about radiation exposure, it is important to realize that the patient may want to know if the proposed benefit outweighs the risks involved.

Guidelines

- Assess the patient for any similar or recent x-ray procedures.
- Evaluate the patient for allergies to iodine dye.
  1. Many types of contrast media are used in radiographic studies. For example, organic iodides and iodized oils are frequently used.
  2. Allergic reactions to iodinated dye may vary from mild flushing, itching, and urticaria to severe, life-threatening anaphylaxis (evidenced by respiratory distress, drop in blood pressure, or shock). In the unusual event of anaphylaxis, the patient is treated with diphenhydramine (Benadryl), steroids, and epinephrine. Oxygen and endotracheal equipment should be on hand for immediate use.
  3. The patient should always be assessed for allergies to iodine dye before it is administered. Inform the radiologist if an allergy to iodinated contrast is suspected. The radiologist may prescribe a Benadryl and steroid preparation to be administered before testing. Usually hypoallergenic nonionic contrast will be used during the test.
  4. After the x-ray procedure, evaluate the patient for delayed reaction to dye (e.g., dyspnea, rashes, tachycardia, hives). This usually occurs within 2 to 6 hours after the test. Treat with antihistamines or steroids.
- Women in their childbearing years should have x-ray examinations during menses or 10 to 14 days after the onset of menses to avoid possible exposure to a fetus.
- Pregnant women should not have x-ray procedures, if possible, because of the risk of damage to the fetus.
- Note if other x-ray studies are being planned; schedule them in the appropriate sequence. For example, x-ray examinations that do not require contrast should precede examinations that do require contrast. X-ray studies using barium should be scheduled after ultrasonography studies.

- Note the necessary dietary restrictions. Studies such as a barium enema and intravenous pyelogram (IVP) are more accurate if the patient is kept NPO for several hours before the test.
- Determine if bowel preparations are necessary. For example, barium enemas and IVPs require bowel-cleansing regimens.
- Determine if signed consent forms are required. These are necessary for most invasive x-ray procedures.
- Remove metal objects such as necklaces and watches because they can hinder visualization of the x-ray field.
- Patient aftercare is determined by the type of x-ray procedure. For example, a patient having a simple chest x-ray study will not require postprocedure care. However, invasive x-ray procedures involving contrast dyes (such as cardiac catheterization) require extensive nursing measures to detect potential complications.

Nuclear scanning

Overview

With the administration of a radionuclide and subsequent detection of the measurement of radiation of a particular organ, functional abnormalities of various body areas such as the brain, heart, lung, and bones can be detected. Because the half-lives of the radioisotopes are short, only minimal radiation exposure occurs.

Guidelines

- Radiopharmaceuticals concentrate in target organs by various mechanisms. For example, some labeled compounds such as hippuran are cleared from the blood and excreted by the kidneys. Some phosphate compounds concentrate in the bone and infarcted tissue. Lung function can be studied by imaging the distribution of inhaled gases or aerosols.
- Note whether the patient has had any recent exposure to radionuclides. The previous study could interfere with the interpretation of the current study.
- Note the patient's age and current weight. This information is used to calculate the amount of radioactive substance to be administered.
- Nuclear scans are contraindicated in pregnant women and nursing mothers.
- Many of the scanning procedures do not require special preparation. However, a few have special requirements.

For example, for bone scanning the patient is encouraged to drink several glasses of water between the time of the injection of the isotope and the actual scanning. For some studies, blocking agents may need to be given to prevent other organs from taking up the isotope.

- For most nuclear scans, a small amount of an organ-specific radionuclide is given orally or injected intravenously. After the radioisotope concentrates in the desired area, the area is scanned. The scanning procedure usually takes place in the nuclear medicine department.
- Instruct the patient to lie still during the scanning.
- Usually encourage the patient to drink extra fluids to enhance excretion of the radionuclide after the test is finished.
- Although the amount of radionuclide excreted in the urine is very low, rubber gloves are sometimes recommended if the urine must be handled. Some hospitals may advise the patient to flush the toilet several times after voiding.

Ultrasound studies

Overview

In diagnostic ultrasonography, harmless high-frequency sound waves are emitted and penetrate the organ being studied. The sound waves bounce back to the sensor and are electronically converted into a picture of the organ. Ultrasonography is used to assess a wide variety of body areas, including the pelvis, abdomen, heart, and pregnant uterus.

Guidelines

- Most ultrasound procedures require little or no preparation. However, the patient having a pelvic sonogram needs a full bladder, and the patient having an ultrasound examination of the gallbladder must be kept NPO before the procedure.
- Ultrasound examinations are usually performed in an ultrasound room; however, they can be performed on the patient unit.
- For ultrasound, a greasy paste is applied to the skin overlying the desired organ. This paste is used to enhance sound transmission and reception because air impedes transmission of sound waves to the body.
- Because of the noninvasive nature of ultrasonography, no special nursing measures are needed after the study except for helping the patient remove the ultrasound paste.

- Ultrasound examinations have no radiation risk.
- Ultrasound examinations can be repeated as many times as necessary without being harmful to the patient. No cumulative effect has been seen.
- Barium has an adverse effect on the quality of abdominal studies. For this reason, schedule ultrasound of the abdomen before barium studies.
- Large amounts of gas in the bowel will not permit visualization of the bowel. This is because bowel gas is a reflector of sound.

Endoscopy procedures

Overview

With the help of a lighted, flexible instrument, internal structures of many areas of the body such as the stomach, colon, joints, bronchi, urinary system, and biliary tree can be directly viewed. The specific purpose and procedure should be reviewed with the patient.

Guidelines

- Preparation for an endoscopic procedure varies with the internal structure being examined. For example, examination of the stomach (gastroscopy) will require the passage of an instrument through the esophagus to the stomach. The patient is kept NPO for 8 to 12 hours before the test to prevent gagging, vomiting, and aspiration. For colonoscopy, an instrument is passed through the rectum and into the colon. Therefore the bowel must be cleansed and free of fecal material to afford proper visualization. Arthroscopic examination of the knee joint is usually done with the patient under general anesthesia, which necessitates routine preoperative care.
- Schedule endoscopic examinations before barium studies.
- Obtain a signed consent for endoscopic procedures.
- Endoscopic procedures are preferably performed in a specially equipped endoscopy room or in the operating room by a physician. However, some kinds can safely be performed at the bedside.
- Air is instilled into the bowel during colon examinations to maintain patency of the bowel lumen and to afford better visualization. This sometimes causes gas pains.
- In addition to visualization of the desired area, special procedures can be performed. Biopsies can be obtained, and

bleeding ulcers can be cauterized. Also, knee surgery can be performed during arthroscopy.

- Specific postprocedure interventions are determined by the type of endoscopic examination performed. All procedures have the potential complication of perforation and bleeding. Most procedures use some type of sedation; safety precautions should be observed until the effects of the sedatives have worn off.

- After colonoscopy and similar studies, the patient may complain of rectal discomfort. A warm tub bath may be soothing.

- Usually keep the patient NPO for 2 hours after endoscopic procedures of the upper gastrointestinal system. Be certain that swallow, gag, and cough reflexes are present before permitting fluids or liquids to be ingested orally.

List of figures

abdominal ultrasound (Abdominal sonogram; Echogram; Ultrasound of the kidney, liver, pancreatobiliary system, gallbladder, pancreas, biliary tree)

Type of test Ultrasound

Normal findings Normal abdominal aorta, liver, gallbladder, bile ducts, pancreas, kidneys, ureters, and bladder

Test explanation and related physiology

Through the use of reflected sound waves, ultrasonography provides accurate visualization of the abdominal aorta, liver, gallbladder, pancreas, bile ducts, kidneys, ureters, and bladder. The technique of ultrasonography requires the emission of high-frequency sound waves from the transducer to penetrate the particular organ being studied. The sound waves are bounced back to the transducer and then electronically converted into a pictorial image (Figure 1). Real-time ultrasound provides an accurate picture of the organ being studied. Doppler ultrasound provides information concerning blood flow to those organs.

The *kidney* is ultrasonographically evaluated to diagnose and locate renal cysts, to differentiate renal cysts from solid renal tumors, to demonstrate renal and pelvic calculi, to document hydronephrosis, and to guide a percutaneously inserted needle for cyst aspiration or biopsy. Ultrasound of the urologic tract is also used to detect malformed or ectopic kidneys and perinephric abscesses. Renal transplantation surveillance is possible per ultrasound. One advantage of a kidney sonogram over intravenous pyelography (see p. 497) is that it can be performed on patients with impaired renal function because no intravenous contrast is required.

The testes and the prostate are discussed on pp. 682 and 746.

Another use of sonography is in the assessment of the *abdominal aorta* for aneurysmal dilation. Sonographic evidence of an aortic aneurysm greater than 5 cm or any size aneurysm that is documented to be significantly enlarging is an indication for abdominal aorta aneurysm resection. Ultrasound is also an ideal way to evaluate aneurysm patients, before and after surgery.

Ultrasound is used in detecting cystic structures of the *liver*

Figure 1 Ultrasound of the abdomen.

(e.g., benign cysts, hepatic abscesses, dilated hepatic ducts) and solid intrahepatic tumors (primary and metastatic). Hepatic ultrasound can also be performed intraoperatively by using a sterile probe. This technique allows for accurate location of small, nonpalpable hepatic tumors or abscesses. The *gallbladder* and *extrahepatic ducts* can be visualized and are examined for evidence of gallstones, polyps, or dilation secondary to obstructive strictures or tumors. The *pancreas* is examined for evidence of tumor, pseudocysts, acute inflammation, chronic inflammation, or pancreatic abscess. Ultrasound of the pancreas is frequently performed serially to document and demonstrate resolution of acute pancreatic inflammatory processes.

Because this study requires no contrast material and has no associated radiation, it is especially useful in patients who are allergic to contrast and in those who are pregnant. While fasting may be preferred, it is not mandatory. (See discussion of pelvic ultrasonography [p. 623] for sonographic evaluation of pelvic organs.)

Interfering factors

- Barium or gas will distort the sound waves and alter test results. Ultrasound tests should be performed before any x-ray testing with barium.
- The accuracy of ultrasonography is very dependent on the skills of the sonographer (the technician who performs the study).

Procedure and patient care

Before

- Explain the procedure to the patient.
- Tell the patient that fasting may or may not be required depending on the organ to be examined. No fasting is required for ultrasonography of the abdominal aorta, kidney, liver, spleen, or pancreas. Fasting, however, is preferred for ultrasound of the gallbladder and biliary tree.

During

- Note the following procedural steps:
  1. The patient is placed on the ultrasonography table in the prone or supine position, depending on the organ to be studied.
  2. A greasy conductive paste is applied to the patient's skin. This paste is used to enhance sound wave transmission and reception.
  3. A transducer is placed over the skin.
  4. Pictures are taken of the reflections from the organs being studied.
- The test is completed in approximately 20 minutes, usually by an ultrasound technologist, and interpreted by a radiologist.
- Tell the patient that no discomfort is associated with the procedure.

After

- Remove the coupling agent (grease) from the patient's abdomen or back.
- Note that if a biopsy is done, refer to biopsy of the specific organ (e.g., liver or kidney biopsy).

Abnormal findings

Kidney

Renal cysts
Renal tumor
Renal calculi
Hydronephrosis
Ureteral obstruction
Perirenal abscess
Glomerulonephritis
Pyelonephritis
Perirenal hematoma

Gallbladder

Polyps
Tumor
Gallstone

Liver

Tumor
Abscess
Intrahepatic dilated bile ducts

Pancreas

Tumor
Cysts
Pseudocysts
Abscess
Inflammation

Bile ducts

Gallstone
Dilation
Stricture
Tumor

Abdominal aorta

Aneurysm

Abdominal cavity

Ascites
Abscess

acetylcholine receptor antibody (AChR Ab, Anti–acetylcholine receptor antibody)

Type of test Blood

Normal findings ≤0.03 nmol/L or negative

Test explanation and related physiology

This antibody may cause a block in neuromuscular transmission by interfering with the binding of AChR sites on the muscle membrane, thereby preventing muscle contraction. It is this phenomenon that characterizes myasthenia gravis (MG). Antibodies to AChR occur in over 85% of patients with acquired MG. Lower levels are seen in patients with only ocular MG. The presence of this antibody is virtually diagnostic of MG, but a negative test does not exclude the disease. The measured titers do not correspond well with the severity of MG in different patients. In an individual patient, however, antibody levels are particularly useful in monitoring response to therapy. As the patient improves, antibody titers decrease.

There are three different AChR antibodies that test for MG. The AChR-*binding* antibody is most commonly used. The AChR-*modulating* antibody is more sensitive. A positive modulating antibody test may indicate subclinical MG, contraindicating the use of curare-like drugs during surgery. The AChR-*blocking* antibody is the least sensitive test (positive in only 61% of patients with MG), but can be quantified more accurately.

Interfering factors

- False-positive results may occur in patients with amyotrophic lateral sclerosis who have been treated with cobra venom.
- False-positive results may be seen in patients with penicillamine-induced, myasthenia-like symptoms.
- Drugs that may cause *increased* levels include muscle paralytic medicines (succinylcholine) and snake venom.
- Immunosuppressive drugs may suppress the formation of these antibodies in patients with subclinical MG.

Procedure and patient care

Before

- Explain the procedure to the patient.
- Tell the patient that no fasting is required.

During

- Collect a venous blood sample in a red-top tube.
- List on the laboratory slip all medications that the patient has taken in the last few days.

After

- Apply pressure or a pressure dressing to the venipuncture site.
- Assess the venipuncture site for bleeding.

Abnormal findings

▲ **Increased titer levels**
    Myasthenia gravis
    Ocular myasthenia gravis
    Thymoma

notes

acid phosphatase (Prostatic acid phosphatase [PAP], Tartrate-resistant acid phosphatase [TRAP])

Type of test Blood

Normal findings
Adult/elderly: 0.11-0.60 U/L (Roy, Brower, Hayden; 37° C)
    or 0.11-0.60 U/L (SI units)
Child: 8.6-12.6 U/ml (30° C)
Newborn: 10.4-16.4 U/ml (30° C)

Test explanation and related physiology
Acid phosphatase is found in many tissues, including liver, red blood cells, bone marrow, and platelets. Highest levels are found in the prostate gland. Determination of the acid phosphatase level is primarily used to diagnose and stage prostatic carcinoma and to monitor the efficacy of treatment. Elevated levels are seen in patients with prostatic cancer that has metastasized beyond the capsule to other parts of the body, especially bone. If the tumor is successfully treated by surgery, acid phosphatase levels decrease in several days. If the tumor is treated by estrogen therapy, enzyme levels return to normal in several weeks. Rising levels of acid phosphatase may indicate a poor prognosis. The most clinically significant isoenzyme is the prostatic acid phosphatase (PAP). It is more accurate than total acid phosphatase in the prostatic cancer patient but less accurate than the prostate-specific antigen (PSA) (see p. 684).

Acid phosphatase is also found at high concentrations in seminal fluid; therefore acid phosphatase tests may be performed on vaginal secretions to investigate alleged acts of rape.

The identification of *tartrate-resistant acid phosphatase (TRAP)* is very helpful in the diagnosis of hairy-cell leukemia (and occasionally other lymphoproliferative diseases). Five percent of patients with hairy-cell leukemia are not tartrate resistant.

Interfering factors
- Alkaline and acid phosphatase are very similar enzymes that differ in the pH at which they are identified. Any condition associated with very high levels of alkaline phosphatase may falsely indicate high acid phosphatase levels.
- Falsely high levels of acid phosphatase may occur in males

after a digital examination or after instrumentation of the prostate (e.g., cystoscopy) because of prostatic stimulation.

- ☛ Drugs that may cause *elevated* levels include androgens (in females) and clofibrate (Atromid S).
- ☛ Drugs that may cause *decreased* levels include fluorides, phosphates, oxalates, and alcohol.

Procedure and patient care

Before

- Explain the procedure to the patient.
- Tell the patient that no food or drink restrictions are associated with this test.
- Remember that some laboratories request they be notified before the blood sample is drawn so that immediate attention (<1 hr) can be given to the sample.

During

- Collect approximately 5 to 10 ml of blood in a red-top tube.
- Avoid hemolysis. Red blood cells contain acid phosphatase.
- Note on the laboratory slip if the patient has had a prostatic examination or instrumentation of the prostate within the last 24 hours.

After

- Apply pressure or a pressure dressing to the venipuncture site.
- Assess the venipuncture site for bleeding.
- Have the test performed without delay or freeze the specimen.
- Do *not* leave the specimen at room temperature for 1 hour or longer, because the enzyme is heat and pH sensitive and its activity will decrease.

Abnormal findings

▲ **Increased levels**

Prostatic carcinoma	Benign prostatic hypertrophy
Multiple myeloma	Prostatitis
Paget's disease	Cancer of the breast and bone
Sickle cell crisis	Cirrhosis
Gaucher's disease	Hyperparathyroidism
Renal impairment	Thrombocytosis
Recent prostate manipulation	Cancer metastasis to the bone

adrenal venography

Type of test X-ray with contrast dye

Normal findings Normal adrenal veins and normal adrenal vein hormone assay

Test explanation and related physiology

Adrenal venography is a radiologic test performed to obtain blood samples from the adrenal vein and to detect adrenal pathology. Once the vein is identified, a catheter can be placed in the vein, and blood selectively obtained from each adrenal vein.

In patients with Cushing's syndrome, the blood is analyzed for plasma cortisol. If the plasma cortisol level in the blood obtained from one side is much higher than that of the other, a unilateral adrenal tumor is causing Cushing's syndrome. If, on the other hand, plasma cortisol levels are bilaterally elevated, one can safely conclude that Cushing's syndrome is caused by bilateral adrenal hyperplasia.

In patients with a pheochromocytoma, the adrenal venous blood is analyzed for catecholamines. If the catecholamine level on one side is much higher than that of the other, a unilateral pheochromocytoma exists on the side with the elevated levels. If blood obtained from both sides is equally elevated, the patient probably has bilateral adrenal pheochromocytoma. If the adrenal venous blood samples are not elevated on either side in a patient who has elevated peripheral blood catecholamine levels, the pheochromocytoma exists outside the adrenal gland (i.e., extra-adrenal pheochromocytoma).

Aldosterone can also be measured in blood obtained from adrenal venous sampling (see p. 31). Unilateral high aldosterone suggests unilateral adrenal gland pathology or renal artery stenosis. High unilateral renin levels with unilateral high aldosterone levels would indicate renal artery stenosis. Bilateral high levels are associated with bilateral adrenal hyperplasia. Androgens and other substances can be studied with this technique.

Contraindications

- Patients with allergies to shellfish or iodinated dye
- Patients with bleeding disorders

- Patients who are pregnant because of radiation exposure to the fetus.

Potential complications

- Allergic reaction to iodinated dye
- Hypoglycemia or acidosis may occur in patients who are taking metformin (Glucophage) and receive iodine dye.
- Adrenal hemorrhage or necrosis caused by the pressure of the dye injection; this may cause Addison's disease (adrenal insufficiency).
- Cellulitis
- Thrombophlebitis
- Bacteremia

Procedure and patient care

Before

- Explain the procedure to the patient.
- Ensure that a written and informed consent for this procedure has been obtained.
- See p. xviii for appropriate interventions concerning the care for patients with iodine allergy.
- Administer propranolol (Inderal), a beta-adrenergic blocker, and phenoxybenzamine (Dibenzyline), an alpha-adrenergic blocker, for the patient with a suspected pheochromocytoma. This prevents a potentially fatal catecholamine-induced hypertensive episode.

During

- Bring the fasting patient to the angiography laboratory (usually in the radiology department).
- Place the patient in the supine position on the x-ray table.
- Note the following procedural steps:
  1. The patient's groin is prepared and draped in a sterile manner.
  2. After the venipuncture site is locally anesthetized, the femoral vein is catheterized.
  3. The catheter is passed into the adrenal vein.
  4. Dye is injected to visualize the adrenal veins and ensure that the catheter is in the adrenal vein.
  5. Blood is obtained and sent to the chemistry laboratory for assays.
- Note that this procedure is usually performed by an angiographer (radiologist) in approximately 1 hour.

■ Tell the patient that the only discomfort is the groin puncture necessary for venous access.

After

■ Evaluate the patient's vital signs frequently for signs of bleeding or hemorrhage.
■ Assess the patient with a suspected pheochromocytoma for signs and symptoms of a hypertensive episode. If such an episode occurs, notify the physician immediately to obtain an order for appropriate alpha- and beta-adrenergic blocking agents.
■ Assess the groin site for redness, pain, swelling, and bleeding with each vital sign check.
■ Apply cold compresses to the puncture site if needed to reduce discomfort or swelling.

 Home care responsibilities

■ After the test, assess the patient for signs of bleeding (increased pulse, decreased B/P).
■ If there is a possibility of pheochromocytoma, carefully monitor the patient's B/P for a hypertensive episode.
■ Assess the groin for redness, swelling, pain, or bleeding.
■ Persons with diabetes taking metformin (Glucophage) should discontinue that medication for 48 hours after testing and monitor glucose more closely.

Abnormal findings

Unilateral adrenal tumor
Bilateral adrenal hyperplasia
Unilateral pheochromocytoma

Bilateral pheochromocytoma
Extraadrenal pheochromocytoma

notes

adrenocorticotropic hormone (ACTH, Corticotropin)

Type of test Blood

Normal findings

AM: 15-100 pg/ml or 10-80 ng/L (SI units)

PM: <50 pg/ml or <50 ng/L (SI units)

Test explanation and related physiology

The serum ACTH study is a test of anterior pituitary gland function that affords the greatest insight into the causes of either Cushing's syndrome (overproduction of cortisol) or Addison's disease (underproduction of cortisol). An elaborate feedback mechanism for cortisol exists to coordinate the function of the hypothalamus, pituitary gland, and adrenal glands. ACTH is an important part of this mechanism. Corticotropin-releasing hormone (CRH) is made in the hypothalamus. This stimulates ACTH production in the anterior pituitary gland. This, in turn, stimulates the adrenal cortex to produce cortisol. The rising levels of cortisol act as a negative feedback and curtail further production of CRH and ACTH.

In the patient with Cushing's syndrome, an elevated ACTH level can be caused by a pituitary or a nonpituitary (ectopic) ACTH-producing tumor, usually in the lung, pancreas, thymus, or ovary. ACTH levels over 200 pg/ml usually indicate ectopic ACTH production. If the ACTH level is below normal in a patient with Cushing's syndrome, an adrenal adenoma or carcinoma is probably the cause of the hyperfunction.

In patients with Addison's disease, an elevated ACTH level indicates primary adrenal gland failure, as in adrenal gland destruction caused by infarction, hemorrhage, or autoimmunity; surgical removal of the adrenal gland; congenital enzyme deficiency; or adrenal suppression after prolonged ingestion of exogenous steroids. If the ACTH level is below normal in a patient with adrenal insufficiency, hypopituitarism is most probably the cause of the hypofunction.

One must be aware that there is a diurnal variation of ACTH levels that corresponds to variation of cortisol levels. Levels in evening (8 to 10 PM) samples are usually one half to two thirds those of morning (4 to 8 AM) specimens. This diurnal variation is lost when disease (especially neoplasm) affects the pituitary or adrenal glands. Likewise, stress can blunt or eliminate this normal diurnal variation.

Interfering factors

- Stress (trauma, pyrogens, or hypoglycemia) and pregnancy can increase levels.
- Recently administered radioisotope scans can affect levels.
- Drugs that may cause *increased* levels include estrogens, ethanol, vasopressin, aminoglutethimide, amphetamines, insulin, metyrapone, and spironolactone.
- Corticosteroids may *decrease* ACTH levels.

Procedure and patient care

Before

- Explain the procedure to the patient. Allow plenty of time to answer questions so that the patient's stress is diminished as much as possible.
- Keep the patient NPO after midnight the day of the test.
- Evaluate the patient for stress factors that would invalidate the test results.
- Evaluate the patient for sleep pattern abnormalities. With a normal sleep pattern, the ACTH level is highest between 4 AM and 8 AM and lowest around 9 PM.

During

- Collect approximately 20 ml of heparinized venous blood in a green-top tube.
- Chill the blood tube to prevent enzymatic degradation of ACTH.

After

- Place the specimen in ice water and send it to the chemistry laboratory immediately. ACTH is a very unstable peptide in plasma and should be stored at −20° C to prevent artificially low values.
- Apply pressure or a pressure dressing to the venipuncture site.

Abnormal findings

▲ **Increased levels**

Addison's disease
   (primary adrenal insufficiency)
Cushing's disease
   (pituitary-dependent
   adrenal hyperplasia)
Ectopic ACTH syndrome
Stress
Adrenogenital syndrome
   (congenital adrenal
   hyperplasia)

▼ **Decreased levels**

Secondary adrenal insuffi-
   ciency (pituitary insuffi-
   ciency)
Cushing's syndrome
Hypopituitarism
Adrenal adenoma or
   carcinoma
Steroid administration

notes

adrenocorticotropic hormone stimulation test with cosyntropin (ACTH stimulation test, Cortisol stimulation test)

Type of test   Blood

Normal findings

Rapid test: cortisol levels increase more than 7 μg/dl above
    baseline
24-hour test: cortisol levels greater than 40 μg/dl
3-day test: cortisol levels greater than 40 μg/dl

Test explanation and related physiology

This test is performed on patients found to have an adrenal
insufficiency. An increase in plasma cortisol levels after the
infusion of an "ACTH-like" drug indicates that the adrenal
gland is normal and capable of functioning if stimulated. In that
case, the cause of the adrenal insufficiency would lie within the
pituitary gland (hypopituitarism, which is called secondary
adrenal insufficiency). If little or no rise in cortisol levels occurs
after the administration of the "ACTH-like" drug, the adrenal
gland is the source of the problem and cannot secrete cortisol.
This is called primary adrenal insufficiency (Addison's disease),
which may be caused by adrenal hemorrhage, infarction,
autoimmunity, metastatic tumor, surgical removal of the adrenal
glands, or congenital adrenal enzyme deficiency.

This test can also be used in the evaluation of patients with
Cushing's syndrome. Patients with Cushing's syndrome caused
by bilateral adrenal hyperplasia have an exaggerated cortisol
elevation in response to the administration of the "ACTH-like"
drug. Those experiencing Cushing's syndrome as a result of
hyperfunctioning adrenal tumors (which are usually autonomous
and relatively insensitive to ACTH) have little or no increase in
cortisol levels over baseline values.

Cosyntropin (Cortrosyn) is a synthetic subunit of ACTH that
has the same corticosteroid-stimulating effect as endogenous
ACTH in healthy persons. During this test cosyntropin is
administered to the patient, and the ability of the adrenal gland
to respond is measured by plasma cortisol levels.

The *rapid stimulation test* is only a screening test. A normal
response excludes adrenal insufficiency. An abnormal response,
however, requires a 1-to 3-day prolonged ACTH stimulation
test to differentiate primary insufficiency from secondary insuffi-

ciency. It should be noted that the adrenal gland can also be stimulated by insulin-induced hypoglycemia as a stressing agent. When insulin is the stimulant, cortisol and glucose levels are measured.

Interfering factor

✔ Drugs that may cause artificially *increased* cortisol levels include corticosteroid, estrogens, and spironolactone.

Procedure and patient care

Before

- Keep the patient NPO after midnight the day of the test.

During

Rapid test

- Obtain a baseline plasma cortisol level. This should be done within 30 minutes of cosyntropin (ACTH-like drug) administration.
- Administer an IV injection of cosyntropin over a 2-minute period.
- Measure plasma cortisol levels 30 and 60 minutes after drug administration.

24-hour test

- Obtain a baseline plasma cortisol level.
- Start an IV infusion of synthetic cosyntropin in 1 L of normal saline.
- Administer the solution at the rate of 2 U/hr for 24 hours.
- After 24 hours, obtain another plasma cortisol level.

3-day test

- Obtain a baseline plasma cortisol level.
- Administer 25 U of cosyntropin IV over an 8-hour period on 2 to 3 consecutive days.
- The plasma cortisol is then measured at 12, 24, 36, 48, 60, and 72 hours after the start of the test.
- Collect plasma for cortisol levels in a red-top tube.

After

- Apply pressure to the venipuncture site.

Abnormal findings

In Adrenal insufficiency
  Increase above normal response (secondary adrenal insufficiency)
    Hypopituitarism
    Exogenous steroid ingestion
    Endogenous steroid production from a nonendocrine tumor
  Normal or below normal response (primary adrenal insufficiency)
    Addison's disease
    Adrenal infarction/hemorrhage
    Metastatic tumor to the adrenal gland
    Congenital enzyme adrenal insufficiency
    Surgical removal of the adrenal gland
In Cushing's syndrome
  Increase above normal response
    Bilateral adrenal hyperplasia
  Normal or below normal response
    Adrenal adenoma
    Adrenal carcinoma
    ACTH-producing nonadrenal tumor
    Chronic steroid use

notes

adrenocorticotropic hormone stimulation test with metyrapone (ACTH stimulation test with metyrapone, Metyrapone)

Type of test   Blood; urine (24-hour)

Normal findings

24-hour urine: baseline excretion of urinary
   17-hydroxycorticosteroid (OCHS) more than doubled
Blood: 11-deoxycortisol increased to 7 µg/dl and cortisol
   10 µg/dl

Test explanation and related physiology

Metyrapone (Metopirone) is a potent blocker of an enzyme involved in cortisol production. Therefore cortisol production is reduced. When this drug is given, the resulting fall in cortisol production should stimulate pituitary secretion of ACTH by way of a negative feedback mechanism. Cortisol precursors (11-deoxycortisol and OCHS) can be detected in the urine or blood. This test is similar to the cosyntropin ACTH stimulation test (see p. 15).

In patients with adrenal hyperplasia caused by pituitary overproduction of ACTH, the cortisol precursors are greatly increased, more than expected in normal patients. This is because the normal adrenal/pituitary feedback response mechanism is still intact. No response to metyrapone occurs in patients with Cushing syndrome resulting from adrenal adenoma or carcinoma because the tumors are autonomous and therefore insensitive to changes in ACTH secretion.

This test is also used to evaluate the pituitary reserve capacity to produce ACTH. It can document that adrenal insufficiency exists as a result of pituitary disease (secondary adrenal insufficiency) rather than primary adrenal pathology. This test should not be performed if primary adrenal insufficiency is likely. Severe, life-threatening adrenal crisis could be precipitated. A normal response to administration of ACTH should be demonstrated before the metyrapone is performed.

Contraindications

- Patients with possible adrenal insufficiency

Potential complications

- Addison's disease and Addisonian crisis, because metyrapone inhibits cortisol production

Interfering factors

- Recent administration of radioisotopes will interfere with test results.
- Chlorpromazine (Thorazine) interferes with the response to metyrapone and should not be administered during the testing.

Procedure and patient care

Before

- Explain the procedure to the patient.
- Obtain a baseline 24-hour urine specimen for 17-OCHS level (see p. 283) for the urine test.
- Obtain a baseline cortisol level (see p. 283) for the blood test.

During

Blood

- Administer 2 to 3 g of metyrapone at 11 PM the night before the blood specimen is to be collected. Collect a blood specimen in the morning.

Urine

- Obtain a 24-hour urine specimen for 17-OCHS level as a baseline. Then collect a 24-hour urine specimen for 17-OCHS level during and again 1 day after the oral administration of 500 to 750 mg of metyrapone, which is given every 4 hours for 24 hours.

After

- Assess the patient for impending signs of Addisonian crisis (muscle weakness, mental and emotional changes, anorexia, nausea, vomiting, hypotension, hyperkalemia, vascular collapse).
- Note that Addisonian crisis is a medical emergency that must be treated vigorously. Basically the immediate treatment includes replenishing steroids, reversing shock, and restoring blood circulation.

Abnormal findings

Increased cortisol precursors
    Adrenal hyperplasia
No change in cortisol precursors
    Adrenal tumor
      ectopic ACTH syndrome
    Secondary adrenal insuffi-
      ciency

notes

agglutinins, febrile/cold

Type of test Blood

Normal findings

Febrile (warm) agglutinins: no agglutination in titers ≤1:80
Cold agglutinins: no agglutination in titers ≤1:16

Test explanation and related physiology

Febrile agglutinins serologic studies are used to diagnose infectious diseases such as salmonellosis, rickettsial diseases, brucellosis, and tularemia. Neoplastic diseases such as leukemias and lymphomas are also associated with febrile agglutinins. Appropriate antibiotic treatment of the infectious agent is associated with a drop in the titer activity of febrile agglutinins.

Cold agglutinins occur in patients who are infected by other agents, most notably *Mycoplasma pneumoniae.* Other diseases include influenza, mononucleosis, rheumatoid arthritis, and lymphomas.

The febrile and cold agglutinins are antibodies that cause RBCs to aggregate at high or low temperatures, respectively. Agglutination occurring at titers greater than 1:16 for cold agglutinins and 1:80 for febrile agglutinins is considered abnormal and diagnostic of the infectious agent the agglutinins represent. High titers of either cold or warm agglutinins can interfere with blood typing, crossmatching, and transfusion.

Temperature regulation is important for the performance of these tests. Under no circumstances should the cold agglutinin specimen be refrigerated or the febrile agglutinin heated.

Interfering factors

☒ Some antibiotics (penicillin and cephalosporins) can interfere with the development of cold agglutinins.

Procedure and patient care

Before
- Explain the procedure to the patient.
- Tell the patient that no fasting is required.

During
- Collect approximately 7 ml of venous blood in a red-top tube (warmed or cooled; see previous discussion).

After
- Apply pressure to the venipuncture site.
- Transport the specimen immediately to the laboratory.

Abnormal findings

▲ **Increased febrile agglutinins**

Salmonellosis infection
Rickettsial disease
Brucellosis
Tularemia
Leukemia
Lymphoma

▲ **Increased cold agglutinins**

Mycoplasma pneumoniae infection
Viral illness
Infectious mononucleosis
Multiple myeloma
Scleroderma
Cirrhosis
Staphylococcemia
Thymic tumor
Influenza
Rheumatoid arthritis
Lymphoma

notes

AIDS serology (Acquired immunodeficiency serology, AIDS screen, Human immunodeficiency virus [HIV] antibody test, Western blot test for HIV and antibody, Enzyme-linked immunosorbent assay [ELISA] for HIV and antibody)

Type of test Blood

Normal findings No evidence of HIV antigen or antibodies

Test explanation and related physiology

Tests used to detect the antibody to HIV, which is the virus that causes AIDS, were first licensed for the screening of blood and plasma donors. The HIV virus is also known as human T-lymphotrophic virus, type III (HTLV-III), or the lymphadenopathy-associated virus (LAV). There are two types of HIV viruses (types 1 and 2). Type 1 is most prevalent in the United States and western Europe. Type 2 is mostly limited to western African nations.

Those at high risk for AIDS include sexually active homosexual and bisexual men and women with multiple partners, IV drug abusers, persons receiving blood products tainted with HIV, and infants exposed to the virus during gestation and delivery.

Because of the medical and social significance of a positive test for HIV antibody, test results must be accurate, and their interpretation correct. Therefore the U.S. Public Health Service has emphasized that an individual can be said to have serologic evidence of HIV infection only after an enzyme immunoassay (EIA) screening test is repeatedly reactive and another test, such as Western blot or immunofluorescence assay, validates the results. However, a positive EIA that is not confirmed by Western blot or immunofluorescence should not be considered negative. Repeat testing is required in 3 to 6 months. A person with a positive HIV test result does not have AIDS until the clinical criteria are fulfilled. The ELISA, which tests for antibodies to HIV in serum or plasma, is the most widely used serologic test for AIDS. It is important to reiterate that ELISA detects *antibodies* to HIV. Because it does not detect viral antigens, it cannot detect infection in its earliest stage, before antibodies are formed. ELISA is used to support the clinical diagnosis of AIDS, screening blood and blood products and testing individuals who believe they may be infected with HIV.

The sensitivity (i.e., probability that the test results will be reactive if the specimen is a true positive) of the ELISA test is approximately 99% for blood from persons infected with HIV for 12 weeks or more. The probability of a false-negative test is remote, except during the first few weeks after infection before detectable antibodies appear.

The specificity (probability that test results will be nonreactive if the specimen is a true negative) of the ELISA test is approximately 99% when repeated. To increase the specificity of serologic tests further, a supplemental test (most often the Western blot) is done to validate repeatedly reactive ELISA results. Sensitivity of the blot test is comparable to or greater than a repeatedly reactive ELISA. The testing sequence of a repeatedly reactive ELISA and a positive Western blot test is highly predictive of HIV infection.

The diagnostic tests described in the preceding paragraphs detect HIV infection based on demonstration of *antibodies* to HIV. Recently it has become possible to diagnose HIV infection by the direct detection of HIV or one of its components. New tests are now available in the research laboratory and are of considerable help when the Western blot results are indeterminate. The simplest of these tests is the *p24 antigen capture assay.* This detects the viral protein p24 in the peripheral blood of HIV-infected individuals, where it exists either as a free antigen or complexed to anti-p24 antibodies.

The p24 antigen may be detectable as early as 2 to 6 weeks after infection. Throughout the course of HIV infection, an equilibrium exists between the p24 antigen and anti-p24 antibodies. During the first few weeks of infection, before the development of an immune response, there is a sharp increase in p24 antigen levels. These levels decline after the development of anti-p24 antibodies. Later in HIV disease, p24 antigen levels become detectable again.

The p24 antigen test is currently being used to assess the antiviral activity of experimental HIV therapies. The p24 antigen test can also be used to diagnose neonatal HIV infection, detect HIV before seroconversion, and determine the progression of AIDS.

Home kits are now available that provide anonymous registration and pretest counseling via toll free telephoning. Sample collection in the privacy of one's home, laboratory processing, and post-test counseling are components of this home testing process.

Interfering factors

- False-positive results can occur in patients who have autoimmune disease, lymphoproliferative disease, leukemia, lymphoma, syphilis, or alcoholism.
- False-negative results can occur in the early incubation stage or end stage of AIDS.

Procedure and patient care

Before

- Explain the procedure to the patient.
- Obtain an informed consent if required by the institution.
- Tell the patient that no fasting or preparation is required.
- Maintain a nonjudgmental attitude toward the patient's sexual practices and allow the patient ample time to express his or her concerns regarding the results.

During

- Observe universal blood and body precautions. Wear gloves when handling blood products from all patients.
- Collect 7 ml of peripheral venous blood in a red-top tube. The blood is usually sent to an outside laboratory for testing.
- If the patient wishes to remain anonymous, use a number with the patient's name and record it accurately.
- Note that if the ELISA test is repeatedly reactive (i.e., test is positive twice consecutively), the Western blot test is performed on the same blood sample.
- If the Western blot test is equivocal, collect a second serum specimen 2 to 4 months later for testing.

After

- Apply pressure to the venipuncture site.
- Inform the patient to observe the venipuncture site for infection. Patients with AIDS are immunocompromised and susceptible to infection.
- Follow the institution's policy regarding test result reporting. Do not give results over the telephone. Remember that positive results may have devastating consequences.
- Explain to the patient that a positive Western blot test merely implies exposure to and presence of the AIDS virus within

the body. It does not mean that the patient has clinical AIDS. Not all patients with positive antibodies will acquire the disease.

- Encourage patients who test positive to identify their sexual contacts so that they can be informed and tested.
- Inform the patient that subsequent sexual contact will put new partners at high risk for contracting AIDS.
- Provide patient education regarding safe sexual practices.

🏠 Home care responsibilities

- Do not give the test results over the telephone.
- Positive results may have devastating consequences, including loss of job, insurance, relationships, and housing.
- Encourage patients who test positive to inform their sexual partners so they can be tested.
- Inform patients who test positive that subsequent sexual contact will put partners at high risk for contracting AIDS.

Abnormal findings

▲   **Increased levels**
AIDS
HIV infection

notes

A

alanine aminotransferase (ALT, Serum glutamic-pyruvic transaminase [SGPT])

Type of test Blood

Normal findings

Adult/child: 5-35 IU/L or 8-20 U/L (SI units)
Elderly: may be slightly higher than adult
Infant: may be twice as high as adult

Test explanation and related physiology

ALT is found predominantly in the liver; lesser quantities are found in the kidneys, heart, and skeletal muscle. Injury or disease affecting the liver parenchyma will cause a release of this hepatocellular enzyme into the bloodstream, thus elevating serum ALT levels. Generally most ALT elevations are caused by liver disease. Therefore this enzyme is not only sensitive but also quite specific in indicating hepatocellular disease. In hepatocellular disease other than viral hepatitis, the ALT/AST ratio (*DeRitis ratio*) is less than 1. In viral hepatitis, the ratio is greater than 1. This is helpful in the diagnosis of viral hepatitis.

Interfering factors

- Previous IM injections may cause elevated levels.
- Drugs that may cause *increased* ALT levels include acetaminophen, allopurinol, aminosalicylic acid (PAS), ampicillin, azathioprine, carbamazepine, cephalosporins, chlordiazepoxide, chlorpropamide, clofibrate, cloxacillin, codeine, dicumarol, indomethacin, isoniazid (INH), methotrexate, methyldopa, nafcillin, nalidixic acid, nitrofurantoin, oral contraceptives, oxacillin, phenothiazines, phenylbutazone, phenytoin, procainamide, propoxyphene, propranolol, quinidine, salicylates, tetracyclines, and verapamil.

Procedure and patient care

Before
- Explain the procedure to the patient.
- Tell the patient that no fasting is required.

During
- Collect approximately 7 to 10 ml of blood in a red-top tube and send it to the laboratory for analysis.

After

- Apply pressure to the venipuncture site. Patients with liver
  dysfunction often have prolonged clotting times.

Abnormal findings

▲   **Increased levels**

Hepatitis
Hepatic necrosis
Hepatic ischemia
Cirrhosis
Cholestasis
Hepatic tumor
Hepatotoxic drugs
Obstructive jaundice

Severe burns
Trauma to striated muscle
Myositis
Pancreatitis
Myocardial infarction
Infectious mononucleosis
Shock

notes

aldolase

Type of test Blood

Normal findings

Adult: 3-8.2 Sibley-Lehninger U/dl or 22-59 mU at 37° C (SI
  units)
Child: approximately two times the adult values
Newborn: approximately four times the adult values

Test explanation and related physiology

Serum aldolase is very similar to the enzymes aspartate aminotransferase AST [SGOT] (see p. 130) CPK (see p. 290).
Aldolase is an enzyme used in the glycolytic breakdown of
glucose. As with AST and creatine phosphokinase, aldolase exists
throughout the body in most tissues. This test is most useful in
indicating muscular or hepatic cellular injury or disease. The
serum aldolase level is very high in patients with muscular
dystrophies, dermatomyositis, and polymyositis. Levels also are
increased in patients with gangrenous processes, muscular
trauma, and muscular infectious diseases (e.g., trichinosis).
Elevated levels are also noted in chronic hepatitis, obstructive
jaundice, and cirrhosis.

Neurologic diseases causing weakness can be differentiated
from muscular causes of weakness with this test. Normal values
are seen in patients with such neurologic diseases as poliomyelitis, myasthenia gravis, and multiple sclerosis. Elevated aldolase
levels are seen in the primary muscular disorders.

Interfering factors

- Previous IM injections may cause elevated levels.
- ✗ Drugs that may cause *increased* aldolase levels include hepa-
  totoxic agents.
- ✗ Drugs that may cause *decreased* levels include phenothiazines.

Procedure and patient care

Before
- Explain the procedure to the patient.
- Note that a short period of fasting usually will provide more
  accurate results.

During
- Collect 7 to 10 ml of blood in a red-top tube.

After

- Apply pressure to the venipuncture site.

Abnormal findings

▲ **Increased levels**

Hepatocellular diseases
(e.g., hepatitis)
Muscular diseases (e.g.,
muscular dystrophy,
dermatomyositis, poly-
myositis)
Muscular trauma (e.g.,
severe crush injuries)
Muscular infections (e.g.,
trichinosis)
Gangrenous processes
(e.g., gangrene of the
bowel)
Myocardial infarction

▼ **Decreased levels**

Late muscular dystrophy
Hereditary fructose intoler-
ance
Muscle-wasting disease

notes

aldosterone

Type of test Blood; urine (24-hour)

Normal findings

Blood

Supine: 3-10 ng/dl or 0.08-0.3 nmol/L (SI units)
Upright
    Female: 5-30 ng/dl or 0.14-0.8 nmol/L (SI units)
    Male: 6-22 ng/dl or 0.17-0.61 nmol/L (SI units)
Newborn: 5-60 ng/dl
    1 week-1 year: 1-160 ng/dl 5-7 years: <5-50 ng/dl
    1-3 years: 5-60 ng/dl 7-11 years: 5-70 ng/dl
    3-5 years: <5-80 ng/dl 11-15 years: <5-50 ng/dl

Urine

2-80 μg/24 hr or 5.5-72 nmol/24 hr (SI units)

Test explanation and related physiology

This test is used to diagnose hyperaldosteronism. Production of aldosterone, a hormone produced by the adrenal cortex, is regulated primarily by the renin-angiotensin system. Secondarily, aldosterone is stimulated by ACTH, low serum sodium levels, and high serum potassium levels. Aldosterone in turn stimulates the renal tubules to absorb sodium (water follows) and secrete potassium into the urine. In this way, aldosterone regulates serum sodium and potassium levels. Because water follows sodium transport, aldosterone also partially regulates water absorption (and plasma volume).

Increased aldosterone levels are associated with primary aldosteronism, in which a tumor (usually an adenoma) of the adrenal cortex (Conn's syndrome) or bilateral adrenal nodular hyperplasia causes increased production of aldosterone. Patients with primary aldosteronism characteristically have hypertension, weakness, polyuria and hypokalemia.

Increased aldosterone levels also occur with secondary aldosteronism caused by nonadrenal conditions. These include the following:

1. Renal vascular stenosis or occlusion
2. Hyponatremia (from diuretic or laxative abuse) or low salt intake
3. Hypovolemia

4. Pregnancy or use of estrogens.
5. Malignant hypertension
6. Potassium loading
7. Edematous states such as congestive heart failure, cirrhosis, or nephrotic syndrome

The aldosterone assay can be done on a 24-hour urine specimen or a plasma blood sample. The advantage of the 24-hour urine sample is that short-term fluctuations are eliminated. Plasma values are more convenient to sample, but they are affected by the short-term fluctuations.

Primary aldosteronism can be diagnosed by demonstrating very little or no rise in serum renin levels during an *aldosterone stimulation test* (using salt restriction as the stimulant). This is because aldosterone is already maximally secreted by the pathologic adrenal gland. Failure to suppress aldosterone with saline infusion (1.5 to 2 L of NSS infused between 8 and 10 AM) *(aldosterone suppression test)* is further evidence of primary aldosteronism. Aldosterone can also be measured in blood obtained from adrenal venous sampling (see p. 9).

Interfering factors

- Strenuous exercise and stress can stimulate adrenocortical secretions and increase aldosterone levels.
- Excessive licorice ingestion can cause decreased levels, because it produces an "aldosterone-like" effect.
- Values are influenced by posture, diet, diurnal variation, and pregnancy.
- Position can significantly affect aldosterone levels.
- Because the test is usually performed using radioimmunoassay, recently administered radioactive medications will affect test results.
- Drugs that may cause *increased* levels include diazoxide (Hyperstat), hydralazine (Apresoline), nitroprusside (Nipride), diuretics, laxatives, potassium, and spironolactone.
- Drugs that may cause *decreased* levels include fludrocortisone (Florinef), propranolol (Inderal), and angiotensin-converting inhibitor (e.g., captopril), as well as licorice.

Procedure and patient care

Before

- Explain the procedure for the blood collection to the patient.
- Note that the patient is asked to be in the upright position.

(at least sitting) for at least 2 hours before the blood is drawn.

- Tell the patient that no fasting is necessary.
- Explain the procedure for collecting a 24-hour urine sample if urinary aldosterone is ordered.
- Give the patient verbal and written instructions regarding dietary and medication restrictions.
- Instruct the patient to maintain a normal sodium diet (approximately 3 g/day) for at least 2 weeks before the blood or urine collection.
- Have the patient ask the physician whether drugs that alter sodium, potassium, and fluid balance (e.g., diuretics, antihypertensives, steroids, oral contraceptives) should be withheld. Test results will be more accurate if these are suspended at least 2 weeks before either the blood or the urine test.
- Inform the patient that renin inhibitors (e.g., propranolol) should not be taken 1 week before the test.
- Tell the patient to avoid licorice for at least 2 weeks before the test because of its aldosterone-like effect.

During blood collection
- Collect approximately 5 to 10 ml of venous blood in a gold-top (serum separator) tube.
- Occasionally, for hospitalized patients, draw the sample with the patient in the supine position *before* he or she arises.
- Obtain the specimen in the morning.
- Note that sometimes a second specimen (upright sample) is collected 4 hours later, after the patient has been up and moving.
- Indicate on the laboratory slip if the patient was supine or standing during the venipuncture.
- Handle the blood specimen gently. Rough handling may cause hemolysis and alter the test results.
- Transport the specimen on ice to the laboratory.
- List on the laboratory slip any medications that can affect test results.

During urine collection
- Instruct the patient to begin the 24-hour urine collection after urinating.
- Discard this specimen and note this time as the start of the 24-hour collection.

- Collect urine micturated over the next 24 hours.
- Instruct the patient to void before defecating so that the urine is not contaminated by feces.
- Remind the patient not to put toilet paper in the collection container.
- Use a preservative with this 24-hour specimen.
- Keep the urine specimen on ice or refrigerated during the 24 hours.
- Collect the last specimen as close as possible to the end of the 24 hours. Add this urine to the container.

After blood collection
- Apply pressure to the venipuncture site.

After urine collection
- Transport the urine specimen promptly to the laboratory.

Abnormal findings

▲ **Increased levels**
  Primary aldosteronism
  Aldosterone-producing
    adrenal adenoma
    (Conn's disease)
  Adrenal cortical nodular
    hyperplasia
  Bartter syndrome

  Secondary aldosteronism
  Hyponatremia
  Hyperkalemia
  Diuretic ingestion result-
    ing in hypovolemia and
    hyponatremia
  Laxative abuse
  Stress
  Malignant hypertension
  Generalized edema
  Renal arterial stenosis
  Pregnancy
  Oral contraceptives
  Hypovolemia or hemor-
    rhage
  Cushing syndrome

▼ **Decreased values**
  Aldosterone deficiency
  Renin deficiency
  Steroid therapy
  Addison's disease
  Patients on a high-
    sodium diet
  Hypernatremia
  Hypokalemia
  Addison's disease
  Toxemia of pregnancy
  Antihypertensive therapy

alkaline phosphatase (ALP)

Type of test Blood

Normal findings

Adult: 30-85 ImU/ml or 42-128 U/L (SI units)
Elderly: slightly higher than adults
Child/adolescent
    <2 years: 85-235 ImU/ml
    2-8 years: 65-210 ImU/ml
    9-15 years: 60-300 ImU/ml
    16-21 years: 30-200 ImU/ml

Test explanation and related physiology

Although ALP is found in many tissues, the highest concentrations are found in the liver, biliary tract epithelium, and bone. The intestinal mucosa and placenta also contain ALP. Detection of this enzyme is important for determining liver and bone disorders. Within the liver, ALP is present in Kupffer's cells. These cells line the biliary collecting system. This enzyme is excreted into the bile. Enzyme levels of ALP are greatly increased in both extrahepatic and intrahepatic obstructive biliary disease and cirrhosis. Other liver abnormalities such as hepatic tumors, hepatotoxic drugs, and hepatitis cause lesser elevations in ALP levels. Reports have indicated that the most sensitive test to indicate metastatic tumor to the liver is ALP.

Bone is the most frequent extrahepatic source of ALP; new bone growth is associated with elevated ALP levels, which explains why ALP levels are high in adolescents. Pathologic new bone growth occurs with osteoblastic metastatic (e.g., breast, prostate) tumors. Paget's disease, healing fractures, rheumatoid arthritis, hyperparathyroidism, and normal-growing bones are sources of elevated ALP levels as well.

Isoenzymes of ALP are sometimes used to distinguish between liver and bone diseases. The detection of isoenzymes can help differentiate the source of the pathology associated with the elevated total ALP. ALP_1 is from the liver. ALP_2 is from the bone.

Interfering factors

- Recent ingestion of a meal can increase ALP levels.
- Drugs that may cause *elevated* ALP levels include albumin

made from placental tissue, allopurinol, antibiotics, azathioprine, colchicine, fluorides, indomethacin, isoniazid (INH), methotrexate, methyldopa, nicotinic acid, phenothiazine, probenecid, tetracyclines, and verapamil.

▼ Drugs that may cause *decreased* levels include arsenicals, cyanides, fluorides, nitrofurantoin, oxalates, and zinc salts.

Procedure and patient care

Before

- Explain the procedure to the patient.
- Tell the patient that no fasting is usually required. Overnight fasting may be required for isoenzymes.

During

- Collect approximately 7 to 10 ml of blood in a red-top tube.

After

- Apply pressure to the venipuncture site. Patients with liver dysfunction often have prolonged clotting times.

Abnormal findings

▲ **Increased levels**

Cirrhosis
Intrahepatic or extrahepatic biliary obstruction
Primary or metastatic liver tumor
Normal pregnancy (third trimester, early postpartum)
Intestinal ischemia or infarction
Metastatic tumor to the bone
Healing fracture
Hyperparathyroidism
Paget's disease
Rheumatoid arthritis
Sarcoidosis
Normal bones of growing children

▼ **Decreased levels**

Hypothyroidism
Malnutrition
Milk-alkali syndrome
Pernicious anemia
Hypophosphatemia
Scurvy (vitamin C deficiency)
Celiac disease
Excess vitamin B ingestion

A

alpha₁-antitrypsin (A1AT, ATT)

Type of test Blood

Normal findings >250 mg/dl or 0.8-2.1 g/L (SI units)

Test explanation and related physiology

Serum alpha₁-antitrypsin (α_1-antitrypsin) determinations are obtained when an individual has a family history of emphysema, because a familial tendency to have a deficiency of this antienzyme exists. Deficient or absent serum levels of this enzyme are found in some patients with the early onset of emphysema. These people usually develop severe, disabling emphysema. A similar deficiency is seen in children with cirrhosis and other liver diseases. ATT is also an acute-phase reactant that is elevated in the face of inflammation, infection, or malignancy. It is not specific as to the source of the inflammatory process.

Deficiencies of ATT can be genetic or acquired. Acquired deficiencies in ATT can occur in patients with protein deficiency syndromes (such as malnutrition, liver disease, nephrotic syndrome, and neonatal respiratory distress syndrome). People with ATT deficiency develop severe panacinar emphysema, although it is usually more severe in the lower third of the lungs in the third or fourth decade of life.

Individuals of the heterozygous state have serum levels of alpha₁-antitrypsin between 50 and 250 mg/dl. Approximately 5% to 14% of the adult population are in the heterozygous state and are considered to be at increased risk for the development of emphysema. Routine serum protein electrophoresis (see p. 686) is a good screening test for ATT deficiency because ATT accounts for about 90% of the protein in the alpha₁ globulin region.

Interfering factors

- Serum levels of alpha₁-antitrypsin increase during pregnancy.
- ✔ Drugs that may cause *increased* levels include oral contraceptives.

Procedure and patient care

Before
- Explain the procedure to the patient.
- Note that no fasting is usually required. Verify this with the laboratory performing the study.

During
- Collect approximately 5 to 10 ml of blood.

After
- Apply pressure to the venipuncture site.
- If the results show the patient is at risk for developing emphysema, begin patient teaching. Include such factors as avoidance of smoking, infection, and inhaled irritants; proper nutrition; adequate hydration; and education about the disease process of emphysema.

Abnormal findings

▲ Increased levels
Acute inflammatory disorders
Chronic inflammatory disorders
Stress
Infection
Thyroid infections

▼ Decreased levels
Early onset of emphysema (in adults)
Neonatal respiratory distress syndrome
Cirrhosis (in children)
Low serum proteins (e.g., nephrotic syndrome, malnutrition, end-stage cancer, protein-losing enteropathy)

notes

alpha-fetoprotein (AFP, α₁-Fetoprotein)

Type of test Blood

Normal findings

Adult: <40 ng/ml or <40 µg/L (SI units)
Child (<1 yr): <30 ng/ml
Ranges are stratified by weeks of gestation and vary according
    to different laboratories.

Test explanation and related physiology

AFP is an oncofetal protein normally produced by the fetal liver and yolk sac. It is the dominant fetal serum protein in the first trimester of life and diminishes to very low levels by the age of 1 year. Increased serum levels of AFP are found in as many as 90% of patients with hepatomas. The higher the AFP level, the greater the tumor burden. A decrease in AFP would be seen if the patient were experiencing a response to antineoplastic therapy. AFP is not specific for hepatomas, although extremely high levels (above 500 ng/ml) are diagnostic for hepatoma. Other neoplastic conditions such as nonseminomatous germ cell tumors and teratomas of the testes, yolk sac and germ cell tumors of the ovaries, and, to a lesser extent, Hodgkin's disease, lymphoma, and renal cell carcinoma are also associated with elevated AFP levels. Noncancerous causes of elevated AFP levels occur in patients with cirrhosis or chronic active hepatitis.

AFP is also helpful in the diagnosis of fetal body wall defects. The most notable of these is neural tube defects (NTDs), which can vary from a small myelomeningocele to anencephaly. Although not widely used in United States, AFP can be used for widespread screening for NTDs.

Other examples of fetal body wall defects would include omphalocele and gastroschisis. Elevated serum AFP levels in pregnancy may also indicate multiple pregnancy, fetal distress, fetal congenital abnormalities, or intrauterine death. Low AFP levels after correction as to age of gestation, maternal weight, race, and presence of diabetes are found in mothers carrying offspring with trisomy 21 (Down syndrome).

Interfering factors

- Recent administration of radioisotopes can affect values.

Procedure and patient care

Before

- If AFP is to be performed on amniotic fluid, follow the Procedure and Patient Care for amniocentesis; see p. 46.)
- Explain the procedure to the patient.
- Tell the patient that no food or fluid restriction is required.

During

- Collect approximately 7 to 10 ml of blood in a red-top tube.

After

- Apply pressure to the venipuncture site.
- Include the gestational age on the laboratory slip.

Abnormal findings

▲ **Increased maternal serum AFP levels**

Neural tube defects (e.g., anencephaly, encephalocele, spina bifida, myelomeningocele)
Abdominal wall defects (e.g., gastroschisis or omphalocele)
Multiple pregnancy
Threatened abortion
Fetal distress or congenital anomalies
Fetal death

▲ **Increased nonmaternal AFP**

Primary hepatocellular cancer (hepatoma)
Germ cell or yolk sac cancer of the ovary
Embryonal cell or germ cell tumor of the testes
Other cancers (e.g., stomach, colon, lung, breast, and lymphoma)
Liver cell necrosis (e.g., cirrhosis or hepatitis)

▼ **Decreased maternal AFP**

Trisomy 21 (Down syndrome)
Fetal wastage

notes

ammonia level

Type of test Blood

Normal findings
Adult: 15-110 µg/dl or 47-65 µmol/L (SI units)
Child: 40-80 µg/dl
Newborn: 90-150 µg/dl

Test explanation and related physiology
Ammonia is used to support the diagnosis of severe liver diseases (fulminant hepatitis or cirrhosis). Ammonia levels are also used in the diagnosis and follow up of hepatic encephalopathy.

Ammonia is a by-product of protein catabolism. Most of the ammonia is made by bacteria acting on proteins present in the gut. By way of the portal vein, ammonia goes to the liver, where it is normally converted into urea and then secreted by the kidneys. With severe hepatocellular dysfunction, ammonia cannot be catabolized. Further, when portal blood flow to the liver is altered (e.g., in portal hypertension), ammonia cannot reach the liver to be catabolized. Ammonia levels in the blood rise. Congenital enzymatic defects in the urea cycle also can cause a rise in ammonia levels. Finally, impaired renal function diminishes excretion of ammonia, and blood levels rise. High levels of ammonia result in encephalopathy and coma. Arterial ammonia levels are more reliable than venous levels but more difficult to obtain and are therefore not routinely used.

Interfering factors
- Hemolysis increases ammonia levels because the RBCs contain about three times the ammonia level content of plasma.
- Muscular exertion can increase ammonia.
- Cigarette smoking can produce significant increases in ammonia levels.
- Ammonia levels may be fictitiously increased if the tourniquet is too tight for too long.
- ☛ Drugs that may cause *increased* ammonia levels include acetazolamide, alcohol, ammonium chloride, barbiturates, narcotics, parenteral nutrition, and diuretics (loop, thiazide).
- ☛ Drugs that may cause *decreased* levels include broad-spectrum

antibiotics (e.g., neomycin), lactulose, levodopa, lactobacillus, and potassium salts.

Procedure and patient care

Before

- Explain the procedure to the patient.
- Note that no fasting is usually required.

During

- Collect approximately 5 to 7 ml of blood in a green-top tube. Note that some institutions require that the specimen be sent to the laboratory in an iced container.
- List on the laboratory slip any drugs that can affect test results.
- Avoid hemolysis and send the specimen promptly to the laboratory.

After

- Apply pressure to the venipuncture site. Many patients with liver disease have prolonged clotting times.

Abnormal findings

▲ **Increased levels**

Primary hepatocellular disease

Reye syndrome

Asparagine intoxication

Portal hypertension

Severe heart failure with congestive hepatomegaly

Hemolytic disease of the newborn (erythroblastosis fetalis)

Gastrointestinal bleeding with mild liver disease

Gastrointestinal obstruction with mild liver disease

Hepatic encephalopathy and hepatic coma

Genetic metabolic disorder of the urea cycle

▼ **Decreased levels**

Essential or malignant hypertension

Hyperornithinemia

amniocentesis (Amniotic fluid analysis)

Type of test   Fluid analysis

Normal findings

Amniotic fluid volume (ml)	*Weeks' gestation*
450	15
750	25
1500	30-35
<1500	Full term

Amniotic fluid appearance: clear; pale to straw yellow
L/S ratio: ≥2:1
Bilirubin : <0.2 mg/dl
No chromosomal or genetic abnormalities
Phosphatidylglycerol (PG) : positive for PG
Lamellar body count: >30,000
Alpha fetoprotein: 2 µg/ml

Test explanation and related physiology

Amniocentesis is performed on women to gather information about the fetus. The following can be evaluated by studying the amniotic fluid:

1. *Fetal maturity status*, especially pulmonary maturity (when early delivery is preferred). Fetal maturity is determined by analysis of the amniotic fluid in the following manner:

   a. *Lecithin/sphingomyelin (L/S) ratio.* The L/S ratio is a measure of fetal lung maturity, which is determined by measuring the phospholipids in amniotic fluid. Lecithin is the major constituent of surfactant, an important substance required for alveolar ventilation. If surfactant is insufficient, the alveoli collapse during expiration. This may result in respiratory distress syndrome (RDS), which is a major cause of death in immature babies. In the immature fetal lung the sphingomyelin concentration in amniotic fluid is higher than the lecithin concentration. At 35 weeks of gestation, the concentration of lecithin rapidly increases, whereas sphingomyelin concentration decreases. An L/S ratio of 2:1 (3:1 in mothers with diabetes) or greater is a highly reliable indication that the fetal lung and therefore the fetus are mature. In such a case, the infant would be unlikely to develop RDS after birth. As the L/S ratio decreases, the risk of RDS increases.

b. *Phosphatidylglycerol (PG)*. This is a minor component (about 10%) of lung surfactant phospholipids. However, since PG is almost entirely synthesized by mature lung alveolar cells, it is a good indicator of lung maturity. In healthy pregnant women, PG appears in amniotic fluid after 35 weeks of gestation, and levels gradually increase until term. The simultaneous determination of the L/S ratio and the presence of PG is an excellent method of assessing fetal maturity based on pulmonary surfactant.

c. *Lamellar body count*. This test to determine fetal maturity is also based on the presence of surfactant. These lamellar bodies represent the storage form of pulmonary surfactant. Lamellar body results are calculated in units of particle density per microliter of amniotic fluid. Some researchers have recommended cutoffs of 30,000/μl and 10,000/μl to predict low and high risk for RDS, respectively. If the count is greater than 30,000, there is 100% chance that the infant's lungs are mature enough to not experience RDS. If the lamellar body count is less than 10,000, the probability of RDS is high (67%). Values between 10,000 and 30,000/μl represent intermediate risk for RDS.

2. *Sex of the fetus*. Sons of mothers who are known to be carriers of X-linked recessive traits would have a 50:50 chance of inheritance.

3. **Genetic and chromosomal aberrations**. Genetic and chromosomal studies performed on cells aspirated within the amniotic fluid can indicate the gender of the fetus (important in sex-linked diseases such as hemophilia) or any of the described genetic and chromosomal aberrations (e.g., trisomy 21).

4. **Fetal status affected by Rh isoimmunization**. Mothers with Rh isoimmunization may have a series of amniocentesis procedures during the second half of pregnancy to assess the level of bilirubin pigment in the amniotic fluid. The quantity of bilirubin is used to assess the severity of hemolysis in Rh-sensitized pregnancy. Amniocentesis is usually initiated at 24 to 25 weeks when hemolysis is suspected.

5. **Hereditary metabolic disorders** such as cystic fibrosis.

6. **Anatomic abnormalities** such as neural tube closure defects

(myelomeningocele, anencephaly, spina bifida). Increased levels of alpha-fetoprotein (AFP) in the amniotic fluid may indicate a neural crest abnormality (see p. 39). Decreased AFP may be associated with increased risk of trisomy 21.

7. *Fetal distress*, detected by meconium staining of the amniotic fluid. This is caused by relaxation of the anal sphincter. In this case, the normally colorless and pale, straw-colored amniotic fluid may be tinged with green. Other color changes may also indicate fetal distress. For example, a yellow discoloration may indicate a blood incompatibility. A yellow-brown opaque appearance may indicate intrauterine death. A red color indicates blood contamination either from the mother or the fetus.

The timing of the amniocentesis varies according to the clinical circumstances. With advanced maternal age and if chromosomal or genetic aberrations are suspected, the test should be done early enough (at 14 to 16 weeks of gestation; at least 150 ml of fluid exists at this time) to allow a safe abortion. If information on fetal maturity is sought, performing the study during or after the thirty-fifth week of gestation is best.

Contraindications

- Patients with abruptio placentae
- Patients with placenta previa
- Patients with a history of premature labor (before 34 weeks of gestation, unless the patient is receiving antilabor medication)
- Patients with an incompetent cervix

Potential complications

- Miscarriage
- Fetal injury
- Leak of amniotic fluid
- Infection (amnionitis)
- Abortion
- Premature labor
- Maternal hemorrhage with possible maternal Rh isoimmunization
- Amniotic fluid embolism
- Abruptio placentae
- Inadvertent damage to the bladder or intestines

Interfering factors

- Fetal blood contamination can cause falsely elevated AFP levels.
- Hemolysis of the specimen can alter results.
- Contamination of the specimen with meconium or blood may give inaccurate L/S ratios.

Procedure and patient care

Before

- Explain the procedure to the patient. Allay any fears and allow the patient to verbalize her concerns.
- Obtain an informed consent from the patient and her spouse.
- Tell the patient that no food or fluid is restricted.
- Evaluate the mother's blood pressure and the fetal heart rate.
- Follow instructions regarding emptying the bladder, which depend on gestational age. Before 20 weeks of gestation, the bladder may be kept full to support the uterus. After 20 weeks, the bladder may be emptied to minimize the chance of puncture.
- Note that the placenta is localized before the study by ultrasound to permit selection of a site that will avoid placental puncture.

During

- Place the patient in the supine position.
- Note the following procedural steps:
  1. The skin overlying the chosen site is prepared and usually anesthetized locally.
  2. A long needle with a stylet is inserted through the midabdominal wall and directed at an angle toward the middle of the uterine cavity (Figure 2).
  3. The stylet is then removed, and a sterile plastic syringe attached.
  4. After 5 to 10 ml of amniotic fluid is withdrawn, the needle is removed.
  5. The specimen is placed in a light-resistant container to prevent breakdown of bilirubin.
  6. The site is covered with an adhesive bandage.
  7. If the amniotic fluid is bloody, the physician must determine whether the blood is maternal or fetal in origin. Kleinhauer-Boetke stain will stain fetal cells pink. Meconium in the fluid is usually associated with a compromised fetus.

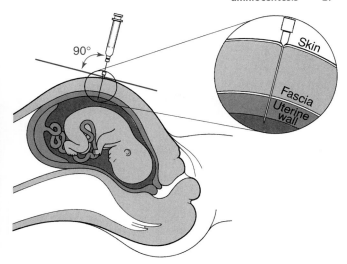

Figure 2 Amniocentesis. Ultrasound scanning is usually used to determine the placental site and to locate a pocket of amniotic fluid. The needle is then inserted. Three levels of resistance are felt as the needle penetrates the skin, fascia, and uterine wall. When the needle is placed within the uterine cavity, amniotic fluid is withdrawn.

  8. *Amniotic fluid volume* is calculated.
- Note that this procedure takes approximately 20 to 30 minutes.
- Tell the patient that the discomfort associated with amniocentesis is usually described as a mild uterine cramping that occurs when the needle contacts the uterus. Some women may complain of a "pulling" sensation as the amniotic fluid is withdrawn.
- Remember that many women are extremely anxious during this procedure.

After
- Place amniotic fluid in a sterile, siliconized glass container and transport it to a special chemistry laboratory for analysis. Sometimes the specimen may be sent by air mail to another commercial laboratory.
- Inform the patient that the results of this study are usually not available for at least 2 weeks.

- For women who have Rh-negative blood, administer RhoGAM because of the risk of immunization from the fetal blood.
- Assess the fetal heart rate after the test to detect any ill effects related to the procedure. Compare this value with the pre-procedural baseline value.
- If the patient felt dizzy or nauseated during the procedure, instruct her to lie on her left side for several minutes before leaving the examining room.
- Observe the puncture site for bleeding or other drainage.
- Instruct the patient to call her physician if she has any fluid loss, bleeding, temperature elevation, abdominal pain or cramping, fetal hyperactivity, or unusual fetal lethargy.

🏠 Home care responsibilities

- Instruct the patient to call her physician if she has any fluid loss, bleeding, temperature elevation, abdominal cramping, or unusual fetal movement.
- Inform the patient that the puncture site should be checked for bleeding or amniotic fluid loss.

Abnormal findings

Hemolytic disease of the newborn

Rh isoimmunization

Neural tube closure defects (e.g., myelomeningocele, anencephaly, spina bifida)

Abdominal wall closure defects (e.g., gastroschisis, omphalocele)

Sacrococcygeal teratoma

Meconium staining

Immature fetal lungs

Hereditary metabolic disorders (e.g., cystic fibrosis, Tay-Sachs disease, galactosemia)

Genetic or chromosomal aberrations (e.g., sickle cell anemia, thalassemia, Down syndrome)

Sex-linked disorders (e.g., hemophilia)

Polyhydramnios

Oligohydramnios

notes

amylase

Type of test Blood; urine

Normal findings
Blood
56-190 IU/L, 80-150 Somogyi units/dl, or 25-125 U/L (SI
units). Values may be slightly increased during normal
pregnancy and in the elderly.
Urine (24-hour)
3-35 IU/hr or 6-30 Wohlgemuth units/ml, up to 5000
Somogyi units/24 hr or 6.5-48.1 U/hr (SI units)

Possible critical values Blood: More than three times the
upper limit of normal, (depending on the method)

Test explanation and related physiology
Serum amylase is an easily and rapidly performed test that is
most specific for pancreatitis. Amylase is normally secreted from
the pancreatic acinar cell into the pancreatic duct and then into
the duodenum. Once in the intestine, it aids the catabolism of
carbohydrates to their component simple sugars. Damage to
acinar cells (as in pancreatitis) or obstruction of the pancreatic
duct flow (as in pancreatic carcinoma) causes an outpouring of
this enzyme into the intrapancreatic lymph system and the free
peritoneum. Blood vessels draining the free peritoneum and
absorbing the lymph pick up the excess amylase. An abnormal
rise in the serum level of amylase occurs within 12 hours of the
onset of disease. Because amylase is rapidly cleared by the kidney,
serum levels return to normal 48 to 72 hours after the initial
insult. Persistent pancreatitis, duct obstruction, or pancreatic
duct leak (e.g., pseudocysts) will cause persistent elevated serum
amylase levels.

Although serum amylase is a sensitive test for pancreatic
disorders, it is not specific. Other nonpancreatic diseases can
cause elevated amylase levels in the serum. For example, in a
bowel perforation, intraluminal amylase leaks into the free
peritoneum and is picked up by the peritoneal blood vessels. This
results in an elevated serum amylase level. Also, a penetrating
peptic ulcer into the pancreas will cause elevated amylase levels.
Duodenal obstruction can be associated with less significant

elevations in amylase. Because salivary glands contain amylase, elevations can be expected in patients with parotiditis (mumps). Amylase is also found in low levels in the ovaries and skeletal muscles. Ectopic pregnancy and severe diabetic ketoacidosis are also associated with hyperamylasemia.

Patients with chronic pancreatic disorders (e.g., chronic pancreatitis) that have previously resulted in pancreatic cell destruction often do not have high amylase levels associated with the above disorders, because less amylase is made within the pancreas.

Urine amylase levels rise after the blood levels. Several days after the onset of the disease process, serum amylase levels may be normal, but urine levels are significantly elevated. Urine amylase is particularly useful in detecting pancreatitis late in the disease course.

As with serum amylase, urine amylase is sensitive but not specific for pancreatic disorders. A comparison of the renal clearance ratio of amylase to creatinine provides more specific diagnostic information than either the urine amylase level or the serum amylase level alone. When the *amylase/creatinine clearance* ratio is 5% or more, the diagnosis of pancreatitis can be made with certainty. With ratios less than 5% in a patient having elevated serum and urine amylase levels, nonpancreatic pathologic conditions should be suspected (e.g., perforated bowel, macroamylasemia).

Interfering factors

- IV dextrose solutions can cause a false-negative result.
- Serum lipemia fictitiously decreases amylase with the current laboratory methods.
- Drugs that may cause *increased* serum amylase levels include aminosalicylic acid (PAS), aspirin, azathioprine, corticosteroids, dexamethasone, ethyl alcohol, glucocorticoids, iodine-containing contrast media, loop diuretics (e.g., furosemide), methyldopa, narcotic analgesics, oral contraceptives, and prednisone.
- Drugs that may cause *decreased* levels include citrates, glucose, and oxalates.

Procedure and patient care

Before
- Explain the procedure to the patient.
- Tell the patient that no fasting is required.

During

Blood

- Collect 5 to 7 ml of venous blood in a red-top tube.
- Indicate on the laboratory slip any medications that may affect test results.

Urine

- Instruct the patient to begin the 24-hour urine collection after urinating. Discard the initial specimen and start the 24-hour timing at that point.
- Collect all urine passed during the next 24 hours.
- A 2-hour spot urine can be sent instead of the 24-hour urine collection.
- Show the patient where to store the urine specimen.
- Keep the specimen on ice or refrigerated during the collection period. No preservative is needed.
- Post the hours for urine collection in a prominent place to prevent accidental discarding of the specimen.
- Instruct the patient to void before defecating so that urine is not contaminated by stool.
- Remind the patient not to put toilet paper in the urine collection container.
- Collect the last specimen as close as possible to the end of the collection period. Add this urine to the container.
- List on the laboratory slip any medications that may affect test results.

After

- Apply pressure to the venipuncture site.

Abnormal findings

▲ **Increased levels**

Acute pancreatitis
Penetrating peptic ulcer
Perforated peptic ulcer
Necrotic bowel
Perforated bowel
Acute cholecystitis
Parotiditis (mumps)
Ectopic pregnancy
Pulmonary infarction
Diabetic ketoacidosis
Chronic relapsing pancreatitis
Duodenal obstruction

amyloid beta protein precursor, soluble (sBPP)

Type of test CSF analysis

Normal findings >450 U/L

Test explanation and related physiology

This test is used to support the clinical diagnosis of Alzheimer's disease and other senile dementias. It has recently been confirmed that the histologic lesions of the brain known as senile plaques (which contain amyloid) and the amyloid in the meningeal blood vessels of patients with Alzheimer's disease consist of this newly described protein. Recent evidence suggests that it may be this protein that exerts neurotoxic effects.

A cerebrospinal fluid (CSF) sample is obtained by lumbar puncture (see p. 539). The soluble BPP is normally found in the CSF of healthy individuals. Low levels may be found in some elderly patients suffering from dementia. Low levels may indicate an alteration in the formation of the amyloid beta protein or its precursors, which is characteristic of Alzheimer's disease.

Procedure and patient care

Before
- Explain the procedure to the patient.
- Refer to the instructions for a lumbar puncture and CSF examination (see p. 539).

During
- Collect a CSF specimen as indicated in the lumbar puncture discussion.

After
- Follow the postprocedure guidelines after a lumbar puncture.

Abnormal findings

▼ **Decreased levels**
   Alzheimer's disease

androstenedione

Type of test Blood

Normal findings <250 ng/dl

Possible critical values >1000 ng/dl

Test explanation and related physiology

Androstenedione is a precursor of cortisol, aldosterone, testosterone, and estrogen. The importance of this hormone is in the diagnosis of virilizing syndromes, especially in the female. In the adrenal glands of females, androstenedione is converted to the above-noted hormones. In the female peripheral tissues and ovaries, androstenedione is converted into testosterone and estrogen. Tumors of the adrenal glands (cancers or adenomas) or ovaries (stroma tumors) can secrete large amounts of androstenedione, which is then converted into a large amount of testosterone relative to normal. In the adult female this can cause virilizing symptoms such as hirsutism, change in voice, and sterility. Children with congenital adrenal hyperplasia have enzyme defects in the conversion of androstenedione to cortisol. Excess androstenedione is built up. As ACTH levels increase, androstenedione production is stimulated, and levels increase still further. Again, this hormone is converted into a relative high level of testosterone by the peripheral tissues. In female children pseudohermaphroditism results. In male children with similar congenital defects, precocious puberty will become obvious. Adult female patients with Cushing's syndrome experience virilization through the same pathophysiologic process.

Patients with polycystic ovary syndrome (Stein-Leventhal syndrome) may also have elevated levels of testosterone precursors, including androstenedione.

Interfering factors

- A radioactive scan performed 1 week before the test may invalidate the test results.
- Drugs that may *increase* levels of androstenedione are corticotropin, clomiphene, and metyrapone.
- Steroids may *decrease* levels of androstenedione.

Procedure and patient care

Before

- Explain the procedure to the patient.
- Tell the patient that the specimen should be collected 1 week before or after the menstrual period.

During

- Collect one red-top tube of venous blood.
- Indicate the date of the last menstrual period on the laboratory form.

After

- Apply pressure to the venipuncture site.

Abnormal findings

▲ **Increased levels**

Adrenal tumor
Congenital adrenal hyperplasia
Ectopic ACTH-producing tumors
Cushing syndrome
Stein-Leventhal syndrome
Ovarian sex cord tumor

▼ **Decreased levels**

Primary or secondary adrenal insufficiency
Ovarian failure
Oophorectomy

notes

angiotensin-converting enzyme (ACE, Serum angiotensin-converting enzyme [SACE])

Type of test Blood

Normal findings 23-57 U/ml (over 20 years of age)

Test explanation and related physiology

ACE is used to detect and monitor the clinical course of sarcoidosis (a granulomatous disease that affects many organs, especially the lungs). Further, it is used to differentiate between sarcoidosis from other granulomatous diseases. It is also used to differentiate between active and dormant sarcoid disease.

Elevated ACE levels are found in a high percentage of patients with sarcoidosis. This test is primarily used in patients with sarcoidosis to evaluate the severity of disease and the response to therapy. Levels are especially high with active pulmonary sarcoidosis and can be normal with inactive (dormant) sarcoidosis. Elevated ACE levels also occur in conditions other than sarcoidosis, including Gaucher's disease (a rare familial lysosomal disorder of fat metabolism), leprosy, alcoholic cirrhosis, active histoplasmosis, tuberculosis, Hodgkin's disease, myeloma, scleroderma, pulmonary embolism, and idiopathic pulmonary fibrosis.

Interfering factors

- Patients under 20 years of age normally have very high ACE levels.
- Hemolysis or hyperlipidemia may factitiously decrease ACE levels.
- ✗ Drugs that may cause *decreased* ACE levels include ACE inhibitor antihypertensives and steroids.

Procedure and patient care

Before
- Explain the procedure to the patient.
- Tell the patient that no fasting is required.

During
- Collect approximately 5 ml of blood in a red-top tube.
- Note on the laboratory slip if the patient is taking steroids.

After

- Apply pressure to the venipuncture site.

Abnormal findings

▲ **Increased levels**

Sarcoidosis
Gaucher's disease
Tuberculosis
Leprosy
Alcoholic cirrhosis
Active histoplasmosis
Hodgkin's disease
Myeloma
Idiopathic pulmonary
  fibrosis

Diabetes mellitus
Primary biliary cirrhosis
Amyloidosis
Hyperthyroidism
Scleroderma
Pulmonary embolism

notes

anion gap (AG, R factor)

Type of test Blood

Normal findings
8-16 mEq/L (if potassium is used in the calculation)
8-12 mEq/L (if potassium is not used in the calculation)

Test explanation and related physiology

The anion gap is the difference between the cations and the anions in the extracellular space (i.e., anion gap = [sodium + potassium] – [chloride + bicarbonate]). In some laboratories the potassium is not measured. The normal value is adjusted downward if potassium is eliminated from the equation. Normally the anion gap is created by the small amounts of anions in the blood such as lactate, phosphates, sulfates, and proteins.

This calculation can help identify the cause of metabolic acidosis. As acids such as lactic acid or ketoacids accumulate in the bloodstream, bicarbonate levels diminish to regulate the pH within the blood. Mathematically, when bicarbonate decreases, the AG increases. If bicarbonate is lost from the extracellular space through diarrhea or increased excretion by a diseased kidney, the AG will increase. In general, most metabolic acidotic states are associated with an increased anion gap. Most metabolic alkalotic states are associated with a reduced anion gap.

Interfering factors

- ☛ Drugs that *increase* AG include carbonic anhydrase inhibitors (e.g. acetazolamide), salicylate, spironolactone, triamterene, and methanol.
- ☛ Drugs that *decrease* AG include carbenicillin, penicillin phosphate, diuretics, antacids, licorice, and carbenoxolone.

Procedure and patient care

Before
- Explain the procedure to the patient.
- Tell the patient that no food or fluid is restricted.

During
- Collect 5 to 10 ml of venous blood in a red- or green-top tube.

- If the patient is receiving an IV infusion, obtain the blood from the opposite arm.
- List on the laboratory slip any drugs that may affect test results.

After

- The sodium, potassium, chloride, and bicarbonate levels are determined by an automated multichannel analyzer. The AG is then calculated as indicated as above.
- Apply pressure to the venipuncture site.

Abnormal findings

▲ **Increased levels**
Lactic acidosis
Diabetic ketoacidosis
Alcoholic ketoacidosis
Starvation
Renal failure
Renal tubular acidosis
Increased gastrointestinal
losses of bicarbonate
(e.g., diarrhea or fistulae)
Hypoaldosteronism

▼ **Decreased levels**
Excess alkali ingestion
Multiple myeloma
Chronic vomiting or
gastric suction
Hyperaldosteronism

notes

antegrade pyelography

Type of test X-ray with contrast dye

Normal findings Normal outline, size, and position of the ureters and bladder

Test explanation and related physiology

Occasionally a kidney with very poor dye excretion following intravenous pyelography (IVP) also cannot be adequately examined by retrograde pyelography either because the ureter is impassable from below (e.g., from obstruction) or because a cystoscopic procedure is clinically contraindicated. For this patient the upper collecting system may be opacified by antegrade pyelography with an injection of contrast material via a percutaneous needle puncture of the renal pelvis or calyx. This test is usually performed when attempts at retrograde catheterization (retrograde pyelography) have been unsuccessful. Antegrade pyelography is specifically indicated in the following conditions:

1. Localization of ureteral obstruction caused by a stricture, nonopaque ureteral stone, or tumor
2. Evaluation of ureteral obstruction after a urinary diversion procedure
3. Hydronephrosis in a child with poor IVP dye excretion to identify ureteropelvic and ureterovesical obstruction

Potential complications

- Hemorrhage from the needle (the kidney is a highly vascular organ)
- Allergic reaction to iodinated dye (this rarely occurs because the dye is not administered intravenously)

Procedure and patient care

Before

- Explain the procedure to the patient. Allay the patient's fears and allow time for the patient to verbalize concerns.
- Obtain an informed consent.
- Check for allergy to iodine or shellfish and inform the physician.

During

- Place the patient in a prone position.
- Note the following procedural steps:
  1. The renal pelvis is localized by ultrasound or fluoroscopy. A dilated collecting system is more easily identified than a normal collecting system.
  2. Skin overlying the desired site is marked and prepared antiseptically.
  3. With the patient under local anesthesia, the skin is incised, and a needle with a stylet is inserted toward the renal pelvis.
  4. With the patient suspending respiration, a smaller, thin-walled needle with a stylet is advanced through the needle into the lumen of the renal pelvis. Flexible tubing connects the syringe to the needle to aspirate urine.
  5. Contrast material is injected to outline the upper collection system to the point of obstruction below.
  6. Posteroanterior, oblique, and anteroposterior x-ray views are taken.
- Note that this test is performed by a radiologist or urologist in less than 1 hour.
- Inform the patient that the only uncomfortable aspect of this test is the local anesthesia used to numb the skin overlying the pelvis.

After

- Apply a small pressure dressing to the incision site.
- Assess the incision site for bleeding.
- Because the kidney is a highly vascular organ, check the vital signs as ordered to detect any evidence of bleeding.
- Note that antibiotic drugs are often recommended for several days to avoid infection, which may be caused by the instrumentation at a level above the ureteral obstruction.
- Evaluate for signs of an allergic reaction to dye (e.g., dyspnea, rash, tachycardia, hives).

🏠 Home care responsibilities

- Check the incision site for bleeding.
- Evaluate the vital signs for evidence of bleeding (increased pulse and decreased BP).
- Antibiotics may be ordered prophylactically after this procedure to avoid infection.

Abnormal findings

Ureteral stone
Ureteral obstruction from tumor or adhesions
Ureteropelvic or ureterovesical obstruction from a stone,
    tumor, or scarring
Congenital or acquired hydronephrosis

notes

anticardiolipin antibodies (aCL antibodies, ACA)

Type of test Blood

Normal findings
Negative
>   <23 g/L for IgG anticardiolipin antibodies
>   <11 mg/L for IgM anticardiolipin antibodies

Test explanation and related physiology

This test is positive in some patients with systemic lupus erythematosus (SLE). *Antiphospholipid antibodies* include *anticardiolipin antibodies* and the *"lupus anticoagulant."* Anticardiolipin antibodies (immunoglobulins G and M to cardiolipin) are found in approximately 40% of patients with SLE. SLE patients who are positive for anticardiolipin antibodies and the lupus anticoagulant are at higher risk for the development of the "antiphospholipid antibody syndrome." The clinical features include venous and arterial thrombosis, neuropsychiatric disorders, recurrent spontaneous abortion, and thrombocytopenia. Both antibodies may be found in drug-induced lupus, in nonautoimmune diseases (e.g., syphilis and acute infection), and in the normal elderly person.

Interfering factors

- Patients who have or had syphilis infections can have a false positive.
- Transient presence of these antibodies can occur in patients with infections, AIDS, inflammation, autoimmune diseases, or cancer.
- False *positive* results have been seen in patients who take medications such as chlorpromazine, procainamide, dilantin, penicillin, hydralazine, and quinidine.

Procedure and patient care

Before
- Explain the procedure to the patient.
- Tell the patient that no fasting is required.

During
- Collect a venous blood sample according to the laboratory protocol.

After
- Apply pressure to the venipuncture site.

Abnormal findings

▲ **Increased levels**

Systemic lupus erythematosus

Thrombosis

Thrombocytopenia

Recurrent fetal loss

Syphilis

Acute infection

Elderly

notes

anticentromere antibody test (Centromere antibody)

Type of test Blood

Normal findings

Negative (if positive, serum will be titrated)

Weak positive: positive at the screening titer (1:40 for HEp -2 cells) (1:20 for kidney cells)

Moderately positive: one dilution above screening titer

Strong positive: two dilutions above screening titer

Test explanation and related physiology

A centromere is the region of the chromosome referred to as the "primary constriction" that divides the chromosome into "arms." During cell division, the centromere exists in the "pole" of the mitotic spindle.

Anticentromere antibodies are a form of *anti-nuclear antibodies*. They are found in a very high percentage of patients with CREST syndrome, a variant of scleroderma. CREST is characterized by calcinosis, Raynaud's phenomenon, esophageal dysfunction, sclerodactyly, and telangiectasia. Anticentromere antibodies, on the contrary, are present in only a small minority of patients with scleroderma, a disease that is difficult to differentiate from CREST. No correlation exists between antibody titer and severity of CREST disease.

Procedure and patient care

Before
- Explain the procedure to the patient.
- Tell the patient that no fasting is usually required.

During
- Collect one red-top tube of venous blood.

After
- Apply pressure to the venipuncture site.

Abnormal finding

Positive

CREST syndrome

antideoxyribonuclease-B titer (Anti-DNase-B [ADB], ADNase-B)

Type of test Blood

Normal findings
Preschool: ≤60 U
School age: ≤170 U
Adult: ≤85 U

Test explanation and related physiology

Like the antistreptolysin O titer (ASO) test (see p. 91), this immunologic test also detects antibodies directed against antigens produced by group A streptococci and is elevated in most patients with acute rheumatic (ARF) fever or poststreptococcal glomerulonephritis. This test is often run concurrently with the ASO; subsequent testing is usually performed to detect differences between the acute and convalescent blood samples. A rise in the titer of two or more dilution increments between acute and convalescent sera is significant and indicates that a streptococcal infection has occurred. The American Heart Association does not recommend performance of this test alone in the evaluation of patients with ARF. It may be more sensitive than ASO, but its results are too variable. ASO is the recommended test, but when done together, is better than either the ASO or ADB alone.

Procedure and patient care

Before
- Explain the procedure to the patient.
- Inform the patient that no fasting is required.

During
- Collect one red-top tube of venous blood.

After
- Apply pressure to the venipuncture site.

Abnormal findings

▲ Increased levels
   Acute rheumatic fever
   Poststreptococcal glomerulonephritis

antidiuretic hormone (ADH, Vasopressin)

Type of test Blood

Normal findings

ADH: 1-5 pg/ml or <1.5 ng/L (SI units)
ADH suppression test (water load test):
    65 % of water load excreted in 4 hours
    80% of water load excreted in 5 hours
    Urine osmolality (in second hour) ≤100 mmol/kg
    Urine to serum (U/S) osmolality ratio >100
    Urine specific gravity <1.003

Test explanation and related physiology

ADH, also known as *vasopressin*, is formed by the hypothalamus and stored in the posterior pituitary gland. It controls the amount of water resorbed by the kidney. ADH release is stimulated by an increase in serum osmolality or a decrease in intravascular blood volume. Physical stress, surgery, and even high levels of anxiety may also stimulate ADH release. With a release of ADH, more water is resorbed from the kidney. This increases the amount of free water within the bloodstream and causes a very concentrated urine. With low ADH levels, water is allowed to be excreted, thereby producing hemoconcentration and a more dilute urine.

Diabetes insipidus (DI) results when ADH secretion is inadequate or when the kidney is unresponsive to ADH stimulation. Inadequate ADH secretion is usually associated with central neurologic abnormalities (neurogenic DI) such as trauma, tumor, inflammation of the brain (hypothalamus), or surgical ablation of the pituitary gland. Patients with DI excrete large volumes of free water within a dilute urine. Their blood is hemoconcentrated, causing them to have a strong thirst.

Primary renal diseases may make the renal collecting system less sensitive to ADH stimulation (nephrogenic DI). Again, in this instance, a dilute urine created by excretion of high volumes of free water may occur. To differentiate neurogenic DI from nephrogenic DI, a *water deprivation ADH stimulation* test is performed. During this test, water intake is restricted, and urine osmolality is measured before and after vasopressin is administered. In neurogenic DI there is no rise in urine osmolality with water restriction, but there is a rise after vasopressin administration. In nephrogenic DI there is no rise in urine osmolality after water deprivation or vasopressin administration. The diagnosis indicated by this test can be corroborated by a serum ADH level. In neurogenic DI ADH levels are low. In nephrogenic DI ADH levels are high.

High serum ADH levels are also associated with the syndrome of inappropriate ADH secretion (SIADH). In response to the inappropriately high level of ADH secretion, water is resorbed by the kidneys greatly in excess of normal amounts. Thus the patient becomes very hemodiluted, and the urine concentrated. Blood levels of important serum ions diminish, causing severe neurologic, cardiac, and metabolic alterations. The most frequent cause of SIADH is the paraneoplastic syndrome, causing ectopic secretion of ADH. The most common tumors associated with SIADH include carcinoma of the lung and thymus; lymphomas; leukemia; and carcinomas of the pancreas, urologic tract, and intestine. SIADH is also associated with pulmonary diseases (e.g., tuberculosis, bacterial pneumonia), severe stress (e.g., surgery, trauma), CNS tumor, infection, or trauma. Patients with myxedema or Addison's disease also can experience SIADH.

The *water load test (ADH suppression test)* is used to differentiate the syndrome of inappropriate ADH (SIADH) from other causes of hyponatremia or edematous states. Usually this test is done concomitantly with measurements of urine and serum osmolality. Patients with SIADH will excrete none or very little of the "water load." Further, their urine osmolality will never be <100, and the urine/serum ratio is >100. Patients with other hyponatremia, edematous states, or chronic renal diseases will excrete up to 80% of the water load and will develop mid-range osmolality results.

Interfering factors

- Patients with dehydration, hypovolemia, and stress may have increased ADH levels.
- Patients with overhydration, decreased serum osmolality, and hypervolemia may have decreased ADH levels.
- Use of a glass syringe or collection tube causes degradation of ADH.
- Drugs that *elevate* ADH levels include acetaminophen, barbiturates, cholinergic agents, estrogen, nicotine, oral hypoglycemic agents, some diuretics (e.g., thiazides), cyclophosphamide, narcotics, and tricyclic antidepressants.

☛ Drugs that *decrease* ADH levels include alcohol, beta-adrenergic agents, morphine antagonists, and phenytoin (Dilantin).

Procedure and patient care

Before

- Explain the procedure to the patient.
- Ensure that the patient is adequately hydrated. Tell the patient to fast for 12 hours.
- Evaluate the patient for high levels of physical or emotional stress.

During

- Collect approximately 7 ml of venous blood in a *plastic* red-top tube with the patient in the sitting or recumbent position.
- Record on the laboratory slip any drugs that may alter test results.

After

- Apply pressure to the venipuncture site.
- Note that the laboratory personnel usually freeze the serum and send it to a reference laboratory for testing.

Abnormal findings

▲ **Increased levels**
SIADH
Nephrogenic diabetes insipidus caused by primary renal diseases
Postoperative days 1 to 3
Severe physical stress (e.g., trauma, pain, prolonged mechanical ventilation)
Hypovolemia
Dehydration
Acute porphyria

▼ **Decreased levels**
Neurogenic (or central) diabetes insipidus
Surgical ablation of the pituitary gland
Hypervolemia
Decreased serum osmolality

anti-DNA antibody test (Antideoxyribonucleic acid antibodies, Antibody to double-stranded DNA, Anti-double-stranded DNA, Anti-ds-DNA, DNA antibody, Native double-stranded DNA)

Type of test Blood

Normal findings

Negative: <70 units
Borderline: 70-200 units
Positive: >200 units

Test explanation and related physiology

The anti-ds-DNA test is useful for the diagnosis and follow-up of systemic lupus erythematosus (SLE). This antibody is found in approximately 65% to 80% of patients with active SLE and rarely in other diseases. High titers are characteristic of SLE. Low to intermediate levels of this antibody may be found in patients with other rheumatic diseases and in those with chronic hepatitis, infectious mononucleosis, and biliary cirrhosis. The anti-DNA titer decreases with successful therapy and increases with an exacerbation of SLE and especially with the onset of lupus glomerulonephritis. The test can return to near negative with dormant SLE.

The anti-DNA antibody is a subtype of the *anti-nuclear antibodies* (ANAs) (see p. 80). There are two types of anti-DNA antibodies. The first and most popular is the antibody against double-stranded DNA (Anti-ds-DNA). The second type is the antibody against single-stranded DNA, Anti-ss-DNA, which is less sensitive and specific for SLE but is positive in other autoimmune diseases. These antibody-antigen complexes that occur with autoimmune disease are not only diagnostic but are major contributors of the disease process. These complexes induce the complement system, which then may cause local or systemic tissue injury.

Interfering factors

- A radioactive scan performed within 1 week before the test may alter the test results.
- Drugs that may cause *increased* levels include hydralazine and procainamide.

Procedure and patient care

Before

- Explain the procedure to the patient.
- Tell the patient that no fasting is required.

During

- Collect one red-top tube of venous blood.

After

- Apply pressure to the venipuncture site.

Abnormal findings

▲ **Increased levels**

Systemic lupus
   erythematosus
Other autoimmune
   diseases (e.g., rheumatic
   fever)

Chronic hepatitis
Infectious mononucleosis
Biliary cirrhosis

notes

anti-extractable nuclear antigens antibody (Anti-ENA,
Antibodies to extractable nuclear antigens, Antiribonucleo-
protein [anti-RNP], Anti-Smith [anti-SM])

Type of test Blood

Normal findings Negative

Test explanation and related physiology

The anti-ENAs are used to assist in the diagnosis of systemic
lupus erythematosus (SLE) and mixed connective tissue disease
(MCTD) and to eliminate other rheumatoid diseases.

Anti-ENAs are a type of *anti-nuclear antibodies* to certain
nuclear antigens that consist of RNA and protein. The ENA
antigen is sometimes referred to as "saline-extracted antigen."
The most common ENAs are Smith (SM) and ribonucleoprotein (RNP).

The *antinuclear Smith (anti-SM)* antibody is present in about
30% of patients with SLE and in about 8% of patients with
MCTDs. However, it is not present in patients with most other
rheumatoid-collagen diseases.

The *antinuclear ribonucleoprotein (anti-RNP)* is reported in
nearly 100% of patients with MCTD and in about 25% of
patients with SLE, discoid lupus, and progressive systemic
sclerosis (scleroderma). In high titer, anti-RNP is suggestive
of MCTD.

There are two other antibodies to ENAs. Anti-SS-A and
anti-SS-B are described on p. 89 and are used mainly in the
diagnostic evaluation of Sjögren's syndrome.

Procedure and patient care

Before
- Explain the procedure to the patient.
- Tell the patient that no fasting is required.

During
- Collect a venous blood sample in a red-top tube.

After
- Apply pressure to the venipuncture site.
- Check the venipuncture site for infection. Patients with
  autoimmune disease have a compromised immune system.

Abnormal findings

▲ **Increased anti-SM antibodies**
Systemic lupus erythematosus

▲ **Increased anti-RNP antibodies**
MCTD
SLE
Discoid lupus scleroderma

notes

antiglomerular basement membrane antibodies
(Anti-GBM antibody, AGBM, Glomerular basement antibody, Goodpasture's antibody)

Type of test

Blood or microscopic examination (lung or renal)

Normal findings

Tissue
Negative: no immunofluorescence noted on the renal or lung
    tissue basement membrane.
Blood
    Negative: <20 units EIA
    Borderline: 20-100 units
    Positive: >100 units

Test explanation and related physiology

This test is used to detect the presence of circulating glomerular basement membrane antibodies commonly present in autoimmune-induced nephritis (Goodpasture syndrome).

Goodpasture syndrome is an autoimmune disease characterized by the presence of circulating antibodies against antigens in the basement membrane of the renal glomerular and the pulmonary alveoli. These immune complexes activate the complement system and thereby cause tissue injury. Patients with this problem usually display a triad of glomerulonephritis (hematuria), pulmonary hemorrhage (hemoptysis), and antibodies to basement membrane antigens. About 60% to 75% of patients with immune- induced glomerular nephritis have the pulmonary complications.

Lung or renal biopsies are required to obtain tissue on which to demonstrate these antibodies with immunohistochemical techniques. Serum assays performed are a faster and more reliable method for diagnosing Goodpasture syndrome, especially in patients in whom renal or lung biopsy may be difficult or contraindicated. Furthermore, serum levels can be used in monitoring response to therapy (plasmapheresis or immunosuppression).

Procedure and patient care

Before
- Explain the procedure to the patient.
- Tell the patient to fast for 8 hours before the test. Water is permitted.
- If a lung biopsy (see p. 548) or renal biopsy (see p. 718) will be used to collect the specimen, explain these procedures to the patient.

During
- Collect one red-top tube of venous blood.

After
- Apply pressure to the venipuncture site.

Abnormal findings

Positive
Goodpasture syndrome
Autoimmune glomerulonephritis
Lupus nephritis

notes

antimitochondrial antibody (AMA)

Type of test Blood

Normal findings No antimitochondrial antibodies (AMAs) at titers >1:5

Test explanation and related physiology

The AMA is used primarily to aid in the diagnosis of primary biliary cirrhosis. AMA is an anticytoplasmic antibody directed against a lipoprotein in the mitochondrial membrane. Normally the serum does not contain AMA at a titer greater than 1:5. AMA appears in 94% of patients with primary biliary cirrhosis. This disease may be an autoimmune disease that occurs predominantly in young or middle-aged women. It has a slow, progressive course marked by elevated liver enzymes (especially alkaline phosphatase and gamma-glutamyl transpeptidase (see pp. 35 and 422) and positive AMA. Liver biopsy (see p. 531) is usually required to confirm the diagnosis because AMA can be positive in patients with chronic active hepatitis, drug-induced cholestasis, autoimmune hepatitis (e.g., scleroderma, systemic lupus erythematosus), extrahepatic obstruction, or acute infectious hepatitis. There are subgroups of AMA. The M-2 subgroup is suspected to be very specific for primary biliary cirrhosis.

Procedure and patient care

Before

- Explain the procedure to the patient.
- Tell the patient that no fasting or special preparation is required.

During

- Collect 7 to 10 ml of venous blood in a red-top tube.

After

- Apply pressure to the venipuncture site.
- Patients with liver disease often have bleeding disorders.

Abnormal findings

▲ **Increased levels**

Primary biliary cirrhosis

Chronic active hepatitis

Systemic lupus erythematosus (SLE)

Syphilis

Drug-induced cholestasis

Autoimmune hepatitis (e.g., scleroderma, SLE)

Extrahepatic obstruction

Acute infectious hepatitis

notes

A

antimyocardial antibodies (AMA)

Type of test Blood

Normal findings Negative (if positive, serum will be titrated)

Test explanation and related physiology

This test is used to detect an autoimmune source of myocardial injury and disease. Antimyocardial antibodies may be detected in rheumatic heart disease, cardiomyopathy, postthoracotomy syndrome, and postmyocardial infarction syndromes. This test is not only used in the detection of an autoimmune cause for these conditions but also for monitoring their response to treatment. Antibodies against heart muscle are also found in 20% to 40% of postcardiac surgery patients and in a smaller number of postmyocardial infarction patients. These antibodies are usually associated with a pericarditis that follows the myocardial injury associated with cardiac surgery or myocardial infarction (Dressler syndrome). AMA has also been detected with cardiomyopathy.

Procedure and patient care

Before

- Explain the procedure to the patient.
- Tell the patient that no fasting or special preparation is necessary.

During

- Collect a venous blood sample in a red-top tube of blood.

After

- Apply pressure to the venipuncture site.

Abnormal findings

▲ Increased values

Rheumatic heart disease
Cardiomyopathy
Postthoracotomy
  syndrome

Postmyocardial
  infarction
Rheumatic fever
Streptococcal infection

antineutrophil cytoplasmic antibody (ANCA)

Type of test Blood

Normal findings Negative

Test explanation and related physiology

This blood test is used to assist in the diagnosis of Wegener's granulomatosis (WG). It also is useful to follow the course of the disease, monitor the response to therapy, and provide early detection of relapse. WG is a regional systemic vasculitis in which the small arteries of the kidneys, lungs, and upper respiratory tract (nasopharynx) are damaged by a granulomatous inflammation. Diagnosis has been made by biopsy of clinically affected tissue. Recently serologic testing has begun to play a key role in the diagnosis of WG and other systemic vasculitis syndromes.

ANCAs are antibodies directed against cytoplasmic components of neutrophils. There are two types of antineutrophil cytoplasmic antibodies. The *C-ANCA* pattern is highly specific (95% to 99%) for WG. When the disease is limited to the respiratory tract, the C-ANCA is positive in only about 65% of patients. Nearly all patients with WG limited to the kidney do not have positive C-ANCA. When WG is inactive, the percentage of positives drops to about 30%.

The second type of ANCA is the *P-ANCA*, which produces a perinuclear pattern of staining in the neutrophil cytoplasm. P-ANCA pattern is found in 50% of patients with WG centered in the kidney. It also occurs in patients with non-WG glomerulonephritis. In patients with ulcerative colitis or sclerosing cholangitis, 75% will have positive P-ANCA.

Procedure and patient care

Before

- Explain the procedure to the patient.
- Tell the patient that no fasting is required.

During

- Collect venous blood in a tube as determined by the laboratory performing the test.

After

- Apply pressure to the venipuncture site.

Abnormal findings

▲ **Increased levels**

WG
Microscopic polyarteritis
Idiopathic crescentic glomerulonephritis
Ulcerative colitis
Primary sclerosing cholangitis
Autoimmune hepatitis
Churg-Strauss vasculitis
Active viral hepatitis
Crohn's disease

notes

antinuclear antibody (ANA)

Type of test Blood

Normal findings No ANA detected in a titer with a dilution >1:20

Test explanation and related physiology

ANA is a group of anti-nuclear antibodies used to diagnose systemic lupus erythematosus (SLE). Because almost all patients with SLE develop autoantibodies, a negative ANA test excludes the diagnosis. Positive results occur in approximately 95% of patients with this disease; however, many other rheumatic diseases are also associated with ANA.

There are several different patterns of fluorescence, seen by the UV microscope. When combined with the specific subtype of ANA, the pattern can increase specificity of the ANA subtypes for the various autoimmune diseases (Figure 3). As the diseases becomes less active because of therapy, the ANA titers can be expected to fall. As one can see from Table 1, none of the ANA subtypes are exclusive for any one autoimmune disease.

TABLE 1 Autoimmune disease and positive ANAs

Autoimmune disease	Positive antibodies
SLE	ANA, SLE prep, dsDNA, ssDNA, anti-DNP, SS-A
Drug-induced SLE	ANA
Sjögren syndrome	RF, ANA, SS-A, SS-B
Scleroderma	ANA, Scl-70, RNA, dsDNA
Raynaud's disease	ACA, Scl-70
Mixed connective tissue disease	ANA, RNP, RF, ssDNA
Rheumatoid arthritis	RF, ANA, RANA, RAP
Primary biliary cirrhosis	AMA
Thyroiditis	Antimicrosomal, antithyroglobulin
Chronic active hepatitis	ASMA

Interfering factors

▪ Drugs that may cause a *false-positive* ANA test include acetazolamide, aminosalicylic acid, chlorprothixene, chlorothiazides, griseofulvin, hydralazine, penicillin, phenylbutazone, phenytoin sodium, procainamide, streptomycin, sulfonamides, and tetracyclines.

▪ Drugs that may cause a *false-negative* test include steroids.

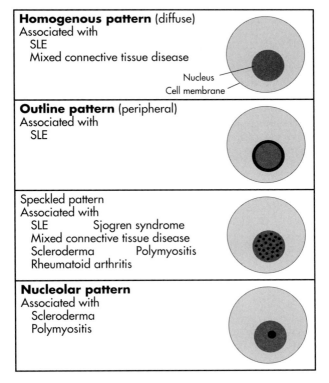

Figure 3 Patterns of immunofluorescent staining of antinuclear antibodies and the diseases with which they are associated. (From Pagana KD, Pagana TJ: *Mosby's manual of diagnostic and laboratory tests,* St Louis, 1998, Mosby.)

Procedure and patient care

Before
- Explain the procedure to the patient.
- Tell the patient that no fasting or preparation is required.

During
- Collect 7 to 10 ml of venous blood in a red-top tube.
- Indicate on the laboratory slip any drugs that may affect the test results.

After
- Apply pressure to the venipuncture site.

Abnormal findings

▲ **Increased levels**

SLE
Rheumatoid arthritis
Chronic hepatitis
Periarteritis (polyarteritis) nodosa
Dermatomyositis
Scleroderma
Infectious mononucleosis
Raynaud's disease
Sjögren syndrome
Other immune diseases
Leukemia
Myasthenia gravis
Cirrhosis

notes

antiscleroderma antibody (Scl-70 antibody, Scleroderma antibody)

Type of test Blood

Normal findings Negative

Test explanation and related physiology

This antibody is diagnostic for scleroderma (progressive systemic sclerosis [PSS]) and is present in 45% of patients with that disease. Scl-70 antibody is an *antinuclear antibody* (see p. 80). PPS (scleroderma) is a multisystem disorder characterized by inflammation with subsequent fibrosis of the small blood vessels in skin and visceral organs, including the heart, lungs, kidneys, and gastrointestinal tract. A collagen-like substance is also deposited into the tissue of these organs. In general, the higher the titer of Scl-70 antibody, the more likely that PSS exists and the more active the disease is. As the diseases becomes less active because of therapy, the Scl-70 antibody titers can be expected to fall.

The absence of this antibody does not exclude the diagnosis of scleroderma. The antibody is rather specific for PSS but is occasionally seen in other autoimmune diseases such as systemic lupus erythematosus, mixed connective tissue disease, Sjögren's syndrome, polymyositis, and rheumatoid arthritis.

Interfering factors

☛ Drugs that may cause *increased* levels include aminosalicylic acid, isoniazid, methyldopa, penicillin, propylthiouracil, streptomycin, and tetracycline.

Procedure and patient care

Before
- Explain the procedure to the patient.
- Tell the patient that no fasting is required.

During
- Collect a venous sample of blood in a red-top tube.

After
- Apply pressure to the venipuncture site.

Abnormal findings

Positive

Scleroderma
CREST syndrome

notes

anti-smooth muscle antibody (ASMA)

Type of test Blood

Normal findings No anti-smooth muscle antibodies (ASMAs) at titers >1:20

Test explanation and related physiology

The ASMA is used primarily to aid in the diagnosis of autoimmune chronic active hepatitis (CAH), which has also been referred to as "lupoid" CAH. ASMA is an *anticytoplasmic antibody* directed against actin, a cytoskeletal protein. Normally the serum does not contain ASMA at a titer greater than 1:20. ASMA is the most commonly recognized autoantibody in the setting of CAH. It appears in 70% to 80% of patients with CAH. Some types of CAH do not have positive ASMA antibodies. This disease may be an autoimmune disease that occurs predominantly in adult women. The clinical presentation of CAH is similar to viral hepatitis. That clinical picture, along with serologic and pathologic criteria, must exist for >6 months to be classified as CAH.

ASMA is not specific for CAH and can be positive in patients with viral infections, malignancy, multiple sclerosis, primary biliary cirrhosis, and *Mycoplasma* infections. Usually the titer of ASMA is low in these diseases. With CAH the titer is usually higher than 1:160. The titers are not helpful in predicting prognosis, nor do they indicate disease response to therapy.

Procedure and patient care

Before
- Explain the procedure to the patient.
- Tell the patient that no fasting or special preparation is required.

During
- Collect 7 to 10 ml of venous blood in a red-top tube.

After
- Apply pressure to the venipuncture site.
- Patients with liver disease can have bleeding disorders.

Abnormal findings

▲ **Increased levels**

CAH
Mononucleosis hepatitis
Primary biliary cirrhosis
Viral hepatitis

Multiple sclerosis
Malignancy
Intrinsic asthma

notes

antispermatozoal antibody (Sperm agglutination and inhibition, Sperm antibodies, Antisperm antibodies, Infertility screen)

Type of test Fluid analysis; blood

Normal findings Negative

Test explanation and related physiology

The antispermatozoal antibody test is an infertility screening test used to detect the presence of sperm antibodies. Antibodies directed toward sperm antigens can result in diminished fertility. This test is commonly used in the evaluation of an infertile couple. Antisperm antibodies may be found in the blood of men with blocked efferent ducts of the testes (a common cause of low sperm counts or poor sperm mobility) and in 30% to 70% of men who have had a vasectomy. Resorption of sperm from the blocked ducts results in the formation of autoantibodies to sperm as a result of sperm antigens interacting with the immune system. The IgA antisperm antibodies to the sperm tail are associated with poor motility and poor penetration of cervical mucus. IgG antisperm antibodies are associated with blockage of sperm-ovum fusion. High titers of IgG autoantibodies are often associated with postvasectomy degeneration of the testes, which explains why 50% of males remain infertile after successful repair of a previous vasectomy.

In men high serum titers of antispermatozoal antibody are considered strong evidence of infertility. Low titers are of unknown significance, as that is not an uncommon finding among normal fertile males. Serum antispermatozoal antibodies are found in nearly 20% of women. However, many of these women become pregnant. Therefore the significance of this antibody in women is uncertain.

Antispermatozoal antibodies can also be detected in the sperm of infertile males and in the cervical mucus of infertile females. It is often necessary to identify these antibodies in the serum and other body fluids in the thorough evaluation of infertility.

Procedure and patient care

Before
- Explain the procedure to the patient.

Sperm specimen
- Inform the man that a semen specimen should be collected after avoiding ejaculation for at least 3 days.
- Give the male patient the proper container for the sperm collection.
- If the specimen is to be collected at home, be certain the patient is told that it must be taken to the laboratory for testing within 2 hours after collection.

During
- Collect a venous blood sample of approximately 7 to 10 ml from both the male and the female patient in red-top tubes.
- For a sperm specimen, collect the ejaculate in a plastic container.
- For a vaginal mucus specimen, collect 1 ml of cervical mucus and place in a plastic vial.

After
- Apply pressure to the venipuncture site.
- For a sperm, blood, or cervical specimen, place the specimen in a plastic vial, freeze, and send to a reference laboratory on dry ice.
- Instruct the couple when and how to obtain the test results.

Abnormal findings

Infertility
Blocked efferent ducts in the testes
Vasectomy

notes

anti-SS-A (Ro), anti-SS-B (La), and anti-SS-C anti-body (Anti-Ro, Anti-La, Sjögren's antibodies)

Type of test Blood

Normal findings Negative

Test explanation and related physiology

These three antinuclear antibodies are used to diagnose Sjögren syndrome. Ro, La, and SS-C antibodies are a subtype of *antinuclear antibodies (ANA)* and react to nuclear antigens extracted from human B lymphocytes. Ro and La result in a speckled immunofluorescent pattern when seen in the UV microscope (see Figure 3, p. 81). Sjögren syndrome is an immunogenic disease characterized by progressive destruction of the lacrimal and salivary exocrine glands leading to mucosal and conjunctival dryness. This disease can occur by itself (primary) or in association with other autoimmune diseases such as systemic lupus erythematosus (SLE), rheumatoid arthritis, and sclero-derma. In the latter case, it is referred to as secondary Sjögren's syndrome.

Anti-SS-A antibodies may be found in approximately 60% to 70% of patients with primary Sjögren syndrome. Anti-SS-B antibodies may be found in approximately half of patients with primary Sjögren syndrome. When anti SS-A and SS-B antibodies are both positive, Sjögren syndrome can be diagnosed. These antibodies are only occasionally found when secondary Sjögren syndrome is associated with rheumatoid arthritis (RA). In fact SS-B is only found in primary Sjögren syndrome. However, anti-SS-C is positive in about 75% of patients with RA or patients with RA and secondary Sjögren syndrome. Therefore these antibodies are also useful in differentiating primary from secondary Sjögren syndrome.

SS-A can also be found in 25% of patients with SLE. This is particularly useful in "ANA (antinuclear antigen)-negative" cases of SLE, because these antibodies are present in the majority of such patients. SS-B is never found in SLE, however. In general, the higher the titer of anti SS antibodies, the more likely that Sjögren syndrome exists, and the more active is the disease. As Sjögren syndrome becomes less active with therapy, the anti SS antibodies titers can be expected to fall.

Procedure and patient care

Before

- Explain the procedure to the patient.
- Tell the patient that no fasting is required.

During

- Collect a venous blood sample in a red-top tube.

After

- Apply pressure to the venipuncture site.

Abnormal findings

Positive

Sjögren syndrome
Rheumatoid arthritis

ANA-negative SLE
Neonatal lupus

notes

antistreptolysin O titer (ASO titer)

Type of test Blood

Normal findings

Adult/elderly: ≤160 Todd units/ml
Newborn: similar to mother's value
  6 months-2 years: ≤50 Todd units/ml
  2-4 years: ≤160 Todd units/ml
  5-12 years: 170-330 Todd units/ml

Test explanation and related physiology

This test is used primarily in determining that a previous *Streptococcus* infection has caused a poststreptococcal disease such as glomerulonephritis, rheumatic fever, bacterial endocarditis, or scarlet fever. Levels are highest in glomerulonephritis and rheumatic fever. The ASO titer is a serologic procedure demonstrating the reaction of the body to infection caused by group A beta hemolytic streptococci bacteria. The *Streptococcus* organism produces an enzyme called streptolysin O, which has the ability to destroy (lyse) red blood corpuscles. Because streptolysin O is antigenic, the body reacts by producing ASO, a neutralizing antibody. ASO appears in the serum 1 week to 1 month after the onset of a streptococcal infection; a high titer is not specific for a certain type of poststreptococcal disease (i.e., rheumatic fever versus glomerulonephritis), but merely indicates that a streptococcal infection is or has been present. When the ASO elevation is seen in a patient with glomerulonephritis or endocarditis, one can safely assume that the disease was caused by streptococcal infection. Serial rising titers of ASO over several weeks, followed by a slow fall in titers, is more supportive of the diagnosis of a previous streptococcal infection than is a single titer. The highest incidence of positive results is during the third week after the onset of acute symptoms of the poststreptococcal disease. By 6 months only about 30% of patients have abnormal titers.

Another immunologic test, *antideoxyribonuclease B (anti-DNase B)* (see p. 65) also detects antigens produced by group A streptococci. The anti-DNase B level is elevated in most patients with acute rheumatic fever and poststreptococcal glomerulonephritis. When ASO and anti-DNase B are performed concurrently, 95% of previous streptococcal infections are detected.

Interfering factors

- Increased beta-lipoprotein levels inhibit streptolysin O and give a falsely high ASO titer.
- Drugs that may cause *decreased* ASO levels include antibiotics and adrenocorticosteroids.

Procedure and patient care

Before
- Explain the procedure to the patient.
- Tell the patient that no fasting is required.

During
- Collect approximately 5 to 10 ml of blood in a red-top tube.
- Avoid hemolysis of the blood specimen.
- Note on the laboratory slip any medications that may affect the test results.

After
- Apply pressure to the venipuncture site.
- Note that repeat ASO testing may be done to determine the highest level of increase.

Abnormal findings

▲ Increased levels
    Streptococcal infection
    Acute rheumatic fever
    Acute glomerulonephritis
    Bacterial endocarditis
    Scarlet fever
    Streptococcal pyoderma

notes

antithrombin III (AT-III, Functional antithrombin III assay, Heparin cofactor, Immunologic antithrombin III, Serine protease inhibitor)

Type of test Blood

Normal findings

Plasma: >50% of control value
Serum: 15% to 34% lower than plasma value
Immunologic: 17-30 mg/dl
Functional: 80% to 120%
   (Values vary according to laboratory methods.)

Test explanation and related physiology

This test is used to evaluate patients suspected of having hypercoagulable states. It is also used to help identify the cause of "heparin resistance" in patients receiving heparin therapy. AT-III is an alpha$_2$ globulin produced in the liver. It inhibits the serum proteases involved in coagulation (II, X, IX, XI, XII). In normal homeostasis the coagulation system results from a balance between AT-III and thrombin. A deficiency of AT-III increases coagulation or the tendency toward thrombosis. A hereditary deficiency of AT-III is characterized by a predisposition toward thrombus formation. This is passed on as an autosomal-dominant abnormality. Individuals with hereditary AT III deficiency typically develop thromboembolic events in their early twenties. These thrombotic events are usually venous. Acquired AT-III deficiency may be seen in patients with cirrhosis, liver failure, advanced carcinoma, nephrotic syndrome, disseminated intravascular coagulation, and acute thrombosis. AT III is also decreased as much as 30% by pregnancy or with the use of exogenous estrogens. AT III provides most of the anticoagulant effect of heparin. Heparin requires AT III to express its effect. Patients who are deficient in AT III may be heparin resistant and require unusually high doses to provide anticoagulation. In general, patients respond to heparin if more than 60% of normal AT III levels exists.

Asymptomatic individuals with an antithrombin deficiency should receive prophylactic anticoagulation to raise their antithrombin levels before any medical/surgical circumstances in which inactivity increases the risk of thrombosis. Increased levels of AT-III may occur in patients with acute hepatitis, obstructive jaundice, vitamin K deficiency, and kidney transplantation.

Interfering factors

☞ Drugs that may cause *increased* levels include anabolic steroids, androgens, oral contraceptives (containing progesterone), and sodium warfarin.

☞ Drugs that may cause *decreased* levels include fibrinolytics, heparin, L-asparaginase, and oral contraceptives (containing estrogen).

Procedure and patient care

Before
- Explain the procedure to the patient.
- Tell the patient that no fasting is required.

During
- Collect a venous blood sample in a blue- or red-top tube.

After
- Apply pressure to the venipuncture site.
- Send the specimen to the laboratory immediately after collection.

Abnormal findings

▲ **Increased levels**
Kidney transplant
Acute hepatitis
Obstructive jaundice
Vitamin K deficiency

▼ **Decreased levels**
Disseminated intravascular coagulation
Hypercoagulation states (e.g., deep vein thrombosis)
Hepatic disorders (especially cirrhosis)
Nephrotic syndrome
Protein-wasting diseases (malignancy)
Hereditary familial deficiency of AT-III

antithyroglobulin antibody (Thyroid autoantibody, Thyroid antithyroglobulin antibody, Thyroglobulin antibody)

Type of test Blood

Normal findings Titer <1:100

Test explanation and related physiology

This test is primarily used in the differential diagnosis of thyroid diseases such as Hashimoto's thyroiditis or chronic lymphocytic thyroiditis (in children). There are several antibodies to various thyroid gland components. Antithyroglobulin occurs when thyroglobulin, which normally exists in the blood (as a thyroid hormone carrier) and in the thyroid acts as an immune stimulating antigen. Autoantibodies are developed and react against the thyroglobulin in the thyroid cells. This leads to thyroid inflammation and destruction.

Although many different thyroid diseases are associated with elevated antithyroglobulin levels, the most frequent is chronic thyroiditis (Hashimoto's thyroiditis in the adult and lymphocytic thyroiditis in children and young adults). The level must be extremely high to confirm the diagnosis of Hashimoto's thyroiditis. This antibody is present in only about 50% of patients with Hashimoto's thyroiditis. Both Hashimoto's and lymphocytic thyroiditis have been associated with other autoimmune (collagen vascular) diseases. The antithyroglobulin test is usually performed in conjunction with the antithyroid microsomal antibody test (see p. 97). When this is done, the specificity and sensitivity are greatly increased.

A small percentage of the normal population have antithyroglobulin antibodies. Normally women tend to have higher levels than men.

Interfering factors

- Normal individuals, especially elderly women, may have antithyroglobulin antibodies.

Procedure and patient care

Before
- Explain the procedure to the patient.
- Tell the patient that no fasting is required.

During
- Collect approximately 3 to 5 ml of blood in a red-top tube.

After
- Apply pressure to the venipuncture site.

Abnormal findings

▲   **Increased levels**

Hashimoto's thyroiditis   Hypothyroidism
Rheumatoid arthritis   Thyroid carcinoma
Rheumatoid-collagen disease   Myxedema
Pernicious anemia
Thyrotoxicosis

notes

antithyroid microsomal antibody (Antimicrosomal antibody, Microsomal antibody, Thyroid autoantibody, Thyroid antimicrosomal antibody)

Type of test Blood

Normal findings Titer <1:100; present in 5% to 10% of healthy people

Test explanation and related physiology

This test is primarily used in the differential diagnosis of thyroid diseases such as Hashimoto's thyroiditis or chronic lymphocytic thyroiditis (in children). Thyroid microsomal antibodies are commonly found in patients with various thyroid diseases. They are found in 70% to 90% of patients with Hashimoto's thyroiditis. Microsomal antibodies are produced in response to microsomes escaping from the thyroid epithelial cells surrounding the thyroid follicle. These escaped microsomes then act as antigens and stimulate the production of antibodies. These immune complexes initiate inflammatory and cytotoxic effects on the thyroid follicle. This test is often performed in conjunction with the antithyroglobulin antibody test (see p. 95). When this is done, the specificity and sensitivity are greatly increased.

Although many different thyroid diseases are associated with elevated antimicrosomal antibody levels, the most frequent is chronic thyroiditis (Hashimoto's thyroiditis in adults and lymphocytic thyroiditis in children and young adults). Both of these chronic inflammatory diseases have been associated with other autoimmune (collagen vascular) diseases. Twelve percent of normal females and 1% of normal males have positive antimicrosomal antibodies.

Procedure and patient care

Before
- Tell the patient that no fasting is required.

During
- Collect approximately 3 to 5 ml of venous blood in a red-top tube.

After
- Apply pressure to the venipuncture site.

Abnormal findings

▲ **Increased values**

Chronic thyroiditis
  (Hashimoto's thyroiditis)
Rheumatoid arthritis
Rheumatoid-collagen
  disease
Pernicious anemia

Thyrotoxicosis
Hypothyroidism
Thyroid carcinoma
Myxedema

notes

apolipoproteins (Apolipoprotein A-I [Apo A-I], Apolipoprotein B [Apo B], Lipoprotein (a) [Lp (a)])

Type of test Blood

Normal findings

Apo A-I
Adult/elderly
  Male: 75-160 mg/dl
  Female: 80-175 mg/dl
Child
  Newborn
    Male: 41-93 mg/dl
    Female: 38-106 mg/dl
  6 months-4 years
    Male: 67-167 mg/dl
    Female: 60-148 mg/dl
  5 to 17 years: 83-151 mg/dl

Apo B
Adult/elderly
  Male: 50-125 mg/dl
  Female: 45-120 mg/dl
Child
  Newborn: 11-31 mg/dl
  6 months-3 years: 23-75 mg/dl
  5-17 years:
    Male: 47-139 mg/dl
    Female: 41-132 mg/dl

Apo A-I/Apo B ratio
Male: 0.85-2.24
Female: 0.76-3.23

Lipoprotein (a)
Caucasian (5th-95th percentile)
  Male: 2.2-49.4 mg/dl
  Female: 2.1-57.3 mg/dl
African-American (5th-95th percentile)
  Male: 4.6-71.8 mg/dl
  Female: 4.4-75 mg/dl

Test explanation and related physiology

This test is used to evaluate the risks of atherogenic disease of the heart and peripheral arteries. These levels may be better indicators of atherogenic risks than lipoproteins such as HDL, LDL, and VLDL (see p. 528). The protein component of those lipoproteins, which plays an important role in lipid transport, is composed of several specific polypeptides called apolipoproteins. Apolipoproteins are also involved in binding lipoproteins to lipoprotein receptors at the cell surface, thus facilitating lipid uptake by cells.

Apolipoprotein A (apo A) is the major polypeptide component of HDL. Apo A has two major forms: apo A-I, which constitutes about 75% of the apo A in HDL, and apo A-II, which constitutes about 20% of the total HDL protein. In general, as HDL levels increase, apo A-I values increase. Since apo A-I reflects the HDL content of the serum and HDL levels are greater in females, apo A-I values are also higher in women than in men. Apo A-I has been proposed to be a better index of atherogenic risk than HDL assay.

Apolipoprotein B (apo B) is the major polypeptide component of LDL and makes up about 80% of that protein. Forty percent of the protein portion of very low–density lipoprotein (VLDL) is composed of apo B. Apo B has been shown to exist in two forms: apo B-100 and apo B-48. Apo B-100 is synthesized in the liver and found in lipoproteins of endogenous origin (VLDL and LDL). Apo B-100 is the principle transport mechanism for endogenous cholesterol. Apo B-100 has an affinity for the LDL receptor located on cell surfaces in peripheral tissues and is involved with cellular deposition of cholesterol. Because of this, some believe that apo B-100 may be a better indicator of atherosclerotic heart disease than LDL. The second apo B component is apo B-48, which is of intestinal origin and found mainly in chylomicrons. Apo B-48 serves to transport ingested lipids through the intestines and into the bloodstream.

Lipoprotein (a) [Lp(a)] (referred to as "lipoprotein little a") is another lipoprotein. The two polypeptide components of Lp(a) are apo (A) and an LDL-like protein containing apo B-100. Recent research has suggested that increased levels of Lp(a) may be an independent risk factor for atherosclerosis. It has been shown that apo (A) is a deformed relative of plasminogen, the precursor of the proteolytic enzyme plasmin, which is responsible for dissolving fiber clots. This strong resemblance between an apolipoprotein and plasminogen may provide a link between lipids, the clotting mechanism, and atherogenesis. Microthrombi containing fibrin on the vessel wall become incorporated into the atherosclerotic plaque. It is suggested that, following endothelial damage, Lp(a) may insinuate itself into the arterial wall, inhibiting the cleavage of fibrin in microthrombi by competing with plasminogen for access for fibrin. Atherosclerotic damage of the arterial wall soon follows, leading to occlusive disease or aneurysm.

Decreased levels of apo A-I and increased levels of apo B-100 are associated with increased risk of coronary heart disease. Reports also indicate that a low ratio of apo A-I to apo B may be a good predictor of coronary heart disease. Individuals with increased concentrations of Lp(a) appear to have a significantly higher risk for coronary heart disease. Quantification of apolipoproteins is beginning to be performed as a routine clinical procedure.

These and other apolipoproteins are associated with the identification of other maladies. For example, the apo E4 gene has been proposed as a risk factor for Alzheimer's disease. Familial hypercholesterolemia, some forms of renal failure, nephrotic syndrome, and estrogen depletion in women over the age of 50 may be associated with increased levels of Lp(a).

Interfering factors

Apo A-I

- Physical exercise may increase apo A-I levels.
- Smoking may decrease levels.
- Diets high in carbohydrates or polyunsaturated fats may decrease apo A-I levels.
- Drugs that may *increase* apo A-I levels include carbamazepine, estrogens, ethanol, lovastatin, niacin, oral contraceptives, phenobarbital, pravastatin, and simvastatin.
- Drugs that may *decrease* apo A-I levels include androgens, beta blockers, diuretics, and progestins.

Apo B

- Diets high in saturated fats and cholesterol may increase apo B levels.
- Drugs that may *increase* apo B levels may include androgens, beta blockers, diuretics, ethanol abuse, and progestins.
- Drugs that may *decrease* apo B levels include cholestyramine, estrogen (postmenopausal women), lovastatin, simvastatin, neomycin, niacin, and thyroxine.

Lipoprotein (a)

☛ Drugs that may *decrease* Lp(a) include estrogens, niacin, neomycin, and stanozolol.

Procedure and patient care

Before

- Explain the procedure to the patient.
- Instruct the patient to fast for 12 to 14 hours before testing. Only water is permitted.
- Inform the patient that smoking is prohibited.

During

- Collect venous blood in a red-top tube.
- Indicate on the laboratory slip any drugs that may affect test results.

After

- Apply pressure to the venipuncture site.

Abnormal findings

▲ **Increased apo A-I**
Familial hyperalpha-
  lipoproteinemia
Pregnancy
Weight reduction

▼ **Decreased apo A-I**
Coronary artery disease
Ischemic coronary disease
Myocardial infarction
Familial hypoalphalipopro-
  teinemia
Fish eye disease
Uncontrolled diabetes
  mellitus
Tangier disease
Nephrotic syndrome
Chronic renal failure
Cholestasis
Hemodialysis

▲ **Increased apo B**
  Hyperlipoproteinemia
    (types IIa, IIb, IV, V)
  Nephrotic syndrome
  Pregnancy
  Hemodialysis
  Biliary obstruction
  Coronary artery disease
  Diabetes
  Hypothyroidism
  Anorexia nervosa

▲ **Increased levels
  of Lp(a)**
  Premature coronary
    artery disease
  Stenosis of cerebral
    arteries
  Uncontrolled diabetes
    mellitus
  Severe hypothyroidism
  Familial hypercholester-
    olemia
  Chronic renal failure
  Estrogen depletion

▼ **Decreased apo B**
  Tangier disease
  Hyperthyroidism
  Malnutrition
  Inflammatory joint
    disease
  Chronic pulmonary
    disease
  Weight reduction
  Chronic anemia
  Reye's syndrome

▼ **Decreased levels
  of Lp(a)**
  Alcoholism
  Malnutrition
  Chronic liver hepa-
    tocellular disease

notes

arterial blood gases (blood gases [ABGs])

Type of test Blood

Normal findings

pH
Adult/child: 7.35-7.45
Newborn: 7.32-7.49
2 months-2 years: 7.34-7.46
pH (venous) 7.31-7.41

Pco_2
Adult/child: 35-45 mm Hg
Child <2 years: 26-41 mm Hg
Pco_2 (venous) 40-50 mm Hg

HCO_3^-
Adult/child: 21-28 mEq/L
Newborn/infant: 16-24 mEq/L

Po_2
Adult/child: 80-100 mm Hg
Newborn: 60-70 mm Hg
Po_2 (venous) 40-50 mm Hg

O_2 saturation
Adult/child: 95% to 100%
  Elderly: 95%
  Newborn: 40% to 90%
  O_2 content (arterial) 15-22 vol %
  O_2 content (venous) 11-16 vol %

Possible critical values

pH: <7.25, >7.55
Pco_2: <20, >60
HCO_3^-: <15, >40
Po_2: <40
O_2 saturation: 75% or lower
Base Excess ±3 mEq/L

Test explanation and related physiology

  Measurement of ABGs provides valuable information in assessing and managing a patient's respiratory (ventilation) and metabolic (renal) acid/base and electrolyte homeostasis. It is also used to assess adequacy of oxygenation. ABGs are used to monitor patients on ventilators, monitor critically ill nonventilator patients, establish preoperative baseline parameters, and enlighten electrolyte therapy.

pH

The pH is inversely proportional to the actual hydrogen ion concentration. Therefore, as the hydrogen ion concentration decreases, the pH increases, and vice versa. The pH is a measure of alkalinity (pH >7.4) and acidity (pH <7.35). In respiratory or metabolic alkalosis, the pH is elevated; in respiratory or metabolic acidosis, the pH is decreased (Table 2).

Pco_2

The Pco_2 is a measure of the partial pressure of CO_2 in the blood. Pco_2 is a measurement of ventilation capability. The faster and more deeply one breathes, the more CO_2 is blown off, and Pco_2 levels drop. Therefore Pco_2 is referred to as the *respiratory* component in acid-base determination because this value is primarily controlled by the lungs. As the CO_2 level increases, the pH decreases. The CO_2 level and the pH are inversely proportional. The Pco_2 in the blood and cerebrospinal fluid is a major stimulant to the breathing center in the brain. As Pco_2 levels rise, breathing is stimulated. If Pco_2 levels rise too high, breathing cannot keep up with the demand to blow off or ventilate. As Pco_2 levels rise further, the brain is depressed, and ventilation decreases further causing coma.

The Pco_2 level is elevated in primary respiratory acidosis and decreased in primary respiratory alkalosis (see Table 2). Because the lungs compensate for primary metabolic acid-base derangements, Pco_2 levels are affected by metabolic disturbances as well. In metabolic acidosis the lungs attempt to compensate by "blowing off" CO_2 to raise pH. In metabolic alkalosis the lungs attempt to compensate by retaining CO_2 to lower pH (Table 3).

Bicarbonate (HCO_3^-) or CO_2 content

Most of the CO_2 content in the blood is HCO_3^-. The bicarbonate ion is a measure of the *metabolic (renal/kidney)* component of the acid-base equilibrium. It is regulated by the kidney. This ion can be measured directly by the bicarbonate value or indirectly by the CO_2 content (see p. 197). As the HCO_3^- level increases, the pH also increases; therefore the relationship of bicarbonate to pH is directly proportional. HCO_3^- is elevated in metabolic alkalosis and decreased in

TABLE 2 Normal values for arterial blood gases and abnormal values in uncompensated acid-base disturbances

Acid-base disturbances	pH	Pco₂ (mm Hg)	HCO₃⁻ (mEq/L)	Common cause
None (normal values)	7.35-7.45	35-45	22-26	
Respiratory acidosis	↓	↑	Normal	Respiratory depression (drugs, central nervous system trauma) Pulmonary disease (pneumonia, chronic obstructive pulmonary disease, respiratory underventilation)
Respiratory alkalosis	↑	↓	Normal	Hyperventilation (emotions, pain, respirator overventilation)
Metabolic acidosis	↓	Normal	↓	Diabetes, shock, renal failure, intestinal fistula
Metabolic alkalosis	↑	Normal	↑	Sodium bicarbonate overdose, prolonged vomiting, nasogastric drainage

TABLE 3 Acid-base disturbances and compensatory mechanisms

Acid-base disturbance	Mode of compensation
Respiratory acidosis	Kidneys will retain increased amounts of HCO_3^- to increase pH.
Respiratory alkalosis	Kidneys will excrete increased amounts of HCO_3^- to lower pH.
Metabolic acidosis	Lungs "blow off" CO_2 to raise pH.
Metabolic alkalosis	Lungs retain CO_2 to lower pH.

metabolic acidosis (see Table 2). The kidneys also are used to compensate for primary respiratory acid-base derangements. For example, in respiratory acidosis the kidneys attempt to compensate by resorbing increased amounts of HCO_3^-. In respiratory alkalosis the kidneys excrete HCO_3^- in increased amounts in an attempt to lower pH through compensation. In diabetic ketoacidosis HCO_3^- ion does decrease because it is directly used to neutralize the plasma diabetic acids (see Table 3).

Po_2

This is an indirect measure of the oxygen content of arterial blood. Po_2 is a measure of the tension (pressure) of oxygen dissolved in the plasma. This pressure determines the force of O_2 to diffuse across the pulmonary alveoli membrane. The Po_2 level is decreased in:

1. Patients who are unable to oxygenate the arterial blood because of O_2 diffusion difficulties (e.g., pneumonia, shock lung, congestive failure)
2. Patients who have premature mixing of venous blood with arterial blood (e.g., in congenital heart disease)
3. Patients who have underventilated and overperfused pulmonary alveoli (Pickwickian syndrome [i.e., obese patients who cannot breathe properly when in the supine position or patients with significant atelectasis])

O_2 saturation

Oxygen saturation is an indication of the percentage of hemoglobin saturated with O_2. When 92% to 100% of the hemoglobin carries O_2, the tissues are adequately provided with O_2, assuming normal O_2 dissociation. As the Po_2 level decreases, the percentage of hemoglobin saturation also decreases. When the Po_2 level drops below 60 mm Hg, small decreases in the Po_2 level cause large decreases in the percentage of hemoglobin saturated with O_2. At O_2 saturation levels of 70% or lower, the tissues are unable to extract enough O_2 to carry out their vital functions.

O_2 saturation is calculated by the blood gas machine using the following formula:

$$\text{Percentage of } O_2 \text{ saturation} = 100 \times \frac{\text{volume of } O_2 \text{ content Hgb}}{\text{volume of } O_2 \text{ Hgb capacity}}$$

Pulse oximetry is a noninvasive method of determining O_2 saturation. This can be done easily and continuously. This machine measures O_2 saturation. It actually measures all forms of oxygen-saturated hemoglobin, including carboxyhemoglobin (which rises during smoke inhalation or some inhalants). Therefore, in cases of carbon monoxide poisoning in which carboxyhemoglobin is high, oximetry will indicate an inaccurately high O_2 saturation. During oximetry monitoring a small cliplike sensor is applied to the tip of the finger or earlobe. The oximeter transmits light from one side and records the amount of light on the other side, thus determining O_2 saturation.

O_2 content

This is a calculated number that represents the amount of O_2 in the blood. The formula for calculation is:

$$O_2 \text{ content} = O_2 \text{ saturation} \times Hgb \times 1.34 + Po_2 \times 0.003$$

Nearly all O_2 in the blood is bound to hemoglobin. O_2 content decreases with the same diseases that diminish Po_2.

Base excess/deficit

This number is calculated by the blood gas machine using the pH, Pco_2, and the hematocrit. It represents the amount of buffering anions in the blood. HCO_3^- is the largest of these. Others include hemoglobin, proteins, and phosphates. Base excess is a way to take all these anions into account when determining acid/base treatment based on the *metabolic* component. Negative base excess (deficit) indicates a metabolic acidosis (e.g., lactic acidosis). A positive base excess indicates metabolic alkalosis or compensation to prolonged respiratory acidosis.

Contraindications

- Negative Allen's test indicating that there is no ulnar artery
- AV fistula proximal to the site of proposed access
- Severe coagulopathy

Potential complications

- Occlusion of the artery used for access
- Penetration of other important structures anatomically juxtaposed to the artery (e.g., nerve)

Interfering factors

- O_2 saturation can be falsely increased with the inhalation of carbon monoxide.
- Respiration can be inhibited by the use of sedative hypnotics or narcotics.

Procedure and patient care

Before

- Explain the procedure to the patient.
- Notify the laboratory before drawing ABGs so that the necessary equipment can be calibrated before the blood sample arrives.
- Perform the Allen test to assess collateral circulation.
- To perform the Allen test, make the patient's hand blanch by obliterating both the radial and the ulnar pulses, and then release the pressure over the ulnar artery only. If flow through the ulnar artery is good, flushing will be seen immediately. The Allen test is then positive, and the radial artery can be used for puncture.
- If the Allen test is negative (no flushing), repeat it on the other arm.
- If both arms give a negative result, choose another artery for puncture.
- Note that the Allen test ensures collateral circulation to the hand if thrombosis of the radial artery should follow the puncture.

During

- Note that arterial blood can be obtained from any area of the body where strong pulses are palpable, usually from the radial, brachial, or femoral artery.
- Cleanse the arterial site.

- Consider applying 0.5 ml of lidocaine in the skin overlying the proposed access site.
- Attach a 20-gauge needle to a syringe containing approximately 0.2 ml of heparin.
- After drawing 3 to 5 ml of blood, remove the needle and apply pressure to the arterial site for 3 to 5 minutes.
- Expel any air bubbles in the syringe.
- Cap the syringe and gently rotate to mix the blood and heparin.
- Indicate on the laboratory slip if the patient is receiving oxygen therapy or is attached to a ventilator.
- Note that an arterial puncture is performed by laboratory technicians, respiratory-inhalation therapists, nurses, or physicians in approximately 10 minutes.
- Tell the patient that the arterial puncture is associated with more discomfort than a venous puncture.

After

- Place the arterial blood on ice and immediately take it to the chemistry laboratory for analysis.
- Apply pressure or a pressure dressing to the arterial puncture site for 3 to 5 minutes to avoid hematoma formation.
- Assess the puncture site for bleeding. Remember that an artery rather than a vein has been stuck.
- If the patient has an abnormal clotting time or is taking anticoagulants, apply pressure for a longer period (approximately 15 minutes).

Abnormal findings

▲ **Increased pH (alkalosis)**
   Metabolic alkalosis
   Hypokalemia
   Hypochloremia
   Chronic and high volume
     gastric suction
   Chronic vomiting
   Aldosteronism
   Mercurial diuretics

   Respiratory alkalosis
   Chronic heart failure
   Cystic fibrosis
   Carbon monoxide poisoning
   Pulmonary emboli
   Shock
   Acute severe pulmonary
     diseases
   Anxiety neuroses
   Pain
   Pregnancy

▼ **Decreased pH
   (acidosis)**
   Metabolic acidosis
   Ketoacidosis
   Lactic acidosis
   Severe diarrhea
   Renal failure

   Respiratory acidosis
   Respiratory failure

▲ **Increased P_{CO_2}**
   Chronic obstructive
     pulmonary disease
     (COPD) (bronchitis,
     emphysema)
   Oversedation
   Head trauma
   Overoxygenation in a
     patient with COPD
   Pickwickian syndrome

▼ **Decreased P_{CO_2}**
   Hypoxemia
   Pulmonary emboli
   Anxiety
   Pain
   Pregnancy

▲ **Increased P_{O_2}, increased O_2 content**
Polycythemia
Increased inspired O_2
Hyperventilation

▼ **Decreased P_{O_2}, decreased O_2 content**
Anemias
Mucus plug
Bronchospasm
Atelectasis
Pneumothorax
Pulmonary edema
Adult respiratory distress
  syndrome
Restrictive lung disease
Atrial or ventricular cardiac
  septal defects
Emboli
Inadequate O_2 in inspired air
  (suffocation)
Severe hypoventilation (e.g.,
  oversedation, neurologic
  somnolence)

▲ **Increased HCO_3^-**
Chronic vomiting
Chronic high volume
  gastric suction
Aldosteronism
Use of mercurial
  diuretics
COPD

▼ **Decreased HCO_3^-**
Chronic and severe
  diarrhea
Chronic use of loop
  diuretics
Starvation
Diabetic ketoacidosis
Acute renal failure

notes

arteriography (Angiography)

Type of test X-ray with contrast dye

Normal findings Normal arterial vasculature

Test explanation and related physiology

With the injection of radiopaque contrast material into arteries, blood vessels can be visualized to determine arterial anatomy, vascular disease, or neoplasms. With a catheter usually placed through the femoral artery and into the desired artery, radiopaque contrast is rapidly injected while x-ray films are obtained. Blood flow dynamics, abnormal blood vessels, vascular anomalies, normal and abnormal vascular anatomy, and tumors are easily seen. With the use of *digital subtraction angiography (DSA)*, bony structures can be obliterated from the picture.

DSA is a sophisticated type of computerized fluoroscopy that, when used with arterial angiography, can better visualize the arteries of the body, especially the carotid and cerebral arteries. It is especially useful when adjacent bone inhibits visualization of the blood vessel to be evaluated. For DSA an image (mask) is made of the area of clinical interest and stored in the computer program. After intraarterial injection of contrast material, subsequent images are made. The computer then subtracts the preinjection "mask" image from the postinjection image. This removes all the undesired images (e.g., bone) and leaves the arterial image of high contrast and quality.

Although nearly all major blood vessels can be visualized through the technique of arteriography, the kidneys, adrenal glands, brain, and abdominal aorta (with lower extremities) are most usually visualized. Coronary arteriography is described under cardiac catheterization (see p. 203).

Renal angiography permits evaluation of blood flow dynamics, demonstration of abnormal blood vessels, and differentiation of a vascular renal cyst from hypervascular renal cancers. Arteriosclerotic narrowing (stenosis) of the renal artery is best demonstrated with this study. The angiographic location of the stenotic area is helpful for the vascular surgeon considering repair. Complete transection of the renal artery by blunt or penetrating trauma can also be seen as total vascular obstruction. Highly vascular renal cancers can produce a "blush" of contrast material during angiography.

The adrenal gland and its arterial system can also be visualized by *adrenal arteriography*. Both benign and malignant tumors of the adrenal gland can be detected easily by this technique. Bilateral adrenal hyperplasia can also be identified.

Cerebral angiography provides radiographic visualization of the cerebral vascular system with the injection of radiopaque dye into the carotid or vertebral arteries. With this procedure, abnormalities of the cerebral circulation such as aneurysms, occlusions, stenosis, or arteriovenous (AV) malformations can be identified. A vascular tumor is seen as a mass containing small, abnormal blood vessels. A nonvascular tumor, abscess, or hematoma appears as a mass distorting the normal vascular contour.

Lower extremity arteriography allows for accurate identification and location of occlusions within the abdominal aorta and lower extremity arteries. After the catheter is placed in the aorta or more selectively into the femoral artery, radiopaque dye is injected. X-ray films are taken in timed sequence to allow radiographic visualization of the arterial system of the lower extremities. Total or near-total occlusion of the flow of dye is seen in arteriosclerotic vascular occlusive disease. Emboli are seen as total occlusions of the artery. Arterial traumas such as lacerations or intimal tears (laceration of the arterial inner lining) likewise appear as total or near-total obstruction of the flow of dye. Aneurysmal dilation of the arteries or its branches also can be seen. Unusual arterial disorders such as Buerger's disease and fibromuscular dysplasia have the classic arterial "beading," which is pathognomonic.

Arterial vascular balloon dilation can be performed if a short segment arterial stenosis is identified. In these instances the wire is placed through the angiocatheter into the area of narrowing. A balloon catheter is inserted over the wire. The dilating balloon is inflated, and the arteriosclerotic plaque is gently and persistently dilated.

Contraindications

- Patients with allergies to shellfish or iodinated dye
- Patients who are uncooperative or agitated
- Patients who are pregnant
- Patients with renal disorders, because iodinated contrast is nephrotoxic
- Patients with a bleeding propensity
- Patients with unstable cardiac disorders

- Patients who are dehydrated, because they are especially susceptible to dye-induced renal failure

Potential complications

- Allergic reaction to iodinated dye
- Hemorrhage from the arterial puncture site used for arterial access
- Arterial embolism from dislodgment of an arteriosclerotic plaque
- Soft tissue infection around the puncture site
- Renal failure, especially in elderly patients who are chronically dehydrated or have a mild degree of renal failure
- Dissection of the intimal lining of the artery causing complete or partial arterial occlusion
- Pseudoaneurysm development as a result of failure of the puncture site to seal
- With adrenal angiography, fatal hypertensive crisis may occur in patients with pheochromocytoma. Propranolol (Inderal), a beta-adrenergic blocker, and phenoxybenzamine (Dibenzyline), an alpha-adrenergic blocker, are given for several days before the study to avoid precipitation of a malignant hypertensive episode.
- In adrenal angiography, hemorrhage of the adrenal gland can occur. This may lead to adrenal insufficiency.
- Hypoglycemia or acidosis may occur in patients who are taking metformin (Glucophage) and receive iodine dye.

Procedure and patient care

Before

- Explain the procedure to the patient. Allay any fears and allow the patient to verbalize concerns.
- Ensure that written and informed consent for this procedure is in the patient's chart.
- Inform the patient that a warm flush may be felt when the dye is injected.
- Assess the possibility of allergies to iodinated dye.
- Determine if the patient has been taking anticoagulants.
- Keep the patient NPO for at least 2 to 8 hours before testing.
- Mark the site of the patient's peripheral pulses with a pen before arterial catheterization. This will permit assessment of the peripheral pulses after the procedure.
- If the patient does not have peripheral pulses before arteriog-

raphy, document that fact so that arterial occlusion will not be suspected on the postangiogram assessment.

- Administer preprocedural medications as ordered.
- If the patient is suspected of having pheochromocytoma, administer propranolol and phenoxybenzamine as ordered to prevent a potentially fatal hypertensive episode.
- Ensure that the appropriate coagulation studies have been performed and are normal.
- For cerebral angiograms, perform a baseline neurologic assessment to compare subsequent assessments. This is to potentially diagnose any strokes that may be precipitated by cerebral arteriography.
- Remove all valuables and dental prostheses.
- Instruct the patient to void before the study because the iodinated dye can act as an osmotic diuretic.
- Inform the patient that bladder distention may cause some discomfort during the study.

During

- Note the following preprocedural steps:
  1. The patient may be sedated before being taken to the angiography room, which is usually within the radiology department.
  2. The patient is placed on the x-ray table in the supine position.
  3. If the femoral artery is to be used, the groin is shaved, prepared, and draped in a sterile manner.
  4. The femoral artery is cannulated, and a wire is threaded up that artery and into or near the opening of the desired artery to be examined (Figure 4).
  5. A catheter is then placed over that wire. The wire and catheter are both placed under fluoroscopic visualization. Because the catheter and wire have a curled tip at the end, both can be manipulated directly into the artery to be studied. The wire is removed.
  6. Through the catheter, iodinated contrast material is injected by the use of an automated injector at a preset, controlled rate. This occurs over several seconds.
  7. Serial x-ray films are taken in timed sequence to show the arterial injection, and subsequent x-ray films are taken to show the venous phase of the injection.
- Note that this procedure is usually performed by an angiographer (radiologist) in approximately 1 to 2 hours.

Figure 4 Catheter insertion for renal angiogram. The angiocatheter with attached syringe is inserted into the femoral artery and advanced into the renal artery.

- During the dye injection, remind the patient that an intense, burning flush may be felt throughout the body but lasts only a few seconds.
- Tell the patient that the most significant discomfort is the groin puncture necessary for arterial access.
- Remind the patient of the discomfort of lying on a hard x-ray table for a long period of time.

- During adrenal angiography monitor blood pressure for evidence of malignant hypertensive storm.

After

- X-ray studies are completed, the catheter is removed, and a pressure dressing is applied to the puncture site.
- Monitor the patient's vital signs for indications of hemorrhage.
- Assess the peripheral arterial pulse in the extremity used for vascular access and compare it with the preprocedural baseline values.
- Perform a neurologic assessment for any signs of catheter-induced embolic stroke syndrome if cerebral arteriography is performed.
- Observe the arterial puncture site frequently for signs of bleeding or hematoma.
- Maintain pressure at the puncture site with a 1- to 2-pound sandbag or an IV bag.
- Keep the patient on bed rest for about 8 hours following the procedure to allow for complete sealing of the arterial puncture site.
- Assess the patient's extremities for signs of loss of blood supply (e.g., loss of pulses, numbness, pallor, tingling, pain, loss of sensory/motor function).
- Note and compare the color and temperature of the extremity with that of the uninvolved extremity.
- Administer mild analgesics for minor discomfort at the arterial puncture site.
- Notify the physician if the patient has severe, continuous pain.
- Have the patient drink fluids to prevent dehydration caused by the diuretic action of the dye.
- Evaluate the patient for delayed allergic reaction to the dye.

Abnormal findings

Adrenal angiography
Pheochromocytoma
Adrenal adenoma
Adrenal carcinoma
Bilateral adrenal hyperplasia

Arteriography of the lower extremity
Arteriosclerotic occlusion
Embolus occlusion
Primary arterial diseases (e.g., fibromuscular dysplasia, Buerger's disease)
Aneurysm
Aberrant arterial anatomy
Tumor neovascularity
Neoplastic arterial compression

Brain arteriography
Vascular aneurysm
Vascular occlusion or stenosis
Vascular AV malformations
Tumor
Abscess
Hematoma
Cerebral vascular thrombosis

Kidney arteriography
Anatomic aberrant blood vessels
Renal cyst
Renal solid tumor
Arthrosclerotic narrowing of the renal artery
Renal vascular causes of hypertension

notes

arthrocentesis with synovial fluid lysis (Synovial fluid analysis, Joint aspiration)

Type of test   Fluid analysis

Normal findings

Synovial fluid: clear and straw colored with few white blood cells (WBCs), no crystals, and a good mucin clot

Chemical test values (e.g., glucose determination): approximating those found in the bloodstream

Test explanation and related physiology

Arthrocentesis is performed to establish the diagnosis of joint infection, arthritis, crystal-induced arthritis (gout and pseudogout), synovitis, or neoplasms involving the joint. This procedure is also used to identify the cause of joint inflammation or effusion, to monitor chronic arthritic diseases, and to inject antiinflammatory medications (usually corticosteroids) into a joint space.

Arthrocentesis is performed by inserting a sterile needle into the joint space of the involved joint to obtain synovial fluid for analysis. Synovial fluid is a liquid found in small amounts within the joints. Aspiration (withdrawal of the fluid) may be performed on any major joint such as the knee, shoulder, hip, elbow, wrist, or ankle.

The fluid sample is examined microscopically and chemically. A culture of the fluid is usually performed. Normal joint fluid is clear, straw colored, and quite viscous due to the hyaluronic acid, which acts as a lubricant. Viscosity is reduced in patients with inflammatory arthritis. Viscosity can be roughly estimated by forcing some synovial fluid from a syringe. Fluid of high viscosity forms a "string" several inches long; fluid of low viscosity drips similar to water.

The synovial fluid glucose value is usually within 10 ml/dl of the serum glucose value. For proper interpretation the synovial fluid glucose and serum glucose samples should be drawn simultaneously after the patient has fasted for 6 hours. The synovial fluid glucose level falls with increasing severity of inflammation. Although lowest in septic arthritis (the synovial fluid glucose value may be less than 50% of the serum glucose value), a low synovial glucose level also may be seen in patients with rheumatoid arthritis. The synovial fluid is also tested for

A

protein, uric acid, and lactate levels. Increased uric acid levels would indicate gout. Increased protein and lactate levels indicate bacterial infection.

Cell counts are also performed on the synovial fluid. Normally the joint fluid contains less than 200 WBCs/mm^3 and 2000 red blood cells (RBCs)/μl. An increased WBC count with a high percentage of neutrophils (over 75%) supports the diagnosis of acute bacterial infectious arthritis. Leukocytes can also occur in other conditions such as acute gouty arthritis and rheumatoid arthritis. The differential white cell count, however, will indicate monocytosis or lymphocytosis with these later-mentioned diseases.

Bacterial and fungal cultures are usually requested and performed when infection is suspected. Gonococci are a cause of joint infection. Smears for acid-fast stains for tubercle bacilli are also performed on the synovial fluid.

The synovial fluid is also analyzed for complement levels (see p. 259). Complement levels are decreased in patients with systemic lupus erythematosus, rheumatoid arthritis, or other immunologic arthritis. These decreased joint complement levels are caused by consumption of the complement induced by the antigen-antibody immune complexes within the joint cavity.

Synovial fluid is also examined under polarized light for the presence of crystals, which permits differential diagnosis between gout and pseudogout (the calcium pyrophosphate dihydrate crystals of pseudogout are birefringent [blue on red background] when examined with a polarized light microscope). Cholesterol crystals occur in rheumatoid arthritis.

Contraindications

- Patients with skin or wound infections in the area of the needle puncture because of the risk of sepsis

Potential complications

- Joint infection
- Hemorrhage in the joint area

Procedure and patient care

Before

- Explain the procedure to the patient.
- Obtain an informed consent if this is the institution's policy.
- Keep the patient NPO after midnight on the day of the test. This is done to prevent alterations of the chemical deter-

minations (e.g., glucose) that may be performed with the study. However, this study may be done more conveniently in a physician's office without the patient fasting.

During

- Have the patient lie on his or her back with the joint fully extended.
- Note the following procedural steps:
  1. The skin is locally anesthetized to minimize pain.
  2. The area is aseptically cleansed, and a needle is inserted through the skin and into the joint space.
  3. Fluid is obtained for analysis. The joint area sometimes may be wrapped with an elastic bandage to compress free fluid within a certain area, thereby ensuring maximal collection of fluid.
  4. If a corticosteroid is to be administered, a syringe containing the steroid preparation is attached to the needle, and the drug is injected.
  5. The needle is removed, and a pressure dressing may be applied to the site.
  6. Sometimes a peripheral venous blood sample is taken to compare chemical tests on the blood with chemical studies on the synovial fluid.
- Note that a physician performs this procedure in an office or at the patient's bedside in approximately 10 minutes.
- Tell the patient that the only discomfort associated with this test is the injection of the local anesthetic.
- Be aware that joint-space pain may worsen after fluid aspiration, especially in patients with acute arthritis.

After

- Assess the joint for any pain, fever, or swelling, which may indicate infection.
- Apply ice to decrease pain and swelling.
- Keep a pressure dressing on the joint to avoid recollection of joint fluid or development of a hematoma.
- Tell the patient to avoid strenuous use of the joint for the next several days.

🏠 Home care responsibilities

- Teach patient to walk on crutches.
- Educate patient to observe for signs of bleeding into the joint (significant swelling, increasing pain, or joint weakness).
- Teach patient to observe for signs of infection of the joint (fever, swelling, redness about the joint, and increasing pain).
- Educate patient to observe for signs of phlebitis. This is not uncommon in a person immobilized by joint pain. The involved leg may get swollen, painful, and edematous.
- Instruct the patient not to drive until approved by the physician.
- Ice should be applied at home to minimize the normal swelling that may occur around the involved joint.

Abnormal findings

Infection
Degenerative arthritis
  (osteoarthritis)
Synovitis
Neoplasm
Joint effusion

Septic arthritis
Systemic lupus erythematosus
Rheumatoid arthritis
Gout
Pseudogout

notes

arthrography (Arthrogram)

Type of test X-ray with contrast dye

Normal findings Normal bursae, menisci, ligaments, and articular cartilage of the joint

Test explanation and related physiology

Arthrography affords radiographic visualization of a joint after the injection of a radiopaque substance, air, or both into the joint cavity to outline the soft tissue structures not normally seen on routine x-ray films. Bones, meniscus, cartilage, and ligaments are clearly visualized with this procedure. Joint derangement and synovial cysts are also diagnosed with arthrography.

Arthrography is usually performed on the knee and shoulder joints; however, it can also be done on other joints such as the ankles, hips, wrists, or temporomandibular joint. This procedure is usually performed on patients with persistent, unexplained joint pain, swelling, or dysfunction.

Contraindications

- Patients who are pregnant
- Patients with active arthritis
- Patients with joint infection

Potential complications

- Infection at the puncture site
- Allergic reaction to the iodinated dye; this rarely occurs because the dye is not administered intravenously.

Procedure and patient care

Before
- Explain the procedure to the patient.
- Obtain an informed consent if required by the institution.
- Tell the patient that no fasting or sedation is required.

During
- Place the patient in the supine position on the examining table.
- Note the following procedural steps:
  1. The skin overlying the joint is aseptically cleansed and anesthetized.

2. A needle is inserted into the joint space.
3. Fluid is aspirated to minimize dilution of the contrast material, which could diminish the quality of the x-ray films.
4. With the needle still in place, the aspirating syringe is removed and a syringe containing dye is inserted.
5. The contrast agent is injected.
6. The needle is removed, and the joint is manipulated to help distribute the contrast material. The patient may be asked to walk several steps or to pass the joint through range-of-motion exercises.
7. X-ray films are taken with the joint held in various positions.

- Note that the physician performs this procedure in approximately 30 minutes.
- Tell the patient that pressure or a tingling sensation may be felt as the contrast medium is injected and that some discomfort in the joint may occur.

After

- Assess the joint for swelling after the test. Apply ice if necessary.
- Administer a mild analgesic (e.g., aspirin, acetaminophen) if the patient has mild discomfort.
- Report any increase in pain or swelling to the physician.
- Inform the patient that crepitant noises (crackling tissue-paper sounds) in the joint may be heard after the test. These symptoms are normal and usually disappear in 1 to 2 days. The sounds are caused by the air injected into the joint during the procedure.

Abnormal findings

Joint derangement
Cysts
Arthritis
Fractured knee meniscus
Muscle tendon tears

Cartilaginous diseases (e.g., chondromalacia)
Ligamentous injury
Synovial tumor
Synovitis

arthroscopy

Type of test Endoscopy

Normal findings Normal ligaments, menisci, and articular surfaces of the joint

Test explanation and related physiology

Arthroscopy is an endoscopic procedure that allows examination of a joint interior with a specially designed endoscope. Arthroscopy is a highly accurate test because it allows direct visualization of an anatomic site (Figure 5). Although this technique can visualize many joints of the body, it is most often used to evaluate the knee for meniscus cartilage or ligament injury. It is also used in the differential diagnosis of acute and chronic disorders of the knee (e.g., arthritic inflammation vs. injury).

Physicians can now perform corrective surgery on the knee through the endoscope. Meniscus removal, spur removal, ligamentous repair, and biopsy are but a few of the procedures that are done through the arthroscope. Arthroscopy provides a safe, convenient alternative to open surgery (arthrotomy) because surgery is done through small trocars that are placed into the joint. Surgical maneuvers are carried out under direct vision of the camera, which is attached to the arthroscope. Because a large incision is avoided, recovery is faster and more comfortable.

Arthroscopy is also used to monitor the progression of disease and the effectiveness of therapy. Visual findings may be recorded by attaching a video camera to the arthroscope. Joints that can be evaluated by the arthroscope include the tarsal, ankle, knee, hip, carpal, wrist, shoulder, and temporomandibular joints.

Contraindications

- Patients with ankylosis
- Patients with local skin or wound infections
- Patients who have recently had an arthrogram

Potential complications

- Infection
- Hemarthrosis
- Swelling

Figure 5 Arthroscopy. The arthroscope is placed within the joint space of the knee. Video arthroscopy requires the availability of a water source to distend the joint space, a light source to see the contents of the joint, and a TV monitor to project the image. Other trocars are used for access of the joint space for other operative instruments.

- Thrombophlebitis
- Joint injury
- Synovial rupture

Procedure and patient care

Before

- Explain the procedure to the patient.
- Ensure that the physician has obtained written consent for this procedure.
- Follow the routine preoperative procedure of the institution.
- Keep the patient NPO after midnight on the day of the test.
- Instruct the patient who will use crutches after the procedure regarding the appropriate crutch gait. The patient should use

crutches after arthroscopy until he or she can walk without limping.

- Shave the hair in the area 6 inches above and below the joint before the test (as ordered).

During

- Place the patient on his or her back on an operating room table.
- Note the following procedural steps:
    1. Local or general anesthesia is used.
    2. The leg is carefully scrubbed, elevated, and wrapped with an elastic bandage from the toes to the lower thigh to drain as much blood from the leg as possible.
    3. A tourniquet is placed on the patient's leg. If the tourniquet is not used, a fluid solution may be instilled into the patient's knee immediately before insertion of the arthroscope to distend the knee and help reduce bleeding.
    4. The foot of the table is lowered so that the patient's knee is at a 45-degree angle.
    5. A small incision is made in the skin around the knee.
    6. The arthroscope (a lighted instrument) is inserted into the joint space to visualize the inside of the knee joint. In the past the surgeon looked directly into the scope. More recently, a video camera is attached to the scope, and the image is projected on a TV monitor.
    7. Although the entire joint can be viewed from one puncture site, additional punctures for better visualization are often necessary.
    8. After the area is examined, biopsy or appropriate surgery can be performed.
    9. Before removing the arthroscope, the joint is irrigated. Pressure is then applied to the knee to remove the irrigating solution.
    10. After a few stitches are placed into the skin, a pressure dressing is applied over the incision site.
- Note that this procedure is performed in the operating room by an orthopedic surgeon in approximately 15 to 30 minutes.
- Tell the patient receiving local anesthesia that he or she may have transient discomfort from the injection of the local anesthetic and the pressure of the tourniquet on the leg.
- Inform the patient that a thumping sensation may be felt as the arthroscope is inserted into the joint and that the joint may be painful for several days.

After

- Assess the patient's neurologic and circulatory status.
- Assess vital signs and observe the patient for signs of infection, including fever, swelling, increased pain, and redness or drainage at the incision site.
- Instruct the patient to elevate the knee when sitting and to avoid overbending the knee so that swelling is minimized.
- Inform the patient that he or she can usually walk with the assistance of crutches; however, this depends on the extent of the procedure and the physician's protocol.
- Tell the patient to minimize use of the joint for several days.
- Examine the incision site for bleeding.
- Apply ice to reduce pain and swelling.
- Inform the patient that the sutures will be removed in approximately 7 to 10 days.

🏠 Home care responsibilities

- Teach patient to walk on crutches.
- Educate patient to observe for signs of bleeding into the joint. (significant swelling, increasing pain, or joint weakness).
- Teach the patient to observe for signs of infection of the joint (fever, swelling, redness about the joint, and increasing pain).
- Educate patient to observe for signs of phlebitis. This is not uncommon in a person immobilized by joint pain. The involved leg may become swollen, painful, and edematous.
- Instruct the patient not to drive until approved by the physician.
- Ice should be applied at home to minimize the normal swelling that may occur around the involved joint.

Abnormal findings

Torn cartilage	Synovitis
Torn ligament	Osteoarthritis
Patellar disease	Rheumatoid arthritis
Patellar fracture	Degenerative arthritis
Chondromalacia	Meniscal disease
Osteochondritis dissecans	Osteochondromatosis
Cyst (e.g., Baker's)	Trapped synovium

aspartate aminotransferase (AST; formerly called Serum glutamic-oxaloacetic transaminase [SGOT])

Type of test Blood

Normal findings

Adult: 8-20 U/L, 5-40 IU/L, or 8-20 U/L (SI units); females
  tend to have slightly lower values than males
Elderly: values slightly higher than adult
Child: values similar to adult
Newborn/infant: 15-60 U/L

Test explanation and related physiology

This test is used in the evaluation of suspected coronary
occlusive heart disease or suspected hepatocellular diseases.
When disease or injury affects the cells of these tissues, the cells
lyse. The AST is released and picked up by the blood, and the
serum level rises. The amount of AST elevation is directly related
to the number of cells affected by the disease or injury. Further,
the elevation depends on the time after the injury that the blood
is drawn. AST is cleared from the blood in a few days. Serum
AST levels become elevated 8 hours after cell injury, peak at 24
to 36 hours, and return to normal in 3 to 7 days. If the cellular
injury is chronic, levels will be persistently elevated.

AST was formerly known as *SGOT*. The AST/SGOT enzyme
is one of the enzymes tested in the cardiac enzyme series.
Although not specific for myocardial injury, when observed with
the enzymes creatine phosphokinase (CPK, see p. 290) and lactic
dehydrogenase (LDH, see p. 511), it is useful in diagnosis of a
myocardial infarction (MI). It aids in determining the timing of a
recent MI and the extent of the MI. In the case of an acute MI,
the AST level rises within 6 to 10 hours after MI, peaks at 12 to
48 hours, and returns to normal in 3 to 4 days, assuming further
cardiac injury does not occur. A second rise in AST would
indicate extension or progression of myocardial injury despite
therapy. Myocardial injuries such as angina, pericarditis, or
rheumatic carditis do not increase the AST level. AST is much
less specific for infarction of myocardial muscle cells.

Because AST also exists within the liver cells, diseases that
affect the hepatocyte cause elevated levels of this enzyme. In
acute hepatitis AST levels can rise 20 times the normal value. In
acute extrahepatic obstruction (e.g., gallstone) AST levels

quickly rise to 10 times the normal and swiftly fall. In cirrhotic patients the level of AST depends on the amount of active inflammation.

Serum AST levels are often compared with alanine aminotransferase (ALT, see p. 27) levels. The AST/ALT ratio is usually greater than 1.0 in patients with alcoholic cirrhosis, liver congestion, and metastatic tumor of the liver. Ratios less than 1.0 may be seen in patients with acute hepatitis, viral hepatitis, or infectious mononucleosis. The ratio is less accurate if AST levels exceed 10 times normal.

Patients with acute pancreatitis, acute renal diseases, musculoskeletal diseases, or trauma may have a transient rise in serum AST. Patients with red blood cell abnormalities such as acute hemolytic anemia and severe burns also can have elevations of this enzyme.

Interfering factors

- Exercise may cause increased levels.
- Drugs that may cause *increased* levels include antihypertensives, cholinergic agents, coumarin-type anticoagulants, digitalis preparations, erythromycin, isoniazid, methyldopa, oral contraceptives, opiates, salicylates, hepatotoxic medications, and verapamil.
- Pyridoxine deficiency (beriberi or pregnancy), severe long-standing liver disease, uremia, or diabetic ketoacidosis may cause decreased levels.

Procedure and patient care

Before

- Explain the procedure to the patient.
- Discuss with the patient the need and reason for frequent venipunctures in diagnosing MI.
- Avoid giving the patient any IM injection.
- If possible, hold drugs that could interfere with test results for 12 hours before the test.

During

- Collect a venous sample of blood in a red-top tube. This is usually done daily for 3 days and then again in 1 week.
- Rotate the venipuncture site.
- Avoid hemolysis.
- Indicate on the laboratory slip any drugs that may cause false-positive results.
- Record the time and date of any IM injection given.

- Record the exact time and date when the blood test is performed. This aids in the interpretation of the temporal pattern of enzyme elevations.

After

- Apply pressure to the venipuncture site.

Abnormal findings

▲ **Increased levels**

Heart diseases
Myocardial infarction
Cardiac operations
Cardiac catheterization
  and angioplasty

Liver diseases
Hepatitis
Hepatic cirrhosis
Drug-induced liver injury
Hepatic metastasis
Hepatic necrosis (initial
  stages only)
Hepatic surgery
Infectious mononucleosis
  with hepatitis
Hepatic infiltrative
  process (e.g., tumor)

Skeletal muscle diseases
Skeletal muscle trauma
Recent noncardiac
  surgery
Multiple traumas
Severe, deep burns
Progressive muscular
  dystrophy
Recent convulsions
Heat stroke
Primary muscle diseases
  (e.g., myopathy, myo-
  sitis)

Other diseases
Acute hemolytic anemia
Acute pancreatitis

▼ **Decreased levels**

Acute renal disease
Beriberi
Diabetic ketoacidosis
Pregnancy
Chronic renal dialysis

barium enema (BE, Lower GI series)

Type of test   X-ray with contrast dye

Normal findings

Normal filling, contour, patency, and positioning of barium in the colon

Normal filling of the appendix and terminal ileum

Test explanation and related physiology

The BE study consists of a series of x-ray films visualizing the colon. It is used to demonstrate the presence and location of polyps, tumors, and diverticula. Anatomic abnormalities (e.g., malrotation) also can be detected. Therapeutically the BE may be used to reduce nonstrangulated ileocolic intussusception in children. Bleeding from diverticula can cease with barium enema.

The BE is occasionally used to assess filling of the appendix. When the clinical picture suggests possible appendicitis, failure of the appendix to fill with barium may support the diagnosis. Although the colon is the main organ evaluated by a BE, reflux of barium into the terminal ileum also allows adequate visualization of the distal part of the small intestine. Diseases that affect the terminal ileum, especially Crohn's disease (regional enteritis), can be identified. Inflammatory bowel disease involving the colon can be detected with BE. Fistulas involving the colon can be demonstrated by BE.

In many instances, air is insufflated into the colon after the instillation of barium. This provides an air contrast to the barium. With air contrast, the colonic mucosa can be much more accurately visualized. This is called an *air-contrast barium enema*. It is used especially when small polyps are suspected. The accuracy of the regular BE in detecting small colonic tumors is approximately 60%; however, the accuracy of an air-contrast BE in detecting small colonic tumors exceeds 85%.

Contraindications

- Patients suspected of a perforation of the colon. In these patients diatrizoate (Gastrografin), a water-soluble contrast medium, is used.
- Patients who are unable to cooperate. This test requires the

patient to hold the barium in the rectum and colon. This is especially difficult for elderly patients.

- Patients with megacolon. Barium may worsen the disease.

Potential complications

- Colonic perforation, especially when the colon is weakened by inflammation, tumor, or infection
- Barium fecal impaction

Interfering factors

- Barium within the abdomen from previous barium tests
- Significant residual stool within the colon. This precludes adequate visualization of the entire bowel wall. Stool may be confused for polyps.
- Spasm of the colon Spasm can mimic the radiographic signs of a cancer. The use of IV glucagon minimizes spasm.

Procedure and patient care

Before

- Explain the procedure to the patient. Encourage the patient to verbalize questions and fears.
- Assist the patient with the bowel preparation, which varies among institutions. In elderly patients this preparation can be exhaustive and even cause severe dehydration. A typical preparation for most adults would include the following actions.

Day before examination

- Give the patient clear liquids for lunch and supper (no dairy products).
- Have the patient drink one glass of water or clear fluid every hour for 8 to 10 hours.
- Administer a cathartic (10 ounces) of magnesium citrate or X-Prep (extract of senna fruit) at 2 PM. In children lesser volumes may be used.
- Administer three 5-mg bisacodyl (Dulcolax) tablets at 7 PM.
- Pediatric Fleet enema the night before testing and repeated 3 hours before testing may be adequate prep for an infant.
- Keep the patient NPO after midnight the day of the test.

Day of examination

- Keep the patient NPO.
- Administer a bisacodyl suppository at 6 AM and/or a cleansing enema.

- Note that pediatric patients will have individualized bowel preparations.
- Note that special preparations will be ordered for patients with an ileostomy or colostomy.
- Determine whether the bowel is adequately cleansed. When the fecal return is similar to clear water, preparation is adequate; if large, solid fecal waste is still being evacuated, preparation is inadequate. Notify the radiologist, who may want to extend the bowel preparation.
- Suggest that the patient take reading material to the x-ray department to occupy the time while expelling the barium.

During

- Note the following procedural steps:
  1. The test begins with placement of a balloon rectal catheter.
  2. The balloon on the catheter is inflated tightly against the anal sphincter to hold the barium within the colon.
  3. The patient is asked to roll in the lateral, supine, and prone positions.
  4. The barium is dripped into the rectum by gravity. The colon of the young child is not able to tolerate the volume and pressure of instillation of barium that an adult can. Both should be reduced.
  5. The barium flow is monitored fluoroscopically.
  6. The colon is thoroughly examined as the barium flow progresses through the large colon and into the terminal ileum.
  7. The barium is drained out.
  8. If an air-contrast BE has been ordered, air is insufflated into the large bowel.
  9. The patient is asked to expel the barium, and a post-evacuation x-ray film is taken.
  10. The standard procedure for administering the barium through a colostomy is to instill the contrast medium through an irrigation cone placed in the stoma. When the x-ray series is completed, the barium is allowed to be expelled from the stoma. A gentle stream of clean water for irrigation is helpful in expelling residual barium.
- Note that this test is usually performed in the radiology department by a radiologist in approximately 45 minutes.

- Inform the patient that abdominal bloating and rectal pressure will occur during instillation of barium.

After

- Ensure that the patient defecates as much barium as possible.
- Inform the patient that bowel movements will be white. When all the barium has been expelled, the stool will return to normal color.
- Suggest the use of soothing ointments on the anal area to minimize any anorectal pain that may result from the aggressive test preparation.
- Encourage ingestion of fluids to avoid dehydration caused by the cathartics.
- Encourage rest after the procedure. The cleansing regimen and BE procedure may be exhausting.
- Note that laxatives may be ordered to facilitate evacuation of barium.
- Be aware of dehydration and electrolyte abnormalities. Instruct the parent to hydrate the child well with electrolyte-containing fluids after the BE.

Abnormal findings

Malignant tumor
Polyps
Diverticula
Inflammatory bowel diseases (e.g., ulcerative colitis, Crohn's disease)
Colonic stenosis secondary to ischemia, infection, or previous surgery
Perforated colon
Colonic fistula
Appendicitis
Extrinsic compression of the colon from extracolonic tumors (e.g., ovarian)
Extrinsic compression of the colon from an abscess
Malrotation of the gut
Colon volvulus
Intussusception
Hernia

notes

barium swallow

B

Type of test X-ray with contrast dye

Normal findings Normal size, contour, filling, patency, and positioning of the esophagus

Test explanation and related physiology

This barium contrast study is a more thorough examination of the esophagus than that provided by most upper GI series (see p. 854). As in most barium contrast studies, defects in normal filling and narrowing of the barium column indicate tumor, strictures, or extrinsic compression from extraesophageal tumors or an abnormally enlarged heart and great vessels. Varices also can be seen as serpiginous, linear-filling defects. Anatomic abnormalities such as hiatal hernia, Shatzski's rings, and diverticula (Zenker's or epiphrenic) can be seen as well.

In patients with esophageal reflux, the radiologist may identify reflux of the barium from the stomach back into the esophagus. Muscular abnormalities such as achalasia, as well as diffuse esophageal spasm, can be easily detected by a barium swallow. If perforations or rupture of the esophagus is suspected, it is best not to use barium. A water-soluble x-ray contrast should be used. If swallowing function is to be evaluated and there is a concern for the potential of aspiration during the test, barium should be used instead of Gastografin. The latter can cause a chemical pneumonitis, whereas the former does not.

Contraindications

- Patients with evidence of bowel obstruction Barium may create a stonelike impaction.
- Patients with a perforated viscus. If barium were to leak, the degree and duration of infection would be much worse. Usually, when perforation is suspected, diatrizoate (Gastrografin), a water-soluble contrast medium, is used.
- Patients whose vital signs are unstable
- Patients who are unable to cooperate for the test

Potential complication

- Barium-induced fecal impaction

Interfering factor

- Food within the esophagus, which prevents adequate visualization

Procedure and patient care

Before

- Explain the procedure to the patient.
- Instruct the patient not to take anything by mouth for at least 8 hours before the testing. Usually the patient is kept NPO after midnight on the day of the test.
- Assess the patient's ability to swallow. If the patient tends to aspirate, inform the radiologist.
- Accompany the hospitalized patient to the x-ray department if vital signs are not stable and the test still needs to be performed.

During

- Note the following procedural steps:
  1. The fasting patient is asked to swallow the contrast medium. Usually this is barium sulfate in a milkshake-like substance; however, if a perforated viscus is possible, Gastrografin is used.
  2. As the patient drinks the contrast through a straw, the x-ray table is tilted to the near-erect position.
  3. The patient is asked to roll into various positions so that the entire esophagus can be adequately visualized.
  4. With fluoroscopy, the radiologist follows the barium column through the entire esophagus.
- Note that this procedure is usually performed in the radiology department by a radiologist in approximately 15 to 20 minutes.
- Tell the patient that no discomfort is associated with this test.

After

- Inform the patient of the need to evacuate all the barium. Cathartics are recommended. Initially stools are white but should return to normal color with complete evacuation.

B

Abnormal findings

Total or partial esophageal
   obstruction
Cancer
Scarred strictures
Lower esophageal rings
Peptic esophageal ulcers
Varices
Peptic or corrosive esophagitis
Achalasia

Esophageal motility disorders
   (e.g., presbyesophagus,
   diffuse esophageal spasm)
Diverticula
Chalasia
Extrinsic compression from
   extraesophageal tumors,
   cardiomegaly, or aortic
   aneurysm

notes

Bence Jones protein

Type of test Urine

Normal findings No Bence Jones protein present

Test explanation and related physiology

The detection of Bence Jones protein in the urine most commonly indicates multiple myeloma (especially when the urine levels are high). The test is used to detect and monitor the treatment and clinical course of multiple myeloma and other similar diseases.

Bence Jones proteins are light chain portions of immunoglobulins found in 75% of the patients with multiple myeloma. These proteins are most notably made by the plasma cells in these patients. They also may be associated with tumor metastases to the bone, chronic lymphocytic leukemias, lymphoma, macroglobulinemia, and amyloidosis.

Normally there is no protein in the urine because the glomerular spaces do not allow filtration of large molecules such as proteins. Bence Jones proteins, however, are very small and are easily filtrated by the kidney and excreted into the urine. Because the Bence Jones protein is rapidly cleared from the blood by the kidney, it is very difficult to detect in the blood; therefore only urine is used for this study. Normally urine should contain no Bence Jones proteins.

Routine urine testing for proteins using reagent strips often does not reflect the type or amount of proteins in the urine. In fact, the strip may even show a completely negative result, despite large amounts of Bence Jones globulins.

Interfering factor

- Dilute urine may yield a false-negative result.

Procedure and patient care

Before
- Explain the procedure to the patient.
- Instruct the patient not to contaminate the urine specimen with toilet paper or stool.

During

- Instruct the patient to collect an early morning specimen of at least 50 ml of uncontaminated urine in a container. It may be helpful to know the amount of these proteins excreted over 24 hours. If so, a 24-hour collection is ordered.

After

- Immediately transport the specimen to the laboratory. If it cannot be taken to the laboratory immediately, refrigerate it, because heat-coagulable proteins can decompose, causing a false-positive test.

Abnormal findings

▲ **Increased levels**

Multiple myeloma (plasmacytoma)
Various metastatic tumors
Chronic lymphocytic leukemia
Amyloidosis
Lymphoma
Waldenstrom's macroglobulinemia

notes

bilirubin, blood

Type of test Blood

Normal findings

Adult/elderly/child

Total bilirubin: 0.1-1 mg/dl or 5.1-17 μmol/L (SI units)

Indirect bilirubin: 0.2-0.8 mg/dl or 3.4-12.0 μmol/L (SI units)

Direct bilirubin: 0.1-0.3 mg/dl or 1.7-5.1 μmol/L (SI units)

Newborn total bilirubin: 1-12 mg/dl or 17.1-20.5 μmol/L (SI units)

Test explanation and related physiology

Bile, which is formed in the liver, has many constituents, including bile salts, phospholipids, cholesterol, bicarbonate, water, and bilirubin. Bilirubin metabolism begins with the breakdown of red blood cells (RBCs) in the reticuloendothelial system (Figure 6). Hemoglobin is released from RBCs and broken down to heme and globin molecules. Heme is then catabolized to form biliverdin, which is transformed to bilirubin. This form of bilirubin is called *unconjugated (indirect) bilirubin*. In the liver indirect bilirubin is conjugated with a glucuronide, resulting in *conjugated (direct) bilirubin*. The conjugated bilirubin is then excreted from the liver cells and into the intrahepatic canaliculi, which eventually lead to the hepatic ducts, the common bile duct, and the bowel.

Jaundice is the discoloration of body tissues caused by abnormally high blood levels of bilirubin. This yellow discoloration is recognized when the total serum bilirubin exceeds 2.5 mg/dl.

Physiologic jaundice of the newborn occurs if the newborn's liver is immature and does not have enough conjugating enzymes. This results in a high circulating blood level of unconjugated bilirubin, which can pass through the blood-brain barrier and deposit in the brain cells of the newborn. This can cause encephalopathy (*kernicterus*).

Once the jaundice is recognized either clinically or chemically, it is important (for therapy) to differentiate whether it is predominantly caused by unconjugated or conjugated bilirubin. This in turn will help differentiate the etiology of the defect. In general, jaundice caused by hepatocellular dysfunction (e.g.,

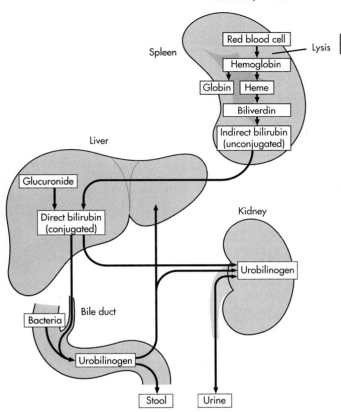

Figure 6 Bilirubin metabolism and excretion. The spleen, liver, kidney, and gastrointestinal tract contribute to this process.

hepatitis) results in elevated levels of unconjugated bilirubin. Jaundice resulting from extrahepatic obstruction of the bile ducts (e.g., gallstones or tumor blocking the bile ducts) results in elevated conjugated bilirubin levels; this type of jaundice usually can be resolved surgically or endoscopically.

The total serum bilirubin level is the sum of the conjugated (direct) and unconjugated (indirect) bilirubin. These are separated out when "fractionation or differentiation" of the total bilirubin to its direct and indirect parts is requested from the laboratory. Normally the unconjugated bilirubin makes up 70% to 85% of the total bilirubin. In patients with jaundice, when more than 50% of the bilirubin is conjugated, it is considered a conjugated hyperbilirubinemia from gallstones, tumor, inflammation, scarring, or obstruction of the extrahepatic ducts. Unconjugated hyperbilirubinemia exists when less than 15% to 20% of the total bilirubin is conjugated. Diseases that typically cause this form of jaundice include accelerated erythrocyte (RBC) hemolysis, hepatitis, or drugs.

Delta bilirubin is a form of bilirubin that is covalently bound to albumin. It has a longer half-life than the other bilirubins; therefore it remains elevated during the convalescent phases of hepatic disorders when the conjugated bilirubin would have already returned to normal. It can be derived by the following calculation: delta bilirubin equals total bilirubin minus the sum of the conjugated and unconjugated bilirubin.

Interfering factors

- Blood hemolysis and lipemia can produce erroneous results.
- Drugs that may cause *increased* levels of total bilirubin include allopurinol, anabolic steroids, antibiotics, antimalarials, ascorbic acid, azathioprine, chlorpropamide (Diabinese), cholinergics, codeine, dextran, diuretics, epinephrine, meperidine, methotrexate, methyldopa, monoamine oxidase inhibitors, morphine, nicotinic acid (large doses), oral contraceptives, phenothiazines, quinidine, rifampin, salicylates, steroids, sulfonamides, theophylline, and vitamin A.
- Drugs that may cause *decreased* levels of total bilirubin include barbiturates, caffeine, penicillin, and salicylates (high-dose).

Procedure and patient care

Before

- Explain the procedure to the patient.
- Note that fasting requirements vary among different laboratories. Some require keeping the patient NPO after midnight the day of the test except for water.

During

- Collect 5 to 7 ml of venous blood in a red-top tube.
- Use a heel puncture for blood collection in infants.
- Prevent hemolysis of blood during phlebotomy.

- Do *not* shake the tube because inaccurate test results may occur.
- Protect the blood sample from bright light. Prolonged exposure (over 1 hour) to sunlight or artificial light can reduce bilirubin content.
- List on the laboratory slip any drugs that may affect test results.

After

- Apply pressure to the venipuncture site. Patients who are jaundiced can have prolonged clotting times.

Abnormal findings

▲ **Increased levels of conjugated (direct) bilirubin**
Gallstones
Extrahepatic duct obstruction (tumor, inflammation, gallstone, scarring, or surgical trauma)
Extensive liver metastasis
Cholestasis from drugs
Dubin-Johnson syndrome
Rotor's syndrome

▼ **Increased levels of unconjugated (indirect) bilirubin**
Erythroblastosis fetalis
Hemolytic jaundice
Large-volume blood transfusion
Resolution of a large hematoma
Hepatitis
Sepsis
Neonatal hyperbilirubinemia
Hemolytic anemia
Crigler-Najjar syndrome
Gilbert syndrome
Pernicious anemia
Cirrhosis
Transfusion reaction
Sickle cell anemia

notes

bleeding time (Ivy bleeding time)

Type of test Blood

Normal findings 1-9 minutes (Ivy method) (Results vary among laboratories.)

Possible critical values >12 minutes

Test explanation and related physiology

The bleeding time test is used to evaluate the vascular and platelet factors associated with hemostasis. It is frequently performed on preoperative patients to ensure adequate hemostasis. When vascular injury occurs, the first hemostatic response is a spastic contraction of the lacerated microvessels. Next, platelets adhere to the wall of the vessel at the area of laceration in an attempt to plug the hole. Failure of either process results in a prolonged bleeding time. If platelets are present in inadequate quantities (usually less than 50,000), if the platelet function is inadequate (as in patients with uremia or with recent ingestion of aspirin), or if vessel constriction is inadequate (such as exists in the elderly or with increased capillary fragility), the bleeding time is prolonged.

For this study a small, standard superficial incision is made in the forearm, and the time required for the bleeding to stop is recorded. This is called the *bleeding time*. Normal values vary according to the method used; the method most often used today is the Ivy bleeding time test.

Because vessel constriction and platelet adherence are not affected by coagulation (intrinsic and extrinsic system), defects in coagulation do not affect the bleeding time. Therefore this test only evaluates platelet function and quantity and vascular constriction capability. It is not an accurate test of platelet number. This can better be quantified by a direct platelet count (see p. 645).

Contraindications

- Patients with low platelet counts
- Patients who are unable to cooperate

- Patients who cannot have a blood pressure cuff placed on the arm (e.g., those with cellulitis)
- Patients with a history of keloid formation
- Patients with senile skin changes
- Patients who have had a mastectomy or axillary lymph node dissection
  Avoid the arm on the affected side.

Potential complications

- Skin infection
- Excessive bleeding from test site

Interfering factors

- Aggressively wiping the site of laceration can prolong the test results.
- Extremes in body temperatures can alter results. High temperatures can prolong results, low body temperatures can fictitiously shorten results.
- Drugs that may cause *increased* bleeding times include anticoagulants, dextran, indomethacin, salicylates, streptokinase, allopurinol, some antibiotics, halothane, nonsteroidal antiinflammatory drugs, urokinase, and warfarin.

Procedure and patient care

Before

- Explain the procedure to the patient.
- Obtain a consent form if required by the institution.
- Tell the patient that no fasting is required.
- Obtain a drug history to detect if the patient has recently had aspirin, anticoagulants, or any other medications that may affect test results.
- Inform the patient that minor discomfort may occur with this test because of the skin laceration.

During

- Note the following procedural steps:
  1. The skin of the inner part of the forearm is cleansed with alcohol or povidone-iodine (Betadine).
  2. A blood pressure cuff is applied on the arm above the elbow, inflated to 40 mm Hg, and maintained at this pressure during the study.
  3. A small laceration is then made 1-mm deep into the skin, and the time is recorded.

4. Bleeding ensues, and the blood is wiped clean at 30-second intervals.
5. When no new bleeding occurs, the time is again noted.
6. The interval from the beginning to the end of bleeding is calculated. This is the bleeding time.
7. The blood pressure cuff is then removed, and an adhesive dressing is applied to the patient's arm.
8. If bleeding persists more than 10 minutes, the test is stopped, and a pressure dressing is applied.

- Indicate on the laboratory slip any medications that may affect test results.
- Note that this test is usually performed by a laboratory technician in less than 10 minutes.
- Inform the patient that minor discomfort may occur with this test because of the skin laceration.

After

- Apply pressure or pressure dressing to the puncture site.
- Assess the puncture site for bleeding.
- Abnormal results should be repeated.

Abnormal findings

▲ **Prolonged times or increased values**

Bone marrow failure
Primary or metastatic tumor infiltration of bone marrow
Disseminated intravascular coagulation
Thrombocytopenia
Hypersplenism
von Willebrand's disease
Collagen vascular disease
Cushing syndrome

Henoch-Schönlein syndrome
Severe liver disease
Clotting factor deficiency
Capillary fragility
Leukemia
Uremia
Bernard-Soulier syndrome
Connective tissue disorder
Hereditary telangiectasia
Glanzmann's thrombasthenia

notes

blood culture and sensitivity

Type of test Blood

Normal findings Negative

Test explanation and related physiology

Blood cultures are obtained to detect the presence of bacteria in the blood. Bacteremia (the presence of bacteria in the blood) can be intermittent and transient, except in endocarditis or suppurative thrombophlebitis. The episode of bacteremia is usually accompanied by chills and fever; thus the blood culture should be drawn when the patient manifests these signs to increase the chances of growing out bacteria on the cultures. It is important that at least two culture specimens be obtained from two different sites. If one produces bacteria and the other does not, it is safe to assume that the bacteria in the first culture may be a contaminant and not the infecting agent. When both cultures grow the infecting agent, bacteremia exists and is caused by the organism that is growing out in the culture. If the patient is receiving antibiotics during the time that the cultures are drawn, the laboratory should be notified. Resin can be added to the culture medium to negate the antibiotic effect in inhibiting growth of the offending bacteria in the culture. If cultures are to be performed while the patient is on antibiotics, the blood culture specimen should be taken shortly before the next dose of the antibiotic is administered. All cultures preferably should be performed before antibiotic therapy is initiated.

Culture specimens drawn through an IV catheter are frequently contaminated, and tests using them should not be performed unless catheter sepsis is suspected. In these situations blood culture specimens drawn through the catheter help to identify the causative agent more accurately than a culture specimen from the catheter tip.

Most organisms require approximately 24 hours to grow in the laboratory, and a preliminary report can be given at that time. Often, 48 to 72 hours are required for growth and identification of the organism. Anaerobic organisms may take longer to grow.

Interfering factors

- Contamination of the blood specimen, especially by skin bacteria, may occur.

Procedure and patient care

Before

- Explain the procedure to the patient.
- Tell the patient that no fasting is required.

During

- Carefully prepare the proposed venipuncture site with povidone-iodine (Betadine). Allow the skin to dry.
- Clean the tops of the Vacutainer tubes or culture bottles with povidone-iodine and allow them to dry. Some laboratories suggest cleaning with 70% alcohol after cleaning with povidone-iodine and air drying.
- Collect approximately 10 to 15 ml of venous blood by venipuncture from each site in a 20-ml syringe.
- Discard the needle on the syringe and replace with a second sterile needle before injecting the blood sample into the culture bottle.
- Inoculate the anaerobic bottle first if both anaerobic and aerobic cultures are needed.
- Mix gently after inoculation.
- Label the specimen with the patient's name, date, time, and tentative diagnosis.
- Indicate on the laboratory slip any medications that may affect test results.

After

- Transport the culture bottles immediately to the laboratory (or at least within 30 minutes).
- Notify the physician of any positive results so that appropriate antibiotic therapy can be initiated.

Abnormal finding

Bacteremia

notes

Type of test Blood

Normal findings

Normal quantity of red and white blood cells (RBCs, WBCs) and platelets

Normal size, shape, and color of RBCs

Normal WBC differential count

Test explanation and related physiology

Examination of the peripheral blood smear can provide a significant amount of information concerning drugs and diseases that affect RBCs and WBCs. Furthermore, other congenital and acquired diseases can be diagnosed by an examination of the peripheral blood smear. When special stains are applied to the blood smear, leukemia, infection, infestation, and other diseases can be identified.

When adequately prepared and examined microscopically by an experienced technologist and pathologist, a smear of peripheral blood is the most informative of all hematologic tests. All three hematologic cell lines, erythrocytes (RBCs), platelets, and leukocytes (WBCs) can be examined. In the peripheral blood, five different types of leukocytes can routinely, be identified: neutrophils, eosinophils, basophils, lymphocytes, and monocytes. The first three are also referred to as granulocytes. Please see discussion in "bone marrow biopsy/aspiration" for more information concerning the various elements of blood.

Microscopic examination of the RBCs can reveal variations in RBC size (anisocytosis), shape (poikilocytosis), color, or intracellular content. Classification of RBCs according to these variables is most helpful in identifying the causes of anemia and the presence of other diseases.

RBC size abnormalities

Microcytes (small RBCs)

Iron deficiency

Hereditary spherocytosis

Thalassemia

Macrocytes (larger size)

Vitamin B_{12} or folic acid deficiency

Reticulocytosis secondary to increased erythropoiesis
(RBC production)
Occasional liver disorder
Postsplenectomy anemia

RBC shape abnormalities

Spherocytes (small and round)
Hereditary spherocytosis
Acquired immunohemolytic anemia
Elliptocytes (crescent or sickle shaped)
Hereditary elliptocytosis
Sickle cell anemia
Leptocytes, or "target cells" (thin cells and with less hemo-
globin)
Hemoglobinopathies
Thalassemia
Spicule cell
Uremia
Liver disease
Bleeding ulcer

RBC color abnormalities

Hypochromic (pale)
Iron deficiency
Thalassemia
Cardiac disease
Hyperchromasia (more colored)
Concentrated hemoglobin, usually caused by dehydra-
tion

RBC intracellular structure

Nucleated (normoblasts) (Usually RBCs do not have a
nucleus, but immature RBCs do. Immature nucleated cells
indicate increased RBC synthesis.)
Anemia
Chronic hypoxemia
"Normal" for an infant
Marrow-occupying neoplasm or fibrotic tissue
Basophilic stippling (refers to bodies enclosed or
included in the cytoplasm of the RBCs)
Lead poisoning
Howell-Jolly bodies (small, round remnants of nuclear mate-
rial remaining within the RBC)
After a surgical splenectomy
Hemolytic anemia
Megaloblastic anemia

Heinz bodies (small, irregular particles of hemoglobin)
    Drug-induced RBC injury
    Hemoglobinopathies
    Hemolytic anemia

The WBCs are examined for total quantity, differential count, and degree of maturity. An increased number of immature WBCs may indicate leukemia or infection. A decreased WBC count indicates failure of marrow to produce WBCs, resulting from drugs, chronic disease, neoplasia, or fibrosis.

Finally, an experienced cell examiner also can estimate platelet number (see p. 631) on a peripheral blood smear.

Procedure and patient care

Before
- Explain the procedure to the patient.
- Tell the patient that no fasting is required.

During
- Collect a drop of blood from a finger stick or heel stick and place it on a slide.
- If necessary, perform a venipuncture and collect the blood in a lavender-top tube.
- Note that a blood smear is first studied with an automated calculator programmed to recognize abnormal blood cell shapes and so on. A more accurate smear is performed by a technologist. Low counts may be "hand counted" to ensure accuracy. The most accurate smear requires review by a pathologist.

After
- Apply pressure to the venipuncture site.

Abnormal findings

See listing under Test Explanation and Related Physiology.

notes

blood typing

Type of test Blood

Normal findings Compatibility

Test explanation and related physiology

With blood typing, ABO and Rh antigens can be detected in the blood of prospective blood donors and potential blood recipients. This test is also used to determine the blood type of expectant mothers and newborns. A description of the ABO system, Rh factors, and blood crossmatching is reviewed below.

ABO system

Human blood is grouped according to the presence or absence of A or B antigens. The surface membrane of group A red blood cells (RBCs) contain A antigens; group B RBCs contain B antigens on their surface; group AB RBCs have both A and B antigens; and group O RBCs have neither A nor B antigens A person's serum does not contain antibodies to match the surface antigen on their RBCs. That is, persons with group A antigens (Type A blood) will not have anti-A antibodies. However, they may have anti B- antibodies. Visa versa is true for persons with group B antigens. Group O blood may have both anti-A and anti-B antibodies. See Table 4. Blood transfusions are actually transplantations of tissue (blood) from one person to another. It is important that the recipient not have antibodies to the donor's RBCs. If this were to occur, there could be a hypersensitivity reaction, which can vary from mild fever to anaphylaxis with severe intravascular hemolysis. If donor ABO antibodies are present against the recipient antigens, usually only minimal reactions occur.

TABLE 4 Blood typing

Blood type	Antigen	Antibody
Group A	A	B
Group B	B	A
Group AB (universal receiver)	A, B	None
Group O (universal donor)	None	A, B

Persons with group O blood are considered "universal donors" because they do not have antigens on their RBCs. People with group AB blood are considered "universal recipients" because they have no antibodies to react to the transfused blood. Group O blood is often transfused in emergent situations in which rapid life-threatening blood loss occurs and immediate transfusion is required. There is no time for crossmatching (about 20 minutes). The chance of a transfusion reaction is least when type O is used.

Rh factors

The presence or absence of Rh antigens on the RBCs surface determines the classification of Rh positive or Rh negative. After ABO compatibility, Rh factor is the next most important antigen affecting the success of a blood transfusion. The major Rh factor is Rh_o (D). There are several minor Rh factors. If Rh_o (D) is absent, the minor Rh antigens are tested. If negative, the patient is considered "Rh negative" (Rh_).

Procedure and patient care

Before

- Explain the procedure to the patient.
- Tell the patient that no fasting is required.

During

- Collect approximately 7 to 14 ml of venous blood in a red-top tube. (This may vary among laboratories.)
- Avoid hemolysis.
- Appropriately label the blood tube before sending it to the laboratory.

After

- Assess the venipuncture site for bleeding.

Abnormal findings

See Test Explanation and Related Physiology.

notes

bone densitometry (Bone mineral content [BMC], Bone absorptiometry, Bone mineral density [BMD])

Type of test X-ray

Normal findings

Normal: <1 standard deviation below normal (>−1)
Osteopenia: 1-2.5 standard deviations below normal
    (−1 to −2.5)
Osteoporosis >2.5 standard deviations below normal (<−2.5)

Test explanation and related physiology

   Bone densitometry is used to determine bone mineral content and density to diagnose osteoporosis as early as possible. Osteoporosis/osteopenia are terms used for bone that becomes weakened and fractures easily. This most commonly occurs in postmenopausal women. However, there are other diseases that are associated with osteoporosis such as malnourishment or osteopenic endocrinopathies (e.g. hyperparathyroidism) in patients.

   The earlier osteoporosis is recognized, the more effective the treatment, and the milder the clinical course. If the diagnosis of osteoporosis is delayed until fractures occur or even until the plain film x-rays identify "thin" bones, the success of treatment is less likely. Because therapy can be expensive and is not without risks, the diagnosis of osteoporosis must be made on the basis of accurate data. Bone densitometry can provide early and accurate measurements of bone strength based on bone density.

   Several groups of bones are routinely evaluated because they accurately represent the entire skeleton. The lumbar spine is the best representative of cancellous bone. The radius is the most easily studied cortical bone. The proximal hip (neck of the femur) is the best representative of mixed (cancellous and cortical) bone. However, specific bone sites can be evaluated if they are particularly symptomatic.

   Dual energy densitometry (absorptiometry) is most commonly used. There are two different types of dual photon energy and therefore two different methods of performing dual energy densitometry. *Dual-photon absorptiometry (DPA)* and *dual-energy x-ray absorptiometry (DEXA)* are most commonly used. Because DPA and DEXA use two photons, more energy is produced so that bones (spine and hip [femoral neck]) surrounded by a lot of soft tissue can be more easily penetrated. The source of the photon is placed on one side of the bone to be studied. The gamma detector is placed on the other side. Increased bone density is associated with increased bone photon absorption and therefore less photon recognition at the site of the gamma detector.

The diagnosis of osteoporosis can be made when vertebral bone density is more than 10% below that expected according to a chart based on sex, age, height, weight, and race. Usually bone density is reported in terms of standard deviation (SD) removed from mean values. T scores compare the patient's results to a group of young healthy adults. Z scores compare the patient's results to a group of age-matched controls. The World Health Organization has defined osteopenia as a bone density value of >1 SD below peak bone mass levels of young women and osteoporosis as a value of >2.5 SD below that same measurement scale. Positive T scores indicate bone stronger than normal. Negative T scores indicate bone weaker than normal.

This test is also used to monitor patients who are undergoing treatment for osteoporosis.

Interfering factors

- Barium may falsely increase the density of the lumbar spine. Bone density measurements should not be performed for about 10 days after barium studies.
- Calcified abdominal aortic aneurysm may falsely increase bone density of the spine.
- Internal fixation devices of the hip or radius will falsely increase bone density of those bones.
- Overlying metal jewelry or other objects may falsely increase bone density of the bones.
- Previous fractures of the bone to be studied can falsely increase bone density of the bone.
- Metallic clips placed in the plane of the vertebra of patients who have had previous abdominal surgery can falsely increase bone density of the bone.
- Prior bone scans can falsely decrease bone density because the photons generated from the bone (as a result of the previously administered bone scan radionuclide) will be detected by the scintillator detector.

Procedure and patient care

Before

- Explain the procedure to the patient
- Tell the patient that no fasting or sedation is required.
- The machine is usually calibrated by the x-ray or nuclear medicine technician before the patient's arrival.
- Ask the patient to remove all metallic objects (e.g., belt buckles, zippers, coins, keys) that might be in the scanning path.

During

- Note the following procedural steps:
  1. The patient lies on an imaging table with the legs supported and placed on a padded box to flatten the pelvis and lumbar spine.
  2. Under the table, a photon generator is slowly successively passed under the lumbar spine.
  3. A scintillator (gamma or x-ray) detector/camera is passed over the patient in a manner parallel to the generator. An image of the lumbar spine and hip bone is obtained by the scintillator camera and projected on a computer monitor.
  4. Next, the foot is applied to a brace that internally rotates the nondominant hip, and the procedure is repeated over the hip. The similar procedure is performed for radius evaluation.
  5. When the radius is examined, the nondominant arm is preferred, unless there is a history of fracture to that bone.
- Note that the data are interpreted by a radiologist or a physician trained in nuclear medicine.
- Note that bone density studies take about 30 to 45 minutes to perform and are free of any discomfort. Only minimal radiation is used for this procedure.

After

- On the computer screen, a small window of the lumbar spine, femoral neck, or distal radius is drawn. The computer calculates the amount of photons not absorbed by the bone. This is called the bone mineral content (BMC). Bone mineral density (BMD) is computed as follows:

$$BMD = \frac{BMC}{\text{surface area of the bone}} \ (gm \cdot cm^2)$$

Abnormal findings

Osteopenia
Osteoporosis

notes

bone marrow biopsy (Bone marrow examination, Bone marrow aspiration)

Type of test Microscopic examination of tissue

Normal findings

Cell type	Range (%)
Myeloblasts	<5
Promyelocytes	1-8
Myelocytes	
Neutrophilic	5-15
Eosinophilic	0.5-3
Basophilic	<1
Metamyelocytes	
Neutrophilic	15-25
Eosinophilic	<1
Basophilic	<1
Mature myelocytes	
Neutrophilic	10-30
Eosinophilic	<5
Basophilic	<5
Mononuclear	
Monocytes	<5
Lymphocytes	3-20
Plasma cells	<1
Megakaryocytes	<5
M/E ratio	<4
Normoblasts	25-50

Normal iron content is demonstrated by staining with Prussian blue

Test explanation and related physiology

Bone marrow examination is an important part of the evaluation of patients with hematologic diseases. Indications for bone marrow examination include the following:

1. To confirm the diagnosis of megaloblastic anemias
2. To diagnose leukemia or myeloma
3. To determine if the marrow is the cause of reduced blood cells in the peripheral bloodstream
4. To document deficient iron stores

5. To document bone marrow infiltrative diseases (neoplasm or fibrosis)
6. Identification of tumor, as staging lymphomas

The bone marrow is located in the central fatty core of cancellous bone (sternum, rib, and pelvis) and the long bones (femur, tibia, and humerus). There the blood-forming cells produce the blood cells and release them into the circulation.

By examination of a bone marrow specimen, the hematologist can fully evaluate hematopoiesis. Examination of the bone marrow reveals the number, size, and shape of the red and white blood cells (RBCs, WBCs) and megakaryocytes (platelet precursors) as these cells evolve through their various stages of development in the bone marrow. Microscopic examination includes estimation of cellularity, determination of the presence of fibrotic tissue or neoplasms (both primary and metastatic), and estimation of iron storage.

To estimate cellularity, the specimen is examined, and the relative quantity of each cell type determined. Leukemias or leukemoid drug reactions are suspected when increased numbers of leukocyte precursors are present. Physiologic marrow leukemoid compensation for infection also will be recognized by finding an increased number of leukocyte precursors. Decreased numbers of marrow leukocyte precursors occur in patients with myelofibrosis, metastatic neoplasia, or agranulocytosis; in elderly patients; and following radiation therapy or chemotherapy.

Increased numbers of marrow RBC precursors occur with polycythemia vera or as physiologic compensation to hypoxemia or hemorrhagic or hemolytic anemias. Decreased numbers of marrow RBC precursors occur with erythroid hypoplasia following chemotherapy, radiation therapy, administration of other toxic drugs, iron deficiency, or marrow replacement by fibrotic tissue or neoplasms.

Increased numbers of platelet precursors (megakaryocytes) are seen in the marrow of patients who are compensating after an episode of acute hemorrhage. They are also seen in some forms of chronic myeloid leukemia. This increase also may be compensatory in patients with secondary hypersplenism associated with portal hypertension or other conditions. In these patients the spleen prematurely extracts platelets from the circulation. Platelet counts decrease, and the marrow compensates by increasing production. Decreased numbers of megakaryocytes occur in patients who have had radiation therapy, chemotherapy, or other drug therapy and in patients with neoplastic or fibrotic marrow infiltrative diseases. Patients with aplastic anemia also have decreased numbers of megakaryocytes.

Increased numbers of lymphocyte precursors occur in chronic, viral, or mycoplasma infections (e.g., mononucleosis), lymphocytic leukemia, and lymphoma. Plasma cells (plasmocytes) are increased in number in patients with multiple myelomas, Hodgkin's disease, hypersensitivity states, rheumatic fever, and other chronic inflammatory diseases.

Estimation of cellularity also can be expressed as a ratio of myeloid (WBC) to erythroid (RBC) cells (M/E ratio). The normal M/E ratio is approximately 3:1. The M/E ratio is greater than normal in those diseases mentioned previously in which increased leukocyte precursors are present or erythroid precursors are decreased. The M/E ratio is below normal when either leukocyte precursors are decreased or erythroid precursors are increased. A more detailed listing of diseases affecting the M/E ratio can be found in most hematology textbooks.

Drug-induced or idiopathic myelofibrosis can be detected by examination of the bone marrow. Using special stains, one can estimate iron stores with a marrow biopsy. Although fibrosis or neoplasia occasionally can be detected in aspiration studies, biopsy is the best method. Leukemias, multiple myelomas, and polycythemia vera can be detected easily in biopsy specimens. Similarly, lymphomas and other metastatic tumors (e.g., cancers of the breast, kidney, and lung) can be seen. Bone marrow biopsy is an important part of staging for lymphomas and Hodgkin's disease.

Contraindications

- Patients with acute coagulation disorders because of the risk of excessive bleeding
- Patients who cannot cooperate and remain still during the procedure

Potential complications

- Hemorrhage, especially if the patient has a coagulopathy
- Infection, especially if the patient is leukopenic
- Sternal fracture as a result of too aggressive application of pressure to the sternum at the time of biopsy
- Inadvertent puncture of the heart or great vessels when the test is performed on the sternum

Figure 7 Bone marrow aspiration. Sampling of the bone marrow is taken from along the posterior superior iliac crest. (From Pagana KD, Pagana TJ: Mosby's manual of diagnostic tests, St Louis, 1998, Mosby.)

Procedure and patient care

Before

- Explain the procedure to the patient.
- Obtain a written and informed consent for this procedure.
- Encourage the patient to verbalize fears, because many patients are anxious concerning this study.
- Assess the coagulation studies. Report any evidence of coagulopathy to the physician.
- Obtain an order for sedatives if the patient appears extremely apprehensive.
- Remind the patient to remain very still throughout the procedure.

During

- Note the following procedural steps for *bone marrow aspiration*, which is performed on the sternum, iliac crest, anterior or posterior iliac spines, and proximal tibia (in children):
  1. The procedure is usually performed at the patient's bedside using local anesthesia.
  2. A preferred site is the posterior iliac crest, with the patient placed prone or on the side (Figure 7).
  3. The area overlying the bone is prepared and draped in a sterile manner.
  4. The overlying skin and soft tissue, along with the periosteum, is infiltrated with lidocaine.
  5. A large-bore needle containing a stylus is slowly ad-

vanced through the soft tissue and into the outer table of the bone.

6. Once inside the marrow, the stylus is removed, and a syringe is attached.
7. One half to 2 ml of bone marrow is aspirated, smeared on slides, and allowed to dry.
8. The slides are sprayed with a preservative and taken to the pathology laboratory.

- Note the following procedural steps for *bone marrow biopsy*:
  1. The skin and soft tissues overlying the bone are incised.
  2. A core biopsy instrument is "screwed" into the bone.
  3. The biopsy specimen is obtained and sent to the pathology laboratory for analysis.
- Note that aspiration is performed by a trained nurse or physician. Bone marrow biopsy is usually performed by a physician. The duration of these studies is approximately 20 minutes.
- Inform the patient that he or she may have some apprehension when pressure is applied to puncture the outer table of the bone during biopsy specimen removal or aspiration.
- Tell the patient that he or she probably will feel pain during lidocaine infiltration and pressure when the syringe plunger is withdrawn for aspiration.

After

- Apply pressure to the puncture site to arrest minimal bleeding. Apply an adhesive bandage.
- Observe the puncture site for bleeding. Ice packs may be used to help control bleeding.
- Assess for tenderness and erythema, which may indicate infection. Report this to the physician.
- Evaluate the patient for signs of shock (increased pulse rate, decreased blood pressure) and pain.
- Normally place the patient on bed rest for 30 to 60 minutes after the test.
- Note that some patients complain of tenderness at the puncture site for several days after this study. Mild analgesics may be ordered.

🏠 Home care responsibilities

- Instruct the patient to observe the puncture site for bleeding.
- Inform the patient that tenderness and erythema may indicate infection. This should be reported to the physician.
- Mild analgesics may be needed for several days after this procedure for complaints of tenderness at the puncture site.

Abnormal findings

Neoplasm
Viral infection
Bacterial infection
Fungal infection
Myelofibrosis
Agranulocytosis
Polycythemia vera
Multiple myelomas
Hodgkin's disease
Hypersensitivity states

Acute hemorrhagic marrow hyperplasia
Anemia
Lymphoma
Chronic inflammatory disease
Leukemia
Rheumatic fever
AIDS

notes

bone scan

Type of test Nuclear scan

Normal findings No evidence of abnormality

Test explanation and related physiology

The bone scan permits examination of the skeleton by a scanning camera after IV injection of a radionuclide material. Usually technetium (Tc)-99m is the radionuclide used. After injection of the Tc, the radiopharmaceutical is taken up by the bone. Gamma rays are emitted from the Tc through the body and detected by a scintillator. The scintillator emits light with each photon it receives from the gamma ray. When these light patterns are arranged in a spatial order, a realistic image of the bones is apparent.

The degree of radionuclide uptake is related to the metabolism of the bone. Normally a uniform concentration should be seen throughout the bones of the body. An increased uptake of isotope is abnormal and may represent tumor, arthritis, fracture, degenerative bone and joint changes, osteomyelitis, bone necrosis, osteodystrophy, and Paget's disease. These areas of concentrated radionuclide uptake are often called *"hot spots"* and are detectable months before an ordinary x-ray film can reveal the pathology. Hot spots occur because new bone growth is usually stimulated around areas of pathology. If pathology exists and there is no new bone formation around the lesion, the scan will not pick up the abnormality.

The major reason a bone scan is performed is to detect metastatic cancer to the bone. All malignancies capable of metastasis may reach the bone, especially those of the prostate, breast, lung, kidney, urinary bladder, and thyroid gland. Bone scans may be serially repeated to monitor tumor response to antineoplastic therapy.

Bone scans also provide valuable information in the evaluation of patients with trauma or unexplained pain. Bone scanning is much more sensitive than routine x-ray films in detecting small and difficult-to-find fractures, especially in the spine, ribs, face, and small bones of the extremities. Bone scans are used to determine the age of a fracture as well. If a fracture line is seen on a plain x-ray film and the uptake around that fracture is not increased on a bone scan, the injury is said to be an "old" fracture, exceeding several months in age.

Although the bone scan is extremely sensitive, unfortunately it is not very specific. Fractures, infections, tumors, and arthritic changes all appear similar in this scan. Bone scans are helpful in identifying infection (osteomyelitis) when plain films fail to identify the classic findings of infection.

Contraindications

- Patients who are pregnant because of the risk of fetal damage
- Patients who are lactating because of the risk of contaminating the infant

Procedure and patient care

Before

- Explain the procedure to the patient.
- Assure patients they will not be exposed to large amounts of radioactivity, because only tracer doses of the isotope are used.
- Tell the patient that no fasting or sedation is required.

During

- Note the following procedural steps:
  1. The patient receives an IV injection of an isotope, usually sodium pertechnetate (technetium-99m) in a peripheral vein.
  2. The patient is encouraged to drink several glasses of water between the time of radioisotope injection and the scanning. This facilitates renal clearance of the circulating tracer not picked up by the bone. The waiting period before scanning is approximately 1 to 3 hours.
  3. The patient is instructed to urinate.
  4. The patient is positioned in the supine position on the scanning table in the nuclear medicine department.
  5. A radionuclide detector is placed over the patient's body and records the radiation emitted by the skeleton.
  6. This information is translated into a two-dimensional view of the skeleton, which is then visualized on Polaroid or x-ray film.
  7. The patient is repositioned in the prone and lateral positions during the test.

- Note that this scan is performed by a nuclear medicine technician in 30 to 60 minutes. It is interpreted by a physician trained in nuclear medicine imaging.
- Tell the patient that the injection of the radioisotope causes slight discomfort.
- Inform patients in significant pain that lying on the hard scanning table can be uncomfortable.

After

- Because only tracer doses of radioisotope are used, remember that no precautions need to be taken to prevent radioactive exposure to other personnel or family present.
- Assure the patient that the radioactive substance is usually excreted from the body within 6 to 24 hours.
- Encourage the patient to drink fluids to aid in the excretion of the radioactive substance.
- Observe the injection site for redness or swelling.

Abnormal findings

Primary or metastatic tumor
  of the bone
Fracture
Degenerative arthritis
Rheumatoid arthritis

Osteomyelitis
Bone necrosis
Renal osteodystrophy
Paget's disease
Osteomyelitis

notes

bone x-ray

B

Type of test X-ray

Normal findings

No evidence of fracture, tumor, infection, or congenital abnormalities

Test explanation and related physiology

X-ray films of the long bones are usually taken when the patient has complaints about a particular body area. Fractures or tumors are readily detected by x-ray studies. In patients who have a severe or chronic infection overlying a bone, an x-ray film may detect the infection involving that bone (osteomyelitis). X-ray studies of the long bones also can detect joint destruction and bone spurring as a result of persistent arthritis. Growth patterns can be followed by serial x-ray studies of a long bone, usually the wrists and hands. Healing of a fracture also can be documented and followed. X-ray films of the joints reveal the presence of joint effusions and soft tissue swelling as well. Calcifications in the soft tissue indicate chronic inflammatory changes of the nearby bursa or tendons. Soft tissue swelling can also be seen on these bone x-rays. Because the cartilage and tendons are not directly visualized, cartilage fractures or sprains or ligamentous injuries cannot be seen.

At least two x-rays at 90-degree angles are required so that the bone region being studied can be visualized from two different angles (usually anterior to posterior and lateral). Some bone studies (e.g., skull, spine, hip) require oblique views to visualize all the parts that need to be seen.

Interfering factors

- Jewelry or clothing can obstruct radiographic visualization of part of the bone to be evaluated.
- Prior barium studies can diminish the full radiographic visualization of some of the bones surrounding the abdomen (e.g., spine, and pelvis).

Procedure and patient care

Before

- Explain the procedure to the patient.
- Handle carefully any injured parts of the patient's body.

- Instruct the patient that he or she will need to keep the extremity still while the x-ray film is being taken. This can sometimes be difficult, especially when the patient has severe pain associated with a recent injury.
- Shield the patient's testes, ovaries, or pregnant abdomen to avoid exposure from scattered radiation.
- Tell the patient that no fasting or sedation is required.

During

- Note that in the x-ray department the patient is asked to place the involved extremity in several positions. An x-ray film is taken of each position.
- Note that this test is routinely performed by a radiologic technologist within several minutes.
- Tell the patient that no discomfort is associated with this test, except possibly from moving the extremity.

After

- Administer an analgesic for relief of pain if indicated.

Abnormal findings

Fractures
Congenital bone disorders
   (e.g., achondroplasia, dysplasia, dysostosis)
Tumors (osteogenic sarcoma,
   Paget's disease, myeloma, or
   metastatic)

Infection/osteomyelitis
Osteoporosis/osteopenia
Joint destruction (arthritis)
Bone spurring
Abnormal growth pattern
Joint effusion
Foreign bodies

notes

B

breast cancer genetic screening (BRCA genetic testing)

Type of test Blood

Normal findings No genetic mutation in the BRCA 1 or 2 gene

Test explanation and related physiology

BRCA (BR = breast, CA = cancer) genes are the first major genes that have been recognized to indicate an increased susceptibility for development of breast cancer. BRCA 1 and 2 have been identified. The BRCA 1 gene exists on chromosome 17. BRCA 2 is on chromosome 13. These genes are responsible for the synthesis of tumor suppression proteins. More than one half of the women with mutations of this gene will develop breast cancer by the age of 50.

BRCA 1 also confers an increased susceptibility for ovarian cancer. In the normal population only 1% of women develop ovarian cancer by age 70. Of women with mutations of the BRCA gene, 44% develop ovarian cancer.

Those who may most benefit from BRCA genetic testing include:
1. Women who have been diagnosed with breast cancer at a very young age
2. Women who have been diagnosed with ovarian cancer and have a personal or family history of breast cancer
3. Women who have a strong family history of ovarian or breast cancer
4. Women who are relatives of those who carry the BRCA genetic mutation
5. Men who are relatives of those who carry the BRCA genetic mutation

The value of testing a select group of women who may be at high risk for BRCA genetic mutations includes:
1. Identification of those who are at high risk for developing breast or ovarian cancer
2. Consideration of interventions for those who test positive for BRCA mutations (e.g., prophylactic mastectomy/oophorectomy)
3. Allow adoption of risk management screening testing
4. Estimation of potential for passing the mutated BRCA gene to offspring

The ethics and disadvantages to this genetic testing are presently being discussed. Patients may face financial discrimination for health or life insurance or employment if the results are positive.

Contraindications

- Patients who are not emotionally able to deal with the results

Procedure and patient care

Before

- Explain the procedure to the patient.
- Tell the patient that no fasting is required.
- It is recommended that all patients who undergo testing should receive genetic counseling.

During

- Collect venous blood in the special collecting tube provided by the specialized central laboratory.

After

- Apply pressure to the venipuncture site.

Abnormal findings

BRCA 1 and 2 genetic mutation

notes

breast scintography (Breast scan, Sestamibi scan, Scintimammography)

Type of test Nuclear

Normal findings Negative: minimal, symmetric bilateral and uniform breast uptake equal to soft tissue uptake.

Test explanation and related physiology

Nuclear scans of the breast using sestamibi are used to identify breast cancer in patients whose dense breast tissue precludes accurate evaluation by conventional mammography. This test has been used as an adjunct in patients with an indeterminate mammogram and in women with lumpy breasts. This scan may miss as many as 10% to 15% of cancers, however. Furthermore, the false-positive rate is about 15%. Areas of benign cellular hyperplasia also trap the radiotracer. Because cellular hyperplasia is a common finding in the breast just before menses, imaging at this time in the menstrual cycle should be avoided.

Breast nuclear scans will not replace the role of mammography in breast imaging. Nor will it ever be an effective screening tool for the early detection of breast cancer among large populations. However, its role as a second-line imaging modality is growing.

This scan may be helpful in staging breast cancer patients. The radiotracer often goes directly to axillary lymph nodes that contain metastatic breast cancer.

Contraindications

- Patients who are pregnant because of the risk of fetal injury
- Patients who are lactating because of the risk of contaminating maternal milk

Procedure and patient care

Before

- Explain the procedure to the patient.
- Assure patients that they will not be exposed to large amounts of radioactivity because only tracer doses of the isotope are used.
- Tell the patient that no fasting or sedation is required.

During

- Note the following procedural steps:
  1. The patient may be positioned in the supine, prone, or sitting position.
  2. 20 mCi of Tc-99m sestamibi is injected intravenously into the arm contralateral to the suspicious breast.
  3. Imaging begins 10 minutes after injection. A scintillator camera is placed over the breast and records the radiation emitted.
  4. This information is translated into a two-dimensional view of the skeleton, which is then visualized on film.
  5. These images are compared to surrounding soft tissue readings.

After

- Because only tracer doses of radioisotope are used, remember that no precautions need to be taken to prevent radioactive exposure to other personnel or family present.
- Assure the patient that the radioactive substance is usually excreted from the body within 6 to 24 hours.
- Encourage the patient to drink fluids to aid in the excretion of the radioactive substance.
- Observe the injection site for redness or swelling.

Abnormal findings

Breast cancer
Hyperplasia of the breast tissue

notes

breast sonogram (Ultrasound mammography)

Type of test Ultrasound

Normal findings No evidence of cyst or tumor

Test explanation and related physiology

This ultrasound examination of the breast is most commonly used to determine if a mammographic abnormality or a palpable lump is a cyst (fluid-filled) or solid tumor (benign or malignant). In diagnostic real-time ultrasound, harmless high-frequency sound waves are emitted and penetrate the breast. The sound waves are bounced back to the sensor and arranged in a pictorial image by electronic conversion. Ultrasound of the breast is a useful test for differentiating cystic and solid breast lesions. It can be used to monitor a cyst to determine if it enlarges or disappears. Ultrasound is especially useful in patients with an abnormal mass on a mammogram to determine if the abnormality is cystic or solid.

Ultrasound of the breast is also useful in the examination of symptomatic women for whom the radiation of mammography is potentially harmful. These include:

1. Pregnant women
   Radiation may be harmful to the fetus.
2. Young women under the age of 25
   These women may experience a greater oncologic risk from the radiation of mammography.
3. Women who have silicone prosthesis–augmented breasts
   The prosthesis can be penetrated by the ultrasound beam. Ordinarily these prostheses would obscure residual tissue on physical examination and x-ray mammography.
4. Women who refuse to have x-ray mammography because of unreasonable fear of diagnostic radiation

Diagnostic accuracy is improved when breast ultrasound is combined with x-ray mammography (see p. 572). Ultrasound can be used to locate a nonpalpable breast abnormality for biopsy or aspiration.

Procedure and patient care

Before

- Explain the procedure to the patient.
- Assure the patient that no discomfort is associated with this study.
- Inform the patient that no fasting or sedation is required before the tests. Instruct the patient not to apply any lotions or powders to the breasts on the examination day.

During

- Note the following procedural steps:
  1. The patient lies in the prone position on the examining table, which contains a tank that holds heated and chlorinated water.
  2. One breast at a time is immersed in the water.
  3. The transducer that produces the ultrasound waves and detects their echoes is positioned at the bottom of the water tank.
  4. Alternatively the patient is placed in the supine position, and the transducer is directly applied to the breast using contact gel to improve sound transmission.
- Note that this test is performed by an ultrasound technician in approximately 15 minutes.
- Although there is no discomfort associated with this procedure, women with back problems or limited flexibility may have difficulty maintaining the position for this procedure.

After

- After the test is completed, the breasts are dried, the conductive paste is removed.

Abnormal findings

Cyst   Fibroadenoma
Hematoma   Fibrocystic disease
Cancer   Abscess

notes

bronchoscopy

Type of test Endoscopy

Normal findings Normal larynx, trachea, bronchi, and alveoli

Test explanation and related physiology

Bronchoscopy permits endoscopic visualization of the larynx, trachea, and bronchi by either a flexible fiberoptic bronchoscope or a rigid bronchoscope. There are many diagnostic and therapeutic uses for bronchoscopy. *Diagnostic* uses of bronchoscopy include:

1. Direct visualization of the tracheobronchial tree for abnormalities (e.g., tumors, inflammation, strictures)
2. Biopsy of tissue from observed lesions
3. Aspiration of "deep" sputum for culture and sensitivity and for cytology determinations
4. Direct visualization of the larynx for identification of vocal cord paralysis, if present.

Therapeutic uses of bronchoscopy include:

1. Aspiration of retained secretions in patients with airway obstruction or postoperative atelectasis
2. Control of bleeding within the bronchus
3. Removal of foreign bodies that have been aspirated
4. Brachytherapy, which is endobronchial radiation therapy using an iridium wire placed via the bronchoscope
5. Palliative laser obliteration of bronchial neoplastic obstruction

The *flexible fiberoptic bronchoscope* has accessory lumens through which cable-activated instruments can be used for removing biopsy specimens of pathologic lesions. Also, the collection of bronchial washings (obtained by flushing the airways with saline solution), pulmonary toilet, and the instillation of anesthetic agents can be carried out through these extra lumens. Double-sheathed, plugged-protected brushes also can be passed through this accessory lumen. Specimens for cytology and bacteriology can be obtained with these brushes. This allows more accurate determination of pulmonary infectious agents. Needles can be placed through the scope to obtain biopsies from tissue immediately adjacent to the bronchi. Laser therapy can now be performed through the bronchoscope to burn out endotracheal lesions.

Contraindications

- Patients with hypercapnia and severe shortness of breath who cannot tolerate interruption of high-flow oxygen
  However, bronchoscopy can be performed through a special oxygen mask or an endotracheal tube so that the patient can receive oxygen if required.
- Severe tracheal stenosis may make it difficult to pass the scope.

Potential complications

- Fever
- Hypoxemia
- Laryngospasm
- Bronchospasm
- Pneumothorax
- Aspiration
- Hemorrhage (after biopsy)

Procedure and patient care

Before

- Explain the procedure to the patient. Allay any fears and allow the patient to verbalize any concerns.
- Obtain informed consent for this procedure.
- Keep the patient NPO for 4 to 8 hours before the test to reduce the risk of aspiration.
- Instruct the patient to perform good mouth care to minimize the risk of introducing bacteria into the lungs during the procedure.
- Remove and safely store the patient's dentures, glasses, or contact lenses before administering the preprocedural medications.
- Administer the preprocedural medications as ordered.
- Reassure the patient that he or she will be able to breathe during this procedure.
- Instruct the patient not to swallow the local anesthetic sprayed into the throat. Provide a basin for expectoration of the lidocaine.

During

- Note the following procedural steps for *fiberoptic bronchoscopy*:

Figure 8 Bronchoscopy. A bronchoscope is inserted through the trachea and into the bronchus.

1. This test is performed by a pulmonary specialist or a surgeon at the bedside or in an appropriately equipped room.
2. The patient's nasopharynx and oropharynx are anesthetized topically with lidocaine spray before the insertion of the bronchoscope.
3. The patient is placed in the sitting or supine position, and the tube is inserted through the nose or mouth and into the pharynx (Figure 8).

4. After the tube passes into the larynx and through the glottis, more lidocaine is sprayed into the trachea to prevent the cough reflex.
5. The tube is passed farther, well into the trachea, bronchi, and first- and second-generation bronchioles, for systematic examination of the bronchial tree.
6. Biopsy specimens and washings are taken if pathology is suspected.
7. If bronchoscopy is performed for pulmonary toilet (removal of mucus), each bronchus is aspirated until clear.

- Note that this procedure is performed by a physician in approximately 30 to 45 minutes.
- Tell the patient that because of sedation no discomfort is usually felt.

After

- Instruct the patient not to eat or drink anything until the tracheobronchial anesthesia has worn off and the gag reflex has returned, usually in approximately 2 hours.
- Observe the patient's sputum for hemorrhage if biopsy specimens were removed. A small amount of blood streaking may be expected and is normal for several hours. Large amounts of bleeding can cause a chemical pneumonitis.
- Observe the patient closely for evidence of impaired respiration or laryngospasm. The vocal cords may go into spasms after intubation. Emergency resuscitation equipment should be readily available.
- Inform the patient that postbronchoscopy fever often develops within the first 24 hours.
- If a tumor is suspected, collect a postbronchoscopy sputum sample for a cytology determination.
- Inform the patient that warm saline gargles and lozenges may be helpful if a sore throat develops.

B

🏠 Home care responsibilities

- Suggest that the patient gargle with saline or soothing mouthwash to minimize a sore throat.
- Fever is not uncommon after bronchoscopy. High persistent fever should be reported immediately.
- Bronchospasm or laryngospasm should be reported immediately to emergency personnel.
- Inform the patient that biopsy or culture reports will be available in 2 to 7 days.

Abnormal findings

Inflammation	Hemorrhage
Strictures	Foreign body
Tuberculosis	Abscess
Cancer	Infection

notes

CA 27.29 and CA 15-3 tumor markers
(Cancer antigen 15-3)

Type of test Blood

Normal findings

CA 27.29: <38 U/ml
CA 15-3: <22 U/ml

Test explanation and related physiology

The CA 15-3 and CA 27.29 antigens are tumor-associated serum markers available for staging breast cancer and monitoring its treatment. CA 15-3 or CA 27.29 levels are high in less than 50% of patients whose presentation is a localized breast cancer or who have a small tumor burden. Of patients with metastatic breast cancer, however, 80% do have elevated CA 15-3 levels, and 65% have elevated CA 27.29 levels; therefore the usefulness of these antigen tests as a screening technique in early breast cancers (the most common cancer of women) is quite limited. These tumor markers are not used for screening patients for breast cancer. Benign breast disease and nonbreast malignancies (such as lung, pancreas, ovary, and prostate) also can cause elevation of these antigen levels.

The use of these antigens should be limited to monitoring the treatment of advanced disease. CA 15-3 was the first breast tumor marker available. It is not FDA approved. CA 27.29 is now used clinically and has received FDA approval.

Interfering factors

- Some of the other benign and malignant diseases associated with elevations of these antigens include: cancer of the lung, ovary, pancreas, prostate, and colon; fibrocytic disease of the breast; cirrhosis; hepatitis.

Procedure and patient care

Before

- Explain the procedure to the patient.
- Tell the patient that no fasting is required.

During
- Collect 7 to 10 ml of venous blood in a red-top tube.
- Have the blood sample sent to a central diagnostic laboratory. The results are available to the local hospital in 7 to 10 days.

After
- Apply pressure to the venipuncture site.

Abnormal finding

▲ **Increased levels**
  Metastatic breast cancer

notes

CA 19-9 tumor marker (Cancer antigen 19-9)

Type of test Blood

Normal findings <37 U/ml

Test explanation and related physiology

CA 19-9 antigen is a tumor marker used in diagnosis, evaluation of a patient's response to treatment, and surveillance of patients with pancreatic or hepatobiliary cancer. CA 19-9 is a carbohydrate antigen that exists on the surface of cancer cells. It is used primarily in the evaluation of patients with pancreatic or hepatobiliary cancers. For example, in the diagnosis of pancreatic carcinoma, the presence of a pancreatic mass or biliary obstruction and greatly elevated CA 19-9 levels would support pancreatic cancer as the diagnosis over benign pancreatitis. Likewise, patients whose presenting symptoms are ascites, jaundice, and elevated CA 19-9 levels would be suspected of having hepatobiliary cancer. But CA 19-9 levels may not be elevated in all patients with pancreatic carcinoma. Approximately 70% of patients with pancreatic carcinoma and 65% of patients with hepatobiliary cancer have elevated levels.

CA 19-9 levels are used in the posttreatment surveillance of those who have had pancreatic or hepatobiliary cancers. In the few patients with pancreatic or biliary cancer who have a positive response to surgery, chemotherapy, or radiation therapy, a decline in serum levels of CA 19-9 will confirm this response. A rapid rise in CA 19-9 levels may be associated with a recurrent or progressive tumor growth. Mildly elevated levels may exist in patients with gastric cancer, colorectal cancer, or hepatoma and even in 6% to 7% of patients with nongastrointestinal malignancies. Patients who have pancreatitis, gallstones, cirrhosis, inflammatory bowel disease, or cystic fibrosis also can have minimally elevated levels of CA 19-9.

Because of its lack of sensitivity and specificity, CA 19-9 is not effective in screening for pancreaticobiliary tumors in the general population.

Procedure and patient care

Before
- Explain the procedure to the patient.
- Tell the patient that no fasting is required.

During
- Collect 7 to 10 ml of blood in a red-top tube.
- Have the blood sent to a central diagnostic laboratory for CA 19-9 determinations. The results are available to the local hospital in 7 to 10 days.

After
- Apply pressure to the venipuncture site.

Abnormal findings

▲ **Increased levels**

Pancreatic carcinoma	Gastric cancer
Hepatobiliary carcinoma	Colorectal cancer
Pancreatitis	Gallstones
Cholecystitis	Cystic fibrosis
Cirrhosis	Lung cancer

notes

CA-125 tumor marker (Cancer antigen-125)

Type of test Blood

Normal findings 0-35 U/ml

Test explanation and related physiology

CA-125 is an extremely accurate marker for nonmucinous epithelial tumors of the ovary. It is elevated in over 80% of women with ovarian cancer. This tumor marker has a high degree of sensitivity and specificity for ovarian cancer and has been of great benefit to clinicians.

The CA-125 serum tumor marker is also used to determine a patient's response to therapy. Serial comparative testing will show a progressive decline in CA-125 levels for patients responding to treatment. Also, CA-125 tumor markers can predict whether or not a second-look (repeat) diagnostic laparotomy will be positive. A second-look laparotomy will detect a residual tumor in 97% of patients whose CA-125 level is greater than 35 U/ml, whereas only 56% of patients with ovarian cancer whose CA-125 level is less than 35 U/ml will have a positive second-look laparotomy. A precipitous fall in CA-125 after two courses of chemotherapy is an accurate predictor of a complete response to chemotherapy and is used as a good prognostic sign.

Finally, CA-125 determinations can be used in posttreatment surveillance of patients with ovarian cancer. In a patient who has had a complete response as a result of radiation therapy, chemotherapy, or surgery, a delayed rise in the CA-125 level is an early predictor of a recurrent tumor in 93% of patients. Abnormal levels can antedate the appearance of obvious recurrent ovarian cancer by 2 to 7 months.

CA-125 is not an effective screening test for the asymptomatic general public because of its lack of specificity. It is used in a "high-risk" population of women who have a strong family history of ovarian cancer. Elevated levels in the general population indicate that either benign or malignant disease is present in 95% of patients.

Other tumors and benign processes can cause elevated CA-125 levels as well. Diseases that affect the peritoneum such as cirrhosis, pancreatitis, peritonitis, endometriosis, and pelvic inflammatory disease can create elevated levels of CA-125. Other malignancies occurring in the female genital tract, pancreas, colon, lung, and breast can also be associated with elevated levels of this protein. Of the normal population, 1% to 2% have CA 125 levels in excess of 35 U/mL.

Interfering factors

- The first trimester of pregnancy and normal menstruation may be associated with mild elevations of CA-125 levels.
- Patients with benign peritoneal diseases (e.g., cirrhosis, endometriosis) have mildly increased levels.

Procedure and patient care

Before
- Explain the procedure to the patient.
- Tell the patient that no fasting or sedation is required.

During
- Collect 7 to 10 ml of blood in a red-top tube.
- Have the blood sent to a central diagnostic laboratory for determination of CA-125 level. The results are available to the local hospital in 3 to 7 days.

After
- Apply pressure to the venipuncture site.

Abnormal findings

▲ Increased levels

Malignant disorders
Cancer of the ovary
Cancer of the pancreas
Cancer of the nonovarian
   female genital tract
Cancer of the breast
Cancer of the colon
Cancer of the lung
Lymphoma
Peritoneal carcinomatosis

Benign disorders
Cirrhosis
Peritonitis
Pregnancy
Endometriosis
Pancreatitis
Pelvic inflammatory disease

notes

calcitonin (Human calcitonin [HCT], Thyrocalcitonin)

Type of test Blood

Normal findings

Basal
  Males: ≤19 pg/ml or ≤19 ng/L (SI units)
  Females: ≤14 pg/ml or ≤14 ng/L (SI units)
Calcium infusion (2.4 mg/kg)
  Males: ≤190 pg/ml or ≤190 ng/L
  Females: ≤130 pg/ml or ≤130 ng/L
Pentagastrin injection (0.5 μg/kg)
  Males: ≤110 pg/ml or ≤110 ng/L
  Females: ≤30 pg/ml or ≤30 ng/L

Test explanation and related physiology

Calcitonin is a hormone secreted by the parafollicular or C cells of the thyroid gland. Its secretion is stimulated by elevated serum calcium levels. The purpose of calcitonin is to contribute to calcium homeostasis. It decreases serum calcium levels by inhibiting bone resorption and increasing calcium excretion by the kidneys.

This test is usually used in the evaluation of patients with or suspected to have medullary carcinoma of the thyroid. Seventy-five percent of these patients have hypersecretion of calcitonin despite normal serum calcium levels. Calcitonin is also useful in monitoring response to therapy and predicting recurrences of medullary thyroid cancer and as a screening test for those with a family history of medullary cancer and therefore at high risk (20%) for medullary cancer. This is a cancer of the thyroid with a familiar tendency; if it is found late, it has a poor prognosis. Routine screening for elevated calcitonin levels can detect medullary cancer early and improve chances for cure. C-cell hyperplasia, a benign calcitonin-producing disease that also has a familial tendency is also associated with elevated calcitonin levels.

Equivocal elevations in calcitonin levels should be followed with further provocative testing using pentagastrin or calcium to stimulate calcitonin secretion. *Pentagastrin stimulation* involves an IV infusion over 5 to 10 seconds, with blood samples drawn before the injection and at 90 seconds, 2 minutes, and 5 minutes following the infusion. The *calcium infusion test* can be performed in a variety of ways but is most commonly administered over a 1-minute interval with baseline and 5- and 10-minute postinfusion blood levels. With medullary cancer of the thyroid, the provocative tests can cause the calcitonin to rise significantly (often greater than 1000 mg/L).

Elevated levels of calcitonin also may be seen in people with cancer of the lung, breast, and pancreas. This is probably a form of paraneoplastic syndrome in which there is an ectopic production of calcitonin by the nonthyroid cancer cells.

Interfering factors

- ⚑ Drugs that may cause *increased* levels include calcium, cholecystokinin, epinephrine, glucagon, pentagastrin, and oral contraceptives.
- Levels are often elevated in normal pregnant females and newborns.

Procedure and patient care

Before

- Explain the procedure to the patient.
- Tell the patient that an overnight fast is required. Water is permitted.

During

- Collect a venous sample of blood in a heparinized green-top or chilled red-top tube according to the laboratory's protocol.
- The specimen should be placed on ice immediately. The blood is frozen and sent to a reference laboratory.

After

- Apply pressure to the venipuncture site.
- Tell the patient that results may not be available for several days.

Abnormal findings

▲ **Increased levels**

Medullary carcinoma of the thyroid

G cell hyperplasia

Oat cell carcinoma of the lung

Breast carcinoma

Pancreatic cancer

Primary hyperparathyroidism

Secondary hyperparathyroidism because of chronic renal failure

Pernicious anemia

Zollinger-Ellison syndrome

Alcoholic cirrhosis

Thyroiditis

notes

calcium (Total/ionized calcium, Ca, Serum calcium)

Type of test Blood; urine

Normal findings

Age	mg/dl	mmol/L
Total calcium		
<10 Days	7.6-10.4	1.9-2.6
Umbilical	9-11.5	2.25-2.88
10 Days-2 years	9-10.6	2.3-2.65
Child	8.8-10.8	2.2-2.7
Adult*	9-10.5	2.25-2.75
Ionized calcium		
Newborn	4.20-5.58	1.05-1.37
2 Mos-18 yrs	4.80-5.52	1.20-1.38
Adult	4.5-5.6	1.05-1.3

*In the elderly values tend to decrease.

Possible critical values

<6 mg/dl (may lead to tetany)
>14 mg/dl (may lead to coma)

Test explanation and related physiology

The serum calcium test is used to evaluate parathyroid function and calcium metabolism by directly measuring the total amount of calcium in the blood. Determination of serum calcium is used to monitor patients with renal failure, renal transplantation, hyperparathyroidism, and various malignancies. It is also used to monitor calcium levels during and after large-volume blood transfusions.

About one half of the total calcium exists in the blood in its free (ionized) form, and about one half exists in its protein-bound form (mostly with albumin). The serum calcium level is a measure of both. As a result, when the serum albumin level is low (as in malnourished patients), the serum calcium level will also be low, and vice versa. As a rule of thumb, the total serum calcium level decreases by approximately 0.8 mg for every 1-g decrease in the serum albumin level. Serum albumin should be measured with serum calcium. An advantage of measuring only the ionized form is that it is unaffected by changes in serum albumin levels.

When the serum calcium level is elevated on at least three

separate determinations, the patient is said to have hypercalcemia. The most common cause of hypercalcemia is hyperparathyroidism. Parathormone (see p. 616) causes elevated calcium levels by increasing gastrointestinal absorption, decreasing urinary excretion, and increasing bone resorption. Malignancy, the second most common cause of hypercalcemia, can cause elevated calcium levels in two main ways. First, tumor metastasis (myeloma, lung, breast, renal cell) to the bone can destroy the bone, causing resorption and pushing calcium into the blood. Second, the cancer (lung, breast, renal cell) can produce a parathyroid hormone–like substance that drives the serum calcium up (ectopic PTH). Excess vitamin D ingestion can increase serum calcium by increasing renal and gastrointestinal absorption. Granulomatous infections such as sarcoidosis or tuberculosis are associated with hypercalcemia.

Hypocalcemia occurs in patients with hypoalbuminemia. The most common causes of hypoalbuminemia are malnutrition (especially in alcoholics) and large-volume IV infusions of crystallize. Large blood transfusions are associated with low serum calcium levels because the citrate additives used in banked blood for anticoagulation bind the free calcium in the recipient's bloodstream. Intestinal malabsorption, renal failure, rhabdomyolysis, alkalosis, and acute pancreatitis (caused by saponification of fat) are also known to be associated with low serum calcium levels. Hypomagnesemia can be associated with refractory hypocalcemia.

Urinary calcium can be measured and is used most commonly to identify and support the diagnosis of hypercalcemia. Excretion of calcium in the urine is increased in all patients with hypercalcemia. Urinary calcium levels are decreased in patients with hypocalcemia. Urinary calcium is not commonly used today because the development of assays for parathyroid hormone has replaced the need for urine calcium measurements to make the diagnosis of hyperparathyroidism. The test is still helpful in determining the cause of recurrent nephrolithiasis.

Interfering factors

- Vitamin D intoxication may cause increased serum calcium levels.
- Excessive ingestion of milk may cause increased levels.
- Serum pH can affect calcium values. A decrease in pH causes increased calcium levels.
- Prolonged tourniquet time will lower pH and factitiously increase calcium levels.

- There is normally a small diurnal variation in calcium, with peak levels occurring around 9 PM.
- Hypoalbuminemia is artifactually associated with decreased levels of total calcium.
- Drugs that may cause *increased* serum levels include calcium salts, hydralazine, lithium, thiazide diuretics, parathyroid hormone (PTH), thyroid hormone, alkaline antacids, Ca salts, ergocalciferol, androgens, and vitamin D.
- Drugs that may cause *decreased* serum levels include acetazolamide, anticonvulsants, asparaginase, aspirin, calcitonin, cisplatin, corticosteroids, heparin, laxatives, loop diuretics, magnesium salts, diuretics, estrogens, albuterol, and oral contraceptives.

Procedure and patient care

Before

- Explain the procedure to the patient.
- Tell the patient that no fasting is required; however, the serum calcium may be part of a multichemical analysis in which fasting is required for the other studies.

During

- Collect approximately 7 ml of venous blood in a red-top tube. Avoid prolonged tourniquet use.
- List on the laboratory slip any medications that may affect test results.

After

- Apply pressure to the venipuncture site.

Abnormal findings

▲ **Increased levels (hypercalcemia)**

Hyperparathyroidism
Nonparathyroid PTH-
  producing tumor (e.g.,
  lung or renal carcinoma)
Metastatic tumor to the
  bone Paget's disease of
  bone
Prolonged immobilization
Milk-alkali syndrome
Vitamin D intoxication
Lymphoma
Granulomatous infections
  (e.g., sarcoidosis and
  tuberculosis)
Addison's disease
Acromegaly
Hyperthyroidism

▼ **Decreased values (hypocalcemia)**

Hypoparathyroidism
Renal failure
Hyperphosphatemia
  secondary to renal
  failure
Rickets
Vitamin D deficiency
Osteomalacia
Malabsorption
Pancreatitis
Fat embolism
Alkalosis

notes

caloric study (Oculovestibular reflex study)

Type of test Electrodiagnostic

Normal findings Nystagmus with irrigation

Test explanation and related physiology

Caloric studies are used to evaluate the vestibular portion of the eighth cranial nerve (CN VIII) by irrigating the external auditory canal with hot or cold water. Normally stimulation with cold water causes rotary nystagmus (involuntary rapid eye movement) away from the ear being irrigated; hot water induces nystagmus toward the side of the ear being irrigated. If the labyrinth is diseased or CN VIII is not functioning (e.g., from tumor compression), no nystagmus is induced. This study aids in the differential diagnosis of abnormalities that may occur in the vestibular system, brain stem, or cerebellum.

Contraindications

- Patients with a perforated eardrum
  Cold air may be substituted for the fluid.
- Patients with an acute disease of the labyrinth (e.g., Ménière's syndrome)
  The test can be performed when the acute attack subsides.

Interfering factors

✱ Drugs such as sedatives and antivertigo agents can alter test results.

Procedure and patient care

Before

- Explain the procedure to the patient.
- Hold solid foods before the test to reduce the incidence of vomiting.

During

- Although the exact procedures for caloric studies vary, note the following steps in a typical test:
  1. Before the test, the patient is examined for the presence of nystagmus, postural deviation (Romberg's sign), and past-pointing. This examination provides the baseline values for comparison during the test.
  2. The ear canal should be examined and cleaned by a physi-

cian before testing to ensure that the water will freely flow to the middle ear area.

3. The ear on the suspected side is irrigated first because the patient's response may be minimal.

4. After an emesis basin is placed under the ear, the irrigation solution is directed into the external auditory canal until the patient complains of nausea and dizziness or nystagmus is seen. Usually this occurs in 20 to 30 seconds.

5. If after 3 minutes no symptoms occur, the irrigation is stopped.

6. The patient is tested again for nystagmus, past-pointing, and Romberg's sign.

7. After approximately 5 minutes, the procedure is repeated on the other side.

- Note that this procedure is usually performed by a physician or technician in approximately 15 minutes.
- Tell the patient that he or she will probably experience nausea and dizziness during the test.

After

- Usually place the patient on bed rest for approximately 30 to 60 minutes until nausea or vomiting subsides.
- Ensure patient safety related to dizziness.

Abnormal findings

Brainstem inflammation, infarction, or tumor
Cerebellar inflammation, infarction, or tumor
Vestibular or cochlear inflammation or tumor
Acoustic neuroma
Eighth nerve neuritis / neuropathy

notes

C

carbon dioxide content (CO_2 content, CO_2 combining power)

Type of test Blood

Normal findings
Adult/elderly: 23-30 mEq/L or 23-30 mmol/L (SI units)
Child: 20-28 mEq/L
Infant: 20-28 mEq/L
Newborn: 13-22 mEq/L

Possible critical values <6 mEq/L

Test explanation and related physiology

The CO_2 content is a measure of CO_2 in the blood. In the peripheral venous blood, this is used to assist in evaluating the pH status of the patient and to assist in evaluation of electrolytes. The serum CO_2 test is usually included with other assessments of electrolytes. It is usually done with a multiphasic testing machine which also measures sodium, potassium, chloride, BUN and creatinine. It is important not to get this test confused with $P{CO_2}$. This CO_2 content measures the H_2CO_3, dissolved CO_2, and bicarbonate ion (HCO_3^-) that exists in the serum. Because the amounts of H_2CO_3 and dissolved CO_2 in the blood are so small, CO_2 content is an indirect measure of HCO_3^- anion. HCO_3^- anion is second in importance to the chloride ion in electrical neutrality (negative charge) of extracellular and intra-cellular fluid; its major role is in acid-base balance.

Levels of HCO_3^- are regulated by the kidneys. Increases occur with alkalosis, and decreases occur with acidosis. See further discussion of this test as it is performed on arterial blood (p. 105). When CO_2 content is measured in the laboratory with other serum electrolytes, air affects the specimen, and the CO_2 partial pressure can be altered. Therefore venous blood speci-mens are not very accurate for true CO_2 content or HCO_3^-. This test is mostly used as a rough guide as to the patients acid/base balance.

Interfering factors
- Underfilling the tube with blood allows CO_2 to escape from the serum specimen and may significantly reduce HCO_3^- values.

☙ Drugs that may cause *increased* serum CO_2 and HCO_3^- levels include aldosterone, barbiturates, bicarbonates, ethacrynic acid, hydrocortisone, loop diuretics, mercurial diuretics, and steroids.

☙ Drugs that may cause *decreased* levels include methicillin, nitrofurantoin (Furadantin), paraldehyde, phenformin hydrochloride, tetracycline, thiazide diuretics, and triamterene.

Procedure and patient care

Before

- Explain the procedure to the patient.
- Tell the patient that no fasting is required.

During

- Collect approximately 7 to 10 ml of venous blood in a red- or green-top tube.

After

- Apply pressure to the venipuncture site.

Abnormal findings

▲ **Increased levels**
   Severe diarrhea
   Starvation
   Severe vomiting
   Aldosteronism
   Emphysema
   Metabolic alkalosis
   Gastric suction

▼ **Decreased levels**
   Renal failure
   Salicylate toxicity
   Diabetic ketoacidosis
   Metabolic acidosis
   Shock
   Starvation

notes

carboxyhemoglobin (COHb, Carbon monoxide)

C

Type of test Blood

Normal findings
Nonsmoker: <3%
Smoker: ≤12%
Newborn: ≥12%

Possible critical values
20% to 30%: Dizziness, headache, disturbances in judgment
30% to 40%: Tachycardia, hyperpnea, hypotension, confusion
50% to 60%: Coma
>60%: Death

Test explanation and related physiology

This test is used to detect carbon monoxide poisoning. This test measures the amount of serum COHb, which is formed by the combination of carbon monoxide (CO) and hemoglobin (Hb). CO combines with Hb 200 times more readily than oxygen (O_2) can combine with Hb (oxyhemoglobin). This results in fewer Hb bonds available to combine with O_2. Further, when CO occupies the O_2 binding sites, the hemoglobin molecule is changed to bind the remaining O_2 more tightly. This greater affinity of CO for Hb and change in O_2 binding strength does not allow the O_2 to readily pass from the RBCs to the tissue. Less O_2 is therefore available for tissue cell respiration. This results in hypoxemia.

CO poisoning is documented by Hb analysis for COHb. A specimen should be drawn as soon as possible after exposure, because CO is rapidly cleared from the Hb by breathing normal air. O_2 saturation studies and oximetry are inaccurate in CO-exposed patients because they measure all forms of oxygen-saturated hemoglobin, including carboxyhemoglobin. In these circumstances the patient's oximetry will be good, yet the patient is hypoxemic.

This test can also be used to evaluate patients with complaints of headache, irritability, nausea, vomiting, and vertigo, who unknowingly may have been exposed to CO. Its greatest use, however, is in patients exposed to smoke inhalation, exhaust fumes, and fires. Other sources of CO include tobacco smoke, petroleum and natural gas fuel fumes, automobile exhaust, unvented natural-gas heaters, and defective gas stoves. The treatment of CO toxicity is administration of high concentrations of O_2 to displace the carboxyhemoglobin.

Procedure and patient care

Before

- Explain the procedure to the patient or family.
- Obtain the patient history related to any possible source of CO inhalation.
- Assess the patient for signs and symptoms of mild CO toxicity (e.g., headache, weakness, dizziness, malaise, dyspnea) and moderate to severe CO toxicity (e.g., severe headache, bright-red mucous membranes, cherry-red blood). Maintain patient safety precautions if confusion is present.

During

- Collect approximately 5 to 10 ml of venous blood in a lavender- or green-top tube.

After

- Apply pressure to the venipuncture site.
- Treat the patient as indicated by the physician. Usually the patient receives high concentrations of O_2.
- Encourage respirations to allow the patient to clear CO from the Hb.

Abnormal findings

Carbon monoxide poisoning

notes

carcinoembryonic antigen (CEA)

Type of test Blood

Normal findings <5 ng/ml or 0-2.5 μg/L (SI units)

Test explanation and related physiology

The CEA is a protein that normally occurs in fetal gut tissue. By birth detectable serum levels disappear. In the early 1960s CEA was found to exist in the bloodstream of adults who had colorectal tumors. Therefore the antigen was thought to be a specific indicator of the presence of colorectal cancer. Subsequently, however, this protein has been found in patients who have a variety of carcinomas (e.g., breast, pancreatic, gastric, hepatobiliary), sarcomas, and even many benign diseases (e.g., ulcerative colitis, diverticulitis, cirrhosis). Chronic smokers also have elevated CEA levels.

Because the CEA level can be elevated in both benign and malignant diseases, it is not considered to be a specific test for colorectal cancer. As a result, CEA is not a reliable screening test for the detection of colorectal cancer in the general population. Its use is limited to determining the prognosis and monitoring the response of tumor to antineoplastic therapy in a patient with cancer. This is especially helpful in patients with breast and gastrointestinal cancers. The CEA level on the initial test is an indicator of tumor burden and prognosis. Smaller and early-staged tumors are likely to have minimal CEA elevations, if not normal CEA levels. A drastic reduction to normal CEA levels is expected with complete eradication of tumor. Therefore this test is used to determine the adequacy of treatment.

This test also is used in the surveillance of patients with cancer. A steadily rising CEA level is occasionally the first sign of tumor recurrence. This makes CEA testing very valuable in the follow-up of patients who have had potentially curative therapy. It is important to note that many patients with advanced breast or gastrointestinal tumors may not have elevated CEA levels.

CEA can also be detected in body fluid other than blood. Its presence in those body fluids indicates metastasis. This antigen is commonly measured in peritoneal fluid or chest effusions. An elevated CEA in these fluids indicates metastasis to the peritoneum or pleural, respectively. Likewise, elevated CEA levels in the CSF would indicate central nervous system metastasis.

Interfering factors

- Smoking
- Benign diseases (e.g., cholecystitis, colitis, diverticulitis)
- Liver diseases (e.g., hepatitis, cirrhosis)

Procedure and patient care

Before

- Explain the procedure to the patient.
- Tell the patient that no fasting is required.

During

- Collect a peripheral blood specimen. The collecting tube varies according to the commercial laboratory. (The two most frequently used laboratories for this test are Abbott Laboratories and Roche Labs.)
- Indicate on the laboratory slip if the patient smokes or has diseases that can affect test results.

After

- Apply pressure to the venipuncture site.

Abnormal findings

▲ Increased levels

Cancer (gastrointestinal, breast, lung, pancreatic, hepatobiliary)

Inflammation (colitis, cholecystitis, pancreatitis, diverticulitis)

Cirrhosis

Peptic ulcer

notes

cardiac catheterization (Coronary angiography, Angiocardiography, Ventriculography)

Type of test X-ray with contrast dye

Normal findings Normal heart-muscle motion, normal coronary arteries, normal great vessels, and normal intracardiac pressures and volumes

Test explanation and related physiology

Cardiac catheterization is used to visualize the heart chambers, arteries, and great vessels. It is used most often to evaluate patients with chest pain. Patients with a positive stress test are also studied to locate the region of coronary occlusion. This test is also used to determine the effects of valvular heart disease. Right heart catheterization is performed to calculate cardiac output. This is the most accurate method to determine cardiac output. Right heart catheterization is also used to identify pulmonary emboli (see pulmonary angiography, p. 695).

For cardiac catheterization, a catheter is passed into the heart through a peripheral vein or artery, depending on whether catheterization of the right or left side of the heart is being performed. Through the catheter pressures are recorded, and radiographic dyes are injected. With the assistance of a computer, cardiac output and other measures of cardiac functions can be determined. Cardiac catheterization is indicated for the following reasons:

1. To identify, locate, and quantitate the severity of atherosclerotic, occlusive coronary artery disease
2. To evaluate the severity of acquired and congenital cardiac valvular or septal defects
3. To determine the presence and degree of congenital cardiac abnormalities such as transposition of great vessels, patent ductus arteriosus, and anomalous venous return to the heart
4. To evaluate the success of previous cardiac surgery or balloon angioplasty
5. To evaluate cardiac muscle function
6. To identify and quantify ventricular aneurysms
7. To identify and locate acquired disease of the great vessels such as atherosclerotic occlusion or aneurysms within the aortic arch

8. To evaluate patients with acute myocardial infarction and facilitate infusion of thrombolytic agents into the occluded coronary arteries

9. To insert a catheter to monitor right-sided heart pressures such as pulmonary artery and pulmonary wedge pressures. (Table 5 provides pressures and volumes used in cardiac monitoring.)

10. To perform dilation of stenotic coronary arteries (angioplasty), place coronary artery stents, or perform laser atherectomy

Cardiac catheterization is performed under sterile conditions. In right-sided heart catheterization, usually the subclavian, brachial, or femoral vein is used for vascular access. In left-sided heart catheterization, usually the right femoral artery is cannulated; alternatively, however, the brachial artery may be chosen (Figure 9). As the catheter is placed into the great vessels of the heart chamber, pressures are monitored and recorded. Blood samples for analysis of O_2 content are also obtained. The catheter is advanced with appropriate guidance into the desired position. After pressures are obtained, angiographic visualization of the heart chambers, valves, and coronary arteries is achieved with the injection of radiographic dye.

Transluminal coronary angioplasty is a therapeutic procedure that can be performed during coronary angiography in medical centers where open heart surgery is available. During this procedure a specific, specially designed balloon catheter is introduced into the coronary arteries and placed across the stenotic area of the coronary artery. This area can then be dilated by controlled inflation of the balloon. The coronary arteriogram is then repeated to document the effects of the forceful dilation of the stenotic area. Coronary arterial stents can be placed at the site of previous stenosis after angioplasty and maintain patency for longer periods of time. Likewise, laser atherectomy of coronary arterial plaques can be performed to more permanently open hard, atheromatous plaques.

Contraindications

- Patients who are unable to cooperate during the test
- Patients who would refuse intervention if an amenable lesion were found
- Patients with an iodine dye allergy who have not received preventive medication for allergy

TABLE 5 Pressures and volumes used in cardiac monitoring

	Description	Normal values
Pressures		
Routine blood pressure	Routine brachial artery pressure	90-140/60-90 mm Hg
Systolic left ventricular pressure	Peak pressure in the left ventricle during systole	90-140 mm Hg
End-diastolic left ventricular pressure	Pressure in the left ventricle at the end of diastole	4-12 mm Hg
Central venous pressure	Pressure in the superior vena cava	2-14 cm H_2O
Pulmonary wedge pressure	Pressure in the pulmonary venules, an indirect measurement of left atrial pressure and left ventricular end-diastolic pressure	Left atrial: 6-15 mm Hg
Pulmonary artery pressure	Pressure in the pulmonary artery	15-28/5-16 mm Hg
Aortic artery pressure	Same as routine blood pressure	

Continued

C

TABLE 5 Pressures and volumes used in cardiac monitoring—cont'd

Volumes

End-diastolic volume (EDV)	Amount of blood present in the left ventricle at the end of diastole	50-90 ml/m^2
End-systolic volume (ESV)	Amount of blood present in the left ventricle at the end of systole	25 ml/m^2
Stroke volume (SV)	Amount of blood ejected from the heart in one contraction (SV = EDV – ESV)	45 ± 12 ml/m^2
Ejection fraction (EF)	Proportion (fraction) of EDV ejected from the left ventricle during systole (EF = SV/ EDV)	0.67 ± 0.07
Cardiac output (CO)	Amount of blood ejected by the heart in 1 minute	3-6 L/min
Cardiac index (CI)	Amount of blood ejected by the heart in 1 minute per square meter of body surface area (CI = CO/body surface area)	2.8-4.2 L/min/^{2} for a patient with 1.5 m^2 of body surface area

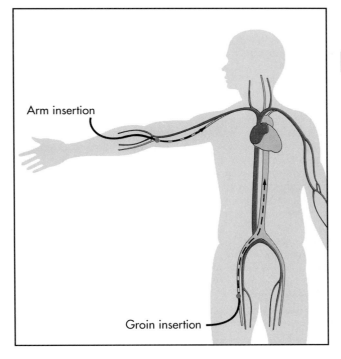

Figure 9 Cardiac catheterization. Brachial (arm) or femoral (groin) arterial insertion for cardiac catheterization. (From Pagana KD, Pagana TJ: *Mosby's manual of diagnostic and laboratory tests,* St Louis, 1998, Mosby.

- Patients who are pregnant, because of radiation exposure to the fetus
- Patients with renal disorders, because iodinated contrast is nephrotoxic
- Patients with a bleeding propensity

Potential complications

- Cardiac arrhythmias (dysrhythmias)
- Perforation of the heart myocardium
- Catheter-induced embolic stroke (cerebrovascular accident) or myocardial infarction
- Complications associated with the catheter insertion site such as arterial thrombosis, embolism, or pseudoaneurysm

- Infection at the catheter insertion site
- Pneumothorax following subclavian vein catheterization of the right side of the heart
- Possible hypoglycemia or acidosis in patients who are taking Glucophage and receive iodine dye

Procedure and patient care

Before

- Explain the procedure to the patient.
- Obtain written permission from the fully informed patient.
- Allay the patient's fears and anxieties regarding this test. Although this test creates tremendous fear in a patient, it is performed often, and complications are rare.
- Instruct the patient to abstain from oral intake for at least 4 to 8 hours before the test.
- Prepare the catheter insertion site by shaving and scrubbing the skin.
- Mark the patient's peripheral pulses with a pen before catheterization. This will facilitate postcatheterization assessment of the pulses at the affected and nonaffected extremities.
- Provide appropriate precatheterization sedation as ordered by the physician.
- Instruct the patient to void before going to the catheterization laboratory.
- Remove all valuables and dental prostheses before transporting the patient to the catheterization laboratory.
- Obtain IV access for delivery of IV fluids and cardiac drugs if necessary.

During

- Take the patient to the cardiac catheterization laboratory.
- Note the following procedural steps:
    1. The chosen catheter insertion site is prepared and draped in a sterile manner.
    2. The desired vessel is punctured with a needle.
    3. A wire is placed through the needle and into the catheter.
    4. The angiographic catheter is threaded on top of the wire.
    5. Once the catheter is in the desired location, the appropriate cardiac pressures and volumes are measured.
    6. Cardiac ventriculography is performed with controlled injection of contrast.

7. Each coronary artery is catheterized. Cardiac angiography is then carried out with a controlled injection of contrast material.

8. During the injection, x-ray films are rapidly made.

9. The patient's vital signs must be monitored constantly during this procedure.

10. If *angioplasty* is performed, the cardiologist appropriately places the catheter and balloon at the stenotic area. Note the following procedural steps:
    a. As the ECG tracing is observed, the balloon is inflated, and the stenotic areas are forcefully dilated.
    b. If signs of myocardial ischemia develop, the balloon is immediately deflated.
    c. Usually inflation of the balloon is continued only for a few seconds.

11. After obtaining all the required information, the catheter is removed.

- Note that this test is usually performed by a cardiologist in approximately 1 hour.
- Tell the patient that during the injection he or she may experience a severe hot flush. This is uncomfortable but lasts only 10 to 15 seconds.
- Note that some patients have a tendency to cough as the catheter is placed into the pulmonary artery.
- Verbally support the patient as the x-ray films are taken, because the loud noises may frighten the patient.

After

- Monitor the patient's vital signs.
- Apply pressure to the site of vascular access.
- Keep the patient on bed rest for 4 to 8 hours to allow for complete sealing of the arterial puncture.
- Keep the affected extremity extended and immobilized with sandbags to decrease bleeding.
- Assess the puncture site for signs of bleeding, hematoma, or absence of pulse.
- Assess the patient's pulses of both extremities. Compare with preprocedural baseline values.
- Encourage the patient to drink fluids to maintain adequate hydration. Dehydration may be caused by the diuretic action of the dye.
- See p. xviii for appropriate interventions concerning the care for patients with iodine allergy.

- Instruct the patient that the test will be reviewed by the cardiologist and the results will be available in 1 or 2 days.

Abnormal findings

Anatomic variation of the cardiac chambers and great vessels
Coronary artery occlusive disease
Ventricular aneurysm
Ventricular mural thrombi
Intracardiac tumor
Aortic root arteriosclerotic or aneurysmal disease
Anomalies in pulmonary venous return
Acquired or congenital septal defects and valvular abnormalities
Pulmonary emboli
Pulmonary hypertension

notes

cardiac exercise stress testing (Stress testing; Exercise testing; Electrocardiograph [ECG] stress testing, exercise testing; Nuclear stress testing, Echo stress testing)

Type of test Electrodiagnostic; nuclear

Normal findings Patient able to obtain and maintain maximal heart rate of 85% for predicted age and gender with no cardiac symptoms or ECG change. No cardiac muscle wall dysfunction present.

Test explanation and related physiology

Stress testing is used in the following situations:

1. To evaluate chest pain in a patient suspected of having coronary disease (Occasionally a person may have significant coronary stenosis that is not apparent during normal physical activity. If, however, the pain can be reproduced with exercise, one may infer that coronary occlusion is present.)
2. To determine the limits of safe exercise during a cardiac rehabilitation program or to assist patients with cardiac disease in maintaining good physical fitness
3. To detect labile or exercise-related hypertension
4. To detect intermittent claudication in patients with suspected vascular occlusive disease in the extremities. (In this situation, the patient may experience leg muscle cramping while performing the exercise.)
5. To evaluate the effectiveness of treatment in patients who take antianginal or antiarrhythmic medications
6. To evaluate the effectiveness of cardiac intervention (such as bypass grafting or angioplasty)

Stress testing is a noninvasive study that provides information about the patient's cardiac function. In stress testing the heart is stressed in some way. The heart is then evaluated during the stress. Changes indicating ischemia indicate coronary occlusive disease. By far the most commonly used method of stress is *exercise stress testing* (bike or treadmill). *Chemical stress testing* methods are becoming more commonly used because of their safety and increased accuracy. A third method, less commonly used, is *pacer stress testing*.

During *exercise stress testing*, the ECG, heart rate, and blood pressure are monitored while the patient engages in some type of physical activity (stress). Two methods of stress testing include pedaling a stationary bike and walking on a treadmill. With the stationary bicycle, the pedaling tension is slowly increased to increase the heart rate. With the treadmill test, the speed and grade of incline are increased. The treadmill test is the most frequently used, because it is the most easily standardized and reproducible. The various grades of exercise are determined by the cardiologist in attendance based on estimation of cardiac function capabilities.

The usual goal of exercise stress testing is to increase the heart rate to just below maximal levels or to the "target heart rate." Usually this target heart rate is 80% to 90% of the maximal heart rate. The test is usually discontinued if the patient reaches that target heart rate or develops any symptoms or ECG changes. The maximal heart rate is determined by a chart that takes into account the patient's age (about 230 minus the patient's age) and gender. The normal maximal heart rate for adults varies from 150 to 200 beats/min; patients taking calcium channel blockers and sympathetic blockers have a lower-than-expected maximal heart rate.

Exercise stress testing is based on the principle that occluded arteries will be unable to meet the heart's increased demand for blood during the testing. This may become obvious with symptoms (e.g., chest pain, fatigue, dyspnea, tachycardia, cardiac arrhythmias [dysrhythmias], fall in blood pressure) or ECG changes (e.g., ST-segment variance >1 mm, increasing premature ventricular contractions, or other rhythm disturbances). An advantage of stress testing is that these symptoms can be stimulated and identified in a safe environment. Besides the electrodiagnostic method of cardiac evaluation, the stressed heart can also be evaluated by nuclear scanning or echocardiography. Findings of ischemia are discussed in following paragraphs.

When exercise testing is not advisable or the patient is unable to exercise to a level adequate to stress the heart (patients with an orthopedic, arthritic, neurologic, or pulmonary limitation), *chemical stress testing* is recommended. Chemical stress testing is becoming increasingly used because of its accuracy and ease of performance. Although chemical stress testing is less physiologic than exercise testing, it is safer and more controllable. *Dipyridamole (Persantine)* is a coronary vasodilator. If one coronary artery is significantly occluded, the coronary blood flow is diverted to the opened vessels.

Adenosine works similarly to dipyridamole. *Dobutamine* is another chemical that can stress the heart. Dobutamine stimulates the heart muscle function. This entails administration of progressively greater amounts of dobutamine over 3-minute intervals. The normal heart muscle increases (augments) its contractility (wall motion). Ischemic muscle has no augmentation. In fact, in time the ischemic area becomes hypokinetic. Infarcted tissue is akinetic. In chemical stress testing the stressed heart is evaluated by nuclear scanning or echocardiography.

Pacing is another method of stress testing. In patients with permanent pacemakers, the rate of capture can be increased to a rate that would be considered a cardiac stress. The heart is then evaluated electrodiagnostically or with nuclear scanning or echocardiography.

The methods of evaluation of the heart are electrophysiologic (ECG) nuclear scanning and echocardiography. These tests are discussed separately (see pp. 354 and 332). Echocardiography is fast becoming the method of choice for urgent and elective cardiac evaluation with or without stress testing.

Contraindications

- Patients with unstable angina
- Patients with severe aortic valvular heart disease
- Patients who cannot participate in an exercise program because of their impaired lung or motor function
- Patients who have recently had a myocardial infarction (In this case, however, limited stress testing can be done.)
- Patients with severe congestive heart failure
- Patients who have severe claudication and cannot walk adequately to stress their hearts

Potential complications

- Fatal cardiac arrhythmias
- Severe angina
- Myocardial infarction
- Fainting

Interfering factors

- Heavy meals before testing can divert blood to the gastrointestinal tract.
- Nicotine from smoking can cause coronary artery spasm.
- Medical problems such as left ventricular hypertrophy, hypertension, valvular heart disease (especially of the aortic valve), left bundle-branch block, severe anemia, hypoxemia, and chronic pulmonary disease can affect results.

▼ Drugs that can affect test results include beta-blockers (e.g., propranolol [Inderal]), calcium channel blockers, digoxin, and nitroglycerine.

Procedure and patient care

Before

- Explain the procedure to the patient.
- Instruct the patient to abstain from eating, drinking, and smoking for 4 hours.
- Inform the patient about the risks of the test and obtain informed consent.
- Instruct the patient to bring comfortable clothing and shoes in which to exercise. Slippers are not acceptable.
- Inform the patient if any medications should be discontinued before testing.
- Obtain a pretest ECG.
- Record the patient's vital signs for baseline values.
- Apply and secure appropriate ECG electrodes.

During

- Note that a physician usually is present during stress testing.
- After the patient begins to exercise, adjust the treadmill machine settings to apply increasing levels of stress at specific intervals. It is helpful to encourage and support the patient at each level of increased stress.
- Encourage patients to verbalize any symptoms.
- Note that during the test the ECG tracing and vital signs are monitored continuously.
- Terminate the test if the patient complains of chest pain, exhaustion, dyspnea, fatigue, or dizziness.
- Note that testing usually takes approximately 45 minutes.
- Inform the patient that the physician in attendance usually interprets the results and will explain them to the patient.

After

- Place the patient in the supine position to rest after the test.
- Monitor the ECG tracing and record vital signs at post-stress intervals, until recordings and values return to pretest levels.
- Remove electrodes and paste.

Abnormal findings

Coronary artery occlusive disease
Exercise-related hypertension
Intermittent claudication
Abnormal cardiac rhythms: stress-induced

notes

cardiac nuclear scanning (Myocardial scan, Cardiac scan, Nuclear cardiac scanning, Heart scan, Thallium scan, MUGA scan, Isonitrile scan, Sestamibi scan)

Type of test Nuclear scan

Normal findings Normal myocardial ejection fraction and coronary perfusion

Test explanation and related physiology

Cardiac nuclear scanning is used to detect myocardial ischemia, infarction, wall dysfunction, and decreased ejection fraction. It is commonly used as the imaging method part of cardiac stress testing (see discussion in cardiac stress testing). Specific indications for cardiac nuclear scanning include:

1. Screening of adults for past and recent infarction
2. Evaluation of patients with chest pain and uninterpretable or equivocal ECG changes caused by drugs, bundle-branch block, or left ventricular hypertrophy
3. Evaluation of myocardial perfusion before and after coronary artery bypass surgery
4. Quantification and surveillance of myocardial infarction
5. Evaluation of medical and surgical therapy for coronary artery perfusion
6. Evaluation of ventricular function in patients with myocardial disease
7. Evaluation of patients receiving cardiotoxic drugs (e.g., adriamycin chemotherapy)

Cardiac radionuclear scanning is a noninvasive and safe method of recognizing alterations of left ventricular muscle function and coronary artery blood distribution. Many different radionuclear materials can be used, most often technetium-99m pertechnetate, thallium-201, or technetium-99m pyrophosphate. When these compounds are injected intravenously and a radiation detector is placed over the heart, an image of the heart can be recorded and photographed.

In evaluating the patency of the coronary arteries, the characteristic abnormality varies according to the type of radiocompound used. When thallium is used, all normal myocardial cells take up the substance and appear on the photoscan. Ischemic or infarcted cells do not take up the substance and appear as "cold spots," devoid of nuclear material and surrounded by normal cells. Technetium Sestamibi (isonitrile) presents a similar picture. It is an even better cardiac imaging agent. Higher-quality images can be obtained on the first pass, providing information similar to angiocardiography. Perfusion images, ventricular function, and gated-pool ejection fractions can all be obtained with a single injection. This is often called a *myocardial perfusion scan*. Furthermore, with the use of isonitrile, an ischemic area will be visible several hours after an ischemic event.

Technetium pyrophosphate is a radionuclide that binds with calcium. When ischemia or early infarction has occurred, intracellular calcium leaks out of the cardiac muscle cells. The calcium in the area of injury is very high. The technetium pyrophosphate binds to that calcium and creates an area of increased radionuclide uptake (hot spot). This is often called a *myocardial infarction scan*. If these patients have chest pain and the pyrophosphate scan is positive, muscle injury can be said to have occurred. This type of scan is also especially helpful if the patient has had chest pain 5 to 10 days before seeing a doctor. Because the pyrophosphate scan stays positive for a long time, the delayed diagnosis of a myocardial infarction can be made.

Using the above radionuclides, cardiac nuclear scanning is used to indicate myocardium ischemia or infarction. Cardiac scanning also can be used to assess myocardial ischemia during stress testing (see p. 211). In some cases, no evidence of diminished blood supply to the myocardium is evident during the resting state. When stressed, however, evidence of myocardial ischemia can become quite obvious and is easily detected by nuclear stress testing. In this form of nuclear cardiac scanning, the radionuclide is injected intravenously at the point of maximal cardiac stress. The radionuclide accumulates in the myocardium in direct proportion to the regional myocardial blood flow. The normal myocardium will have much greater radionuclide activity than the ischemic myocardium. When this stress scan is compared to a resting cardiac nuclear scan, exercise-induced ischemia can be seen. This test is not only beneficial in detecting coronary occlusive disease, but is also successful in assessing postoperative patency of a coronary bypass graft.

For an evaluation of myocardial function, technetium pertechnetate or technetium-labeled albumin is used to measure the part of blood ejected from the ventricle during one cardiac cycle (*ejection fraction*). Normally over 65% of the blood is ejected from the ventricle during systole. Values less than this indicate decreased contractility of the heart caused by ischemia, infarction, or cardiomyopathy. Computers can be synchronized with the electrocardiogram (ECG) during scanning. The amount of blood ejected during systole also can be calculated based on the size of the heart at end-systole and end-diastole. This form of determination of ventricular function is called *gated pool imaging* or the *gated pool ejection fraction*. *Multigated acquisition (MUGA) scan* is another name for this test based on the name of the computer machinery originally required for this determination.

This computer-assisted gated (synchronized) cardiac scan can also allow the myocardial wall to be photographed while in motion. This allows visualization of the myocardium during several cardiac cycles, and contractility of the myocardium can be determined. This imaging technique is called nuclear ventriculography and can provide the same information as radiographic ventriculography, which is performed during cardiac catheterization (see p. 203); however, the nuclear scans are noninvasive and much safer. Ischemic areas are seen to be hypokinetic on scan. Infarcted area are akinetic on scan. This is also evident after stress during a cardiac stress test.

Single-photon emission (the radionuclear materials discussed in previous paragraphs emit single photons) computed tomography (SPECT) has been used to visualize the heart from many different angles. These images are then reconstructed using techniques similar to CT scanning, and three-dimensional images of the physiologic cardiac processes are obtained. Areas of myocardial ischemia can be seen with far greater resolution and more accurately quantified.

Contraindications

- Patients who are uncooperative
- Patients who are pregnant, because of fetal exposure to radio-nuclide material

Interfering factors

- Myocardial trauma
- Recent nuclear scans (e.g., thyroid or bone scan)
- Drugs such as long-acting nitrates

Procedure and patient care

Before
- Explain the procedure to the patient.
- Instruct the patient that a short fasting period may be required.

During
- Take the patient to the nuclear medicine department.
- Note the following procedural steps:
  1. An IV injection of radionuclide material is performed.
  2. Depending on the radionuclide used, scanning is performed 15 minutes to 4 hours later.
  3. A gamma ray detector is placed over the precordium.
  4. The patient is placed in a supine position, then in the lateral position, and then in both the right and left oblique positions.
  5. The gamma-ray scanner records the image of the heart, and a photograph is immediately developed.
  6. For a *thallium exercise stress test*, radioactive thallium is injected during exercise when the patient reaches a maximum heart rate. The patient then lies on a table, and scanning is done. A repeat scan may be done 3 to 4 hours later.
  7. If an *isonitrile stress test* is needed, the patient is injected and scanned 30 to 60 minutes later for the resting phase. Four hours later, cardiac stress testing is done. After a second injection, scanning is repeated. Milk and a muffin are usually given after each isonitrile injection to facilitate clearing of the radionuclide from the hepatobiliary system.
- Tell the patient that the only discomfort associated with this test is the venipuncture required for injection of the radioisotope.
- Note that myocardial scans are usually performed in less than 30 minutes by a nuclear medicine technician.

After
- Because only tracer doses of radioisotopes are used, note that no precautions need to be taken against radioactive exposure to personnel or family.
- Encourage the patient to drink fluids to aid in the excretion of the radioactive substance.
- Apply pressure or a pressure dressing to the venipuncture site.

- If stress testing was performed, evaluate the patient's vital signs at frequent intervals (as indicated).

Abnormal findings

Coronary artery occlusive disease

Decreased myocardial function associated with ischemia, myocarditis, cardiomyopathy, or congestive heart failure

notes

carotid duplex scanning

Type of test Ultrasound

Normal findings Carotid artery free of plaques and stenosis

Test explanation and related physiology

Carotid duplex scanning is a noninvasive, ultrasound test used on the extracranial carotid artery to detect occlusive disease directly. It is recommended for patients with headaches and with neurologic symptom such as transient ischemic attacks (TIA), hemiparesis, paresthesia, acute speech or visual deficits.

The duplex scan can measure the amplitude and the wave form of the carotid arterial pulse. Furthermore, a two-dimensional image of the carotid artery can be produced. As a result, one can directly visualize possibly stenotic or occluded arteries and the arterial flow disruption.

Procedure and patient care

Before
- Explain the procedure to the patient.
- Tell the patient that no special preparation is required.
- Assure the patient that the study is painless.

During
- Place the patient in the supine position with the head supported to prevent lateral motion.
- Note the following procedural steps:
    1. A water-soluble gel is used to couple the sound from the transducer to the skin surface.
    2. Images of the carotid artery and pulse waveform are obtained.
- Note that this test is performed by an ultrasound technologist in the ultrasound or radiology department in approximately 15 to 30 minutes.
- Tell the patient that no discomfort is associated with this test.

After
- Remove the water-soluble gel from the patient.

Abnormal findings

Carotid artery occlusive disease

ceruloplasmin (Cp)

Type of test Blood

Normal findings
Adults: 23-43 mg/dl
Neonates: 2-13 mg/dl

Test explanation and related physiology
Ceruloplasmin is an alpha$_2$-globulin that binds copper for transport within the bloodstream after it is absorbed from the gastrointestinal tract. Ceruloplasmin is decreased in most instances of Wilson's disease, which is an inherited disorder. Patients who are homozygous for this disease make very little ceruloplasmin. High unbound copper blood levels result and are toxic to tissues. The copper is deposited in the eye, brain, liver, and kidney. Wilson's disease is fatal unless early treatment is instituted. If this disease is identified before significant copper deposits affect major organs, the ravages of the disease can be avoided. Cp levels are obtained in children at high risk for the disease. Teenagers and young adults with hepatitis, cirrhosis, or recurrent neuromuscular incoordination (signs compatible with Wilson's disease) should also have this test. Early detection is important, because therapy is effective in most cases.

Cp is also an "acute-phase reactant" that becomes elevated during stress, infection, and pregnancy. However, it rises more slowly than other acute-phase reactants such as C-reactive protein and erythrocyte sedimentation rate.

Interfering factors
- Values are increased during pregnancy.
- Drugs that may cause *increased* levels include estrogen, birth control pills, tamoxifen, methadone, and phenytoin.

Procedure and patient care
Before
- Explain the procedure to the patient.
- Tell the patient that no fasting is required.

During
- Collect venous blood in a red-top tube.
- Keep the specimen on ice.

After

- Apply pressure or a pressure dressing to the venipuncture site.
- Medical follow-up and genetic counseling are indicated when Wilson's disease is confirmed.

Abnormal findings

▲ **Increased levels**

Pregnancy
Thyrotoxicosis
Cancer
Acute inflammatory reactions (e.g., infection, rheumatoid arthritis)
Biliary cirrhosis
Copper intoxication

▼ **Decreased levels**

Wilson's disease
Normal infants (<6 months)
Nephrotic syndrome
Sprue
Kwashiorkor
Menkes' (kinky-hair) syndrome
Hyperalimentation

notes

chest x-ray (CXR, Chest radiography)

Type of test X-ray

Normal findings Normal lungs and surrounding structures

Test explanation and related physiology

The chest x-ray film is important in the complete evaluation of the pulmonary and cardiac systems. This procedure is often part of the general admission screening workup in adult patients. Much information can be provided by the chest x-ray film. One can identify or follow (by repeated chest x-ray films) the following:

1. Tumors of the lung (primary and metastatic), heart (myxoma), chest wall (soft-tissue sarcomas), and bony thorax (osteogenic sarcoma)
2. Inflammation of the lung (pneumonia), pleura (pleuritis), and pericardium (pericarditis)
3. Fluid accumulation in the pleura (pleural effusion), pericardium (pericardial effusion), and lung (pulmonary edema)
4. Air accumulation in the lung (chronic obstructive pulmonary disease) and pleura (pneumothorax)
5. Fractures of the bones of the thorax or vertebrae
6. Diaphragmatic hernia
7. Heart size, which may vary depending on cardiac function
8. Calcification, which may indicate large-vessel deterioration or old lung granulomas
9. Location of centrally placed intravenous access devices

Most chest x-ray films are taken with the patient standing. The sitting or supine position also can be used, but x-ray films taken with the patient in the supine position will not demonstrate fluid levels. A *posteroanterior* (PA) view, with the x-rays passing through the back of the body (posterior) to the front of the body (anterior), is taken first. Then a *lateral* view, with the x-rays passing through the patient's side, is taken.

Oblique views may be taken with the patient turned at different angles as the x-rays pass through the body. *Lordotic* views provide visualization of the apices (rounded upper portions) of the lungs and are usually used for detection of tuberculosis. *Decubitus* films are taken with the patient in the recumbent lateral position to localize fluid, which becomes dependent within the pleural space (pleural effusion).

Chest x-ray studies are best performed in the radiology department. Studies using a portable x-ray machine may be done at the bedside and are often performed on critically ill patients who cannot leave the nursing unit.

Contraindications

- Patients who are pregnant

Interfering factors

- Conditions (e.g., severe pain) that prevent the patient from taking and holding a deep breath
- Scarring from previous lung surgery, which makes interpretation difficult
- Obesity, which requires more x-ray to penetrate the body to provide a readable picture

Procedure and patient care

Before

- Explain the procedure to the patient.
- Tell the patient that no fasting is required.
- Instruct the patient to remove clothing to the waist and to put on an x-ray gown.
- Inform the patient to remove all metal objects (e.g., necklaces, pins) so that they do not block visualization of part of the chest.
- Tell the patient that he or she will be asked to take a deep breath and hold it while the x-ray films are taken.
- Instruct men to ensure that their testicles are covered and women to have their ovaries covered, with a lead shield to prevent radiation-induced abnormalities.

During

- After the patient is correctly positioned, tell him or her to take a deep breath and hold it until the x-ray films are taken.
- Note that x-ray films are taken by a radiologic technologist in several minutes.
- Inform the patient that no discomfort is associated with chest radiography.

After

- Note that no special care is required following the procedure.

Abnormal findings

Lung

Lung tumor (primary or
  metastatic)
Pneumonia
Pulmonary edema
Pleural effusion
Chronic obstructive pulmo-
  nary disease
Pneumothorax
Atelectasis
Tuberculosis
Lung abscess
Congenital lung diseases
  (hypoplasia)
Pleuritis
Foreign bodies (chest, bron-
  chus, or esophagus)

Heart

Cardiac enlargement
Pericarditis
Pericardial effusion

Chest wall

Soft tissue sarcoma
Osteogenic sarcoma
Fracture (ribs or thoracic
  spine)
Thoracic spine scoliosis
Metastatic tumor to the bony
  thorax

Diaphragm

Diaphragmatic/hiatal hernia

Mediastinum

Aortic calcinosis
Enlarged lymph nodes
Dilated aorta
Thymoma
Lymphoma
Substernal thyroid
Widened mediastinum

notes

Chlamydia

Type of test Microscopic examination or blood test

C

Normal findings

Negative culture

Antibodies: Immunoglobulin test ≤1:640

Test explanation and related physiology

There are many *Chlamydia* species that cause various diseases within the human body. *Chlamydia psittaci* causes respiratory tract infections and occurs with close contact with infected birds. *C. pneumoniae*, another species, causes pneumonia. *C. trachomatis* infection is probably the most frequently occurring sexually transmitted disease in developed countries. Infections of the genitalia are most common, followed by those of the conjunctiva, pharynx, urethra, and rectum. Lymphogranuloma venereum was the first form of venereal disease recognized as a *C. trachomatis* infection. The second serotype of *C. trachomatis* causes the eye disease trachoma, which is the most common form of preventable blindness. A third serotype produces genital and urethral infections different from lymphogranuloma. This later type is transmitted by direct contact of the infant with the mother's cervix during vaginal delivery or by direct contact during sexual activity. *Chlamydia* may be associated with cases of pelvic inflammatory disease, particularly in adolescents. Most women colonized with *Chlamydia* are asymptomatic.

Chlamydia infection is thought to be the most prevalent sexually transmitted disease in the United States. Strategies to control its spread include screening all at-risk groups, particularly sexually active adolescents and those with other sexually transmitted disease, for disease.

The *Chlamydia* organism can be detected in many different ways. It seems to be most accurately demonstrated by tissue culture. Although these cultures require a special cell culture line, which takes several days, they are used as the gold standard against which other methods of detection of *Chlamydia* are measured. It is now possible to detect the antigen by direct fluorescent antibody slide staining and enzyme-linked immunosorbent assay (ELISA) technique. The sensitivity and specificity of these newer techniques are lower than culture techniques, however.

Interfering factors

- Women presently having their routine menses.
- Patients undergoing antibiotic therapy.

Procedure and patient care

Before

- Explain the procedure to the patient.
- Note that many different methods are used to perform chlamydial tests.

During

- Collect venous blood in a red-top tube.
- Acute and convalescent serum should be drawn 2 to 3 weeks apart.
- A conjunctival smear is obtained by swabbing the eye lesion with a cotton-tipped applicator or scraping with a sterile ophthalmic spatula and smearing on a clean glass slide.
- Sputum cultures (see p. 784) are used to check for *C. psittaci* respiratory infections.
- Note the following procedural steps for *cervical culture*:
  1. The female patient should refrain from douching and bathing in a tub before the cervical culture is performed.
  2. The patient is placed in the lithotomy position.
  3. A nonlubricated vaginal speculum is inserted to expose the cervix.
  4. The mucus is removed from the squamocolumnar junction of the cervix.
  5. A sterile, cotton-tipped swab is inserted into the endocervical canal and moved from side to side for 30 seconds to obtain the culture.
- Note the following procedural steps for *urethral culture*:
  1. The urethral specimen should be obtained from the man before voiding.
  2. A culture is taken by inserting a sterile thin swab gently into the urethra for about 3 to 4 cm.
- Note that these tests are performed by a physician or nurse in several minutes.
- Tell the patient that minimal discomfort is associated with these procedures.

After
- Treat patients who have positive smears with antibiotics.
- Tell affected patients to have their sexual partners examined.

Abnormal findings

Chlamydia infections

notes

chloride, blood (Cl)

Type of test Blood

Normal findings

Adult/elderly: 90-110 mEq/L or 98-106 mmol/L (SI units)
Child: 90-110 mEq/L
Newborn: 96-106 mEq/L
Premature infant: 95-110 mEq/L

Possible critical values <80 or >115 mEq/L

Test explanation and related physiology

This test is performed as a part of *multiphasic testing* in what is usually called "electrolytes." By itself, not much information is obtained. However, with interpretation of the other electrolytes, chloride can give an indication of acid-base balance and hydrational status.

Chloride is the major extracellular anion. Its main purpose is to maintain electrical neutrality, mostly as a salt with sodium. It follows sodium (cation) losses and accompanies sodium excesses to maintain electrical neutrality. For example, when aldosterone encourages sodium resorption, chloride follows to maintain electrical neutrality. Because water moves with sodium and chloride, chloride also impacts on water balance. Finally, chloride also serves as a buffer to assist in acid-base balance. As carbon dioxide (and H^+ cation) increases, bicarbonate must move from the intracellular space to the extracellular space. To maintain electrical neutrality, chloride will shift back into the cell.

Hypochloremia and hyperchloremia rarely occur alone and are usually part of parallel shifts in sodium or bicarbonate levels (see p. 105). Signs and symptoms of hypochloremia include hyperexcitability of the nervous system and muscles, shallow breathing, hypotension, and tetany. Signs and symptoms of hyperchloremia include lethargy, weakness, and deep breathing.

Interfering factors

- Excessive infusions of saline can result in *increased* chloride levels.
- �rx Drugs that may cause *increased* serum chloride levels include acetazolamide, ammonium chloride, androgens, chlorothi-

azide, cortisone preparations, estrogens, guanethidine, hydro-chlorothiazide, methyldopa, and nonsteroidal antiinflammatory drugs.
* Drugs that may cause *decreased* levels include aldosterone, bicarbonates, corticosteroids, cortisone, hydrocortisone, loop diuretics, thiazide diuretics, and triamterene.

Procedure and patient care

Before
- Explain the procedure to the patient.
- Tell the patient that no fasting is required.

During
- Collect 5 to 10 ml of venous blood in a red- or green-top tube.

After
- Apply pressure or a pressure dressing to the venipuncture site.

Abnormal findings

▲ **Increased levels (hyperchloremia)**

Dehydration
Renal tubular acidosis
Excessive infusion of normal saline
Cushing's syndrome
Eclampsia
Multiple myeloma
Kidney dysfunction
Metabolic acidosis
Hyperventilation
Anemia
Respiratory alkalosis
Hyperparathyroidism

▼ **Decreased levels (hypochloremia)**

Overhydration
Congestive heart failure
Syndrome of inappropriate secretion of antidiuretic hormone
Vomiting
Chronic gastric suction
Chronic respiratory acidosis
Salt-losing nephritis
Addison's disease
Burns
Metabolic alkalosis
Diuretic therapy
Hypokalemia
Aldosteronism
Respiratory acidosis

cholesterol

Type of test Blood

Normal findings Vary with age and testing center

Adult/elderly: <200 mg/dl or <5.20 mmol/L (SI units)
Child: 120-200 mg/dl
Infant: 70-175 mg/dl
Newborn: 53-135 mg/dl

Test explanation and related physiology

Cholesterol is the main lipid associated with arteriosclerotic vascular disease. However, cholesterol is required for the production of steroids, sex hormones, bile acids, and cellular membranes. Most of the cholesterol we eat comes from foods of animal origin. The liver metabolizes the cholesterol to its free form, and cholesterol is transported in the bloodstream by lipoproteins. Nearly 75% of the cholesterol is bound to low-density lipoproteins (LDLs) (see p. 528), and 25% is bound to high-density lipoproteins (HDLs) (see p. 528). Therefore cholesterol is the main component of LDLs and only a minimal component of HDLs and very low-density lipoproteins. It is the LDL that is most directly associated with increased risk of coronary heart disease (CHD).

The purpose of cholesterol testing is to identify patients at risk for arteriosclerotic heart disease. Cholesterol testing is usually done as a part of *lipid profile* testing, which also evaluates lipoproteins (see p. 528) and triglycerides (see p. 845), because by itself cholesterol is not a totally accurate predictor of heart disease. There is considerable overlap in what are considered "normal" and "high-risk" levels. "Normal" levels have been derived from a group of patients who have no obvious evidence of CHD. However, these findings may not be accurate as these patients may have preclinical CHD and may not truly reflect a "no risk" population.

Because of these significant variabilities, elevated results should be corroborated by repeating the study. The two results should be averaged to obtain an accurate cholesterol for risk assessment.

Because the liver is required to make cholesterol, low serum cholesterol levels are indicative of severe liver diseases. Further,

C

TABLE 6 Total cholesterol as an indicator of risk of CHD (mg/100 ml [SI units: mmol/L])*

Age	Low risk	Moderate risk	High risk
2-19	<170 (4.4)	171-185	>185 (4.8)
20-29	<200 (5.5)	201-220	>220 (5.7)
30-39	<220 (5.7)	221-240	>240 (6.2)
>40	<240 (6.2)	241-260	>260 (6.8)

*When cholesterol testing is combined with lipoproteins, risk of CHD can be more accurately calculated.
From Pagana KD, Pagana TJ: *Mosby's manual of diagnostic and laboratory tests,* St Louis, 1998, Mosby.

TABLE 7 Cholesterol to HDL ratio as an indicator of risk of CHD

Risk	Ratio	
	Male	Female
½ Average	3.4	3.3
Average	5.0	4.4
2× Average	10.0	7.0
3× Average	24.0	11.0

From Pagana KD, Pagana TJ: *Mosby's manual of diagnostic and laboratory tests,* St Louis, 1998, Mosby.

because our main source of cholesterol is our diet, malnutrition is also associated with low cholesterol levels. Certain illnesses can affect cholesterol levels. For example, patients with an acute myocardial infarction may have as much as a 50% reduction in cholesterol level for as many as 6 to 8 weeks.

In 1984 the National Institutes of Health developed a consensus in regard to total cholesterol levels and risk of CHD (Table 6). The cholesterol-to-HDL ratio has been used to assess the risk of CHD (Table 7). Familial hyperlipidemias and hyperlipoproteinemias are often associated with high cholesterol.

Interfering factors

- Pregnancy is usually associated with elevated cholesterol levels.

- Oophorectomy increases levels.
- Recumbent position is associated with decreased levels.
- Drugs that may cause *increased* levels include adrenocortico-tropic hormone, anabolic steroids, beta-adrenergic blocking agents, corticosteroids, epinephrine, oral contraceptives, phenytoin (Dilantin), sulfonamides, thiazide diuretics, cyclosporine, and vitamin D.
- Drugs that may cause *decreased* levels include allopurinol, androgens, bile salt-binding agents, captopril, chlorprop-amide, clofibrate, colchicine, colestipol, erythromycin, isoniazid, liothyronine (Cytomel), lovastatin (Mevacor), monoamine oxidase inhibitors, neomycin (oral), niacin, and nitrates.

Procedure and patient care

Before

- Instruct the patient to fast 12 to 14 hours after eating a low-fat diet before testing. Only water is permitted.
- Indicate to the patient that dietary intake at least 2 weeks before testing will affect results.
- Tell the patient that no alcohol should be taken 24 hours before the test.

During

- Collect 5 to 10 ml of blood in a red-top tube.
- Indicate on the laboratory slip any drugs that may affect cholesterol levels.
- Finger stick method is also often used in mass screening.

After

- Apply pressure to the venipuncture site.
- Instruct patients with high levels regarding a low-cholesterol diet, exercise, and appropriate body weight.

Abnormal findings

▲ **Increased levels**

Hypercholesterolemia

Hyperlipidemia

Hypothyroidism

Uncontrolled diabetes
mellitus

Nephrotic syndrome

Pregnancy

High-cholesterol diet

Xanthomatosis

Hypertension

Myocardial infarction

Atherosclerosis

Biliary cirrhosis

Stress

Nephrosis

▼ **Decreased levels**

Malabsorption

Malnutrition

Hyperthyroidism

Cholesterol-lowering
medication

Pernicious anemia

Hemolytic anemia

Sepsis

Stress

Liver disease

Acute myocardial in-
farction

notes

cholinesterase (CHS, Pseudocholinesterase, Cholinesterase RBC, Red cell cholinesterase, Acetylcholinesterase)

Type of test Blood

Normal findings
0.5-1.5 mg/dl or 5-15 mg/L (SI units)
7-19 U/ml or 7-19 kU/L (SI units)
Values vary with laboratory test methods.

Test explanation and related physiology

This test is done to identify patients with pseudocholinesterase deficiency before anesthesia or to identify patients who may have been exposed to phosphate poisoning. Cholinesterases hydrolyze acetylcholine and also other choline esters and thereby regulate nerve impulse transmission at the nerve synapse and neuromuscular junction. There are two types of cholinesterases: acetylcholinesterase, also known as "true cholinesterase," and pseudocholinesterase. True cholinesterase exists primarily in the red blood cell and nerve tissue. It is not in the serum. Pseudocholinesterase, on the other hand, exists in the serum. Deficiencies in either of these enzymes can be acquired or congenital.

Because succinylcholine (a muscle relaxant commonly used during anesthesia induction) is inactivated by pseudocholinesterase, people with an inherited pseudocholinesterase enzyme deficiency exhibit increased prolonged effects of succinylcholine. Prolonged muscle paralysis and apnea occur after anesthesia. This situation can be avoided by measuring serum cholinesterase (pseudocholinesterase) directly on all patients with a family history of prolonged apnea after surgery.

A common form of acquired cholinesterase deficiency, either true or pseudocholinesterase, is caused by overexposure to pesticides or organophosphates. Persons with jobs associated with chronic exposure to these chemicals are often monitored by the frequent testing of cholinesterase levels. Other potential causes include chronic liver diseases, malnutrition, and hypoalbuminemia.

Interfering factors

- Pregnancy decreases test values.
- Drugs that may cause *decreased* values include atropine, caffeine, codeine, estrogens, morphine sulfate, neostigmine,

oral contraceptives, phenothiazines, theophylline, quinidine, and vitamin K.

Procedure and patient care

Before

- Explain the procedure to the patient.
- Tell the patient that no fasting is required.
- If the test is done to identify the presurgical patient who may be at risk for cholinesterase deficiency, be sure the test is done several days before the planned surgery.
- It may be recommended to withhold medications that could alter test results for 12 to 24 hours before the test.

During

- Collect a venous blood sample in a red-top tube.
- Include a listing of all medications taken by the person with the laboratory requisition slip.

After

- Apply pressure or a pressure dressing to the venipuncture site.

Abnormal findings

▲ **Increased Levels**
Reticulocytosis
Hyperlipidemia
Nephrosis
Diabetes

▼ **Decreased levels**
Poisoning from organic phosphate insecticides
Hepatocellular disease
Persons with congenital enzyme deficiency
Malnutrition

notes

chorionic villus sampling (CVS, Chorionic villus biopsy [CVB])

Type of test Cell analysis

Normal findings No genetic or biochemical disorders

Test explanation and related physiology

CVS is performed on women whose unborn child may be at risk for a life-threatening or significant life-altering genetic defects. This would include women who:

- Are over the age of 35 to 40 years at the time of pregnancy
- Have had frequent spontaneous abortions
- Have had previous pregnancies with fetuses or infants with chromosomal or genetic defects (e.g., Down syndrome)
- Have a genetic defect in themselves (e.g., hemoglobinopathies)

The CVS test can be performed between 8 and 12 weeks of gestation for the early detection of genetic and biochemical disorders. Because CVS detects congenital defects early, first-trimester therapeutic abortions can be performed if indicated and desired.

For this study, a sample of chorionic villi from the chorion frondosum, which is the trophoblastic origin of the placenta, is obtained for analysis. These villi are present from 8 to 12 weeks on and reflect fetal chromosome, enzyme, and deoxyribonucleic acid content, thus permitting a much earlier diagnosis of prenatal problems than amniocentesis (see p. 43), which cannot be done before 14 to 16 weeks. Further, the cells derived by chorionic villus sampling are more easily grown in tissue culture for karyotyping (determination of chromosomal/genetic abnormalities). The cells obtained at amniocentesis take a longer time to grow in culture, further adding to the delay in obtaining answers. Although amniocentesis is a safer procedure, the information obtained is available much later in the pregnancy. At this late point, therapeutic abortion for severe genetic defects is more difficult.

This procedure requires significant experience to be performed safely. If the physician does not feel competent to safely perform the procedure, amniocentesis is safer and should be performed a few weeks later.

Potential complications

- Accidental abortion
- Infection
- Bleeding
- Fetal limb deformities

Procedure and patient care

Before

- Explain the procedure to the patient.
- Be certain that the physician has obtained a signed consent for the procedure.
- Tell the patient that no food or fluid restrictions are necessary.
- Encourage the patient to drink at least 1-2 glasses of fluid before testing.
- Instruct the patient not to urinate for several hours before testing. A full bladder is an excellent reference point for pelvic ultrasound.
- Assess the vital signs of the mother and the fetal heart rate of the fetus before testing. These are baseline studies that should be repeated during and on completion of the test.

During

- Note the following procedural steps:
  1. The patient is placed in the lithotomy position.
  2. A cannula is inserted into the cervix and uterine cavity (Figure 10).
  3. Under ultrasound guidance the cannula is rotated to the site of the developing placenta.
  4. A syringe is attached, and suction is applied to obtain several samples of villi.
  5. As many as three or more samples may be obtained to get sufficient tissue for accurate sampling.
  6. If ultrasound indicates that the trophoblastic tissue is remote from the cervix, a transabdominal approach similar to that described for amniocentesis (p. 43) may be used.
- Note that this procedure is performed by an obstetrician in approximately 30 minutes.
- Inform the patient that discomfort associated with this test is similar to that of a Pap smear.

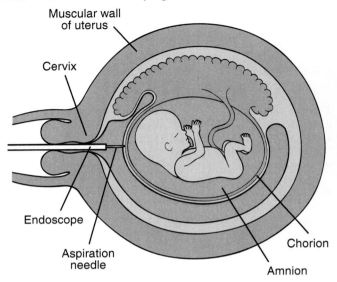

Figure 10 Chorionic villus sampling. Diagram of an 8-week pregnancy showing endoscopic aspiration of extraplacental villi.

After

- Note that some Rh-negative patients may receive RhoGAM. RhoGAM is given because of the risk of Rh incompatibility from the fetal blood, which could threaten the fetus.
- Monitor the vital signs and check the patient for signs of bleeding.
- Schedule the patient for an ultrasound in 2 to 4 days to affirm the continued viability of the fetus.
- Assess the vaginal area for discharge and drainage; note the color and amount.
- Assess and educate the patient for signs of spontaneous abortion (e.g., cramps, bleeding).
- Inform the patient how she can obtain the results from her physician. Make sure she understands that the results are usually not available for several weeks. (Results may be available much sooner at major medical centers that perform this test.)

- Inform the patient about genetic counseling services if needed.

🏠 Home care responsibilities

- Instruct the patient to immediately report signs of spontaneous abortion (e.g., cramps and bleeding).
- Educate the mother to identify and report signs of endometrial infection (vaginal discharge, fever, crampy abdominal pain).

Abnormal findings

Genetic and biochemical disorders

notes

chromosome karyotype (Blood chromosome analysis, Chromosome studies, Cytogenetics, Karyotype)

Type of test Blood

Normal findings

Female: 44 autosomes + 2 X chromosomes; karyotype: 46,XX
Male: 44 autosomes + 1 X, 1 Y chromosome; karyotype: 46,XY

Test explanation and related physiology

This test is used to study an individual's chromosome makeup to determine chromosomal defects associated with disease or the risk of developing disease. The term *karyotyping* refers to the arrangement and pairing of cell chromosomes in order from the largest to the smallest to analyze their number and structure. Variations in either can produce numerous developmental abnormalities and diseases. A normal karyotype of chromosomes consists of a pattern of 22 pairs of autosomal chromosomes and a pair of sex chromosomes: XY for the male and XX for the female. Chromosomal karyotype abnormalities can be congenital or acquired. These karyotype abnormalities can occur because of duplication, deletion, translocation, reciprocation, or genetic rearrangement.

Chromosome karyotyping is useful in evaluating congenital anomalies, mental retardation, growth retardation, delayed puberty, infertility, hypogonadism, primary amenorrhea, ambiguous genitalia, chronic myelogenous leukemia, neoplasm, recurrent miscarriage, prenatal diagnosis of serious congenital diseases (especially in situations of advanced maternal age), Turner syndrome, Klinefelter syndrome, Down syndrome, and other suspected genetic disorders. The products of conception also can be studied to determine the cause of stillbirth or miscarriage.

Procedure and patient care

Before

- Explain the procedure to the patient.
- Determine how the specimen will be collected. Obtain preparation guidelines from the laboratory if indicated.
- Many patients are fearful of the test results and require considerable emotional support.
- In some states informed consent is required.

During

- Specimens for chromosome analysis can be obtained from numerous sources. Leukocytes from a peripheral venipuncture are the most easily and most often used for this study.
- Bone marrow biopsies and surgical specimens also can sometimes be used as sources for analysis.
- During pregnancy specimens can be collected by amniocentesis (see p. 43) and chorionic villus sampling (see p. 238).
- Fetal tissue or products of conception can be studied as well to determine the reason for the loss of the pregnancy.
- Smears and stains of buccal mucosal cells are less costly but not as accurate as other tissue for karyotyping.

After

- Aftercare depends on how the specimen was collected.
- Inform the patient that test results are generally not available for several months.
- If an abnormality is identified, often the entire family line must be tested. This can be exhaustive and expensive.
- If the test results show an abnormality, encourage the patient to verbalize his or her feelings. Provide emotional support.

Abnormal findings

Congenital anomalies
Mental retardation
Growth retardation
Delayed puberty
Infertility
Hypogonadism
Primary amenorrhea
Ambiguous genitalia

Chronic myelogenous leukemia
Neoplasm
Recurrent miscarriage
Down syndrome
Tay-Sachs disease
Sickle cell anemia
Turner syndrome
Klinefelter syndrome

notes

clostridial toxin assay (*Clostridium difficile*, Antibiotic-associated colitis assay; Pseudomembranous colitis toxic assay)

Type of test Stool

Normal findings Negative (no *Clostridium* toxin identified)

Test explanation and related physiology

Clostridium difficile bacterial infection of the intestine may occur in patients who are immunocompromised or taking broad-spectrum antibiotics (e.g., clindamycin, ampicillin, and cephalosporins). The infection results from depression of the normal flora of the bowel through the administration of antibiotics. This increases the number of *C. difficile* bacteria within the intestines. The overgrowth of *C. difficile* causes diarrhea, which is usually watery and voluminous. Abdominal cramps, fever, and leukocytosis are noted in most patients. Occasionally a patient presents with abdominal bloating and fever without diarrhea. Symptoms usually begin 4 to 10 days after the initiation of antibiotic therapy.

The clostridial bacterium releases a toxin that causes necrosis of the colonic epithelium. The detection of this toxin in the stool is therefore diagnostic of clostridial enterocolitis (pseudomembranous colitis). *C. difficile* can also be diagnosed by obtaining colonic-rectal tissue for this toxin. Finally, stool cultures (p. 788) for *C. difficile* can be performed. The patient must wait longer for stool culture results to be available than for results of the toxin assay.

Procedure and patient care

Before

- Explain the method of stool collection to the patient. Be matter-of-fact to avoid embarrassment to the patient.
- Instruct the patient not to mix urine and toilet paper with the stool specimen.
- Handle the specimen carefully, as though it were capable of causing infection. If the nurse is assisting with the specimen collection, gloves should be worn.

During

- Ask the patient to defecate into a clean container. A rectal swab cannot be used because it collects inadequate amounts of stool.
- Note that a stool specimen also can be collected by proctoscopy.
- Place the specimen in a closed container and transport it to the laboratory to prevent deterioration of the toxin.
- If the specimen cannot be processed immediately, refrigerate it.

After

- Maintain enteric isolation precautions on all patients until appropriate therapy is completed.

Abnormal findings

Antibiotic-related (pseudomembranous) *C. difficile* colitis

notes

clot retraction test (Whole-blood clot retraction test)

Type of test Blood

Normal findings
50% to 100% clot retraction in 1 to 2 hours
Complete retraction within 24 hours

Test explanation and related physiology
The clot retraction test is used to evaluate bleeding disorders. Clot retraction is prolonged in thrombocytopenia (i.e., decreased platelet count), and Glanzmann's thrombasthenia (abnormal platelet function). Blood is collected in a tube free of anticoagulants. The time required to form a clot and for the edges of the clot to retract from the sides of the glass tube is the clot retraction time. The clot should be separate from the clear serum. It should maintain its shape (a mold of the glass tube) after being removed from the tube. If the platelet count is reduced or the function of the platelets is inadequate, the clot may only be weakly formed and may have very little if any retraction from the tube side walls. On removal, the clot is shapeless and dissipates. Clot retraction is rarely used today because of availability of accurate platelet counts and more accurate methods of determining platelet dysfunction.

If fibrinolysins are present, no clot retraction will occur. This test is only reliable if the hematocrit and fibrinogen (factor I) concentrations are within normal limits.

If the hematocrit is high (polycythemia or hemoconcentration), clot retraction is reduced. If fibrinogen is reduced, clot retraction is shortened. Poor whole-blood clot retraction also occurs in patients with thrombasthenia (abnormal platelets) and Waldenström's macroglobulinemia.

Contraindications
- Patients with low platelet counts
- Patients with hypofibrinogenemia
- Patients taking aspirin

Interfering factors
- Uremia
- Drugs that may alter test results include aspirin and nonsteroidal antiinflammatory agents.

Procedure and patient care

Before

- Explain the procedure to the patient.
- Tell the patient that no fasting is required.

During

- Avoid excessive probing during venipuncture if a coagulation disorder is suspected.
- Collect approximately 5 to 7 ml of venous blood in a red-top tube.
- Avoid hemolysis.
- Indicate on the laboratory slip if the patient is taking aspirin or a nonsteroidal antiinflammatory agent.

After

- Transport the specimen to the laboratory within 1 hour of collection.
- Apply pressure or a pressure dressing to the venipuncture site.

Abnormal findings

▲ **Increased clot retraction**

Severe anemia
Hypofibrinogenemia

▼ **Decreased or poor clot retraction**

Thrombocytopenia
    von Willebrand's disease
Thrombasthenia (abnormal platelets)
Waldenström's macroglobulinemia

notes

coagulating factors concentration (Factor assay, Coagulating factors, Blood-clotting factors)

Type of test Blood

Normal findings

Factor	*Normal value (% of "normal")*
II	80-120
V	50-150
VII	65-140
VIII	55-145
IX	60-140
X	45-155
XI	65-135
XII	50-150

Test explanation and related physiology

These tests measure the quantity of each specific factor suspected to be responsible for suspected defects in hemostasis. Testing is available to measure the quantity of the factors listed above. When these factors exist in concentrations below their "minimal hemostatic level," clotting is impaired. These minimal hemostatic levels vary according to the factor involved.

Deficiencies of these factors may be a result of inherited genetic defects, acquired diseases, or drug therapy. Common medical conditions associated with decreased factor concentrations are listed in Table 8. It is important to identify the exact factor or factors involved in the coagulating defect so that appropriate blood component replacement can be administered.

The hemostasis and coagulation system is a homeostatic balance between factors encouraging clotting and those encouraging clot dissolution (see Figure 11). See Table 9 for a list of factor names and routine coagulation test abnormalities associated with factor deficiency.

Fibrinogen (Factor I, p. 414), like many other of the coagulation proteins, is considered an acute reactant protein and is elevated in many severe illnesses. It is also considered a risk factor for coronary heart disease and stroke.

Prothrombin is a vitamin K-dependent vitamin. Its production in the liver requires vitamin K. This vitamin is fat soluble and is dependent on bile for absorption. Bile duct obstruction or mal-

TABLE 8 Conditions thay may result in coagulation factor excess or deficiency

Factor	Increased (excess)	Decreased (deficiency)
I (Fibrinogen)	Acute inflammatory reactions Trauma Coronary heart disease Cigarette smoking	Liver disease (hepatitis or cirrhosis) DIC Fibrinolysis Congenital deficiency
II (Prothrombin)	ND	Vitamin K deficiency Liver disease Congenital deficiency Warfarin ingestion
V (Proaccelerin)	ND	Liver disease DIC Fibrinolysis
VII (Proconvertin [stable factor])	ND	Congenital deficiency Vitamin K deficiency Liver disease Warfarin ingestion
VIII (Antihemophilic factor)	Acute inflammatory reactions Trauma/stress Pregnancy	Hemophilia A Congenital deficiency DIC Autoimmune disease

C

Continued

TABLE 8 Conditions thay may result in coagulation factor excess or deficiency—cont'd

Factor	Increased (excess)	Decreased (deficiency)
von Willebrand factor	ND	von Willebrand's disease Congenital deficiency Autoimmune disease
IX (Christmas factor)	ND	Congenital deficiency Hemophilia B Liver disease Nephrotic syndrome Warfarin ingestion DIC Vitamin K deficiency
X (Stuart factor)	ND	Congenital deficiency Liver disease Warfarin ingestion Vitamin K deficiency
XII (Hageman factor)	ND	Congenital deficiency Vitamin K deficiency Liver disease Warfarin ingestion DIC

ND, there is no common disease state noted to be associated with an excess of this factor; *DIC,* disseminated intravascular coagulation.

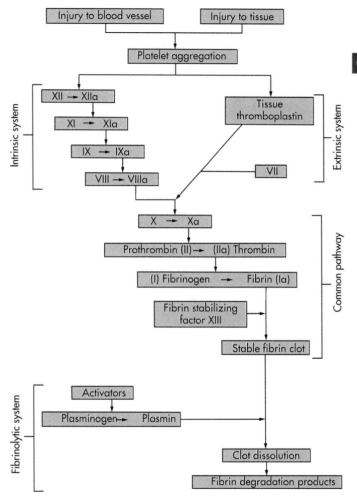

Figure 11 Hemostasis and fibrinolysis. Injury to a blood vessel surface or tissue initiates platelet aggregation. The intrinsic or extrinsic system is activated and then activates the common pathway or fibrin formation. Finally, fibrin is physiologically dissolved by the fibrinolytic system.

TABLE 9 List of minimum concentration of coagulating factors required for fibrin production

Factor	Name	Quantitation minimum hemostatic level (mg/dl)	Abnormal coagulation tests associated with deficiency	Blood components to provide specific factor
I	Fibrinogen	60-100		C, FFP, FWB
II	Prothrombin	10-15	PT	P, WB, FFP FWB
III	Tissue factor or Thromboplastin	QNA	PT	
IV	Calcium	see calcium, p. 191		
V	Proaccelerin	5-10	PT, APTT	FFP, FWB
VII	Stable factor	5-20	PT	P, WB, FFP, FWB
VIII	Antihemophilic factor	30	APTT	C, FFP, VIII CONC
IX	Christmas factor	30	APTT	FFP, FWB
X	Stuart factor	8-10	PT, APTT	P, WB, FFP, FWB
XI	Plasma thromboplastin antecedent	25	APTT	P, WB, FFP, FWB
XII	Hageman factor	yes	APTT, WBC	
XIII	Fibrin stabilizing factor	no		

APTT, activated partial thromboplastin time; *PT*, prothrombin time; *WBC*, whole blood clotting; *C*, cryoprecipitate; *FFP*, fresh frozen plasma; *FWB*, fresh whole blood (less than 24 hours old); *P*, unfrozen banked plasma; *WB*, banked whole blood; *VII CONC*, factor VIII concentrate.

absorption causes a vitamin K deficiency and results in reduced quantity of prothrombin and other vitamin K-dependent factors (VII, IX, X). It usually takes about 3 weeks before body stores of vitamin K are exhausted.

Factor VIII is actually a complex molecule with two components. The first component is related to hemophilia A and is involved in the hemostatic mechanism as described in previous paragraphs. The second component is the von Willebrand factor and is related to von Willebrand disease. This second component is involved in platelet adhesion and aggregation. Patients with factor XII deficiency have been observed to have an increased risk of myocardial infarction and venous thrombosis.

Interfering factors

- Many of these proteins are heat sensitive, and their levels are decreased the longer the specimen is kept at room temperatures.
- Pregnancy or the use of contraceptive medication can increase levels of several of these factors, especially VIII and IX. A mild deficiency can be masked.
- Many of these protein coagulation factors are "acute reactant" proteins. Acute illness, stress, exercise, or inflammation can raise levels.

Procedure and patient care

Before
- Explain the procedure to the patient.
- Tell the patient that no fasting is required.

During
- Collect approximately 7 to 10 ml of venous blood in a blue-top tube.

After
- Apply pressure to the venipuncture site.
- Deliver the blood specimen to the laboratory as soon as possible.

Abnormal findings

Table 8 lists conditions that may result in a coagulation factor excess or deficiency.

colonoscopy

Type of test Endoscopy

Normal findings Normal colon

Test explanation and related physiology

With fiberoptic colonoscopy, the entire colon from anus to cecum can be examined in most patients. As with sigmoidoscopy, benign and malignant neoplasms, polyps, mucosal inflammation, ulceration, and sites of active hemorrhage can be visualized. Diseases such as cancer, polyps, ulcers, and arteriovenous (AV) malformations also can be visualized. Cancers, polyps, and inflammatory bowel diseases can be biopsied through the colonoscope with cable-activated instruments; and sites of active bleeding can be coagulated with the use of laser, electrocoagulation, and injection of sclerosing agents.

This test is recommended for patients who have obvious or occult blood in the stools, lower gastrointestinal bleeding, or a change in bowel habits or are at high risk for colon cancer. The latter group includes patients with a strong personal or family history of colon cancer, polyps, or ulcerative colitis. It is recommended for patients who have abdominal pain and is used as a surveillance tool for patients who have had colorectal cancer, inflammatory bowel disease, or polyposis.

Contraindications

- Patients who are uncooperative
  As in all studies that require technical finesse, patient cooperation is essential to successful completion of the test.
- Patients whose medical condition is not stable
  This test requires sedation, which may induce hypotension in the medically unstable patient.
- Patients who are bleeding profusely from the rectum
  The viewing lens will become covered with blood clots, preventing visualization of the lower intestinal tract.
- Patients with a suspected perforation of the colon
- Patient with toxic megacolon
  These patients may worsen with the test preparation.
- Patients with a recent colon anastomosis (within the last 14 to 21 days)
  The anastomosis may break down with significant insufflation of CO_2.

Potential complications

- Bowel perforation
- Persistent bleeding from a biopsy site
- Oversedation, resulting in respiratory depression

Interfering factors

- Poor bowel preparation
- The stool immediately obstructs the lens and precludes adequate visualization of the colon.
- Active bleeding
- Blood obstructs the lens system and precludes adequate visualization of the colon.

Procedure and patient care

Before

- Explain the procedure to the patient.
- Fully inform the patient about the risks of the procedure and obtain an informed consent.
- Instruct the patient as to the appropriate bowel preparation. One type is the *2-day bowel preparation*, which uses clear liquids for 2 days, along with a strong cathartic such as magnesium citrate and bisacodyl (Dulcolax). On the day of examination, an enema is given. A *1-day preparation* using a glycol (COLyte) bowel preparation has become more widely used. After the patient ingests a gallon of COLyte, enemas are not usually needed. The 1 gallon should be consumed within 4 hours if possible. Lemonade powder may be added to the glycol cathartic.
- Avoid an oral bowel preparation in patients with upper gastrointestinal obstruction, suspected acute diverticulitis, or recent bowel resectional surgery.
- Assure patients that they will be appropriately draped to avoid unnecessary embarrassment.
- Administer appropriate preendoscopy sedation, usually meperidine (Demerol) and diazepam (Valium). Often atropine is ordered to minimize patient secretions.

During

- Note the following procedural steps:
  1. IV access is obtained.
  2. After a rectal examination indicates adequate bowel preparation, the patient is sedated.

3. The patient is placed in the lateral decubitus position, and the colonoscope is placed into the rectum.

4. Under direct visualization, the colonoscope is directed to the cecum. Often a significant amount of manipulation is required to obtain this position.

5. As in all endoscopy, air is insufflated to distend the bowel for better visualization.

6. Complete examination of the large bowel is carried out.

7. Polypectomy, biopsy, and other endoscopic surgery is performed after appropriate visualization.

8. When the laser or coagulator is used, the air is removed, and carbon dioxide is used as an insufflating agent to avoid explosion.

- Note that this test is performed by a physician trained in gastrointestinal endoscopy in approximately 30 to 60 minutes.
- Tell the patient that minimal discomfort is associated with the test.

After

- Explain to patients that air has been insufflated into the bowel. They may experience flatulence or gas pains.
- Examine the abdomen for evidence of colon perforation (abdominal distention and tenderness).
- Assess the patient's vital signs. Watch for a decrease in blood pressure and an increase in pulse as an indication of hemorrhage.
- Inspect the stools for gross blood.
- Notify the physician if the patient develops increased pain or significant gastrointestinal bleeding.
- Allow the patient to eat when fully alert if no evidence of bowel perforation exists.
- Encourage the patient to drink a lot of fluids when intake is allowed. This will make up for the dehydration associated with the bowel preparation.

	🏠 Home care responsibilities

- Observe for increasing abdominal pain, which may indicate bowel perforation.
- Inform the patient that frequent, bloody bowel movements may indicate poor hemostasis if biopsy or polypectomy was performed.
- Observe for abdominal bloating and inability to pass flatus, which may indicate colon obstruction if a neoplasm was identified.
- Assess for weakness and dizziness, which may indicate orthostasis and hypovolemia due to dehydration.
- Evaluate for fever and chills, which may indicate a bowel perforation.

Abnormal findings

Colon cancer
Colon polyps
Inflammatory bowel disease (e.g., ulcerative or Crohn's colitis)
AV malformations
Hemorrhoids
Ischemic or postinflammatory strictures
Diverticulosis

notes

colposcopy

Type of test Endoscopy

Normal findings Normal vagina and cervix

Test explanation and related physiology

Colposcopy provides an in situ macroscopic examination of the vagina and cervix with a colposcope, which is a macroscope with a light source and a magnifying lens. With this procedure, tiny areas of dysplasia, carcinoma in situ, and invasive cancer that would be missed by the naked eye can be visualized; and biopsy specimens can be obtained. The study is performed on patients with abnormal vaginal epithelial patterns, cervical lesions, or suspicious Pap smear results and on those exposed to diethylstilbestrol in utero. It may be a sufficient substitute to cone biopsy (removal and examination of a cone of tissue from the cervix) in evaluating the cause of abnormal cervical cytologic findings.

It is important to realize that colposcopy is useful only in identifying a suspicious lesion. Definitive diagnosis requires biopsy of the tissue. One of the major advantages of this procedure is that of directing the biopsy to the area most likely to be truly representative of the lesion. A biopsy performed without colposcopy may not necessarily be representative of the lesion's true pathologic condition, resulting in a significant risk of missing a serious lesion.

The patient will need to have diagnostic conization if:

1. Colposcopy and endocervical curettage do not explain the problem or match the cytologic findings of the Pap smear within one grade.
2. The entire transformation zone is not seen.
3. The lesion extends up the cervical canal beyond the vision of the colposcope.

The need for up to 90% of cone biopsies is eliminated by an experienced colposcopist. Endocervical curettage may routinely accompany colposcopy to detect unknown lesions in the endocervical canal.

Contraindications

- Patients with heavy menstrual flow

Interfering factor

- Failure to cleanse the cervix of foreign materials (e.g., creams, medications) may impair visualization.

Procedure and patient care

C

Before

- Explain the procedure to the patient.
- Obtain informed consent if required by the institution.

During

- Note the following procedural steps:
  1. The patient is placed in the lithotomy position, and a vaginal speculum is used to expose the vagina and cervix.
  2. After the cervix is sampled for cytologic findings, it is cleansed with a 3% acetic acid solution to remove excess mucus and cellular debris. The acetic acid also accentuates the difference between normal and abnormal epithelial tissues.
  3. The colposcope is focused on the cervix, which is then carefully examined.
  4. Usually the entire lesion can be outlined, and the most atypical areas selected for biopsy specimen removal.
- Note that colposcopy is performed by a physician in approximately 5 to 10 minutes.
- Tell the patient that some women complain of pressure pains from the vaginal speculum and that momentary discomfort may be felt if biopsy specimens are obtained.

After

- Inform the patient that she may have vaginal bleeding if biopsy specimens were taken. Suggest that she wear a sanitary pad.
- Instruct the patient to abstain from intercourse and not to insert anything (except a tampon) into the vagina until healing of a biopsy is confirmed.
- Inform the patient when and how to obtain the results of this study.

Abnormal findings

Dysplasia
Carcinoma in situ
Invasive cancer
Cervical lesions

complement assay

Type of test Blood

Normal findings

Total complement: 75-160 U/ml or 75-160 U/L (SI units)
C3: 55-120 mg/dl or 0.55-1.20 g/L (SI units)
C4: 20-50 mg/dl or 0.20-0.50 g/L (SI units)

Test explanation and related physiology

Measurements of complement are used primarily to diagnose angioedema and to monitor the activity of disease in patients with systemic lupus erythematosus nephritis, membranoproliferative nephritis, or poststreptococcal nephritis.

Serum complement is a group of globulin proteins that act as enzymes. These enzymes facilitate the immunologic and inflammatory response. The total complement, sometimes labeled CH 50, is made up of nine major components: C1 through C9. Besides these major components, there are some subcomponent and "inhibitor" components involved in the system. Once activated, complement acts to increase vascular permeability, allowing antibodies and white blood cells (WBCs) to be delivered to the area of the immune/antigen complex. Complement also acts to increase chemotaxis (attracting WBCs to the area), phagocytosis, and immune adherence of the antibody to antigen. These processes are vitally important in the normal inflammatory response.

Reduced complement levels can be congenital, as in hereditary angioedema. Hereditary angioedema is a congenital lack of a C1 "inhibitor" (often called C1 esterase). The complement system is overly activated, and the complement components are "consumed" or used up. Serum levels fall.

In the chronic presence of antibody/antigen complexes, the complement system is overly activated, and the complement components are "consumed" or used up. Serum levels fall. Diseases associated with these immune complexes include serum sickness, lupus erythematosus, infectious endocarditis, renal transplant rejection, vasculitis, and some forms of glomerulonephritis. As these diseases are successfully treated, complement levels can be expected to return to normal.

Complement components are increased following the onset of

various acute or chronic inflammatory diseases or acute tissue damage. This is very similar to an "acute reaction" protein.

Interfering factors

- C3 is very unstable at room temperatures.

Procedure and patient care

Before

- Explain the procedure to the patient.
- Tell the patient that no fasting or special preparations are required.

During

- Collect 7 to 10 ml of venous blood in a red-top tube.

After

- Apply pressure to the venipuncture site.

Abnormal findings

▲ Increased levels
  Rheumatic fever (acute)
  Myocardial infarction (acute)
  Ulcerative colitis
  Cancer

▼ Decreased levels
  Cirrhosis
  Autoimmune disease (e.g., systemic lupus erythematosus)
  Serum sickness (immune complex disease)
  Glomerulonephritis
  Lupus nephritis
  Renal transplant rejection (acute)
  Protein malnutrition
  Anemia
  Malnutrition
  Hepatitis
  Rheumatoid arthritis
  Sjögren's syndrome
  Severe sepsis

notes

complete blood count and differential count (CBC and diff)

The CBC and differential count are a series of tests of the peripheral blood that provide a tremendous amount of information about the hematologic system and many other organ systems. They are inexpensively, easily, and rapidly performed as a screening test. The CBC and differential count include automated measurement of the following studies, which are discussed separately:

Red blood cell count (RBC, see p. 708)
Hemoglobin (Hgb, see p. 465)
Hematocrit (Hct, see p. 463)
Red blood cell indices (RBC indices, see p. 711)
  Mean corpuscular volume (MCV)
  Mean corpuscular hemoglobin (MCH)
  Mean corpuscular hemoglobin concentration (MCHC)
White blood cell count (WBC) and differential count (see p. 893)
  Neutrophils (polynucleated cells or "polys," segmented cells or "segs," band cells, stab cells)
  Lymphocytes
  Monocytes
  Eosinophils
  Basophils
Blood smear (see p. 151)
Platelet count (see p. 645)

notes

computed tomography of the abdomen
(CAT scan of the abdomen, CT scan of the abdomen)

C

Type of test X-ray with contrast dye

Normal findings No evidence of abnormality

Test explanation and related physiology

The CT scan of the abdomen is a noninvasive, yet very accurate, x-ray procedure used to diagnose pathologic conditions such as tumors, cysts, abscesses, inflammation, perforation, bleeding, obstruction, aneurysms, and calculi of the abdominal and retroperitoneal organs. The CT scan image results from passing x-rays through the abdominal organs at many angles. The variation in density of each tissue allows for a variable penetration of the x-rays. Each density is given a numeric value called a *density coefficient*, which is digitally computed into shades of gray. This is then displayed on a television screen as thousands of dots in various shades of gray. The final display appears as an actual photograph of the anatomic area sectioned by x-rays. The image can be enhanced by repeating the CT scan after IV administration of iodine containing contrast dye. These images can be recorded on Polaroid or x-ray film.

Liver tumors, abscesses, trauma, cysts, and anatomic abnormalities can be seen; and pancreatic tumors, pseudocysts, inflammation, calcification, bleeding, and trauma can be detected. The kidneys and urinary outflow tract are well visualized.

Renal tumors and cysts, ureteral obstruction, calculi, and congenital renal and ureteral abnormalities are easily seen with the use of IV contrast injection. Extravasation of urine secondary to trauma or obstruction can also be demonstrated easily. Adrenal tumors and hyperplasia are best diagnosed with this technique. Some radiology literature indicates that the histology of the tumor can be suggested based on the density coefficients shown on the scan.

Although the bowel can be better visualized by an upper GI series, small bowel follow-through, or barium enema, large tumors and perforations of the bowel can be identified with the CT scan, especially when oral contrast is ingested. The spleen can be well visualized for hematoma, laceration, fracture, tumor infiltration, and splenic vein thrombosis with CT scanning. The retroperitoneal lymph nodes can be evaluated. These are usually present, but all nodes with a diameter greater than 2 cm are considered abnormal. The abdominal aorta and its major branches can be evaluated for aneurysmal dilation and intramural thrombi, and the pelvic structures (including the uterus, ovaries, tubes, prostate, and rectum) and musculature can be evaluated for tumors, abscesses, infection, or hypertrophy. Ascites and hemoperitoneum can easily be demonstrated with the CT scan.

With the development of new and faster scanners, dynamic scanning can be performed during arterial injection of dye to the organ being studied. Dynamic scanning can indicate blood flow and degree of vascularity of an organ or part of an organ in the abdomen. This is called *dynamic CT scanning*. (See CT portography, p. 274, as an example.)

The CT scan can be used to aspirate fluid from the abdomen or one of the abdominal organs. This fluid can be sent for cultures and other studies. The CT scan can also be used to guide biopsy needles into areas of abdominal tumors to obtain tissue of study. Catheters for drainage of intraabdominal abscess can be placed with CT guidance.

The CT scan is an important part of staging and monitoring of many tumors before and after therapy. Tumors of the colon, rectum, liver, breast, lung, prostate, ovary, uterus, kidney, lymph and adrenal commonly recur in the abdomen. Recurrence can be detected early with the CT scan.

Contraindications

- Patients who are allergic to iodinated dye or shellfish
- Patients who are pregnant
- Patients whose vital signs are unstable
- Patients who are very obese, usually over 300 pounds
- Patients who are claustrophobic

Potential complications

- Allergic reaction to iodinated dye
  See p. xviii for appropriate interventions concerning the care for patients with iodine allergy.
- Acute renal failure from dye infusion
  Adequate hydration before the infusion may reduce this likelihood.
- Hypoglycemia or acidosis may occur in patients who are taking Glucophage and receive iodine dye.

Interfering factors

- Presence of metallic objects (e.g., hemostasis clips)
- Retained barium from previous studies
- Large amounts of fecal material or gas in the bowel

Procedure and patient care

Before

- Explain the procedure to the patient. The patient's cooperation is necessary, because he or she must lie still during the procedure.
- Obtain informed consent if required by the institution.
- Assess the patient for allergies to iodinated dye or shellfish.
- Show the patient a picture of the CT machine. Encourage the patient to verbalize his or her concerns because some patients may have claustrophobia. Most patients who are mildly claustrophobic can be scanned after appropriate premedication with antianxiety drugs.
- Keep the patient NPO for at least 4 hours before the test if oral contrast is to be administered; however, this test can be performed on an emergency basis on patients who have recently eaten.
- Note that this procedure is usually performed by a radiologist in less than 30 minutes. If dye is administered, the procedure time may be doubled, because the CT scan is done both with and without contrast dye.
- Tell the patient that the discomforts associated with this study include lying still on a hard table and the peripheral venipuncture. Mild nausea is a common sensation when contrast dye is used. An emesis basin should be readily available. Some patients may experience a salty taste, flushing, and warmth during the dye injection.

During

- Note the following procedure for the abdominal CT scan:
  1. The patient is taken to the radiology department and placed on the CT scan table.
  2. The patient then is placed in an encircling body scanner (gantry). The x-ray tube travels around the gantry and takes pictures of the various levels of the abdomen and pelvis. Any motion causes blurring and streaking of the final picture. Therefore the patient is asked to remain motionless during x-ray exposure. Television monitoring equipment allows for immediate display of the

CT scan image, which is then recorded on an x-ray film. In a separate room the technicians manipulate the CT scan table, affecting the level of the abdomen that is scanned.

3. Through audio communication, the patient is instructed to hold his or her breath during x-ray exposure.

- Remember that oral and IV iodinated x-ray contrast dye provides better results for this test. One can accurately differentiate the gastrointestinal organs from the other abdominal organs with oral contrast. Likewise, the vessels and ureters are contrasted with the surrounding structures with use of IV dye. Sometimes contrast is given rectally to visualize the pelvic organs.

After

- Encourage the patient to drink fluids to avoid dye-induced renal failure and promote dye excretion.
- Inform the patient that diarrhea may occur after ingestion of the oral contrast.
- Evaluate the patient for delayed reaction to dye.

Abnormal findings

Liver
Tumor
Abscess
Bile duct dilation

Pancreas
Tumor
Pseudocyst
Inflammation
Bleeding

Spleen
Hematoma
Fracture
Laceration
Tumor
Venous thrombosis

Gallbladder/biliary system
Gallstones
Tumor
Bile duct dilation

Kidneys
Tumor
Cyst
Ureteral obstruction
Calculi
Congenital abnormalities

Adrenal
Adenoma
Cancer
Pheochromocytoma
Hemorrhage
Myelolipoma hyperplasia

GI tract
Perforation
Tumor
Inflammatory bowel disease
Diverticulitis
Appendicitis

Uterus, tubes, ovaries
Tumor
Abscess
Infection
Hydrosalpinx
Cyst
Fibroid

Prostate
Hypertrophy
Tumor

Retroperitoneum
Tumor
Lymphadenopathy

Other
Abdominal aneurysm
Ascites, hemoperitoneum
Abscess

C

notes

computed tomography of the brain (CT scan of the brain, Computerized axial transverse tomography [CATT])

Type of test X-ray with contrast dye

Normal findings No evidence of pathologic conditions

Test explanation and related physiology

Computed tomography of the brain consists of a computerized analysis of multiple tomographic x-ray films taken of the brain tissue at successive layers, providing a three-dimensional view of the cranial contents. The CT image provides a view of the head as if one were looking down through its top. The variation in density of each tissue allows for variable penetration of the x-ray beam. An attached computer calculates the amount of x-ray penetration of each tissue and displays this as shades of gray. The image is placed on a television screen and photographed. The final result is a series of actual anatomic pictures of coronal sections of the brain.

The CT scan is used in the differential diagnosis of intracranial neoplasms, cerebral infarctions, ventricular displacement or enlargement, cortical atrophy, cerebral aneurysms, intracranial hemorrhage and hematoma, and arteriovenous (AV) malformation. Information about the ventricular system can also be obtained by CT scanning. Multiple sclerosis and other degenerative abnormalities can be identified also.

Visualization of a neoplasm, previous infarction, or any pathologic process that destroys the blood-brain barrier may be enhanced by IV injection of an iodinated contrast dye. CT scans may be repeated frequently to monitor the progress of any disease or to monitor the healing process. In many cases, CT scanning has eliminated the need for more invasive procedures such as cerebral arteriography and pneumoencephalography. In many localities, MRI scanning of the brain has replaced the use of CT scans of the brain.

Contraindications

- Patients who are allergic to iodinated dye or shellfish
- Patients who are claustrophobic
- Patients who are pregnant
- Patients whose vital signs are unstable
- Patients who are very obese, usually over 300 pounds

Potential complications

- Allergic reaction to iodinated dye
  See p. xviii for appropriate interventions concerning the care for patients with iodine allergy.
- Acute renal failure from dye infusion Adequate hydration beforehand may reduce this likelihood.
- Hypoglycemia or acidosis may occur in patients who are taking Glucophage and receive iodine dye.

Procedure and patient care

Before

- Explain the procedure to the patient. The patient's cooperation is necessary, because he or she must lie still during the procedure.
- Obtain informed consent if required by the institution.
- Show the patient a picture of the CT machine and encourage the patient to verbalize his or her concerns, because some patients may have claustrophobia. Most patients who are mildly claustrophobic can be scanned after appropriate premedication with antianxiety drugs.
- Keep the patient NPO for 4 hours before the study, because contrast dye may cause nausea. It is not usually known before the test if enhanced visualization by dye injection will be indicated. If contrast will not be used, food and fluids may be taken.
- Instruct the patient that wigs, hairpins, clips, or partial dental plates cannot be worn during the procedure because they hamper visualization of the brain.
- Assess the patient for allergies to iodinated dye or shellfish. Tell the patient that he or she may hear a "clicking" noise as the scanning machine moves around the head.

During

- Note the following procedure for the brain CT scan. The patient lies in the supine position on an examining table with the head resting on a snug-fitting rubber cap within a water-filled box. The patient's head is enclosed only to the hairline (as in a hair dryer). The face is not covered, and the patient can see out of the machine at all times. Sponges are placed along the side of the head to ensure that the patient's head does not move during the study. The scanner passes an x-ray beam through the brain from one side to the other. The machine then rotates 1 degree, and the procedure is repeated at each degree through a 180-degree arc. The machine is then moved, and the entire procedure is repeated through a total of three to seven planes.

- Remember that an iodinated dye will usually then be used. A peripheral IV line is started, and the iodine dye is administered through it. The entire scanning process is repeated.

- Note that this procedure is performed by a radiologist in less than 1 hour. If dye is administered, the procedure time is doubled, because the CT scan is done with and without the contrast dye.

- Tell the patient that the discomforts associated with this study include lying still on a hard table and peripheral venipuncture. Mild nausea is a common sensation when contrast dye is used. An emesis basin should be readily available. Some patients may experience a salty taste, flushing, and warmth during the dye injection.

After

- Encourage the patient to drink fluids, because dye is excreted by the kidneys and causes diuresis.
- See p. xviii for appropriate interventions concerning the care for patients with iodine allergy.

Abnormal findings

Intracranial neoplasm
Cerebral infarction
Ventricular displacement
Ventricular enlargement
Cortical atrophy
Cerebral aneurysm
Intracranial hemorrhage

Hematoma
AV malformation
Meningioma
Multiple sclerosis
Hydrocephalus
Abscess

notes

computed tomography of the chest (Chest CT scan)

Type of test   X-ray with contrast dye

Normal findings   No evidence of pathologic conditions

Test explanation and related physiology

Computed tomography of the chest is a noninvasive yet very accurate x-ray procedure for diagnosing and evaluating pathologic conditions such as tumors, nodules, hematomas, parenchymal coin lesions, cysts, abscesses, pleural effusion, and enlarged lymph nodes affecting the lungs and mediastinum. Tumors, cysts, and fractures of the chest wall and pleura can also be seen. When an IV contrast material is given, vascular structures can be identified, and a diagnosis of aortic or other vascular abnormality can be made. With oral contrast, the esophagus and upper structures can be evaluated for tumor and other conditions. This procedure provides a cross-sectional view of the chest and is especially useful in detecting small differences in tissue densities, demonstrating lesions that cannot be seen with conventional radiology and tomography. The mediastinal structures can be visualized in a manner that cannot be equaled with conventional x-ray and tomographic scans.

The x-ray image results from using a body scanner (x-ray tube held in a circular gantry) to deliver x-rays through the patient's chest at many different angles. The variation in density of each tissue allows for a variable penetration of the x-rays. Each density is given a numeric value called a *coefficient*, which is digitally computed into shades of gray. This is then displayed on a television screen as thousands of dots in various shades of gray. The final display appears as an actual photograph of the anatomic area sectioned by the x-rays.

Contraindications

- Patients who are pregnant
- Patients who are allergic to iodinated dye or shellfish
- Patients who are claustrophobic
- Patients who are very obese, usually over 300 pounds
- Patients whose vital signs are unstable

Potential complications

- Allergic reaction to iodinated dye. See p. xviii for appropriate interventions concerning the care for patients with iodine allergy.
- Acute renal failure from dye infusion Adequate hydration beforehand may reduce this likelihood.
- Hypoglycemia or acidosis may occur in patients who are taking Glucophage and receive iodine dye.

Procedure and patient care

Before

- Explain the procedure to the patient. The patient's cooperation is necessary, because he or she must lie still during the procedure.
- Obtain informed consent if required by the institution.
- Assess the patient for allergies to iodinated dye or shellfish.
- Show the patient a picture of the CT machine and encourage the patient to verbalize concerns regarding claustrophobia. Most patients who are mildly claustrophobic can tolerate this study after appropriate premedication with antianxiety drugs.
- Keep the patient NPO for 4 hours before the test in the event that contrast dye is administered.

During

- Note the following procedure for the chest CT scan. The patient is taken to the radiology department and asked to remain motionless in a supine position, because any motion will cause blurring and streaking of the final picture. An encircling x-ray camera (body scanner) takes pictures at varying intervals and levels over the chest area. Television equipment allows for immediate display, and the image is recorded on Polaroid or x-ray film. Occasionally IV dye is administered to enhance the chest image, and the x-ray studies are repeated.
- Note that this procedure is performed by a radiologist in 30 to 45 minutes. If dye is administered, the procedure time may be doubled, because the CT scan is done with and without contrast dye.
- Tell the patient that the discomforts associated with this study include lying still on a hard table and peripheral venipuncture. Mild nausea is a common sensation when contrast dye is used. An emesis basin should be readily available. Some

patients may experience a salty taste, flushing, and warmth during the dye injection.

After

- Encourage patients who received dye injection to increase their fluid intake, because the dye is excreted by the kidneys and causes diuresis.
- See p. xviii for appropriate interventions concerning the care for patients with iodine allergy.

Abnormal findings

Pulmonary tumor
Inflammatory nodules
Granuloma
Cyst
Pleural effusion
Enlarged lymph nodes
Aortic aneurysm
Postpneumonic scanning

Pneumonitis
Esophageal tumor
Hiatal hernia
Mediastinal tumor (e.g.,
   lymphoma, thymoma)
Primary or metastatic chest
   wall tumor

notes

computed tomography portogram (CT portogram)

Type of test X-ray with contrast dye

Normal findings No evidence of liver abnormalities

Test explanation and related physiology

A CT scan of the abdomen (see p. 263) is inaccurate in identifying tumors in the liver smaller than 2 cm. A CT portogram can routinely accurately identify abnormalities in the liver as small as 5 mm. The difference between a CT scan of the liver and a CT portogram is in the manner in which the contrast dye is injected. In a routine CT scan dye is injected through a peripheral vein. In a CT portogram, dye is injected through a catheter that is placed in the splenic artery. The dye passes through the spleen and into the splenic vein and subsequently into the portal vein and its tributaries. However, hepatic tumors and cysts do not take up dye. These lesions appear as a filling defect (dark spots) in the liver. Therefore use of this test is limited to identification of suspected smaller neoplasms involved in the liver. It is used in cancer patients who are suspected to have liver metastasis. The number and location of these metastatic lesions are best visualized with a CT portogram.

Contraindications

- Patients with allergies to shellfish or iodinated dye
- Patients who are uncooperative or agitated
- Patients who are pregnant
- Patients with renal disorders, because iodinated contrast is nephrotoxic
- Patients with a bleeding propensity
- Patients with unstable cardiac disorders
- Patients who are dehydrated, because they are especially susceptible to dye-induced renal failure

Potential complications

- Allergic reaction to iodinated dye. See p. xviii for appropriate interventions concerning the care for patients with iodine allergy.
- Hemorrhage from the arterial puncture site used for arterial access

- Arterial embolism from dislodgment of an arteriosclerotic plaque
- Soft tissue infection around the puncture site
- Renal failure, especially in elderly patients who are chronically dehydrated or have a mild degree of renal failure
- Pseudoaneurysm development as a result of failure of the puncture site to seal
- Hypoglycemia or acidosis may occur in patients who are taking Glucophage and receive iodine dye.

Procedure and patient care

Before

- Explain the procedure to the patient. Allay any fears and allow the patient to verbalize concerns.
- Ensure that written and informed consent for this procedure is in the patient's chart.
- Determine if the patient has been taking anticoagulants.
- Keep the patient NPO for at least 2 to 4 hours before testing.
- Mark the site of the patient's peripheral pulses with permanent ink before arterial catheterization. This will permit assessment of the peripheral pulses after the procedure.

During

- Note the following preprocedural steps:
  1. The patient may be sedated before being taken to the angiography room, which is usually within the radiology department.
  2. The patient is placed on the x-ray table in the supine position.
  3. If the femoral artery is to be used, the groin is shaved, prepared, and draped in a sterile manner.
  4. The femoral artery is cannulated, and a wire is threaded up that artery and into or near the opening of the splenic artery.
  5. A catheter is placed over that wire and into the splenic artery.
  6. The patient is transferred to the CT scan unit, which is usually also in the x-ray department.
  7. Through the catheter, iodinated contrast material is injected into the splenic artery.
  8. CT scan images are taken subsequent to the injection.

- Note that the placement of the arterial catheter takes about 30 minutes and is minimally uncomfortable. This is done by a physician.
- Inform the patient that CT scan imaging takes about 15 minutes and is not uncomfortable. This is done by a technician.

After

- After x-rays are completed, the catheter is removed, and a pressure dressing is applied to the puncture site.
- Monitor the patient's vital signs for indications of hemorrhage.
- Assess the peripheral pulse in the extremity used for vascular access and compare it with the preprocedural baseline values.
- Maintain pressure at the puncture site with a 1- to 2-pound sandbag or an IV bag for several hours.
- Keep the patient on bed rest for about 4 to 8 hours following the procedure to allow for complete sealing of the arterial puncture site.
- See p. xviii for appropriate interventions concerning the care for patients with iodine allergy.

Abnormal findings

Hepatic tumor
Hepatic cyst
Hepatic hemangioma

notes

contraceptive localization (Intrauterine device [IUD] localization)

Type of test Ultrasound

Normal findings An IUD contraceptive device is located within the endometrial cavity.

Test explanation and related physiology

When a woman is unable to visualize or palpate the string of an IUD, ultrasound is indicated to determine whether the IUD has perforated the uterus, been expulsed, or been incorporated with an intrauterine pregnancy. IUDs have a particular type-specific morphology and can be easily recognized with ultrasound.

If an IUD can be seen on the abdominal x-ray film but cannot be shown to be in the endometrial cavity by ultrasound, one must strongly suspect that the IUD has perforated the uterus.

Interfering factors

- Patients who have had recent GI contrast studies, because barium creates severe distortion of reflective sound waves.
- Patients with air-filled bowel loops, because gas does not transmit sound waves well.
- Failure to fill the bladder, which is often used as a reference point for pelvic sonography.

Procedure and patient care

Before

- Explain the procedure to the patient.
- Give the patient 3 to 4 glasses (200 to 300 ml) of water or other liquid 1 hour before the examination and instruct her not to void until after the procedure is completed. This will allow the bladder to fill and be used as a reference point.
- Tell the patient that no fasting or sedation is required.

During

- Note the following procedural steps:
  1. The patient is taken to the ultrasound room and placed in the supine position on the examination table.
  2. The ultrasonographer, usually a radiologist, applies a greasy, conductive paste to the abdomen to enhance sound transmission and reception.

3. A transducer is passed vertically and horizontally over the skin.
4. Pictures are taken of the sound waves, and a real image is produced.

- Note that this procedure is performed in approximately 20 minutes.
- Inform the patient that no discomfort is associated with this study other than having a full bladder and the urge to void.

After

- Remove the lubricant from the patient's skin.
- Provide an opportunity for the patient to void.

Abnormal findings

Perforation of the uterus
Expulsion of the IUD
Incorporation of the IUD within an intrauterine pregnancy

notes

Coombs' test, direct (Direct antiglobulin test)

Type of test Blood

Normal findings Negative; no agglutination

Test explanation and related physiology

This test is performed to identify hemolysis (lysis of RBCs) or to investigate hemolytic transfusion reactions. Most of the antibodies to RBCs are directed against the ABO/Rh blood grouping antigens, such as that which occurs in hemolytic anemia of the newborn (erythroblastosis fetalis) or transfusion of incompatible blood. When a transfusion reaction occurs, the Coombs' test can detect the patient's antibodies coating the transfused RBCs. Therefore the Coombs' test is very helpful in evaluating suspected transfusion reactions.

Non-"blood grouping" antigens can develop on the RBC membrane and stimulate formation of antibodies. Drugs such as levodopa or methyldopa cause this. Also, in some diseases antibodies not originally directed against the patient's RBCs can attach to the RBCs and cause hemolysis that is detected by the direct Coombs' test. Examples include antibodies developed in reaction to drugs such as penicillin, autoantibodies formed in various autoimmune diseases, and antibodies developed in some patients with advanced cancer (e.g., lymphoma). Frequently the inciting factor for the production of these autoantibodies against RBCs can be unassociated with any identifiable disease, and the resulting hemolytic anemia is therefore called *idiopathic*.

The direct Coombs' test demonstrates if the patient's RBCs have been attacked by antibodies in the patient's own bloodstream. Coombs' serum is a solution containing antibodies to human globulin (antibodies). Coombs' serum is mixed with the patient's RBCs. If the RBCs had antibodies on them, agglutination of the patient's RBCs will occur. The greater the quantity of antibodies against RBCs, the more clumping occurs. This test is read as *positive*, with clumping on a scale of trace to +4. If the RBCs are not coated with autoantibodies against RBCs (immunoglobulins), agglutination will not occur; this is a *negative* test.

Interfering factors

- Drugs that may cause false-positive results include ampicillin, captopril, cephalosporins, chlorpromazine (Thorazine), chlor-

propamide, hydralazine, indomethacin (Indocin), insulin, isoniazid (INH), levodopa, methyldopa (Aldomet), penicillin,
phenytoin (Dilantin), procainamide, quinidine, quinine,
rifampin, streptomycin, sulfonamides, and tetracyclines.

Procedure and patient care

Before

- Explain the procedure to the patient.
- Tell the patient that no fasting is required.

During

- Collect approximately 5 to 7 ml of venous blood in a red- or
  lavender-top tube.
- Use venous blood from the umbilical cord to detect the presence of antibodies in the newborn.
- List on the laboratory slip all medications that the patient has
  taken in the last few days.

After

- Apply pressure to the venipuncture site.

Abnormal findings

Autoimmune hemolytic anemia
Transfusion reaction
Erythroblastosis fetalis
Lymphoma
Lupus erythematosus
Mycoplasmal infection
Infectious mononucleosis

notes

Coombs' test, indirect (Blood antibody screening)

Type of test Blood

Normal findings Negative; no agglutination

Test explanation and related physiology

The indirect Coombs' test detects circulating antibodies against RBCs. The major purpose of this test is to determine if the patient has minor serum antibodies (other than the major ABO/Rh system) to RBCs that he or she is about to receive by blood transfusion. Therefore this test is the "screening" part of the "type and screen" routinely performed for blood compatibility testing (crossmatching in the blood bank). This test is also used to detect other agglutinins such as cold agglutinins, which are associated *Mycoplasmal* infections.

Unlike the direct Coombs' test that is performed on the patient's RBCs, this test is performed on the patient's serum. In this test a small amount of the recipient's serum is added to donor RBCs containing known antibodies on their surface. This is the first stage. In the second stage of the test, Coombs' serum is added. Coombs' serum is a solution containing antibodies to human globulin (antibodies). If antibodies exist in the patient's serum, agglutination occurs. In blood transfusion screening, visible agglutination indicates that the recipient has antibodies to the donor's RBCs. If the recipient has no antibodies against the donor's RBCs, agglutination will not occur; transfusion should then proceed safely and without any transfusion reaction. Circulating antibodies against RBCs also may occur in an Rh-negative pregnant woman who is carrying an Rh-positive fetus.

Interfering factors

- ✠ Drugs that may cause false-positive results include antiarrhythmics, antituberculins, cephalosporins, chlorpromazine (Thorazine), insulin, levodopa, methyldopa (Aldomet), penicillins, phenytoin (Dilantin), quinidine, sulfonamides, and tetracyclines.

Procedure and patient care

Before

- Explain the procedure to the patient.
- Tell the patient that no fasting is required.

During

- Collect approximately 7 ml of venous blood in a red-top tube.
- List on the laboratory slip all medications that the patient has taken in the last few days.

After

- Apply pressure to the venipuncture site.
- Remember that, if this antibody screening test is positive, antibody identification is then done.

Abnormal findings

Incompatible cross-matched blood
Maternal anti-Rh antibodies
Erythroblastosis fetalis
Acquired hemolytic anemia
Presence of specific cold agglutinin antibody

notes

cortisol, blood and urine (Hydrocortisone, Serum cortisol)

Type of test Blood; urine

Normal findings

Blood
Adult/elderly
    8 AM: 6-28 µg/dl or 170-625 nmol/L (SI units)
    4 PM: 2-12 µg/dl or 80-413 nmol/L (SI units)
Child
    8 AM: 15-25 µg/dl
    4 PM: 5-10 µg/dl
Newborn: 1-24 µg/dl

Urine (24-hour)
Adult/elderly: 10-100 µg/24 hr or 27-276 nmol/day (SI units)
Adolescent: 5-55 µg/24 hr
Child: 2-27 µg/24 hr

Test explanation and related physiology

An elaborate feedback mechanism for cortisol exists to coordinate the function of the hypothalamus, pituitary gland, and adrenal glands. Cortisol is a potent glucocorticoid released from the adrenal cortex. This hormone effects the metabolism of carbohydrates, proteins and fats. It especially has a profound effect on glucose serum levels.

The best method of evaluating adrenal activity is by directly measuring plasma cortisol levels. Normally, cortisol levels rise and fall during the day; this is called the diurnal variation. Cortisol levels are highest around 6 to 8 AM and gradually fall during the day to their lowest point around midnight.

Sometimes the earliest sign of adrenal hyperfunction is only the loss of this diurnal variation, even though the cortisol levels are not yet elevated. For example, individuals with Cushing's syndrome often have top-normal plasma cortisol levels in the morning and do not exhibit a decline as the day proceeds. High levels of cortisol indicate Cushing's syndrome, and low levels of plasma cortisol are suggestive of Addison's disease.

For this test, blood is usually collected at 8 AM and again at around 4 PM. One would expect the 4 PM value to be one third to two thirds of the 8 AM value. Normal values may be transposed in individuals who have worked during the night and slept during the day for long periods of time. Cortisol levels can also be evaluated in a 24-hour urine test.

Interfering factors

- Pregnancy is associated with increased levels.
- Physical and emotional stress can artificially elevate cortisol levels.
- Recent radioisotope scans can affect test results.
- Drugs that may cause *increased* serum levels include estrogen, oral contraceptives, amphetamines, cortisone, and spironolactone (Aldactone).
- Drugs that may cause *decreased* serum levels include androgens, aminoglutethimide, betamethasone, danazol, lithium, levodopa, metyrapone, and phenytoin (Dilantin).

Procedure and patient care

Before

- Explain the procedure to the patient to minimize anxiety.
- Assess the patient for signs of physical stress (e.g., infection, acute illness) or emotional stress and report these to the physician.

During

Blood

- Collect approximately 7 to 10 ml of venous blood in a red- or green-top tube in the morning after the patient has had a good night's sleep.
- Collect another blood sample at about 4 PM.
- Indicate on the laboratory slip the time of the venipuncture and any drugs that may affect test results.

Urine

- Begin the 24-hour collection after the patient urinates. Discard this specimen.
- Collect all urine passed by the patient during the next 24 hours.
- Note that it is not necessary to measure each urine specimen.
- Remind the patient to void before defecating so that the urine is not contaminated by feces.
- Tell the patient not to put toilet paper in the collection container.
- Encourage the patient to drink fluids during the 24 hours unless this is contraindicated for medical purposes.

- Collect the last specimen as close as possible to the end of the 24-hour period. Add this to the collection.
- Place the 24-hour urine collection in a plastic container and keep on ice. Use a preservative.

After

- Apply pressure to the venipuncture site.

Abnormal findings

▲ **Increased levels**
  Cushing's disease
  Adrenal adenoma or carcinoma
  Ectopic ACTH-producing tumors
  Hyperthyroidism
  Obesity
  Stress

▼ **Decreased levels**
  Congential adrenal hyperplasia
  Addison's disease
  Hypopituitarism
  Hypothyroidism
  Liver disease

notes

C-peptide (Connecting peptide insulin, Insulin C-peptide, Proinsulin C-peptide)

Type of test Blood

Normal findings 0.78-1.89 ng/ml or 0.26-0.62 nmol/L (SI units)

Test explanation and related physiology

In the islet of Langerhans of the pancreas, the chains of proinsulin are broken down to form insulin and C-peptide. Because C peptide has a longer half-life than insulin, more C-peptide exists in the peripheral circulation. In general, C-peptide levels correlate with insulin levels in the blood. The capacity of the pancreatic beta cells to secrete insulin can be evaluated by directly measuring either insulin or C-peptide. In most cases, direct measurement of insulin is more accurate. C-peptide levels, however, more accurately reflect islet cell function in the following situations:

1. Patients with diabetes who are treated with exogenous insulin and who have anti-insulin antibodies.

2. Patients who secretly administer insulin to themselves (factitious hypoglycemia). Insulin levels will be elevated. Direct insulin measurement in these patients tends to be high because the insulin measured is the self-administered exogenous insulin. But C-peptide levels in that same specimen will be low because *exogenously* administered insulin suppresses *endogenous* insulin (and C-peptide) production.

3. Diabetic patients who are taking insulin. This is done to see if the diabetic patient is in remission and may not need exogenous insulin.

Further, C-peptide is used in evaluating patients who are suspected of having an insulinoma. In patients with an autonomous secreting insulinoma, C-peptide levels are high. Further, C-peptide can be used to monitor treatment for insulinoma. A rise in C-peptide levels indicates a recurrence or progression of the insulinoma. Likewise, some clinicians use C-peptide testing as an indicator of the adequacy of therapeutic surgical pancreatectomy in patients with pancreatic tumors. C-peptide can also be used to diagnose "insulin resistance" syndrome.

Interfering factors

- Because the majority of C-peptide is degraded in the kidney, renal failure can cause increased levels.
- Drugs that may cause *increased* levels of C-peptide include oral hypoglycemic agents (e.g., sulfonylureas).

Procedure and patient care

Before

- Explain the procedure to the patient.
- Instruct the patient to fast for 8 to 10 hours before the test. Only water is permitted.

During

- Collect venous blood in one red-top tube.

After

- Apply pressure or a pressure dressing to the venipuncture site.

Abnormal findings

▲ **Increased levels**
Insulinoma
Renal failure
Pancreas transplant

▼ **Decreased levels**
Factitious hypoglycemia
Radical pancreatectomy
Diabetes mellitus

notes

C-reactive protein test (CRP)

Type of test Blood

Normal findings <0.8 mg/dl

Test explanation and related physiology

C-reactive protein is a nonspecific, acute-phase reactant used to diagnose bacterial infectious disease and inflammatory disorders such as acute rheumatic fever and rheumatoid arthritis. CRP levels do not consistently rise with viral infections. CRP is an abnormal protein produced primarily by the liver during an acute inflammatory process. A positive test result indicates the presence, but not the cause, of an acute inflammatory reaction. The synthesis of CRP is initiated by antigen-immune complexes, bacteria, fungi, and trauma. CRP is functionally analogous to immunoglobulin G, except that it is not antigen specific. CRP interacts with the complement system.

The CRP test is a more sensitive and rapidly responding indicator than the erythrocyte sedimentation rate (ESR, see p. 369). In an acute inflammatory change, CRP shows an earlier and more intense increase than ESR; with recovery, the disappearance of CRP precedes the return of ESR to normal. The CRP also disappears when the inflammatory process is suppressed by salicylates or steroids.

This test is also useful in evaluating patients with an acute myocardial infarction. The level of CRP correlates with peak levels of the MB isoenzyme of creatine kinase (see p. 290), but CRP peaks occur 1 to 3 days later. Failure of CRP to normalize may indicate ongoing damage to the heart tissue. Levels are not elevated in patients with angina.

This test also may be used after surgery to detect wound infections. CRP levels increase within 4 to 6 hours after surgery and generally begin to decrease after the third postoperative day. Failure of the levels to fall is an indicator of complications such as infection or pulmonary infarction.

Interfering factors

- An intrauterine device may cause positive test results because of tissue stress.
- Drugs that may cause *increased* levels include oral contraceptives.

☛ Drugs that may cause *decreased* levels include nonsteroidal antiinflammatories, salicylates, and steroids.

Procedure and patient care

Before
- Explain the procedure to the patient.
- Tell the patient that fasting usually is not required; however, some laboratories require a 4- to 12-hour fast. Water is permitted.

During
- Collect one red-top tube of venous blood.

After
- Apply pressure or a pressure dressing to the venipuncture site.

Abnormal findings

▲ **Increased levels**

Arthritis
Acute rheumatic fever
Reiter's syndrome
Crohn's disease
Vasculitis syndrome
Lupus erythematosus
Tissue infarction or
 damage
Acute myocardial infarction
Pulmonary infarction
Kidney transplant rejection

Bone marrow transplant
 rejection
Soft tissue trauma
Bacterial infection
Postoperative wound
 infection
Urinary tract infection
Tuberculosis
Malignant disease

notes

creatine phosphokinase (CPK, CP, Creatine kinase [CK])

Type of test Blood

Normal findings

Total CPK

Adult/elderly
  Male: 12-70 U/ml or 55-170 U/L (SI units)
  Female: 10-55 U/ml or 30-135 U/L (SI units)
Values are higher after exercise.
Newborn: 68-580 U/L (SI units)

Isoenzymes

CPK-MM: 100%
CPK-MB: 0%
CPK-BB: 0%

Test explanation and related physiology

CPK is found predominantly in the heart muscle, skeletal muscle, and brain. Serum CPK levels are elevated whenever injury occurs to these muscle or nerve cells. CPK levels can rise within 6 hours after damage. If damage is not persistent, the levels peak at 18 hours after injury and return to normal in 2 to 3 days.

To test specifically for myocardial muscle injury, electrophoresis is performed to detect the three *CPK isoenzymes*: CPK-BB (CPK1), CPK-MB (CPK2), and CPK-MM (CPK3). The CPK-MB isoenzyme part appears to be specific for myocardial cells. CPK-MB levels rise 3 to 6 hours after infarction occurs. If there is no further myocardial damage, the level peaks at 12 to 24 hours and returns to normal 12 to 48 hours after infarction. CPK-MB levels do not usually rise with transient chest pain caused by angina, pulmonary embolism, or congestive heart failure. One can expect to see a rise in CPK-MB in patients with unstable angina, shock, malignant hyperthermia, myopathies, or myocarditis. Very small amounts of CPK-MB also exist in skeletal muscle. Severe injury to skeletal muscle can be significant enough to raise the CPK-MB isoenzyme above normal. To avoid the misdiagnosis of myocardial injury, a *relative index* is calculated to determine whether myocardial injury has occurred. This relative index is a mathematic calculation of the ratio of

CPK-MB to total CPK. A relative index of >2.5 is highly suggestive of myocardial injury.

The CPK-MB isoenzyme level is helpful in both quantifying the degree of myocardial infarction and timing the onset of infarction. With the more frequent use of thrombolytic therapy for myocardial infarction, the CPK-MB isoenzyme is often used to determine appropriateness of thrombolytic therapy. High CPK-MB levels would suggest that significant infarction has already occurred, thereby precluding the benefit of thrombolytic therapy.

Because the CPK-BB isoenzyme is predominantly found in the brain and lung, injury to either of these organs (e.g., cerebrovascular accident, pulmonary infarction) is associated with elevated levels of this isoenzyme.

The CPK-MM isoenzyme normally comprises almost all of the circulatory total CPK enzymes in healthy people. When the total CPK level is elevated as a result of increases in CPK-MM, injury to or disease of the skeletal muscle is present. Examples of this include myopathies, vigorous exercise, multiple IM injections, electroconvulsive therapy, cardioversion, chronic alcoholism, or surgery. Because CPK is made only in the skeletal muscle, the normal value of total CPK (and therefore CPK-MM) varies according to a person's muscle mass. Large muscular people may normally have a CPK level in the high range of normal.

Each isoenzyme has been found to have isoforms. The CPK-MM isoforms MM1 and MM3 are most useful for cardiac disease. A MM3/MM1 ratio of greater than 1 suggests acute myocardial injury. The CPK-MB ratio of MB2/MB1 greater than 1 also indicates acute myocardial injury.

Creatine phosphokinase is the main cardiac enzyme studied in patients with heart disease. Because its blood clearance and metabolism are well known, its frequent determination (on admission, at 12 hours and 24 hours) can accurately reflect timing, quantity, and resolution of a myocardial infarction.

Interfering factors

- IM injections can cause elevated CPK levels.
- Strenuous exercise and recent surgery may cause increased levels.
- Early pregnancy may produce decreased levels.
- Drugs that may cause *increased* levels include amphotericin B, ampicillin, some anesthetics, anticoagulants, aspirin, clofibrate, dexamethasone (Decadron), furosemide (Lasix), capto-

pril, colchicine, alcohol, lovastatin, lithium, lidocaine, propranolol, succinylcholine, and morphine.

Procedure and patient care

Before

- Explain the procedure to the patient.
- Discuss with the patient the need and reason for frequent venipuncture in diagnosing myocardial infarction.
- Avoid IM injections in patients with cardiac disease. These injections may falsely elevate the total CPK level.
- Tell the patient that no food or fluid restrictions are necessary.

During

- Collect a venous blood sample in a red-top tube. This is usually done daily for 3 days and then at 1 week.
- Rotate the venipuncture sites.
- Avoid hemolysis.
- Record the time and date of any IM injection.
- Record the exact time and date of venipuncture on each laboratory slip. This aids in the interpretation of the temporal pattern of enzyme elevations.

After

- Apply pressure to the venipuncture site.

Abnormal findings

▲ **Increased levels of total CPK**
   Diseases or injury affecting the heart muscle, skeletal muscle, and brain

▲ **Increased levels of CPK-BB isoenzyme**
   Diseases affecting the central nervous system
   Adenocarcinoma (especially breast and lung)
   Pulmonary infarction

▲ **Increased levels of CPK-MB isoenzyme**
   Acute myocardial infarction
   Cardiac aneurysm surgery
   Cardiac defibrillation
   Myocarditis
   Ventricular arrhythmias
   Cardiac ischemia

▲ **Increased levels of CPK-MM isoenzyme**
   Rhabdomyolysis
   Muscular dystrophy
   Myositis
   Recent surgery
   Electromyography
   IM injections
   Crush injuries
   Delirium tremens
   Malignant hyperthermia
   Recent convulsions
   Electroconvulsive therapy
   Shock
   Hypokalemia
   Hypothyroidism

notes

creatinine, blood (Serum creatinine)

Type of test Blood

Normal findings
Adult
  Female: 0.5-1.1 mg/dl or 44-97 μmol/L (SI units)
  Male: 0.6-1.2 mg/dl

Elderly: decrease in muscle mass may cause decreased values
Adolescent: 0.5-1.0 mg/dl
Child: 0.3-0.7 mg/dl
Infant: 0.2-0.4 mg/dl
Newborn: 0.3-1.2 mg/dl

Possible critical values >4 mg/dl (indicates serious impairment in renal function)

Test explanation and related physiology

This test measures the amount of creatinine in the blood. Creatinine is a catabolic product of creatine phosphate, which is used in skeletal muscle contraction. The daily production of creatine, and subsequently creatinine, depends on muscle mass, which fluctuates very little. Creatinine, as with blood urea nitrogen (BUN, see p. 857), is excreted entirely by the kidneys and therefore is directly proportional to renal excretory function. Thus, with normal renal excretory function, the serum creatinine level should remain constant and normal. Only renal disorders such as glomerulonephritis, pyelonephritis, acute tubular necrosis, and urinary obstruction, will cause an abnormal elevation in creatinine. There are slight increases in creatinine levels after meals, especially after ingestion of large quantities of meat. Furthermore, there may be some diurnal variation in creatinine—nadir at 7 AM and peak at 7 PM.

The serum creatinine test, as with the BUN, is used to diagnose impaired renal function. Unlike the BUN, however, the creatinine level is affected very little by hepatic function. The serum creatinine level has much the same significance as the BUN level but tends to rise later. Therefore elevations in creatinine suggest chronicity of the disease process. In general, a doubling of creatinine suggests a 50% reduction in the glomerular filtration rate. The creatinine level is interpreted in conjunction with the BUN. These tests are referred to as *renal function studies.*

Interfering factors

✘ Drugs that may *increase* creatinine values include aminoglycosides (e.g., gentamicin), cimetidine, heavy-metal chemotherapeutic agents (e.g., cisplatin), and other nephrotoxic drugs such as cephalosporins (e.g., cefoxitin).

Procedure and patient care

Before

- Explain the procedure to the patient.
- Tell the patient that no fasting is required.

During

- Collect approximately 5 ml of blood in a red-top tube.
- For pediatric patients, blood is usually drawn from a heel stick.

After

- Apply pressure to the venipuncture site.

Abnormal findings

▲ **Increased levels**
  Glomerulonephritis
  Pyelonephritis
  Acute tubular necrosis
  Urinary tract obstruction
  Reduced renal blood flow
    (e.g., shock, dehydration,
    congestive heart failure,
    atherosclerosis)
  Diabetic nephropathy
  Nephritis
  Rhabdomyolysis
  Acromegaly
  Gigantism

▼ **Decreased levels**
  Debilitation
  Decreased muscle mass
    (e.g., muscular dystro-
    phy, myasthenia gravis)

notes

creatinine clearance

Type of test   Urine (24-hour); blood

Normal findings

<Adult (40 years)

    Male: 90-139 ml/min or 0.87-1.34 ml/sec/m^2

    Female: 80-125 ml/min or 0.77-1.20 ml/sec/m^2

Values decrease 6.5 ml/min/decade of life because of decline in glomerular filtration rate (GFR).

Newborn: 40-65 ml/min

Test explanation and related physiology

Creatinine is a catabolic product of creatine phosphate, which is used in skeletal muscle contraction. The daily production of creatinine depends on muscle mass, which fluctuates very little. Creatinine is entirely excreted by the kidneys and therefore is directly proportional to the glomerular filtration rate (GFR; i.e., the number of milliliters of filtrate made by the kidneys per minute). The creatinine clearance (CC) is a measure of the glomerular filtration rate.

The CC depends on the amount of blood present to be filtered and the ability of the glomeruli to act as a filter. The amount of blood present for filtration is decreased in renal artery atherosclerosis, dehydration, or shock. The ability of the glomeruli to act as a filter is decreased by diseases such as glomerulonephritis, acute tubular necrosis, and most other primary renal diseases. Significant bilateral obstruction to urinary outflow affects glomerular filtration (CC) only after it is long-standing.

When one kidney alone becomes diseased, the opposite kidney, if normal, has the ability to compensate by increasing its filtration rate. Therefore, with unilateral kidney disease or nephrectomy, a decrease in CC is not expected if the other kidney is normal.

Several nonrenal factors may influence CC. With each decade of age, the CC decreases 6.5 ml/min because of a decrease in the GFR. Urine collections are timed, and incomplete collections will falsely decrease CC. Muscle mass varies among people. Decreased muscle mass will give lower CC values. Likewise, ingestion of large meat meals will temporarily increase CC.

The CC test requires a 24-hour urine collection and a serum

creatinine level. Creatinine clearance is then computed using the following formula:

$$\text{Creatinine clearance} = \frac{UV}{P}$$

where

U = Number of milligrams per deciliter of creatinine excreted in the urine over 24 hours

V = Volume of urine in milliliters per minute

P = Serum creatinine in milligrams per deciliter

A 24-hour urine collection for creatinine is often measured along with other urine collections to assess the completeness of other 24-hour collections. In patients with normal creatinine, the CC should indicate whether all the urine has been collected for the 24 hours.

Interfering factors

- Exercise may cause increased creatinine values.
- Incomplete urine collection may give a falsely lowered value.
- Pregnancy increases creatinine clearance.
- A diet high in meat content can transiently cause elevation of the creatinine clearance.
- Drugs that may cause *increased* levels include aminoglycosides (e.g., gentamicin), cimetidine, heavy-metal chemotherapeutic agents (e.g., cisplatin), and nephrotoxic drugs such as cephalosporins (e.g., cefoxitin).

Procedure and patient care

Before

- Explain the procedure to the patient.
- Tell the patient that no special diet is usually required.
- Note that some laboratories instruct the patient to avoid cooked meat, tea, coffee, or drugs on the day of the test. Check with the laboratory.

During

- Instruct the patient to begin the 24-hour urine collection after voiding. Discard the initial specimen and start the 24-hour timing as of that point.
- Collect all the urine passed during the next 24 hours.
- Show the patient where to store the urine specimen.

- Keep the specimen on ice or refrigerated during the 24 hours.
- Indicate the starting time on the urine container and laboratory slip.
- Post the hours for the urine collection in a noticeable place to prevent accidental discharge of a specimen.
- Instruct the patient to void before defecating so that urine is not contaminated by feces.
- Remind the patient not to put toilet paper in the collection container.
- Encourage the patient to drink fluids during the 24 hours unless this is contraindicated for medical purposes.
- Instruct the patient to avoid vigorous exercise during the 24 hours, because exercise may cause an increased creatinine clearance.
- Collect the last specimen as close as possible to the end of the 24-hour period. Add this urine to the container.
- Make sure a venous blood sample is drawn in a red-top tube during the 24-hour collection.
- Mark the patient's age, weight, and height on the requisition sheet.

After
- Transport the urine specimen promptly to the laboratory.
- Apply pressure to the venipuncture site.

Abnormal findings

▲ **Increased levels**
Exercise
Pregnancy
High cardiac output
syndromes

▼ **Decreased levels**
Impaired kidney function
(e.g., renal artery atherosclerosis, glomerulonephritis, acute tubular necrosis)
Conditions causing
decreased GFR (e.g.,
congestive heart failure,
cirrhosis with ascites,
shock, dehydration)

notes

cryoglobulin

Type of test Blood

Normal findings No cryoglobulins detected

Test explanation and related physiology

Cryoglobulins are abnormal globulin protein complexes that exist within the blood of patients with various diseases. These proteins precipitate reversibly at low temperatures and redissolve with rewarming. They can precipitate within the blood vessel of the fingers when exposed to cold temperatures. This precipitation causes sludging of the blood within those blood vessels. These patients may have symptoms of purpura, arthralgia, or Raynaud's phenomenon (pain, cyanosis, coldness of the fingers).

These proteins exist in varying degrees, depending on the disease entity with which they are associated. Serum levels greater than 5 mg/ml are associated with multiple myeloma, macroglobulinemia, and leukemia. Globulin levels between 1 and 5 mg/ml are associated with rheumatoid arthritis. Levels less than 1 mg/ml can be associated with systemic lupus erythematosus, rheumatoid arthritis, infectious mononucleosis, viral hepatitis, endocarditis, cirrhosis, and glomerulonephritis. Idiopathic or primary cryoglobulinemia is not associated with any primary disease process.

For this test the blood sample is taken to the chemistry laboratory, where it is refrigerated for 72 hours. After that time the specimen is evaluated for precipitation. If precipitation is identified, it is measured and recorded. The tube is then rewarmed, and the specimen is reexamined for dissolution of that precipitation. If precipitation of the refrigerated specimen is identified and dissolved on rewarming, cryoglobulins are present.

Procedure and patient care

Before

- Explain the procedure to the patient.
- Inform the patient that an 8-hour fast may be required. This will minimize turbidity of the serum caused by ingestion of a recent (especially fatty) meal. Turbidity may make the detection of precipitation rather difficult.

During

- Collect 10 ml of venous blood in a red-top tube that has been prewarmed to body temperature.

After

- Apply pressure to the venipuncture site.
- If cryoglobulins are found to be present, warn the patient to avoid cold temperatures and contact with cold objects to minimize Raynaud's symptoms. Tell the patient to wear gloves in cold weather.

Abnormal findings

Connective tissue disease (e.g., lupus erythematosus, Sjögren's syndrome, rheumatoid arthritis)

Lymphoid malignancies (e.g., multiple myeloma, leukemia, Waldenstrom's macroglobulinemia, or lymphoma)

Acute and chronic infections (e.g., infectious mononucleosis, endocarditis, poststreptococcal glomerulonephritis)

Liver disease (e.g., hepatitis, cirrhosis)

notes

cutaneous immunofluorescence biopsy
(Immunofluorescence skin biopsy, Skin biopsy antibodies, Skin immunohistopathology)

Type of test Microscopic examination of skin tissue

Normal findings Normal skin histology

Test explanation and related physiology

This test of inflamed skin is performed to evaluate and diagnose immunologic mediated dermatitis. It is indicated when an immunologic source for a skin rash is suspected. For this study, a skin biopsy is obtained and evaluated by immunofluorescence. Deposition of human immunoglobulins and complement components is determined by immunofluorescent patterns. This test is useful in detecting immune complexes, complement, and immunoglobulin deposition in systemic and discoid lupus erythematosus, pemphigus, bullous pemphigoid, and dermatitis herpetiformis. This test is also used to confirm the histopathology of skin lesions and to follow the results of treatment.

Procedure and patient care

Before
- Explain the procedure to the patient.
- Obtain an informed consent.

During
- A 4-mm punch biopsy or tissue excision is obtained.

After
- Apply a dry, sterile dressing over the biopsy site.
- Tell the patient that results may not be available for several days.
- Deliver the specimen on ice immediately to the laboratory after the biopsy is taken.

Abnormal findings

Systemic lupus erythematosus
Discoid lupus erythematosus
Pemphigus
Bullous pemphigoid
Dermatitis herpetiformis

cystography (Cystourethrography, Voiding cystography, Voiding cystourethrography)

Type of test X-ray with contrast dye

Normal findings Normal bladder structure and function

Test explanation and related physiology

Filling the bladder with radiopaque contrast material provides visualization of the bladder for radiographic study. Either fluoroscopic or x-ray films demonstrate bladder filling and collapse after emptying. Filling defects or shadows within the bladder indicate primary bladder tumors. Extrinsic compression or distortion of the bladder is seen with pelvic tumor (e.g., rectal, cervical) or hematoma (secondary to pelvic bone fractures). Extravasation of the dye is seen with traumatic rupture, perforation, and fistula of the bladder. Vesicoureteral reflux (abnormal backflow of urine from bladder to ureters), which can cause persistent or recurrent pyelonephritis, also may be demonstrated during cystography. Although the bladder is visualized during an intravenous pyelogram (see p. 497), primary pathologic bladder conditions are best studied by cystography.

Contraindications

- Patients with urethral or bladder infection or injury

Potential complications

- Urinary tract infection
  This may result from catheter placement or the instillation of contaminated contrast material.
- Allergic reaction to iodinated dye
  This rarely occurs because the dye is not administered intravenously.

Procedure and patient care

Before
- Explain the procedure to the patient.
- Obtain informed consent if required by the institution.
- Give clear liquids for breakfast on the morning of the test.
- Assure the patient that he or she will be draped to prevent unnecessary exposure.
- Insert a Foley catheter if ordered.

C

During

- Note the following procedural steps:
  1. The patient is taken to the radiology department and placed in a supine or lithotomy position.
  2. Unless the catheter is already present, one is placed.
  3. Through the catheter, approximately 300 ml of air or radiopaque dye (much less for children) is injected into the bladder.
  4. The catheter is clamped.
  5. X-ray films are taken.
  6. If the patient is able to void, the catheter is removed, and the patient is asked to urinate while films are taken of the bladder and urethra (voiding cystourethrogram).
- Ensure that males wear a lead shield over the testes to prevent irradiation of the gonads.
- Remember that female patients cannot be shielded without blocking bladder visualization.
- Note that a radiologist performs the study in approximately 15 to 30 minutes.
- Tell the patient that this test is moderately uncomfortable if bladder catheterization is required.

After

- Assess the patient for signs of urinary tract infection.
- Encourage the patient to drink fluids to eliminate the dye and to prevent accumulation of bacteria.

Abnormal findings

Bladder tumor
Pelvic tumor
Hematoma
Bladder trauma
Vesicoureteral reflux

notes

cystometry (Cystometrogram [CMG], urethral pressure profile [UPP], Urethral pressure measurements])

Type of test Manometric

Normal findings
Normal sensations of fullness and temperature
Normal pressures and volumes
Maximal cystometric capacity
    Male: 350-750 ml
    Female: 250-550 ml
Intravesical pressure when bladder is empty: usually
    <40 cm H_2O
Detrusor pressure: <10 cm H_2O

Maximal urethral pressures in normal patients (cm H_2O):

Age	Male	Female
<25 years	37-126	55-103
25-44 years	35-113	31-115
45-64 years	40-123	40-100
>64 years	35-105	35-75

Test explanation and related physiology
The purpose of cystometry is to evaluate the motor and sensory functions of the bladder when incontinence is present or neurologic bladder dysfunction is suspected. A graphic recording of pressure exerted at varying phases of the filling of the urinary bladder is produced. A pressure/volume relationship of the bladder is made. This urodynamic study assesses the neuromuscular function of the bladder by measuring the efficiency of the detrusor muscle, intravesical pressure and capacity, and the bladder's response to thermal stimulation.

Cystometry can determine whether bladder pathology is caused by neurologic, infectious, or obstructive diseases. Cystometry is indicated to elucidate the causes for frequency and urgency, especially before surgery on the urologic outflow tract. Cystometry is also part of the evaluation for incontinence, persistent residual urine, vesicoureteral reflux, neurologic disorders, sensory disorders, and the effect of certain drugs on bladder function.

Urethral pressure profile (UPP) is often performed during

cystometry. The UPP indicates the intraluminal pressure along the length of the urethra with the bladder at rest. Indications for this urodynamic investigation include the following:

1. Assessment of prostatic obstruction
2. Assessment of stress incontinence in females
3. Assessment of postprostatectomy sequelae of incontinence
4. Assessment of the adequacy of external sphincterotomy
5. Analysis of the effects of drugs on the urethra
6. Analysis of the effects of stimulation on urethral flow
7. Assessment of the adequacy of implanted artificial urethral sphincter devices

Contraindications

- Urinary tract infections because of the possibility of false results and the potential for the spread of infection

Procedure and patient care

Before

- Explain the purpose and the procedure to the patient.
- Tell the patient that no fluid or food restrictions are needed.
- Assure the patient that he or she will be draped to prevent unnecessary exposure.
- Assess the patient for signs and symptoms of urinary tract infection.
- Instruct the patient not to strain while voiding, because the results can be skewed.
- If the patient has a spinal cord injury, transport him or her on a stretcher. The test will then be performed with the patient on the stretcher.

During

- Note the following procedural steps:
  1. Cystometry, usually performed in a urologist's office or a special procedure room, begins with the patient being asked to void.
  2. The amount of time required to initiate voiding and the size, force, and continuity of the urinary stream are recorded. The amount of urine, the time of voiding, and the presence of any straining, hesitancy, or terminal urine dribbling are also recorded.
  3. The patient is placed in a lithotomy or supine position.
  4. A retention catheter is inserted through the urethra and into the bladder.
  5. Residual urine volume is measured and recorded.

6. Thermal sensation is evaluated by the instillation of approximately 30 ml of room temperature saline solution into the bladder followed by an equal amount of warm water. The patient reports any sensations.

7. This fluid is withdrawn from the bladder.

8. The urethral catheter is connected to a cystometer (a tube used to monitor bladder pressure).

9. Sterile water, normal saline solution, or carbon dioxide gas is slowly introduced into the bladder at a controlled rate, usually with the patient in a sitting position.

10. Patients are asked to indicate the first urge to void and then when they have the feeling that they must void. The bladder is full at this point.

11. The pressures and volumes are plotted on a graph.

12. The patient is asked to void, and the maximal intravesical voiding pressure is recorded.

13. The bladder is drained for any residual urine.

14. If no additional studies are to be done, the urethral catheter is removed.

15. For urethral pressures, fluid or gas is instilled through the catheter, which is withdrawn while pressures along the urethral wall are obtained.

- Throughout the study, ask the patient to report any sensations such as pain, flushing, sweating, nausea, bladder filling, and an urgency to void.

- Note that certain drugs may be administered during the cystometric examination to distinguish between underactivity of the bladder because of muscle failure and underactivity associated with denervation. Cholinergic drugs (e.g., bethanechol [Urecholine]) may be given to enhance the tone of a flaccid bladder. Anticholinergic drugs (e.g., atropine) may be given to promote relaxation of a hyperactive bladder. If these drugs are to be given, the catheter is left in place. The drugs are given, and the examination is repeated 20 to 30 minutes later using the first test as a control value.

- Note that this test is performed by a urologist in approximately 45 minutes.

- Explain to the patient that the only discomfort is that associated with the urethral catheterization.

After

- Observe the patient for any manifestations of infection (e.g., elevated temperature, chills).
- Examine the urine for hematuria. Notify the physician if the hematuria persists after several voidings.
- Provide a warm sitz bath or tub bath for the patient's comfort if desired.

Abnormal findings

Neurogenic bladder
Bladder obstruction
Bladder infection
Bladder hypertonicity
Diminished bladder capacity
Prostatic obstruction secondary to benign prostatic hypertrophy or cancer
Urinary incontinence

notes

cystoscopy (Endourology)

Type of test Endoscopy

Normal findings Normal structure and function of the urethra, bladder, ureters, and prostate (in males)

Test explanation and related physiology

Cystoscopy provides direct visualization of the urethra and bladder through the transurethral insertion of a cystoscope into the bladder (Figure 12). Cystoscopy is used *diagnostically* to allow:

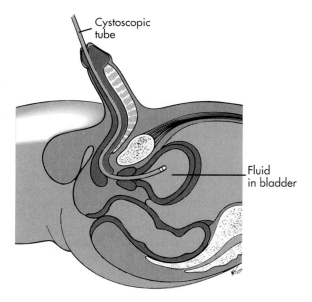

Figure 12 Cystoscopic examination of the male bladder. The cystoscope is passed through the urethra into the bladder. Although shown here as a flexible scope, usually the scope is rigid. Through the scope fluid is instilled to maintain bladder distention. (From Beare PG, Myers JM: Principles and practice of adult health nursing, ed 2, St Louis, 1994, Mosby.)

1. Direct inspection and biopsy of the prostate, bladder, and urethra
2. Collection of a separate urine specimen directly from each kidney by the placement of ureteral catheters
3. Measurement of bladder capacity and determination of ureteral reflux
4. Identification of bladder and ureteral calculi
5. Placement of ureteral catheters (Figure 13) for retrograde pyelography (see p. 734)
6. Identification of the source of hematuria

Cystoscopy is used *therapeutically* to provide:

1. Resection of small, superficial bladder tumors
2. Removal of foreign bodies and stones

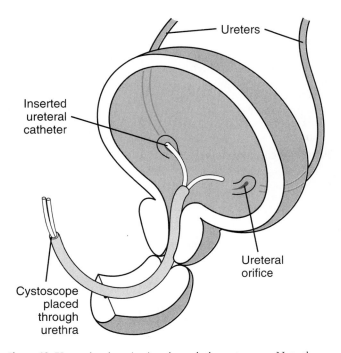

Figure 13 Ureteral catheterization through the cystoscope. Note the ureteral catheter inserted into the right orifice. The left ureteral catheter is ready to be inserted.

3. Dilation of the urethra and ureters
4. Placement of catheters to drain urine from the renal pelvis
5. Coagulation of bleeding areas
6. Implantation of radium seeds into a tumor
7. Resection of hypertrophied or malignant prostate gland overgrowth
8. Placement of ureteral stents for identification of ureters during pelvic surgery

The cystoscope consists primarily of an obturator and a telescope. The obturator is used to insert the cystoscope atraumatically. After the cystoscope is within the bladder, the obturator is removed, and the telescope is passed through the cystoscope. The lens and lighting system of the telescope permit adequate visualization of the lower genitourinary tract. Transendoscopic instruments such as forceps, scissors, needles, and electrodes are used when appropriate. *Endourology* refers to endoscopic surgery performed on the bladder and urethra during cystoscopy.

Cystoscopy is important in the evaluation of hematuria, chronic infection, suspected stones, and radiographic filling defects. On inspection, the urethra may show inflammation or structural causes of obstruction (e.g., stricture, neoplasia, prostatic hypertrophy). If the obstruction is functional rather than structural (e.g., detrusor-bladder neck dyssynergia), no site of obstruction will be demonstrated by endoscopy.

Potential complications

- Perforation of the bladder
- Sepsis by seeding the bloodstream with bacteria from infected urine
- Hematuria
- Urinary retention

Procedure and patient care

Before

- Explain the procedure to the patient.
- Ensure that an informed consent is obtained.
- If enemas are ordered to clear the bowel, assist the patient as needed and record the results.
- Encourage the patient to drink fluids several hours before the procedure to maintain a continuous flow of urine for collection and to prevent multiplication of bacteria that may be introduced during this technique.

- If the procedure will be done with the patient under local anesthesia, allow a liquid breakfast.
- If the procedure will be performed with the patient under general anesthesia, follow routine precautions. Keep the patient NPO after midnight on the day of the test. Fluids may be given intravenously.
- Administer the preprocedural medications as ordered 1 hour before the study. Sedatives decrease the spasm of the bladder sphincter, decreasing the patient's discomfort.

During
- Note the following procedural steps:
  1. Cystoscopy is usually performed in the operating room but also can be done in the urologist's office.
  2. The patient is placed in the lithotomy position with his or her feet in stirrups.
  3. The external genitalia are cleansed with an antiseptic solution such as povidone-iodine (Betadine).
  4. A local anesthetic is instilled into the urethra if general anesthesia has not been used.
  5. The cystoscope is inserted, and the desired diagnostic or therapeutic studies are performed.
- Instruct the patient to lie very still during the entire procedure to prevent trauma to the urinary tract.
- Tell the patient that he or she will have the desire to void as the cystoscope passes the bladder neck.
- When the procedure is completed, keep the patient on bed rest for a short time.
- Note that, if endourology is performed, the urethra will also be evaluated.
- Note that this procedure is performed by a urologist in approximately 25 minutes.
- When local anesthesia is used, inform the patient of the associated discomfort (much more than with urethral catheterization).

After
- Instruct the patient not to walk or stand alone immediately after the legs have been removed from the stirrups. The orthostasis that may result from standing erect may cause dizziness and fainting.
- Assess the patient's ability to void for at least 24 hours after the procedure. Urinary retention may be secondary to edema caused by instrumentation.

- Note the urine color. Pink-tinged urine is common. The presence of bright-red blood or clots should be reported to the physician.
- Monitor the patient for complaints of back pain, bladder spasms, urinary frequency, and burning on urination. Warm sitz baths and mild analgesics may be ordered and given. Sometimes belladonna and opium (B&O) suppositories are given to relieve bladder spasms. Warm, moist heat to the lower abdomen may help to relieve pain and to promote muscle relaxation.
- Encourage increased intake of fluids. A dilute urine decreases dysuria. Fluids also maintain a constant flow of urine to prevent stasis and the accumulation of bacteria in the bladder.
- Check and record the patient's vital signs as ordered. Watch for a decrease in blood pressure and an increase in pulse as an indication of hemorrhage.
- Observe for signs and symptoms of sepsis (elevated temperature, flush, chills, decreased blood pressure, increased pulse).
- Note that antibiotics are occasionally ordered 1 day before and 3 days following the procedure to reduce the incidence of bacteremia that may occur with instrumentation of the urethra and bladder.
- Encourage the patient to use cathartics, especially after cystoscopic surgery. Increases in intraabdominal pressure caused by constipation may initiate severe lower urologic bleeding.
- If postprocedure irrigation is ordered, have the patient use an isotonic solution containing mannitol, glycine, or sorbitol to prevent fluid overhydration in the event any of the irrigation is absorbed through opened venous sinuses in the bladder.
- If a catheter is left in after the procedure, provide catheter care instructions.

C

┌───┐
🏠 Home care responsibilities

- Watch for signs of urinary retention for 24 to 48 hours.
- Watch for signs of bleeding. Pink urine is normal; clots are not.
- Report symptoms of increasing lower abdominal pain immediately.
- Use warm sitz baths or B&O suppositories to reduce bladder spasms.
- Encourage patient to drink lots of fluids.
- Watch for fever, shaking chills, or prolonged dysuria as possible signs of urinary tract infection.
- If ordered, stress the importance of post-procedure antibiotics.
└───┘

Abnormal findings

Lower urologic tract tumor
Stones in the ureter or bladder
Prostatic hypertrophy
Prostate cancer
Inflammation of the bladder and urethra
Urethral/ureteral stricture
Prostatitis
Vesical neck contracture

notes

cytomegalovirus (CMV)

Type of test   Blood

Normal findings   No virus isolated

Test explanation and related physiology

CMV is part of the viral family that includes herpes simplex, Epstein-Barr, and varicella-zoster viruses. CMV infection is widespread and common. Infections usually occur in the fetus, during early childhood, and in the young adult. Certain populations are at increased risk. Male homosexuals, transplant patients, and AIDS patients are particularly susceptible. Infections are acquired by contact with body secretions or urine. Blood transfusions are a common form of spread for CMV. Most patients with acute disease have no or very few (mononucleosis-like) symptoms.

Cytomegalovirus is the most common congenital infection. Pregnant mothers can get the disease during their pregnancy, or an old previous CMV infection can become reactivated. Approximately 10% of infected newborns exhibit permanent damage, usually mental retardation and auditory damage. Fetal infection can cause microcephaly, hydrocephaly, cerebral palsy, mental retardation, or death. The term TORCH (toxoplasmosis, other, rubella, cytomegalovirus, herpes) has been applied to infections with recognized detrimental effects on the fetus.

Virus culture is the most definitive method of diagnosis. However, a culture cannot differentiate an acute infection from a chronic, inactive infection. Antibodies reveal much more information about the activity of the infection. CMV IgG antibody levels persist for years after infection. Identification of IgM antibodies, however, indicates a relatively recent infection. There are three different CMV antigens that can be detected immunologically. They are called early, intermediate-early, and late antigens and indicate onset of infection. A fourfold increase in CMV titer in paired sera drawn 10 to 14 days apart is usually indicative of an acute infection.

Procedure and patient care

Before

- Explain the procedure to the patient.

During

- For culture specimens, a urine, sputum, or mouth swab is the specimen of choice. Fresh specimens are essential.
- The specimens are cultured in a virus laboratory, which takes about 3 to 7 days.
- For antibody or antigen titer, draw 4 to 7 ml of blood in a gold- or red-top tube.
- Collect a specimen from the mother with suspected acute infection as early as possible.
- Collect the convalescent specimen 2 to 4 weeks later.

After

- Apply pressure to the venipuncture site.

Abnormal finding

CMV infection

notes

D-dimer test (Fragment D-dimer, Fibrin degradation fragment)

Type of test Blood

Normal findings

Negative (no D-dimer fragments present)
<250 ng/ml or <250 µg/L (SI units)

Test explanation and related physiology

The fragment D-dimer assesses both thrombin and plasmin activity. D-dimer is a fibrin degradation fragment that is made through fibrinolysis. As plasmin acts on the fibrin polymer clot, fibrin degradation products and D-dimer are produced. The D-dimer assay provides a highly specific measurement of the amount of fibrin degradation that occurs. Normal plasma does not have detectable amounts of fragment D-dimer.

This test provides a simple and confirmatory test for disseminated intravascular coagulation (DIC). Positive results of the D-dimer assay correlate with positive results of fibrin degradation products (FDPs) (see p. 412). Although the D-dimer assay is more specific than the FDP assay, it is less sensitive. Therefore combining the FDP and the D-dimer provides a highly sensitive and specific test for recognizing DIC in a patient.

Levels of D-dimer can also increase when a fibrin clot is lysed by thrombolytic therapy. Thrombotic problems such as deep-vein thrombosis, pulmonary embolism, sickle cell anemia, and thrombosis of malignancy are also associated with high D-dimer levels.

Procedure and patient care

Before

- Explain the procedure to the patient.
- Tell the patient that no fasting is required.

During

- Collect a venous blood sample in a blue-top tube.

After

- Apply pressure to the venipuncture site.
- Assess the venipuncture site for bleeding. Remember that, if the patient is receiving anticoagulants or has coagulopathies, the bleeding time will be increased.

Abnormal findings

▲ **Increased levels**
Fibrinolysis
During thrombolytic or defibrination therapy with tissue
  plasminogen activator
Deep-vein thrombosis
Pulmonary embolism
Arterial thromboembolism
DIC
Vaso-occlusive crisis of sickle cell anemia
Pregnancy
Malignancy
Surgery

notes

delta-aminolevulinic acid (Aminolevulinic acid [ALA], Delta-ALA)

Type of test Urine (24-hour)

Normal findings 1-7 mg/24 hr or 11.1-57.2 μmol/24 hr (SI units)

Possible critical values >20 mg/24 hr

Test explanation and related physiology

As the basic precursor for the porphyrins (see p. 657), delta-ALA is needed for the normal production of porphobilinogen, which ultimately leads to heme synthesis in erythroid cells. Heme is used in the synthesis of hemoglobin. Genetic disorders (porphyria) are associated with a lack of a particular enzyme vital to heme metabolism. These disorders are characterized by an accumulation of porphyrin products in the liver or red blood cells. The liver porphyrias are much more common. Symptoms of liver porphyrias include abdominal pain, neuromuscular signs and symptoms, constipation, and occasionally psychotic behavior. Acute intermittent porphyria (AIP) is the most common form of the liver porphyrias; this is caused by a deficiency in uroporphyrinogen-I-synthase (also called porphobilinogen deaminase).

Most patients with AIP have no symptoms (latent phase) until the acute phase is precipitated by medication or some other factors (see uroporphyrinogen). The acute phase is highlighted by symptoms of abdominal and muscular pain, nausea, vomiting, hypertension, mental symptoms (anxiety, insomnia, hallucinations, and paranoia), sensory loss, and urinary retention. Hemolytic anemia also may occur with these acute attacks. These acute symptoms are associated with increased serum and urine levels of porphyrin precursors (aminolevulinic acid, porphyrins, and porphobilinogens).

In lead intoxication, heme synthesis is similarly diminished by the inhibition of ALA dehydrase. This enzyme assists in the conversion of ALA to porphobilinogen. As a result of lead poisoning, ALA accumulates in the blood and urine.

Interfering factors

☡ Drugs that may cause *increased* ALA levels include penicillin, barbiturates, and griseofulvin.

Procedure and patient care

Before
- Explain the procedure to the patient.

During
- Instruct the patient to begin a 24-hour urine collection after voiding. Discard the initial specimen and start the 24-hour timing at that point.
- Collect all urine passed during the next 24 hours.
- Show the patient where to store the urine container.
- Keep the specimen on ice or refrigerated during the 24 hours.
- Keep the urine in a light-resistant container with a preservative.
- Indicate the starting time on the urine container and on the laboratory slip.
- Post the hours for the urine collection in a noticeable place to prevent accidental discarding of the specimen.
- Instruct the patient to void before defecating so that urine is not contaminated by feces.
- Remind the patient not to put toilet paper in the collection container.
- Encourage the patient to drink fluids during the 24 hours unless this is contraindicated for medical purposes.
- Collect the last specimen as close as possible to the end of the 24-hour period. Add this to the urine collection.
- If the patient has a Foley catheter in place, cover the drainage bag to prevent exposure to light.
- Indicate on the laboratory slip any drugs that may affect test results.

After
- Apply pressure to the venipuncture site.
- Transport the urine specimen promptly to the laboratory.

Abnormal findings

▲ **Increased levels**
    Porphyria
    Lead intoxication
    Chronic alcoholic disorders
    Diabetic ketoacidosis

notes

Type of test Blood; urine (24-hour)

Normal findings

D

Prolonged method

Low dose: >50% reduction of plasma cortisol and
  17-hydroxycorticosteroid (17-OCHS) levels
High dose: 50% reduction of plasma cortisol and 17-OCHS
  levels

Rapid method

Normal: nearly 0 cortisol levels

Test explanation and related physiology

An elaborate feedback mechanism for cortisol exists to
coordinate the function of the hypothalamus, pituitary gland,
and adrenal glands. The DST is based on pituitary adrenocorticotropic hormone (ACTH) secretion being dependent on the
plasma cortisol feedback mechanism. As plasma cortisol levels
increase, ACTH secretion is suppressed; as cortisol levels
decrease, ACTH secretion is stimulated. Dexamethasone is a
synthetic steroid (similar to cortisol) that normally should
suppress ACTH secretion. Under normal circumstances, this
results in reduced stimulation to the adrenal glands and
ultimately a drop of 50% or more in plasma cortisol and
17-OCHS levels. This important feedback system does not
function properly in patients with Cushing's syndrome.

In Cushing's syndrome caused by bilateral adrenal hyperplasia
(Cushing's disease), the pituitary gland is reset upward and
responds only to high plasma levels of cortisol or its analogs. In
Cushing's syndrome caused by adrenal adenoma or cancer
(which acts autonomously), cortisol secretion continues, despite
a decrease in ACTH. When Cushing's syndrome is caused by an
ectopic ACTH-producing tumor (as in lung cancer), that tumor
is also considered autonomous and will continue to secrete
ACTH despite high cortisol levels. Again, no decrease occurs in
plasma cortisol. Knowledge of the following defects in the
normal cortisol-ACTH feedback system is the basis for understanding the DST:

Cushing's syndrome caused by:
    Bilateral adrenal hyperplasia
        Low dose: no change
        High dose: >50% reduction of plasma cortisol and
            17-OCHS levels
    Adrenal adenoma or carcinoma
        Low dose: no change
        High dose: no change
    Ectopic ACTH-producing tumor
        Low dose: no change
        High dose: no change

The DST also may identify depressed persons likely to respond to electroconvulsive therapy or antidepressants rather than to psychologic or social interventions. ACTH production will not be suppressed after administration of low-dose dexamethasone in these patients.

The *prolonged* DST can be performed over a 6-day period on an outpatient basis. The *rapid* DST is easily and quickly performed and is used primarily as a screening test to diagnose Cushing's syndrome. It is less accurate and informative than the prolonged DST, but, when its results are normal, the diagnosis of Cushing's syndrome can safely be excluded. The ease with which the rapid DST can be performed makes it useful in clinical medicine.

Interfering factors

- Physical and emotional stress can elevate ACTH release and obscure interpretation of test results.
- Drugs that can affect test results include barbiturates, estrogens, oral contraceptives, phenytoin (Dilantin), spironolactone (Aldactone), steroids, and tetracyclines.

Procedure and patient care

Before

- Explain the procedure (prolonged or rapid test) to the patient.
- Obtain the patient's weight as a baseline for evaluating side effects of steroids.

During

Prolonged test

- Obtain a baseline 24-hour urine collection for corticosteroids (urine 17-OHCS [see p. 482] or urinary cortisol [see p. 283]).
- Collect blood for determination of baseline plasma cortisol levels (see p. 283) if indicated.
- Collect 24-hour urine specimens daily over a 6-day period. Because 6 continuous days of urine collections are needed, no urine specimens are discarded, except for the first voided specimen on day 1, after which the collection begins.
- On day 3 administer a low dose (0.5 mg) of dexamethasone by mouth every 6 hours for a total of 2 mg.
- On day 5 administer a high dose (2 mg) of dexamethasone by mouth every 6 hours for a total of 8 mg.
- Administer the dexamethasone with milk or an antacid to prevent gastric irritation.
- Remember that the urine samples for cortisol and 17-OCHS do not need a preservative.
- Note that the creatinine content is measured in all the 24-hour urine collections to demonstrate their accuracy and adequacy.
- Keep the urine specimens refrigerated or on ice during the collection period.

Rapid test

- Give the patient 1 mg of dexamethasone by mouth at 11 PM.
- Administer the dexamethasone with milk or an antacid to prevent gastric irritation.
- If ordered, administer a barbiturate to sedate the patient and ensure a good night's sleep.
- At 8 AM the next morning, draw blood for determination of the plasma cortisol level before the patient arises.
- If no cortisol suppression occurs after 1 mg of dexamethasone, administer a higher dose (8 mg) to suppress ACTH production. This is referred to as the *overnight 8-mg dexamethasone suppression test.*

After

- Evaluate the patient for evidence of gastric irritation.
- Assess the patient for steroid-induced side effects by monitoring weight, glucose levels, and potassium levels.
- Send specimens to the laboratory promptly.

Abnormal findings

Cushing's syndrome
Cushing's disease
Ectopic ACTH-producing
  tumors

Adrenal adenoma or carcinoma
Bilateral adrenal hyperplasia
Mental depression
Hyperthyroidism

notes

2,3-diphosphoglycerate (2,3-DPG in erythrocytes)

D

Type of test Blood

Normal findings

$12.3 \pm 1.87 \; \mu$mol/g of hemoglobin
$4.2 \pm 0.64 \; \mu$mol/ml of erythrocytes

Levels are lower in newborns and even lower in premature infants.

Test explanation and related physiology

This test is used in the evaluation of nonspherocytic anemia. 2,3-DPG is a by-product of the glycolytic respiratory pathway of the RBC. A congenital enzyme deficiency in this vital pathway alters the RBC shape and survival significantly. Anemia is the result. Another result of the enzyme deficiency is reduced synthesis of 2,3-DPG. Since 2,3-DPG controls oxygen transport from the RBCs to the tissues, deficiencies of this enzyme result in alterations of the RBC-oxygen dissociation curve that controls release of oxygen to the tissues. Many anemias not due to 2,3-DPG deficiency are associated with increased levels of 2,3-DPG as a compensatory mechanism.

Usually 2,3-DPG levels increase in response to anemia or hypoxic conditions (e.g., obstructive lung disease, congenital cyanotic heart disease, after vigorous exercise). Increases in 2,3-DPG decrease the oxygen binding to hemoglobin so that oxygen is more easily released to the tissues when needed (lower arterial PO_2). Levels of 2,3-DPG are decreased as a result of inherited genetic defects. This genetic defect parallels that of sickle cell anemia and hemoglobin C diseases.

Interfering factors

- Levels may be increased after vigorous exercise.
- High altitudes may increase 2,3-DPG levels.
- Banked blood has decreased amounts of 2,3-DPG.
- Acidosis decreases 2,3-DPG levels.

Procedure and patient care

Before

- Explain the procedure to the patient.
- Tell the patient that no fasting is required.

During
- Collect a venous blood sample in a red-top tube.

After
- Apply pressure to the venipuncture site.

Abnormal findings

▲ **Increased levels**
Anemia
Hypoxic heart (e.g.,
   cyanotic heart disease)
   or lung (e.g., chronic
   obstructive pulmonary
   disease) diseases
Hyperthyroidism
Chronic renal failure
Pyruvate kinase deficiency

▼ **Decreased levels**
Polycythemia
Acidosis
Post massive blood trans-
   fusion
2,3-DPG disease
Respiratory distress syn-
   drome

notes

disseminated intravascular coagulation screening
(DIC screening)

Type of test Blood

Normal findings No evidence of DIC

D

Test explanation and related physiology

This is a group of tests used to detect disseminated intravascular coagulation. Many pathologic conditions can instigate or are associated with DIC. The more common ones include bacterial septicemia, amniotic fluid embolism, retention of a dead fetus, malignant neoplasia, liver cirrhosis, extensive surgery (especially on the liver), postextracorporeal heart bypass, extensive trauma, severe burns, and transfusion reactions.

In DIC, the entire clotting mechanism is inappropriately triggered. This results in significant systemic or localized intravascular formation of fibrin clots. Consequences of this futile clotting are intravascular sludging and excessive bleeding caused by consumption of the platelets and clotting factors that have been used in intravascular clotting. The fibrinolytic system is also activated to break down the clot formation and the fibrin

TABLE 10 Disseminated intravascular coagulation screening tests

Test	Result
Bleeding time (p. 146)	Prolonged
Platelet count (p. 645)	Decreased
Prothrombin time (p. 691)	Prolonged
Partial thromboplastin time (p. 618)	Prolonged
Coagulation factors (p. 248)	Decreased factors I, II, V, VIII, X and XIII
Fibrin degradation products (p. 412)	Increased
Red blood smear (p. 151)	Damaged red blood cell
Euglobulin lysis time (p. 387)	Normal or prolonged
D-dimer (p. 316)	Increased

From Pagana KD, Pagana TJ: Mosby's manual of diagnostic and laboratory tests, St Louis, 1998, Mosby.

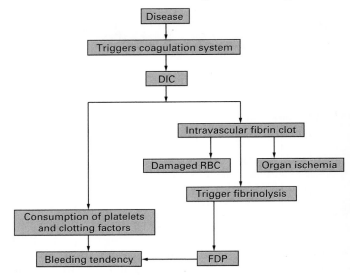

Figure 14 Pathology of disseminated intravascular coagulation *(DIC)*, which may result in bleeding tendency, organ ischemia, and hemolytic anemia. *RBC,* red blood cell; *FDP,* fibrin degradation product.

involved in the intravascular coagulation. This fibrinolysis results in the formation of fibrin degradation products (FDPs), which by themselves act as anticoagulants; these FDPs only serve to enhance the bleeding tendency.

Organ injury can occur as a result of the intravascular clots, which cause microvascular occlusion in various organs. This may cause serious anoxic injury in affected organs. Also, red blood cells passing through partly plugged vessels are injured and subsequently hemolyzed. The result may be ongoing hemolytic anemia. Figure 14 summarizes DIC pathophysiology and effects.

When a patient with a bleeding tendency is suspected to have DIC, a series of readily performed laboratory tests should be done (Table 10). With these tests, the hematologist can make the appropriate diagnosis confidently. All these tests are discussed separately within this book.

Abnormal finding

DIC

Doppler studies, vascular

D

Type of test Ultrasound

Normal findings

Venous

A normal Doppler venous signal with spontaneous respiration

Normal venous system without evidence of occlusion

Arterial

Normal arterial Doppler signal with systolic and diastolic
  components

No reduction in blood pressure in excess of 20 mm Hg compared with the normal extremity

A normal ankle-to-brachial arterial blood pressure index of 0.85
  or greater

No evidence of arterial occlusion

Test explanation and related physiology

Doppler studies are used to identify occlusion of the veins or
arteries. Although this discussion is limited to the extremities,
this technology is also performed on the carotid artery (see p.
221) and on the arterial system of the viscera (e.g., liver, kidney
and bowel.) In the extremity, arterial doppler studies are used on
patients with suspected arterial insufficiency (such as claudication, poorly healing skin ulcer, cold pale leg, pulseless extremity,
or rest pain). Venous ultrasound is used to evaluate the patency
of the venous system in patients with a swollen painful leg,
venous varicosities of the upper or lower extremity, or an
edematous extremity. *Venous* patency is demonstrated through
Doppler ultrasound by detecting moving red blood cells (RBCs)
within the vein. The Doppler transducer directs an ultrasound
beam at the vein. Moving RBCs scatter the frequency of the
beam. The change in frequency of the sound wave reflected back
to the transducer is proportional to the velocity of the blood
flow. Venous doppler studies are not accurate for venous
occlusive disease of the lower calf.

With single mode *arterial* Doppler studies, one can identify
and locate peripheral arteriosclerotic occlusive disease of the
extremities. This can be done with a single mode ultrasound by
slowly deflating blood pressure cuffs placed on the calf and ankle.
The systolic pressure in the various arteries of the extremities can
be accurately measured by detecting the first evidence of blood

flow with the Doppler transducer. The extremely sensitive Doppler ultrasound detector can recognize the "swishing" sound of even the most minimal blood flow. Normally there is a minimal drop in systolic blood pressure from the arteries of the arms to those of the legs. If the drop in blood pressure exceeds 20 mm Hg, occlusive disease is believed to exist immediately proximal to the area tested.

Arterial studies can also be performed by duplex Doppler scanning. The duplex concept is based on the ability to define the arterial walls within a two-dimensional image and uses a pulse Doppler probe to evaluate flow velocities and direction within the artery. This technique can measure the amplitude and waveform of the vascular pulse. Furthermore, a two-dimensional image of the artery can be produced. As a result, one can directly visualize possibly stenotic or occluded arteries and the arterial flow disruption. Lower extremity arterial bypass graft patency can also be assessed by Doppler ultrasound.

Interfering factors

- Venous or arterial occlusive disease proximal to the site of testing
- Cigarette smoking, because nicotine can cause constriction of the peripheral arteries and alter the results

Procedure and patient care

Before

- Explain the procedure to the patient.
- Inform the patient that this is a painless procedure.
- Remove all clothing from the extremity to be examined.
- Instruct the patient to abstain from cigarette smoking for at least 30 minutes before the test.

During

- Note the following procedural steps:
  Venous Doppler studies
  1. A conductive gel is applied to the skin overlying the venous system of the extremity in multiple areas.
  2. Usually, for the lower extremity, the deep venous system is identified in the ankle, calf, thigh, and groin.
  3. The characteristic "swishing" sound of the Doppler indicates a patent venous system. Failure to detect this signal indicates venous occlusion.

4. Usually both the superficial and venous systems are evaluated.

Arterial Doppler studies

1. These are performed with the use of blood pressure cuffs, which are placed around the thigh, calf, and ankle.
2. A conductive paste is applied to the skin overlying the artery distal to the cuffs.
3. The proximal cuff is inflated to a level above systolic blood pressure in the normal extremity.
4. The Doppler ultrasound transducer is placed immediately distal to the inflated cuff.
5. The pressure in the cuff is slowly released.
6. The highest pressure at which blood flow is detected by the characteristic "swishing" Doppler signal is recorded as the blood pressure of that artery.
7. The test is repeated at each successive level.
8. When the ankle pressure is divided by the arm (brachial artery) pressure, this is known as the AB index. If the *AB index* is less than 0.85, significant arterial occlusive disease exists within the extremity.

- Note that these studies are usually performed in the vascular laboratory or radiology department and take approximately 30 minutes.

After

- Encourage the patient to verbalize his or her fears in terms of test results.
- Remove the transducer gel from the extremity.
- Inform the patient that the physician must interpret the studies and that results will be available in a few hours.

Abnormal findings

Venous occlusion, secondary to thrombosis or thrombophlebitis
Venous varicosities
Small or large vessel arterial occlusive disease
Spastic arterial disease (e.g., Raynaud's phenomenon)
Small vessel arterial occlusive disease (as in diabetes)
Embolic arterial occlusion
Arterial aneurysm

echocardiography (Cardiac echo, Heart sonogram, Transthoracic echocardiography [TTE])

Type of test   Ultrasound

Normal findings

Normal position, size, and movement of the cardiac valves and
heart muscle wall
Normal directional flow of blood within the heart chambers

Test explanation and related physiology

Echocardiography is a noninvasive ultrasound procedure used
to evaluate the structure and function of the heart. In diagnostic
ultrasonography, a harmless, high-frequency sound wave emitted
from a transducer penetrates the heart. Sound waves are
bounced off the heart structures and reflected back to the
transducer as a series of echoes. These echoes are amplified and
displayed on an oscilloscope. Tracings also can be recorded on
moving graph paper or videotape. The study usually includes
M-mode recordings, two-dimensional recordings, and a Doppler
study.

M-mode echocardiography is a linear tracing of the motion of
the heart structures over time. This allows the various cardiac
structures to be located and studied regarding their movement
during a cardiac cycle.

Two-dimensional echocardiography angles a beam within one
sector of the heart. This produces a picture of the spatial
anatomic relationships within the heart.

A recent addition has been *color Doppler echocardiography*.
This test detects the pattern of the blood flow and measures
changes in velocity of blood flow within the heart and great
vessels. Turbulent blood or altered velocity and direction of
blood flow can be identified by changes in color. This is seen in a
photograph. In most Doppler ultrasound color flow imaging,
blue and red represent the direction of a given stream of blood;
the various hues from dull to bright represent varying blood
velocities. The most useful application of the color flow imaging
is in determining the direction and turbulence of blood flow
across regurgitant or narrowed valves. Doppler color flow
imaging also may be helpful in assessing proper functioning of
prosthetic valves.

Echocardiography, in general, is used in the diagnosis of a

pericardial effusion, valvular heart disease (e.g., mitral valve prolapse, stenosis, regurgitation), subaortic stenosis, myocardial wall abnormalities (e.g., cardiomyopathy), infarction, and aneurysm. Cardiac tumors (e.g., myxomas) are easily diagnosed with ultrasound. Atrial and ventricular septal defects and other congenital heart diseases are also recognized by ultrasound. Finally, postinfarction mural thrombi are readily apparent with this testing.

Echocardiography is also used in *cardiac stress testing*. It is fast becoming the method of choice in heart imaging for stress testing. During an exercise or chemical cardiac stress test, ischemic muscle areas are evident as hypokinetic areas within the myocardium. Echocardiography is being used with increased frequency in emergent and urgent evaluations of patients with chest pains. If the myocardium is normal and without areas of hypokinesia, no coronary artery occlusive disease is suspected. If, however a hypokinetic or akinetic area is noted, ischemia or infarction has occurred, and the chest pain is cardiac in origin.

It is now possible to perform echocardiography via the esophagus using a probe mounted on an endoscope. This is referred to as *transesophageal echocardiography, TEE* (see p. 841).

Contraindications

- Patients who are uncooperative

Interfering factors

- Chronic obstructive pulmonary disease (COPD)
  Patients who have severe COPD have a significant amount of air and space between the heart and the chest cavity. Air space does not conduct ultrasound waves well.
- Obesity
  In obese patients the space between the heart and the transducer is greatly enlarged; therefore accuracy of the test is decreased.

Procedure and patient care

Before

- Assure the patient that this is a painless study.
- Complete the request for the echocardiogram, including the pertinent patient history.

During

- Note the following procedural steps:
  1. The patient is placed in the supine position.
  2. Electrocardiographic (ECG) leads are placed (see p. 335).
  3. A gel, which allows better transmission of sound waves, is placed on the chest wall immediately under the transducer.
  4. Ultrasound is directed to the heart, and appropriate tracings are obtained.
- Note that this procedure usually takes approximately 45 minutes and is performed by an ultrasound technician in a darkened room within the cardiac laboratory or radiology department.
- Tell the patient that no discomfort is associated with this study but that the transmission gel is usually cooler than body temperature.

After

- Remove the gel from the patient's chest wall.
- Inform the patient that the physician must interpret the study and that the results will be available in a few hours.

Abnormal findings

Valvular stenosis
Valvular regurgitation
Mitral valve prolapse
Pericardial effusion
Ventricular or atrial mural
  thrombi

Myxoma
Poor ventricular muscle
  motion
Septal defects
Ventricular hypertrophy
Endocarditis

notes

E

electrocardiography (Electrocardiogram [ECG, EKG])

Type of test Electrodiagnostic

Normal findings Normal heart rate (60-100 beats/min), rhythm, and wave deflections

Test explanation and related physiology

The ECG is a graphic representation of the electrical impulses that the heart generates during the cardiac cycle. These electrical impulses are conducted to the body's surface, where they are detected by electrodes placed on the patient's limbs and chest. The monitoring electrodes detect the electrical activity of the heart from a variety of spatial perspectives. The ECG lead system is composed of several electrodes that are placed on each of the four extremities and at varying sites on the chest. Each combination of electrodes is called a *lead*.

A *12-lead ECG* provides a comprehensive view of the flow of the heart's electrical currents in two different planes. There are six limb leads (combination of electrodes on the extremities) and six chest leads (corresponding to six sites on the chest). Leads I, II, and III are considered the standard *limb* leads. Lead I records the difference in electrical potential between the left arm (LA) and the right arm (RA). Lead II records the electrical potential between the RA and the left leg (LL). Lead III reflects the difference between the LA and the LL. The right leg (RL) electrode is an inactive ground in all leads. There are three *augmented* limb leads: aV_R, aV_L, and aV_F (a, augmented; V, vector [unipolar]; R, right arm; L, left arm; F, left foot or leg). The augmented leads measure the electrode potential between the center of the heart and the right arm (aV_R), the left arm (aV_L), and the left leg (aV_F). The six standard chest, or precordial, leads (V_1, V_2, V_3, V_4, V_5, V_6) are recorded by placing electrodes at six different positions on the chest, surrounding the heart.

In general, it is said that leads II, III and aV_F look at the inferior part of the heart. Leads aV_L and I look at the lateral part of the heart. Leads V_2-V_4 look at the anterior part of the heart.

The ECG is recorded on special paper with a graphic back of horizontal and vertical lines for rapid measurement of time intervals (X coordinate) and voltages (Y coordinate). Time duration is measured by vertical lines 1 mm apart, each

Figure 15 Electrocardiography. **A,** Normal ECG deflections during depolarization and repolarization of the atrium and ventricles. **B,** Principle ECG intervals between P, QRS, and T waves.

representing 0.04 second. Voltage is measured by horizontal lines 1 mm apart. Five 1-mm squares equal 0.5 mV.

The normal ECG pattern is composed of waves arbitrarily designated by the letters *P, Q, R, S,* and *T.* The Q, R, and S waves are grouped together and described as the QRS complex. The significance of the waves and time intervals is as follows (Figure 15).

P wave. This represents atrial electrical depolarization associated with atrial contraction. It represents electrical activity associated with the spread of the original impulse from the sinoatrial (SA) node through the atria. If the P waves are absent or altered, the cardiac impulse originates outside the SA node.

PR interval. This represents the time required for the impulse to travel from the SA node to the atrioventricular (AV) node. If this interval is prolonged, a conduction delay exists in the AV node (e.g., a first-degree heart block). If the PR interval is shortened, the impulse must have reached the ventricle through a "shortcut" (as in Wolff-Parkinson-White syndrome).

QRS complex. This represents ventricular electrical depolarization associated with ventricular contraction. This complex consists of an initial downward (negative) deflection (Q wave), a large upward (positive) deflection (R wave), and a small downward deflection (S wave). A widened QRS complex indicates abnormal or prolonged ventricular depolarization time (as in a bundle-branch block).

ST segment. This represents the period between the completion of depolarization and the beginning of repolarization of the ventricular muscle. This segment may be elevated or depressed in transient muscle ischemia (e.g., angina) or in muscle injury (as in the early stages of myocardial infarction).

T wave. This represents ventricular repolarization (i.e., return to neutral electrical activity).

U wave. This deflection follows the T wave and is usually quite small. It represents repolarization of the Purkinje nerve fibers within the ventricles.

Through the analysis of these waveforms and time intervals, valuable information about the heart may be obtained. The ECG is used primarily to identify abnormal heart rhythms (arrhythmias [dysrhythmias]) and to diagnose acute myocardial infarction, conduction defects, and ventricular hypertrophy. It is important to note that the ECG may be normal, even in the presence of heart disease.

For some patients at high risk for malignant ventricular arrhythmias, a *signal-averaged ECG (SAECG)* can be performed. This test averages several hundred QRS waveforms to detect late potentials that are likely to lead to ventricular arrhythmias. SAECGs have been a useful precursor to electrophysiologic studies (see p. 354) because they can identify patients with unexplained syncope who may have ventricular tachycardias induced by the electrophysiologic study. SAECGs can be performed by the bedside in 15 to 20 minutes and must be ordered separately from a standard ECG.

Interfering factors

- Inaccurate placement of the electrodes
- Electrolyte imbalances
- Poor contact between the skin and the electrodes
- Movement or muscle twitching during the test
- Drugs that can affect results include digitalis, quinidine, and barbiturates

Procedure and patient care

Before

- Explain the procedure to the patient.
- Tell the patient that no food or fluid restriction is necessary.
- Assure the patient that the flow of electric current is *from*

the patient. He or she will feel nothing during this procedure.

- Expose only the patient's chest and arms. Keep the abdomen and thighs adequately covered.

During

- Note the following procedural steps:
  1. The skin areas designated for electrode placement are prepared by using alcohol swabs or sandpaper to remove skin oil or debris. Sometimes the skin is shaved if the patient has a large amount of hair.
  2. Electrode paste is applied to ensure electrical conduction between the skin and the electrodes.
  3. The four limb leads are usually held in place by straps that encircle the extremity. Newer machines have clamps that can easily be opened and applied to the extremity.
  4. Many cardiologists recommend that arm electrodes be placed on the upper arm, because fewer muscle tremors are detected there.
  5. The chest leads are applied either one at a time, three at a time, or six at a time, depending on the type of ECG machine. These leads are positioned as follows:

     V_1: in the fourth intercostal space (4ICS) at the right sternal border

     V_2: in 4ICS at the left sternal border

     V_3: midway between V_2 and V_4

     V_4: in 5ICS at the midclavicular line

     V_5: at the left anterior axillary line at the level of V_4 horizontally

     V_6: at the left midaxillary line on the level of V_4 horizontally

- List medications the patient is taking on the ECG request form.
- Note that cardiac technicians, nurses, or physicians perform this procedure in less than 5 minutes at the bedside or in the cardiology clinic.
- Tell the patient that, although this procedure carries no discomfort, he or she must lie still in the supine position without talking while the ECG is recorded.

After

- Remove the electrodes from the patient's skin and wipe off the electrode gel.
- Indicate on the ECG strip or request slip if the patient was

experiencing chest pain during the study. The pain may be correlated to an arrhythmia on the ECG.

Abnormal findings

Arrhythmia
Acute myocardial infarction
Myocardial ischemia
Old myocardial infarction
Conduction defects
Conduction system disease
Wolff-Parkinson-White
  syndrome

Ventricular hypertrophy
Cor pulmonale
Pulmonary embolus
Electrolyte imbalance
Pericarditis

E

notes

electroencephalography (Electroencephalogram [EEG])

Type of test Electrodiagnostic

Normal findings Normal frequency, amplitude, and characteristics of brain waves

Test explanation and related physiology

The EEG is a graphic recording of the electrical activity of the brain. EEG electrodes are placed on the scalp over multiple areas of the brain to detect and record electrical impulses within the brain. This study is invaluable in the investigation of epileptic states, in which the focus of seizure activity is characterized by rapid, spiking waves seen on the graph. Patients with cerebral lesions (e.g., tumors, infarctions) have abnormally slow EEG waves, depending on the size and location of the lesion. Because this study determines the overall activity of the brain, it can be used to evaluate trauma and drug intoxication and also to determine cerebral death in comatose patients.

The EEG also can be used to monitor cerebral blood flow during surgical procedures. For example, during carotid endarterectomy, the carotid vessel must be temporarily occluded. When this surgery is performed with the patient under general anesthesia, the EEG can be used for the early detection of cerebral tissue ischemia, which would indicate that continued carotid occlusion will result in a cerebrovascular accident (stroke) syndrome. Temporary shunting of the blood during the surgery is then required.

Interfering factors

- Fasting may cause hypoglycemia, which could modify the EEG pattern.
- Drinks containing caffeine (e.g., coffee, tea, cocoa, cola) interfere with the test results.
- Body and eye movements during the test can cause changes in the brain wave patterns.
- Drugs that may affect test results include sedatives.

Procedure and patient care

Before
- Explain the procedure to the patient.
- Assure the patient that this test cannot "read the mind" or detect senility.
- Assure the patient that the flow of electrical activity is *from* the patient. He or she will not feel anything during the test.
- Instruct the patient to wash his or her hair the night before the test. No oils, sprays, or lotion should be used.
- Check if the physician wants to discontinue any medications before the study. (Anticonvulsants should be taken unless contraindicated by the physician.)
- Instruct the patient if sleeping time should be shortened the night before the test. Adults may not be allowed to sleep more than 4 or 5 hours, and children not more than 5 to 7 hours if a sleep EEG will be done.
- *Do not* administer any sedatives or hypnotics before the test because they will cause abnormal waves on the EEG.
- Inform the patient not to fast before the study. Fasting may cause hypoglycemia, which could alter test results.
- Instruct the patient not to drink any coffee, tea, cocoa, or cola on the morning of the test because of their stimulating effect.
- Tell the patient that he or she needs to remain still during the test. Any movement, including opening the eyes, will create interference and alter the EEG recording.

During
- Note the following procedural steps:
  1. The EEG is usually performed in a specially constructed room that is shielded from outside disturbances.
  2. The patient is placed in a supine position on a bed or reclining on a chair.
  3. Sixteen or more electrodes are applied to the scalp with electrode paste in a uniform pattern over both sides of the head, covering the prefrontal, frontal, temporal, parietal, and occipital areas.
  4. One electrode may be applied to each earlobe for grounding.
  5. After the electrodes are applied, the patient is instructed to lie still with his or her eyes closed.

6. The technician continuously observes the patient during the EEG recording for any movements that could alter results.

7. Approximately every 5 minutes, the recording is interrupted to permit the client to move if desired.

- In addition to the resting EEG, note that the following *activating procedures* can be performed:

  1. The patient is *hyperventilated* (asked to breathe deeply 20 times a minute for 3 minutes) to induce alkalosis and cerebral vasoconstriction, which can activate abnormalities.

  2. *Photostimulation* is performed by flashing a light over the patient's face with the eyes opened or closed. Photostimulated seizure activity may be seen on the EEG.

  3. *A sleep EEG* may be performed to aid in the detection of some abnormal brain waves that are seen only if the patient is sleeping (e.g., frontal lobe epilepsy). The sleep EEG is performed after orally administering methyprylon (Noludar) or chloral hydrate (Noctec). A recording is performed while the patient is falling asleep, while the patient is asleep, and while the patient is waking.

- Note that this study is performed by an EEG technician in approximately 45 minutes to 2 hours.

- Tell the patient that no discomfort is associated with this study, other than possibly missing sleep.

After

- Help the patient to remove the electrode paste. The paste may be removed with acetone or witch hazel.
- Instruct the patient to shampoo the hair.
- Ensure safety precautions until the effects of any sedatives have worn off. Keep the bed's siderails up.
- Tell the patient that one who has had a sleep EEG should not drive home alone.

Abnormal findings

Seizure disorders (e.g., epilepsy)
Brain tumor
Brain abscess
Head injury
Cerebral death

Encephalitis
Intracranial hemorrhage
Cerebral infarct
Narcolepsy
Alzheimer's disease

---

electromyography (EMG)

Type of test Electrodiagnostic

Normal findings No evidence of neuromuscular abnormalities

Test explanation and related physiology

By placing a recording electrode into a skeletal muscle, one can monitor the electrical activity of a skeletal muscle in a way very similar to electrocardiography. The electrical activity is displayed on an oscilloscope as an electrical waveform. An audioelectrical amplifier can be added to the system so that both the appearance and sound of the electrical potentials can be analyzed and compared simultaneously. EMG is used to detect primary muscular disorders, along with muscular abnormalities caused by other system diseases (e.g., nerve dysfunction, sarcoidosis, paraneoplastic syndrome).

Spontaneous muscle movement such as fibrillation and fasciculation can be detected during EMG. When seen, these waves indicate injury or disease of the nerve innervating that muscle or spastic myotonic muscle disease. Reduced amplitude size of the electrical waveform is indicative of a primary muscle disorder (e.g., polymyositis, muscular dystrophies, various myopathies). A progressive decrease in amplitude of the electrical waveform is a classic sign of myasthenia gravis. A decrease in the number of muscle fibers able to contract is seen with peripheral nerve damage. This study is usually done in conjunction with nerve conduction studies (see p. 348) and also may be called *electromyoneurography.*

Contraindications

- Patients receiving anticoagulant therapy
- Patients with extensive skin infection

Potential complication

- Rarely, hematoma at the needle insertion site

Interfering factors

- Edema, hemorrhage, or thick subcutaneous fat can interfere with test results.
- Patients with excessive pain may have false results.

Procedure and patient care

Before

- Explain the procedure to the patient. Allay any fears and allow the patient to express concerns.
- Obtain informed consent if required by the institution.
- Tell the patient that fasting is not usually required; however, some facilities may restrict stimulants (coffee, tea, cocoa, cola, cigarettes) for 2 to 3 hours before the test.
- If serum enzyme tests (e.g., AST [SGOT], CPK, LDH) are ordered, the specimen should be drawn before EMG or 5 to 10 days after the test, because the EMG may cause misleading elevations of these enzymes.
- Premedication or sedation is usually avoided because of the need for patient cooperation.

During

- Note the following procedural steps:
  1. This study is usually done in an EMG laboratory.
  2. The patient's position depends on the muscle being studied.
  3. A needle that acts as a recording electrode is inserted into the muscle being examined.
  4. A reference electrode is placed nearby on the skin surface.
  5. The patient is asked to keep the muscle at rest.
  6. The oscilloscope display is viewed for any evidence of spontaneous electrical activity such as fasciculation or fibrillation.
  7. The patient is asked to contract the muscle slowly and progressively.
  8. The electrical waves produced are examined for their number, form, and amplitude.
- Note that the EMG is performed by a physical therapist, physiatrist, or neurologist in approximately 20 minutes.
- Tell the patient that this test is moderately uncomfortable. Slight pain may occur with the insertion of the needle electrode.

After

- Observe the needle site for hematoma or inflammation.
- Provide pain medication if needed.

Abnormal findings

Polymyositis
Muscular dystrophy
Myopathy
Traumatic injury
Hyperadrenalism
Hypothyroidism
Paraneoplastic syndrome
  (e.g., lung cancer)
Sarcoidosis
Guillain-Barré syndrome
Myasthenia gravis

Peripheral nerve injury,
  entrapment, or compression
Spinal cord injury or disease
Acetylcholine blockers (e.g.,
  curare, snake venom)
Multiple sclerosis
Diabetic neuropathy
Anterior poliomyelitis
Muscle denervation
Amyotrophic lateral sclerosis

E

notes

electromyography of the pelvic floor sphincter
(Pelvic floor sphincter electromyography, Pelvic floor sphincter EMG, Rectal EMG procedure)

Type of test   Electrodiagnostic

Normal findings

Increased EMG signal during bladder filling

Silent EMG signal on voluntary micturition

Increased EMG signal at the end of voiding

Increased EMG signal with voluntary contraction of the anal sphincter

Test explanation and related physiology

This test uses the placement of electrodes on or in the pelvic floor musculature to evaluate the neuromuscular function of the urinary or anal sphincter. It is performed most often in patients who have urinary or fecal incontinence. The pathology causing the muscle weakness can be muscular or neurologic. With sphincter EMG, these two causes can be separated.

The main benefit of this study is to evaluate the external sphincter (skeletal muscle) activity during voiding. This test is also used to evaluate the bulbocavernous reflex and voluntary control of external sphincter or pelvic floor muscles. The pelvic floor sphincter EMG also aids in the investigation of "functional" or "psychologic" disturbances of voiding. Fecal incontinence caused by muscular dysfunction can also be evaluated by rectal sphincter EMG.

Recordings may be made from surface or needle electrodes within the muscle; surface electrodes are most often used. These electrodes allow for observation of and change in the muscle activity before and during voiding.

Patient cooperation is essential. If the patient does not cooperate, the interpretation of the test results will be difficult.

Contraindications

- Patients who cannot cooperate during the procedure

Procedure and patient care

Before

- Explain the procedure to the patient.
- Inform the patient that cooperation is essential.

During

- Note the following procedural steps:
  1. Two electrodes are placed at the 2 o'clock and 10 o'clock positions on the perianal skin to monitor the pelvic floor musculature during voiding.
  2. The third electrode is usually placed on the thigh and serves as a ground.
  3. Electrical activity is recorded with the bladder empty and the patient relaxed.
  4. Reflex activity is evaluated by asking the patient to cough and by stimulating the urethra and trigone by gently tugging on an inserted Foley catheter (bulbocavernous reflex).
  5. Voluntary activity is evaluated by asking the patient to contract and relax the sphincter muscle.
  6. The bladder is filled with sterile water at room temperature at a rate of 100 ml/min.
  7. The EMG responses to filling and detrusor hyperreflexia (if present) are recorded.
  8. Finally, when the bladder is full and with the patient in a voiding position, the filling catheter is removed, and the patient is asked to urinate. In the normal patient the EMG signals build during bladder filling and cease promptly on voluntary micturition, remaining silent until the pelvic floor contracts at the end of voiding.
  9. The electrical waves produced are examined for their number and form.
- Note that a urologist performs this study in less than 30 minutes.
- Explain to the patient that this study is slightly more uncomfortable than urethral catheterization.

After

- If needle electrodes were used, observe the needle site for hematoma or inflammation.

Abnormal findings

Neuromuscular dysfunction of lower urinary sphincter
Pelvic floor muscle dysfunction of the anal sphincter

electroneurography (ENG, Nerve conduction studies)

Type of test Electrodiagnostic

Normal findings

No evidence of peripheral nerve injury or disease
(Conduction velocity is usually decreased in the elderly.)

Test explanation and related physiology

Electroneurography, or nerve conduction studies, allow for
the detection and location of peripheral nerve injury or disease.
By initiating an electrical impulse at one site (proximal) of a
nerve and recording the time required for that impulse to travel
to a second site (distal) of the same nerve, the conduction
velocity of any impulse in that nerve can be determined. This
study is usually done in conjunction with electromyography (see
p. 343) and also may be called *electromyoneurography*.

The normal value for conduction velocity varies from one
nerve to another. Individual variation also exists. It is always
best to compare the conduction velocity of the suspected side
with the contralateral nerve conduction velocity. In general, a
range of normal conduction velocity will be approximately 50
to 60 m/sec.

Traumatic transection or contusion of a nerve will usually
cause maximal slowing of conduction velocity in the affected side
as compared with the normal side. Neuropathies, both local and
generalized, also will cause a slowing of conduction velocity. A
velocity greater than normal does not indicate a pathologic
condition.

Because conduction velocity may require contraction of a
muscle as an indication of an impulse arriving at the recording
electrode, primary muscular disorders may cause a falsely slow
nerve conduction velocity. This "muscular" variable is eliminated if one evaluates the suspected pathologic muscle group
before performing nerve conduction studies. This muscular
factor can be evaluated by measuring *distal latency* (i.e., the time
required for stimulation of the distal end of the nerve to cause
muscular contraction). Once the distal latency is calculated, the
nerve conduction study is then performed normally by stimulat-

ing the proximal part of the nerve bundle. Conduction velocity can then be determined by the following equation:

$$\text{Conduction velocity (in meters per second)} = \frac{\text{Distance in (meters)}}{\text{Total latency} - \text{Distal latency}}$$

Interfering factor

- Patients in severe pain may have false results.

Procedure and patient care

Before

- Explain the procedure to the patient. Allay any fears and allow the patient to express concerns.
- Obtain informed consent if required by the institution.
- Tell the patient that no fasting or sedation is usually required.

During

- Note the following procedural steps:
    1. This test can be performed in a nerve conduction laboratory or at the patient's bedside.
    2. The patient's position depends on the area of suspected peripheral nerve injury or disease.
    3. A recording electrode is placed on the skin overlying a muscle innervated solely by the relevant nerve.
    4. A reference electrode is placed nearby.
    5. All skin-to-electrode connections are ensured by using electrical paste.
    6. The nerve is stimulated by a shock-emitting device at an adjacent location.
    7. The time between nerve impulse and muscular contraction (distal latency) is measured in milliseconds on an EMG machine.
    8. The nerve is similarly stimulated at a location proximal to the area of suspected injury or disease.
    9. The time required for the impulse to travel from the site of initiation to muscle contraction (total latency) is recorded in milliseconds.
    10. The distance between the site of stimulation and the recording electrode is measured in centimeters.
    11. Conduction velocity is converted to meters per second and is computed as in the previous equation.
- Note that this test takes approximately 15 minutes and is performed by a physiatrist or a neurologist.

- Tell the patient that this test is uncomfortable in that a mild shock is required for nerve impulse stimulation.

After
- Remove the electrode gel from the patient's skin.

Abnormal findings

Peripheral nerve injury or disease
Carpal tunnel syndrome
Herniated disc disease

Poliomyelitis
Diabetic neuropathy
Myasthenia gravis
Guillain-Barré syndrome

notes

electronystagmography

Type of test Electrodiagnostic

Normal findings
Normal nystagmus response
Normal oculovestibular reflex

Test explanation and related physiology

Electronystagmography is used to evaluate nystagmus (involuntary rapid eye movement) and the muscles controlling eye movement. By measuring changes in the electrical field around the eye, this study can make a permanent recording of eye movement at rest, with a change in head position, and in response to various stimuli. The test delineates the presence or absence of nystagmus, which is caused by the initiation of the oculovestibular reflex. Nystagmus should occur when initiated by positional, visual, or caloric (see p. 195) stimuli. Unlike caloric studies in which nystagmus is usually determined visually, with ENG the direction, velocity, and degree of nystagmus can be recorded electrically.

If nystagmus does not occur with stimulation, the vestibular-cochlear apparatus, cerebral cortex (temporal lobe), auditory nerve, or brain stem is abnormal. Tumors, infection, ischemia, and degeneration can cause such abnormalities. When put together with the entire clinical picture, the pattern of nystagmus helps in the differentiation between central and peripheral vertigo. This test is used in the differential diagnosis of lesions in the vestibular system, brain stem, and cerebellum.

This study also may help evaluate unilateral hearing loss and vertigo. Unilateral hearing loss may be caused by middle ear problems or nerve injury. If the patient experiences nystagmus with stimulation, the auditory nerve is working, and hearing loss can be blamed on the middle ear.

Contraindications

- Patients with perforated eardrums, who should not have water irrigation
- Patients with pacemakers

Interfering factors

- Blinking of the eyes can alter test results.
- Drugs that can alter results include sedatives, stimulants, and antivertigo agents.

Procedure and patient care

Before

- Explain the procedure to the patient.
- Instruct the patient not to apply facial makeup before the test because electrodes will be taped to the skin around the eyes.
- Hold solid food before the test to reduce the likelihood of vomiting.
- Instruct the patient not to drink caffeine or alcoholic beverages for approximately 24 to 48 hours (as ordered) before the test.
- Check with the physician regarding withholding any medications that could interfere with the test results.

During

- Note the following procedural steps:
  1. This procedure is usually performed in a darkened room with the patient seated or lying down on an examining table.
  2. If there is any wax in the ear, it is removed.
  3. Electrodes are taped to the skin around the eyes.
  4. Various procedures are used to stimulate nystagmus, such as pendulum tracking, changing head position, changing gaze position, and caloric tests (see p. 195).
  5. Several recordings are made with the patient at rest and to demonstrate patient response to various procedures (e.g., blowing air into the ear, irrigating the ear with water).
  6. Nystagmus response is compared with the expected ranges, and the results are recorded as normal, borderline, or abnormal.
- Note that this procedure is performed by a physician or audiologist in approximately 1 hour.
- Tell the patient that nausea and vomiting may occur during the test.

After

- Consider prescribing bed rest until nausea, vertigo, or weakness subsides.

Abnormal findings

Brain stem lesions
Cerebellum lesions
VIII cranial nerve injury

Vestibular system lesions
Congenital disorder
Demyelinating disease

notes

E

electrophysiologic study (EPS, Cardiac mapping)

Type of test Electrodiagnostic; manometric

Normal findings Normal conduction intervals, refractive periods, and recovery times

Tilt-table testing

<20 mm Hg decrease in systolic blood pressure and <10 mm increase in diastolic blood pressure. Heart rate increase should be less than 10 beats/min.

Test explanation and related physiology

In this invasive procedure, multiple electrode catheters are fluoroscopically placed through a peripheral vein and into the right atrium and/or ventricle or, less often, through an artery into the left atrium and/or ventricle. With close cardiac monitoring, the electrode catheters are used to pace the heart and potentially induce arrhythmias. Defects in the heart conduction system can then be identified; arrhythmias that are otherwise inapparent also can be induced, identified, and treated. The effectiveness of the antiarrhythmic drugs (e.g., lidocaine, phenytoin, quinidine) can be assessed by determining the electrical threshold required to induce arrhythmias.

EPS can be also be therapeutic. With the use of radiofrequency, sites with documented low thresholds for inducing arrhythmias can be obliterated to stop the arrhythmias.

The *tilt-table test* is sometimes performed with an electrophysiologic cardiac study and is a provocative test used to diagnose vasopressor syncope syndrome. Patients with this syndrome usually demonstrate symptomatic hypotension and syncope within a few to 30 minutes of being tilted upright by approximately 60 to 80 degrees. The tilt-table test is often used to assess the efficacy of prophylactic pacing in some patients with vasopressor syncope. It is also used to evaluate the impact of posture with some forms of tachyarrhythmias. Normally a minimal drop in systolic blood pressure, rise in diastolic blood pressure, and increase in heart rate occur in the tilted position. Patients with vasopressor syncope demonstrate these changes in an exaggerated fashion and become lightheaded and dizzy on assuming the tilted position.

Contraindications

- Patients who are uncooperative
- Patients with acute myocardial infarction

Potential complications

- Cardiac arrhythmias leading to ventricular tachycardia or fibrillation
- Perforation of the myocardium
- Catheter-induced embolic cerebrovascular accident (stroke) or myocardial infarction
- Peripheral vascular problems
- Hemorrhage
- Phlebitis at the venipuncture site

Interfering factors

- Patients with dehydration or hypovolemia demonstrate similar changes in blood pressure and heart rate with tilt-table testing. This is especially true in elderly patients.
- Patients on antihypertensive medications or diuretics also may demonstrate similar changes when placed in the tilt position.
- Drugs that may interfere with test results include analgesics, sedatives, and tranquilizers.

Procedure and patient care

Before

- Instruct the patient to fast for 6 to 8 hours before the procedure. Usually fluids are permitted until 3 hours before the test.
- Obtain an informed consent from the patient.
- Encourage the patient to verbalize any fears regarding this test.
- Shave and prepare the catheter insertion site.
- Collect a blood sample for potassium or drug levels if indicated.
- Obtain peripheral IV access for the administration of drugs.
- Often, an arterial line is placed to accurately monitor blood pressure during tilt-table testing.
- Inquire as to whether the patient has had excessive fluid loss (diarrhea or vomiting) in the previous 24 hours.
- Record antihypertensive or diuretic medicines that the patient may be taking.

During

- Note the following procedural steps:

Electrophysiologic study

1. After being transported to the cardiac catheterization laboratory, the patient has electrocardiographic (ECG) leads attached.
2. The catheter insertion site, usually the femoral vein, is prepared and draped in a sterile manner.
3. Under fluoroscopic guidance the catheter is passed to the atrium and ventricle.
4. Baseline surface intracardiac ECGs are recorded.
5. Various parts of the cardiac electroconduction system are stimulated by atrial or ventricular pacing.
6. Mapping of the electroconduction system and its defects is performed.
7. Arrhythmias are identified.
8. Drugs may be administered to assess their efficacy in preventing EPS-induced arrhythmias.
9. Because dangerous arrhythmias can be prolonged, cardioversion must be immediately available.
10. Not only are vital signs and the heart monitored, the patient is constantly engaged in light conversation to assess mental status and consciousness.

Tilt-table test

1. The patient lies supine on a horizontal tilt table.
2. Obtain the patient's blood pressure and pulse as baseline values before tilting is carried out.
3. Monitor these vital signs during the procedure.
4. Question the patient as to the presence of symptoms of dizziness and lightheadedness.
5. The table is progressively tilted to 60 to 80 while the patient is being monitored. Alternatively, the patient is asked to sit or stand.

- Tell the patient that he or she may experience palpitations, light-headedness, or dizziness when arrhythmias are induced. Report these sensations to the physician. For most patients this is an anxiety-producing experience.
- Inform the patient that discomfort from catheter insertion is minimal.

After

- Keep the patient on bed rest for approximately 6 to 8 hours.
- Evaluate the venous/arterial access site for swelling and bleeding.
- Monitor the patient's vital signs for at least 2 to 4 hours for hypotension and arrhythmias. Additional monitoring is especially important for certain medications that the patient received during the test. For example, if the patient received quinidine, he or she should be monitored for hypotension and abdominal cramping.
- Continue cardiac monitoring to identify arrhythmias. Transfer arrangements to a monitored unit may be necessary.
- Cover the area with sterile dressings if the electrical catheter is left in place for subsequent studies.

Abnormal findings

Electroconduction defects
Cardiac arrhythmia
Sinoatrial node defects (e.g., sick sinus syndrome)
Atrioventricular node defects and heart blocks
Vasomotor syncope syndrome

notes

endometrial biopsy

Type of test Microscopic examination of tissue

Normal findings

No pathologic conditions
Presence of a "secretory-type" endometrium 3 to 5 days before
  normal menses

Test explanation and related physiology

An endometrial biopsy can determine whether ovulation has
occurred. A biopsy specimen taken 3 to 5 days before normal
menses should demonstrate a "secretory-type" endometrium on
histologic examination if ovulation and corpus luteum formation
have occurred. If not, only a preovulatory "proliferative-type"
endometrium will be seen.

Occasionally an endometrial biopsy is performed to indicate
estrogen's effect in patients with suspected ovarian dysfunction
or absence. Similarly, adequate circulating progesterone levels
can be determined by identifying secretory endometrium.
Another major use of endometrial biopsy is to diagnose
endometrial cancer, tuberculosis, polyps, or inflammatory conditions and to evaluate uterine bleeding.

Contraindications

- Patients with infections (e.g., trichomonal, candidal, or suspected gonococcal) of the cervix or vagina
- Patients in whom the cervix cannot be visualized (e.g.,
  because of abnormal position or previous surgery)

Potential complications

- Perforation of the uterus
- Uterine bleeding
- Interference with early pregnancy
- Infection

Procedure and patient care

Before

- Explain the procedure to the patient.
- Ensure that written and informed consent for this procedure
  is obtained from the patient.
- Tell the patient that no fasting or sedation is usually required.

During

- Note the following procedural steps:
  1. The patient is placed in the lithotomy position, and a pelvic examination is performed to determine the position of the uterus.
  2. The cervix is exposed and cleansed.
  3. A biopsy instrument is inserted into the uterus; and specimens are obtained from the anterior, posterior, and lateral walls. This can be performed as a part of a D&C or hysteroscopy (p. 489).
  4. The specimens are placed in a solution containing 10% formalin solution and sent to the pathologist for histologic examination.
- Note that this procedure is performed by an obstetrician/gynecologist in approximately 10 to 30 minutes.
- Tell the patient that this procedure may cause momentary discomfort (menstrual-type cramping).

After

- Assess the patient's vital signs at regular intervals for the next 48 hours. Any temperature elevation should be reported to the physician, because this procedure may activate pelvic inflammatory disease.
- Advise the patient to wear a pad, because some vaginal bleeding is to be expected. Instruct the patient to call her physician if excessive bleeding (requiring more than one pad per hour) occurs.
- Inform the patient that douching and intercourse are not permitted for 72 hours after the biopsy specimen removal.
- Instruct the patient to rest during the next 24 hours and to avoid heavy lifting to prevent uterine hemorrhage.

🏠 Home care responsibilities

- Instruct the patient to report any temperature elevation to her physician because this procedure may activate pelvic inflammatory disease (PID).
- Advise the patient to wear a sanitary pad after this procedure. Tell the patient to call her physician for excessive bleeding (< pad per hour).
- Tell the patient to avoid heavy lifting after this procedure to prevent increased intra-abdominal pressure and possible uterine bleeding.

Abnormal findings

Anovulation
Tumor
Tuberculosis
Polyps
Inflammatory condition

notes

endoscopic retrograde cholangiopancreatography
(ERCP, ERCP of the biliary and pancreatic ducts)

Type of test Endoscopy

Normal findings

Normal size of biliary and pancreatic ducts
No obstruction or filling defects within the biliary or pancreatic
   ducts

Test explanation and related physiology

With the use of a fiberoptic endoscope, ERCP provides radiographic visualization of the bile and pancreatic ducts. This is especially useful in patients with jaundice. If a partial or total obstruction of those ducts exists, characteristics of the obstructing lesion can be demonstrated. Stones, benign strictures, cysts, ampullary stenosis, anatomic variations, and malignant tumors can be identified. Only ERCP and percutaneous transhepatic cholangiography (PTHC) can provide direct visualization of the biliary and pancreatic ducts. PTHC (see p. 627) is an invasive procedure with significant morbidity; ERCP is associated with much less morbidity but must be performed by an experienced endoscopist.

In contrast to an oral cholecystogram or an IV cholangiogram, which does not visualize the biliary tree when high levels of bilirubin are present, the biliary ducts of jaundiced patients can be visualized by ERCP. As a result, this test is extremely important in the evaluation of patients with jaundice.

Incision of the papillary muscle in the ampulla of Vater can be performed through the scope at the time of ERCP. This incision widens the distal common duct so that common bile duct gallstones can be removed. Stents can be placed through strictured bile ducts with the use of ERCP, and the bile of jaundiced patients can be internally drained. Pieces of tissue and brushings of the common bile duct can be obtained by ERCP for pathologic review. Manometric studies of the sphincter of Oddi and pancreaticobiliary ducts can be performed at the time of ERCP. These are used to investigate unusual function abnormalities of these structures.

Contraindications

- Patients who are uncooperative
  Cannulation of the ampulla of Vater requires that the patient lie very still.
- Patients whose ampulla of Vater is not accessible endoscopically because of previous upper gastrointestinal surgery (e.g., gastrectomy patients whose duodenum containing the ampulla is surgically separated from the stomach)
- Patients with esophageal diverticula
  The scope can fall into a diverticulum and perforate its wall.
- Patients with known acute pancreatitis

Potential complications

- Perforation of the esophagus, stomach, or duodenum
- Gram-negative sepsis
  This results from introducing bacteria through the biliary system and into the blood. Usually this occurs in patients who have obstructive jaundice.
- Pancreatitis
  This results from pressure of the dye injection.
- Aspiration of gastric contents into the lungs
- Respiratory arrest as a result of oversedation

Interfering factor

- Barium within the abdomen as a result of a previous upper GI series or barium enema x-ray studies precludes adequate visualization of the biliary and pancreatic ducts.

Procedure and patient care

Before

- Explain the procedure to the patient.
- Obtain informed consent from the patient.
- Inform the patient that breathing will not be compromised by the insertion of the endoscope.
- Keep the patient NPO as of midnight the day of the test.
- Administer appropriate premedication (e.g., midazolam [Versed] and atropine) if ordered.

During

- Note the following procedural steps:
  1. A flat plate of the abdomen is taken to ensure that any barium from previous studies will not obscure visualization of the bile duct.

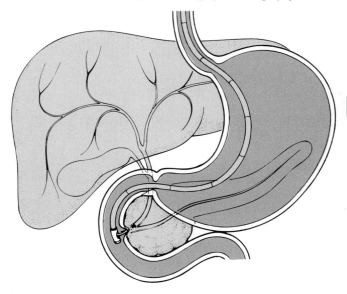

Figure 16 Endoscopic retrograde cholangiopancreatography. The fiberoptic scope is passed into the duodenum. Note the small catheter being advanced into the biliary duct.

2. The patient is placed in the supine position or on the left side.
3. The patient is usually sedated with a narcotic and a sedative/hypnotic.
4. The pharynx is sprayed with a local anesthetic (lidocaine [Xylocaine]) to inactivate the gag reflex and to lessen the discomfort caused by the passage of the scope.
5. A side-viewing fiberoptic duodenoscope is inserted through the oral pharynx and passed through the esophagus and stomach and into the duodenum (Figure 16).
6. Glucagon is often administered intravenously to minimize the spasm of the duodenum and to improve visualization of the ampulla of Vater.
7. Through the accessory lumen within the scope, a small

catheter is passed through the ampulla and into the common bile or pancreatic ducts.

8. Radiographic dye is injected, and x-ray films are taken.

- Note that the test usually takes approximately 1 hour and is performed by a physician trained in endoscopy. The x-ray films are interpreted by the radiologist.
- Tell the patient that no discomfort is associated with the dye injection but that minimal gagging may occur during the initial introduction of the scope into the oral pharynx.

After

- Do *not* allow the patient to eat or drink until the gag reflex returns.
- Observe the patient closely for development of abdominal pain, nausea, and vomiting. This may herald the onset of ERCP-induced pancreatitis.
- Observe safety precautions until the effects of the sedatives have worn off.
- Monitor the patient for signs of respiratory depression. Medication (e.g., naloxone [Narcan]) should be available to counteract serious respiratory depression. Resuscitative equipment should also be present.
- Assess the patient for signs and symptoms of septicemia, which may indicate the onset of ERCP-induced cholangitis.
- Inform the patient that he or she may be hoarse and have a sore throat for several days. Drinking cool fluids and gargling will help to relieve some of this soreness.

🏠 Home care responsibilities

- A sore throat is expected. A soothing mouth wash gargle may help.
- Notify the physician immediately if increasing abdominal pain, nausea or vomiting occurs. These may be the early signs of pancreatitis or gastroduodenal perforation.
- Notify the physician immediately of fever or shaking chills. This may indicate possible cholangitis.
- Encourage the patient to eat lightly for the next 12 to 24 hours.

Abnormal findings

Tumor, strictures, or gallstones of the common bile duct

Sclerosing cholangitis

Biliary sclerosis

Cysts of the common bile duct

Tumor, strictures, or inflammation of the pancreatic duct

Pseudocyst of the pancreatic duct

Chronic pancreatitis

Anatomic biliary or pancreatic duct variations

Cancer of the duodenum or ampulla

E

notes

Epstein-Barr virus titer (EBV)

Type of test Blood

Normal findings

Titers ≤1:10 are nondiagnostic.

Titers of 1:10 to 1:60 indicate infection at some undetermined time.

Titers of 1:320 or greater suggest active infection.

Fourfold increase in titer in paired sera drawn 10 to 14 days apart is usually indicative of an acute infection.

Test explanation and related physiology

EBV infects 80% of the U.S. population. Once infection occurs, the virus becomes dormant but can be reactivated later. EBV infection can produce infectious mononucleosis (IM). Mononucleosis is seen most often in children, adolescents, and young adults. Clinical features include those of acute fatigue, fever, sore throat, lymphadenopathy, and splenomegaly. Laboratory findings of lymphocytosis, atypical lymphocytes, and the development of transient serum heterophil antibodies are found in patients with acute EBV infection. Most patients with infectious mononucleosis recover uneventfully and return to normal activity within 4 to 6 weeks. In Africa EBV has been associated with Burkitt's lymphoma. In China EBV infection has been associated with nasopharyngeal carcinoma.

After recovery from primary EBV infection, a lifelong latent EBV-carrier status is established. In the last several years, specific immunologic tests to identify EBV activity indicate that latent EBV can reactivate and become associated with a constellation of chronic signs and symptoms resembling infectious mononucleosis. Clinical manifestations of chronic EBV are variable and include nonspecific symptoms, such as profound fatigue, pharyngitis, myalgia, arthralgia, low-grade fever, headache, paresthesia, and loss of abstract thinking.

Serologic tests are the only way to make the diagnosis of EBV. The heterophil agglutination slide test (monospot test) is explained on p. 580. Other, more specific immunologic tests indicate more precisely the timing of the infection (Table 11). The viral capsid antigen-antibodies (VCAs) can be IgG or IgM. The EBV nuclear antigen (EBNA) is located in the nuclei of the infected lymphocyte. Another EBV antigen is called the early

TABLE 11 Serologic studies and the timing of infections

Serologic study	Appears/disappears	Clinical significance
Mono spot heterophil	5 days/2 weeks	Acute or convalescent infection
VCA-IgM	7 days/3 months	Acute or convalescent infection
VCA-IgG	7 days/exists for life	Acute, convalescent, or old infection
EBNA-IgG	3 weeks/exists for life	Old infection
EA-D	7 days/2 weeks	Acute or convalescent infection

E

antigen (EA). There are two EA antigens. One is spread diffusely about the cytoplasm of the infected cell (EA-D), and the other is restricted to only one area of the cytoplasm (EA-R). The EA-D is commonly found in nasopharyngeal cancer. The EA-R is commonly found in Burkitt's lymphoma.

The interpretation of EBV antibody tests is based on the following assumptions:

1. Once the person becomes infected with EBV, the anti-VCA antibodies appear first.
2. Anti-EA (EA-D or EA-R) antibodies appear next or are present with anti-VCA antibodies early in the course of illness. An anti-EA antibody titer greater than 80 in a patient 2 years after acute infectious mononucleosis indicates chronic EBV syndrome.
3. As the patient recovers, anti-VCA and anti-EA antibodies decrease, and anti-EBNA antibodies appear. Anti-EBNA antibody persists for life and reflects a past infection.
4. After the patient is well, anti-VCA and anti-EBNA antibodies are always present but at lower ranges. Occasionally anti-EA antibody also may be present after the patient recovers.

If an acute infection is suspected to have occurred more than a few weeks before testing, the monospot may be negative. Detecting anti VCA-IgG or EBNA will not be helpful because it indicates that an EBV infection has occurred sometime in the patient's life—not necessarily the recent syndrome. But detecting anti VCA-IgM would indicate that the syndrome of complaint the patient experienced a few weeks earlier was due to EBV.

Procedure and patient care

Before

- Explain the procedure to the patient.
- Tell the patient that no fasting or special preparation is required.

During

- Collect 5 to 10 ml of venous blood in a red-top tube.
- Record the day of onset of illness on the laboratory slip.
- Obtain serum samples as soon as possible after the onset of the illness.
- Obtain a second blood specimen 14 to 21 days later.

After

- Apply pressure to the venipuncture site.

Abnormal findings

Infectious mononucleosis
Chronic fatigue syndrome
Chronic EBV carrier state
Burkitt's lymphoma
Nasopharyngeal cancer

notes

erythrocyte sedimentation rate (ESR, Sed rate test)

Type of test Blood

Normal findings

Westergren method
Male: up to 15 mm/hr
Female: up to 20 mm/hr
Child: up to 10 mm/hr
Newborn: 0-2 mm/hr

Test explanation and related physiology

ESR is a measurement of the rate with which the red blood cells (RBCs) settle in saline or plasma over a specified time period. It is nonspecific and therefore not diagnostic for any particular organ disease or injury. Because acute and chronic infection, inflammation (collagen-vascular diseases), advanced neoplasm, and tissue necrosis or infarction increase the protein (mainly fibrinogen) content of plasma, RBCs have a tendency to stack up on one another, increasing their weight and causing them to descend faster. Therefore in these diseases the ESR is increased. ESR is considered an "acute-phase" or a "reactant" protein (i.e., it occurs as a reaction to acute illnesses as described previously).

The test can be used to detect occult disease. Many physicians use the ESR test in this way for routine patient evaluation for vague symptoms. Other physicians regard this test as so nonspecific that it is useless as a routine study. The ESR test occasionally can be helpful in differentiating disease entities or complaints. For example, in the patient with chest pain, the ESR will be increased with myocardial infarction but will be normal with angina.

The ESR is a fairly reliable indicator of the course of disease and therefore can be used to monitor disease therapy, especially for inflammatory autoimmune diseases such as temporal arteritis or polymyalgia rheumatica. In general, as the disease worsens, the ESR increases; as the disease improves, the ESR decreases. If the results of the ESR are equivocal or inconsistent with the clinical impressions, the C-reactive protein test (see p. 288) is often performed.

Interfering factors

- Artificially low results can occur when the collected specimen is allowed to stand longer than 3 hours before the testing.
- Pregnancy (second and third trimester) can cause elevated levels.
- Menstruation can cause elevated levels.
- Polycythemia is associated with decreased ESR.
- ✶ Drugs that may cause *increased* ESR levels include dextran, methyldopa (Aldomet), oral contraceptives, penicillamine, procainamide, theophylline, and vitamin A.
- ✶ Drugs that may cause *decreased* levels include aspirin, cortisone, and quinine.

Procedure and patient care

Before

- Explain the procedure to the patient.
- Hold medications that may affect test results if indicated.

During

- Collect approximately 5 to 10 ml of venous blood in a lavender-top tube.

After

- Apply pressure to the venipuncture site.
- Transport the specimen immediately to the laboratory.

Abnormal findings

▲ **Increased levels**
  Chronic renal failure
  Malignant diseases
  Bacterial infection
  Inflammatory diseases
  Necrotic tissue diseases
  Hyperfibrinogenemia
  Macroglobulinemia
  Severe anemias such as
    iron deficiency or B_{12}
    deficiency

▼ **Decreased levels**
  Sickle cell anemia
  Spherocytosis
  Hypofibrinogenemia
  Polycythemia vera

esophageal function studies (Esophageal manometry, Esophageal motility studies)

Type of test Manometric

Normal findings

Lower esophageal sphincter pressure: 10-20 mm Hg
Swallowing pattern: Normal peristaltic waves
Acid reflux: Negative
Acid clearing: <10 swallows
Bernstein test: Negative

Test explanation and related physiology

Esophageal function studies include the following:
1. Determination of the *lower esophageal sphincter* (LES) pressure (manometry).
2. Graphic recording of esophageal swallowing waves, or *swallowing pattern* (manometry).
3. Detection of reflux of gastric acid back into the esophagus (acid reflux).
4. Detection of the ability of the esophagus to clear acid (acid clearing).
5. An attempt to reproduce symptoms of heartburn (Bernstein test).

Manometry studies

Two manometry studies are used in assessing esophageal function: (1) measurement of LES pressure, and (2) graphic recording of swallowing waves (motility). The LES is a sphincter muscle that acts as a valve to prevent reflux of gastric acid into the esophagus. Free reflux of gastric acid occurs when the sphincter pressures are low. An example of such a disorder in adults is gastroesophageal reflux; in children it is called chalasia (incompetent or relaxed LES).

With increased sphincter pressure, as found in patients with achalasia (failure of the LES to relax normally with swallowing) and diffuse esophageal spasms, food cannot pass from the esophagus into the stomach. Increased LES pressures are noted on manometry. In achalasia few if any swallowing waves are detected. In contrast, diffuse esophageal spasm is characterized by strong, frequent, asynchronous, and nonpropulsive waves.

Acid reflux with pH probe

Acid reflux is the primary component of gastroesophageal reflux. Patients with an incompetent LES will regurgitate gastric acid into the esophagus. This will then cause a drop in pH testing done by the pH probe. With the newer and smaller catheters, 24-hour pH monitoring can be performed. Episodes of acid reflux are evident. If they coincide with patient symptoms of chest pain, esophagitis can be incriminated.

Acid clearing

Patients with normal esophageal function can completely clear hydrochloric acid from the esophagus in less than 10 swallows. Patients with decreased esophageal motility (frequently caused by severe esophagitis) require a greater number of swallows to clear the acid.

Bernstein test (acid perfusion)

The Bernstein test is simply an attempt to reproduce the symptoms of gastroesophageal reflux. If the patient suffers pain with the instillation of hydrochloric acid into the esophagus, the test is positive and proves that the patient's symptoms are caused by reflux esophagitis. If the patient has no discomfort, a cause other than esophageal reflux must be sought to explain the patient's discomfort.

Contraindications

- Patients who cannot cooperate
- Patients who are medically unstable

Potential complication

- Aspiration of gastric contents

Interfering factors

- Eating shortly before the test may affect results.
- Drugs such as sedatives can alter test results.

Procedure and patient care

Before

- Explain the procedure to the patient.
- Instruct the patient not to eat or drink anything for at least 8 hours before the test.
- Allay any fears and allow the patient to verbalize concerns. Be sensitive to the patient's fears about choking during the procedure.

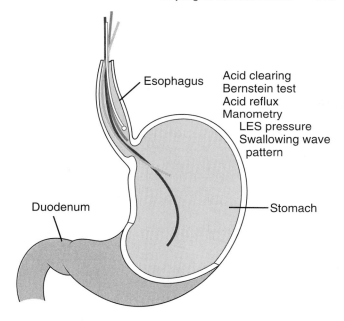

Figure 17 Esophageal function studies demonstrating placement of manometry tubes and a pH probe within the esophagus. *LES,* lower esophageal sphincter.

During

- Note the following procedural steps:
  1. Esophageal studies are usually performed in the endoscopy laboratory.
  2. The fasting, unsedated patient is asked to swallow two or three very tiny tubes. The tubes are equipped so that pressure measurements can be taken at 5-cm intervals (Figure 17).
  3. The outer ends of the tubes are attached to a pressure transducer.
  4. All tubes are passed into the stomach; then three tubes are slowly pulled back into the esophagus. A rapid and extreme increase in the pressure readings indicates the high-pressure zone of the LES.
  5. The LES pressure is recorded.

6. With all tubes in the esophagus, the patient is asked to swallow. Motility wave patterns are recorded.
7. The pH indicator probe is placed in the esophagus.
8. The patient's stomach is filled with approximately 100 ml of 0.1-N hydrochloric acid. A decrease in the pH of the esophageal pH probe indicates gastroesophageal reflux.
9. Hydrochloric acid is instilled into the esophagus, and the patient is asked to swallow. The number of swallows is counted to determine acid clearing. More than 10 swallows to clear the acid (as determined by the pH probe) indicates decreased esophageal motility.
10. Finally, 0.1-N hydrochloric acid and saline solution are alternately instilled into the esophagus for the Bernstein test. The patient is not told which solution is being infused. If the patient volunteers symptoms of discomfort while the acid is running, the test is considered positive. If no discomfort is recognized, the test is negative.

- Note that these tests are performed by an esophageal technician in approximately 30 minutes.
- Inform the patient that the test results are interpreted by a physician and will be available in a few hours.
- Tell the patient that, except for some initial gagging when swallowing the tubes, these tests are not uncomfortable.

After

- Inform the patient that it is not unusual to have a mild sore throat after placement of the tubes.

Abnormal findings

Presbyesophagus

Diffuse esophageal spasm

Chalasia

Achalasia

Gastroesophageal reflux

Reflux esophagitis

notes

esophagogastroduodenoscopy (EGD, Upper gastrointestinal [UGI] endoscopy, Gastroscopy)

Type of test Endoscopy

Normal findings Normal esophagus, stomach, and duodenum

Test explanation and related physiology

Endoscopy enables direct visualization of the upper gastrointestinal (GI) tract by means of a long, flexible, fiberoptic-lighted scope. The esophagus, stomach, and duodenum are examined for tumors, varices, mucosal inflammations, hiatal hernias, polyps, ulcers, and obstructions. The endoscope has one to three channels. The first channel is used for viewing, the second for insufflation of air and aspiration of fluid, and the third for passing cable-activated instruments to perform a biopsy of suspected pathologic tissue. Probes also can be passed through the third channel to allow for coagulation or injection of sclerosing agents to areas of active GI bleeding. A laser beam can pass through the endoscope to perform endoscopic surgery (e.g., obliteration of tumors or polyps, control of bleeding), and the fiberoptics of endoscopy are so refined that video images and "still pictures" can be taken.

This test is used to visualize the lumen of the esophagus, stomach, and duodenum. It is used to evaluate patients with dysphagia, weight loss, early satiety, upper abdominal pain, "ulcer symptoms" or dyspepsia. It is also used to detect esophageal varices in alcoholics. Suspicious barium swallow or upper GI x-ray findings can be corroborated by EGD.

With endoscopy, one can not only evaluate the esophagus, stomach, and duodenum, but with the use of an extralong fiberoptic endoscope, one can also visualize and perform a biopsy of tissue in the upper small intestinal tract. This procedure is referred to as *enteroscopy*. Abnormalities of the small intestine such as arteriovenous (AV) malformations, tumors, enteropathies (e.g., celiac disease), and ulcerations can be diagnosed with enteroscopy.

Besides being much more sensitive and specific than an upper GI series in diagnosing diseases of the esophagus, stomach, and duodenum, EGD also can be used therapeutically. An experienced endoscopist often can control active GI bleeding by electrocoagulation, laser coagulation, or the injection of sclerosing agents such as alcohol. Also, with the endoscope, benign and malignant strictures can be dilated to reestablish patency of the upper GI tract. Biliary stents and a percutaneous gastrostomy can be placed with the use of EGD. The role of endoscopic surgery is expanding in light of its dramatic success and minimal morbidity.

Contraindications

- Patients who cannot cooperate fully
  As in all studies that require technical finesse, patient cooperation is essential for successful, safe, and accurate test completion.
- Patients with severe upper GI bleeding
  The viewing lens will become covered with blood clots, preventing adequate visualization. If the stomach can be lavaged and aspirated to clear the blood clots, however, EGD can be performed.
- Patients with esophageal diverticula
  The scope can easily fall into the diverticulum and perforate the wall of the esophagus.
- Patients with suspected perforation
  The perforation can be worsened by the insufflation of pressurized air into the GI tract.
- Patients who have had recent GI surgery
  The anastomosis may not be able to withstand the pressure of the required air insufflation. This may lead to anastomotic disruption.

Potential complications

- Perforation of the esophagus, stomach, and duodenum
- Bleeding from a biopsy site
- Pulmonary aspiration of gastric contents
- Oversedation from the medication administered during the test
- Hypotension induced by the sedative medication
  Usually, however, the patient already has some significant element of hypovolemia or dehydration.
- Local IV phlebitic reaction to the injection of sclerosing sedative medication

Interfering factors

- Food in the stomach
- Excessive GI bleeding

Procedure and patient care

Before

- Explain the procedure to the patient.
- Obtain informed consent if required by the institution.
- Instruct the patient to abstain from eating as of midnight the day of the test.
- Reassure the patient that this test is not painful. Tell the patient that the throat will be anesthetized with a spray to depress the gag reflex.
- Encourage the patient to verbalize fears. Provide support.
- Remove the patient's dentures and eyewear before testing.
- Remind the patient that he or she will not be able to speak during the test but that respiration will not be affected.
- Instruct the patient not to bite down on the endoscope.
- Instruct the patient as to appropriate oral hygiene, because the tube will be passed through the mouth.

During

- Note the following procedural steps:
  1. The patient is placed on the endoscopy table in the left lateral decubitus position.
  2. The throat is topically anesthetized with viscous lidocaine (Xylocaine) or another anesthetic spray. This is to decrease the gag reflex caused by passage of the endoscope.
  3. The patient is usually sedated. This minimizes anxiety and allows the patient to experience a "light" sleep.
  4. The endoscope is gently passed through the mouth and finally into the esophagus; once in the esophagus, visualization can be performed.
  5. Air is insufflated to distend the upper GI tract for adequate visualization.
  6. The esophagus, stomach, and duodenum are evaluated.
  7. During *enteroscopy* the upper small bowel is visualized, and a biopsy is performed if needed.
  8. Biopsy or any endoscopic surgery is performed with direct visualization.
  9. On completion of direct inspection and surgery, the excess air and GI secretions are aspirated through the scope.
- Note that the test is performed in the endoscopy laboratory by a physician trained in GI endoscopy and takes approximately 20 to 30 minutes.
- Tell the patient that the test is mildly uncomfortable.

After

- Inform the patient that he or she may have hoarseness or a sore throat after the test.
- Withhold any fluids until the patient is completely alert and the swallowing reflex returns to normal, usually 2 to 4 hours.
- Observe the patient's vital signs. Evaluate the patient for bleeding, fever, abdominal pain, dyspnea, or dysphagia.
- Inform the patient that he or she may experience some post-endoscopic bloating, belching, and flatulence.
- Observe safety precautions until the effects of the sedatives have worn off.
- Inform the patient that the sedation may cause some retro-grade and antegrade amnesia for a few hours.

🏠 Home care responsibilities

- A sore throat is expected after EGD. A soothing mouth wash may help.
- Notify the doctor immediately if bleeding, fever, abdominal pain, dyspnea, or dysphagia occurs.
- Inform the patient that it is normal to have some bloating, belching, and flatulence after the procedure.

Abnormal findings

Tumor (benign or malignant) of the esophagus, stomach, or duodenum
Esophageal diverticula
Hiatal hernia
Esophagitis, gastritis, duodenitis
Gastroesophageal varices

Peptic ulcer
Peptic stricture and subsequent scarring
Extrinsic compression by a cyst or tumor outside the upper GI tract
Source of upper GI bleeding

notes

estrogen fractions (estriol excretion)

Type of test Urine (24-hour); blood

Normal findings

	Serum	Urine μg/24 hours
Estradiol		
Child <10 years old	<15 pg/ml	0-6
Adult male	10-50 pg/ml	0-6
Adult female		
Follicular phase	20-350 pg/ml	0-13
Midcycle peak	150-750 pg/ml	4-14
Luteal phase	30-450 pg/ml	4-10
Postmenopause	<20 pg/ml	0-4
Estriol		
Male or child <10 years old	N/A	1-11
Female, adult		
Follicular phase	N/A	0-14
Ovulatory phase	N/A	13-54
Luteal phase	N/A	8-60
Postmenopausal	N/A	0-11
Female, pregnant		
1st trimester	<38 ng/ml	0-800
2nd trimester	38-140 ng/ml	800-12,000
3rd trimester	31-460 ng/ml	5,000-12,000
Total estrogen		
Male or child <10 years old	N/A	4-25
Female, nonpregnant	N/A	4-60
Female, pregnant		
1st trimester	N/A	0-800
2nd trimester	N/A	800-5,000
3rd trimester	N/A	5,000-50,000

Possible critical values Values 40% below the average of two previous values demand immediate evaluation of fetal well-being.

Test explanation and related physiology

There are three major estrogens. E_1 (estrone) is predominantly produced in the ovary. In females there is a feedback mechanism for the secretion for E_1. Low levels of E_1 stimulate the hypothalamus to produce gonadotropin-releasing factors. These hormone factors stimulate the pituitary to produce follicle-stimulating hormone (FSH) and luteinizing hormone (LH). LH and FSH stimulate the ovary to produce E_1, which peaks during the ovulatory phase of the menstrual cycle. This hormone is measured most often to evaluate menopausal status, sexual maturity and gynecomastia or feminization syndromes or as a tumor marker for patients with certain ovarian tumors. E_1 is the most active endogenous estrogen in the nonpregnant female. E_2 (estradiol-17 beta) and estrone production and actions are similar to E_1.

E_3 (estriol) is the major estrogen in the pregnant female. Serial urine and blood studies for estriol excretion provide an objective means of assessing placental function and fetal normality in high-risk pregnancies. Excretion of estriol increases around the eighth week of gestation and continues to rise until shortly before delivery. Estriol is produced in the placenta from estrogen precursors, which are made by the fetal adrenal gland and liver. The measurement of excreted estriol is an important index of fetal well-being. Rising values indicate an adequately functioning fetoplacental unit. Decreasing values suggest fetoplacental deterioration (failing pregnancy, dysmaturity, preeclampsia/eclampsia, complicated diabetes mellitus, encephaly, fetal death) and require prompt reassessment of the pregnancy. If the estriol levels fall, early delivery of the fetus may be indicated.

Serial studies usually begin at approximately 28 to 30 weeks of gestation and are then repeated weekly. The frequency of these estriol determinations can be increased as needed to evaluate a high-risk pregnancy. Collection may be done daily. Although the first collection is the baseline value, all collection results are compared with previous ones, because decreasing values suggest fetal deterioration. Some physicians suggest using an average of three previous values as a control value.

Estriol excretion studies can be done using 24-hour urine tests or blood studies. A serially increasing estriol/creatinine ratio is a favorable sign in pregnancy. Plasma estriol determinations also can be used to evaluate the fetoplacental unit. The blood estriol is an accurate reflection of the current status of the placenta and fetus. The advantage of the plasma estriol determination is that it is more easily obtained than a 24-hour urine specimen and less affected by medications.

Unfortunately only severe placental distress will decrease urinary estriol sufficiently to reliably predict fetoplacental stress. Furthermore, plasma and urinary estriol levels are normally associated with significant daily variation, which may confuse serial results. Maternal illnesses such as hypertension, preeclampsia, anemia, and impaired renal function can also factitiously decrease urinary estriol levels. Because these problems create a high number of false-positive and false-negative findings, most clinicians now use nonstress fetal monitoring (see p. 405) to indicate fetal-placental health.

Interfering factors

- Recent administration of radioisotopes may alter test results.
- Glycosuria and urinary tract infections can increase urine estriol levels.
- ☑ Drugs that may *increase* levels include adrenocorticosteroids, ampicillin, estrogen-containing drugs, phenothiazines, and tetracyclines.
- ☑ Drugs that may *decrease* levels include clomiphene.

Procedure and patient care

Before

- Explain the procedure to the patient.
- If the patient is going to collect the 24-hour urine specimen at home, give her the collection bottle (with a preservative) and instruct her to keep the urine refrigerated.
- Tell the patient that no food or fluid restrictions are needed.

During

Blood
- Collect approximately 5 ml of venous blood in a red-top tube.

24-hour urine
- Instruct the patient to begin the 24-hour urine collection after voiding. Discard the initial specimen and start the 24-hour timing at that point.
- Collect all urine passed during the next 24 hours. Make sure the patient knows where to store the urine container.
- Keep the specimen on ice or refrigerated during the 24-hour collection period.

- Indicate the starting time on the urine container and laboratory slip.
- Post the hours for the urine collection in a prominent place to prevent accidental discarding of the specimen.
- Instruct the patient to void before defecating so that the urine is not contaminated by feces.
- Remind the patient not to put toilet paper in the collection container.
- Encourage the patient to drink fluids during the 24 hours.
- Collect the last specimen as close as possible to the end of the 24-hour period. Add this urine to the collection.
- List any drugs that may affect test results on the laboratory slip.

After
- Apply pressure to the venipuncture site.
- Transport the 24-hour urine specimen promptly to the laboratory.
- Inform the patient how and when to obtain the results of this study.

Abnormal findings

▲ **Increased levels**
Feminization syndromes
Precocious puberty
Ovarian tumor
Testicular tumor
Adrenal tumor
Normal pregnancy
Hepatic cirrhosis
Necrosis of the liver
Hyperthyroidism

▼ **Decreased levels**
Failing pregnancy
Turner syndrome
Hypopituitarism
Primary and secondary hypogonadism
Stein-Leventhal syndrome
Menopause
Anorexia nervosa

notes

estrogen receptor assay (ER assay, ERA, Estradiol receptor)

Type of test Microscopic examination

Normal findings

Negative: ≤10 fmol/mg of protein
Positive: >10 fmol/mg of protein

Test explanation and related physiology

The ER assay is useful in determining the prognosis and treatment of breast cancer. The assay is used to determine whether a tumor is likely to respond to endocrine therapy or removal of the ovaries or adrenal gland. Tumors with a positive ER assay are more than twice as likely to respond to endocrine therapy than an ER-negative tumor. Hormone receptor assays should be done on all primary or recurrent breast carcinomas. Levels tend to be higher in postmenopausal than in premenopausal women. In general, ER-positive tumors have a better prognosis than ER-negative tumors. ER status is now being evaluated on other gynecologic tumors, but its exact role in these patients has yet to be defined.

Slightly over 50% of patients with breast carcinoma who are ER-positive respond to endocrine therapy (e.g., tamoxifen, estrogens, androgens, oophorectomy, adrenalectomy). The response is greater when the progesterone receptors (see p. 678) are also positive. Patients whose breast cancers lack these hormone receptors (i.e., are ER negative) have a much lower chance of tumor response to hormone therapy and may not be candidates for this form of treatment.

Specimens are obtained by the pathologist from surgical specimens. One gram of tissue is required. More recently, an ER assay can be performed by immunohistochemical methods on fixed, paraffin-embedded tissue or microscope slides. With these newer methods, much less tissue is required.

Interfering factors

- Delay in tissue fixation may cause deterioration of receptor proteins and produce lower values.
- Hormones should be discontinued before breast biopsy is performed. Antiestrogen preparations (e.g., tamoxifen

[Nolvadex]) during the past 2 months may cause false-negative ER assays.

✠ Exogenous hormones that are taken for contraceptive purposes or menopausal estrogens may produce lower receptor values.

Procedure and patient care

Before

- Explain the procedure to the patient.
- Instruct patient to discontinue hormones before breast biopsy is performed.
- Before biopsy a gynecologic history is obtained, including menopausal status and exogenous hormone use.

During

- The surgeon obtains tumor tissue.
- This tissue is placed on ice and immediately transferred to the pathology department.
- Part of the tissue is used for routine histology, and at least 1 g is frozen.
- The frozen specimen is sent (in dry ice) to a central laboratory for ER analysis.
- If immunohistochemical methods of ER assays are used, the specimen is fixed as soon as it arrives at the laboratory.

After

- Results are usually available in 2 weeks.

Abnormal findings

Nonapplicable

notes

ethanol (Ethyl alcohol, Blood alcohol, Blood EtOH)

Type of test Blood; urine; gastric; breath

Normal findings None

Possible critical values >300 mg/dl

Test explanation and related physiology

Ethanol depresses the central nervous system and may lead to coma and death. This test is usually performed to evaluate alcohol-impaired driving or overdose. Proper collection, handling, and storage of blood alcohol are important for medicolegal cases involving sobriety. The blood test is the specimen of choice. Blood is taken from a peripheral vein in living patients and from the aorta in cadavers. Ethanol also can be detected in the urine, in gastric contents, or by breath analyzer.

Blood alcohol levels between 50 to 100 mg/dl (0.05% to 0.10% weight/volume) are considered legal intoxication. At this level, flushing, slowing of reflexes, and impaired visual activity are noted. Depression of the central nervous system occurs with levels over 100 mg/dl, and fatalities are reported with levels over 400 mg/dl.

Interfering factors

- Elevated blood ketones (as with diabetic ketoacidosis) can cause false elevation of blood and breath test results.

Procedure and patient care

Before

- Explain the procedure to the patient.
- Follow the institution's protocol if the specimen will be used for legal purposes.

During

- Use a povidone-iodine wipe instead of an alcohol wipe for cleansing the venipuncture site.
- Collect a venous blood sample in a gray- or red-top tube according to the agency's protocol.
- If a gastric or urine specimen is indicated, approximately 20 to 50 ml of fluid is necessary.

- Breath analyzers are taken at the end of expiration after a deep inspiration.

After

- Apply pressure to the venipuncture site.
- Follow the agency's protocol regarding specimen collection.
- The exact time of specimen collection should be indicated. Also, in some instances signatures of the collector and a witness may be needed for legal evidence.

Abnormal findings

Alcohol intoxication or overdose

notes

euglobulin lysis time (Euglobulin clot lysis, Fibrinolysis/euglobulin lysis)

Type of test Blood

Normal findings 90 minutes to 6 hours

Possible critical values <1 hour, indicating excessive fibrinolytic activity (danger of bleeding)

Test explanation and related physiology

The euglobulin lysis test is used to identify systemic fibrinolysis. Fibrinolysis is an important part of normal hemostasis. Clots are constantly being made and dissolved. The fibrinolytic system is responsible for clot dissolution. When this system is abnormally activated by drugs or protein fibrinolysins, a fibrin clot that had been formed will be dissolved immediately, resulting in a bleeding tendency. Primary fibrinolysins are abnormal proteins that are associated with disease such as malignancy, shock or sepsis. Secondary fibrinolysins, on the other hand, are a normal part of hemostasis and clot dissolution. However, they can be abnormally activated during disseminated intravascular coagulation. Plasmin is the main secondary fibrinolysin normally active in clot dissolution (see Figure 11, p. 251). Drugs such as streptokinase and urokinase, used in therapeutic clot lysis (thrombolytic therapy of coronary, cerebral and other organ arterial/venous blood clots), are also considered secondary fibrinolysins. Euglobulin lysis time can detect either primary or secondary fibrinolysis.

Euglobulin lysis time is performed by adding the patient's plasma to a blood clot of a normal person. The clot is observed for 6 to 24 hours. The time measured from clot formation to clot lysis is referred to as the *euglobulin lysis time*. The occurrence of clot lysis before 1 hour is considered abnormal. This test also may be used to monitor streptokinase or urokinase therapy in patients with acute myocardial infarction.

Interfering factors

- Vigorous exercise, increasing age, and hyperventilation may cause increased fibrinolysis.

- Postmenopausal women and normal newborns may have decreased fibrinolysis.
- Decreased fibrinogen levels may result in a falsely shortened lysis time because of the reduced amount of fibrin to be lysed.
- Patients who are obese may have decreased fibrinolysis.
- Drugs that may cause *increased* fibrinolysis include steroids and adrenocorticotropic hormone.

Procedure and patient care

Before
- Explain the procedure to the patient.
- Instruct the patient not to exercise before the blood sample is collected.
- Tell the patient that no fasting is required.

During
- Collect approximately 5 ml of blood in a blue-top tube.
- Avoid excessive agitation of the blood sample.
- Deliver the blood specimen to the laboratory immediately on ice.

After
- Apply pressure to the venipuncture site.

Abnormal findings

▲ **Increased fibrinolysis (shortened euglobulin lysis time)**
Incompatible blood transfusion
Cirrhosis
Obstetric complications (e.g., antepartum hemorrhage, septic abortion, hydatidiform mole, amniotic embolism)
Malignancies (e.g., leukemia, cancer of the prostate or pancreas)
Shock (hemorrhagic or septic)
Streptokinase or urokinase administration for thrombolytic therapy
Extensive vascular trauma or surgery
Disseminated intravascular coagulation

▼ **Decreased fibrinolysis (increased lysis time)**
Prematurity
Diabetes

Type of test Electrodiagnostic

Normal findings No neural conduction delay

Test explanation and related physiology

EP studies are indicated for patients who are suspected of having a sensory deficit but are unable to or are unreliable in indicating recognition of a stimulus. These may include infants, comatose patients, or patients with inability to communicate. These tests are also used to evaluate specific areas of the cortex that receive incoming stimulus from the eyes, ears, and lower/upper extremity sensory nerves. They are used to monitor natural progression or treatment of deteriorating neurologic diseases. Finally, they are also used to identify histrionic or malingering patients who have sensory deficit complaints.

EP studies focus on changes and responses in brain waves that are evoked from stimulation of a sensory pathway. The study of EPs grew out of early work with the electroencephalogram (EEG) (see p. 340). The EEG measures "spontaneous" brain electrical activity, whereas the sensory EP study measures minute voltage changes produced in response to a specific stimulus such as a light pattern, a click, or a shock. In contrast to the EEG, which records signals that reach amplitudes of up to 50 to 100 mV, EP signals are usually less than 5 mV. Because of this, they can only be detected with an averaging computer. The computer averages out (or cancels) unwanted random waves to sum the evoked response that occurs at a specific time after a given stimulus.

Evoked potential studies allow one to measure and assess the entire sensory pathway from the peripheral sensory organ all the way to the brain cortex (recognition of the stimulus). These tests are also used to monitor progressive neurologic diseases (e.g., multiple sclerosis).

Clinical abnormalities are usually detected by an increase in *latency*, which refers to the delay between the stimulus and the wave response. Normal latency times are calculated depending on body size, position of the body where the stimulus is applied, conduction velocity of axons in the neural pathways, number of synapses in the system, location of nerve generators of EP components (brain stem or cortex), and presence of central nervous system pathology. Conduction delays indicate damage or disease anywhere along the neural pathway from the sensory organ to the cortex. Sensory stimuli used for the EP study can be visual, auditory, or somatosensory. The sensory stimulus chosen depends on what sensory system is suspected to be pathologic (e.g., questionable blindness, deafness, or numbness). Also, the sensory stimulus chosen may depend on the area of brain where pathology is suspected (auditory stimuli checks the brain stem and temporal lobes of the brain; visual stimuli test the optic nerve, central neural visual pathway, and occipital parts of the brain; and somatosensory stimuli check the peripheral nerves, spinal cord, and parietal lobe of the brain). Increased latency (i.e., abnormally prolonged time from the time of stimulus to the time of brain EEG recognition) indicates pathology of the sensory organ or the specific neural pathway as described earlier.

Visual-evoked responses (VERs) are usually stimulated by a strobe light flash, reversible checkerboard pattern, or retinal stimuli. Ninety percent of patients with multiple sclerosis show abnormal latencies in VERs, a phenomenon attributed to demyelination of nerve fibers. In addition, patients with other neurologic disorders (e.g., Parkinson's disease) show an abnormal latency with VERs. The degree of latency seems to correlate with the severity of the disease. Abnormal results also may be seen in patients with lesions of the optic nerve, optic tract, visual center, and the eye itself. Absence of binocularity, which is a neurologic developmental disorder in infants, can be detected and evaluated by VERs. Eyesight problems or blindness can be detected in infants through VERs or *electroretinography*. This test also can be used during eye surgery to provide a warning of possible damage to the optic nerve. The gross visual acuity of infants can even be checked via VERs.

Auditory brain stem–evoked potentials (ABEPs) are usually stimulated by clicking sounds to evaluate the central auditory pathways of the brain stem. Either ear can be evoked to detect lesions in the brain stem that involve the auditory pathway without affecting hearing. One of the most successful applications of ABEPs has been screening low–birth weight newborns and other infants for hearing disorders. Recognition of deafness enables infants to be fitted with corrective devices as soon as possible before learning to speak (to prevent speech pathology).

ABEPs also have great therapeutic implications in the early detection of posterior fossa brain tumors.

Somatosensory-evoked responses (SERs) are usually stimulated by sensory stimulus to an area of the body. The time is then measured for the current of the stimulus to travel along the nerve to the cortex of the brain. SERs are used to evaluate patients with spinal cord injuries and to monitor spinal cord functioning during spinal surgery. They are also used to monitor treatment of diseases (e.g., multiple sclerosis), to evaluate the location and extent of areas of brain dysfunction after head injury, and to pinpoint tumors at an early stage. These tests can also be used to identify malingering or hysterical numbness. For example, the latency is normal in these patients, despite the fact they indicate numbness.

One of the main benefits of EPs is their objectivity, because voluntary patient response is not needed. This makes EPs useful with nonverbal and uncooperative patients. This objectivity permits the distinction of organic from psychogenic problems. This is invaluable in settling lawsuits concerning workmen's compensation insurance.

Procedure and patient care

Before

- Explain the procedure to the patient.
- Instruct the patient to shampoo his or her hair before the test.
- Tell the patient that no fasting or sedation is required.

During

- Note that the position of the electrode depends on the type of EP study to be done:
  1. For *VERs* electrodes are placed on the scalp along the vertex and the cortex lobes. Stimulation occurs by using a strobe light, checkerboard pattern, or retinal stimuli.
  2. *ABEPs* are stimulated with clicking noises or tone bursts delivered via earphones. The responses are detected by scalp electrodes placed along the vertex and on each earlobe.
  3. *SERs* are stimulated using electrical stimuli applied to nerves at the wrist (medial nerve) or knee (peroneal nerve). The response is detected by electrodes placed over the sensory cortex of the opposite hemisphere on the scalp.

- Note that this study is performed by a physician in less than 30 minutes.
- Tell the patient that little discomfort is associated with this study.

After

- Remove the gel used for the adherence of the electrodes.

Abnormal findings

Prolonged latency for ABEP

Demyelinating diseases (e.g., multiple sclerosis)
Tumor—acoustic neuroma
Cerebrovascular accident (stroke)
Auditory nerve damage
Deafness

Abnormal latency for SER

Spinal cord injury
Cervical disc disease
Spinal cord demyelinating diseases
Peripheral nerve injury, transection, or disease
Parietal cortical tumor or CVA

Prolonged latency for VER

Parkinson's disease
Demyelinating diseases (e.g., multiple sclerosis)
Optic nerve damage
Ocular disease or injury
Blindness
Optic tract disease
Occipital lobe tumor or CVA
Absence of binocularity
Visual field defects

notes

fecal fat (Fat absorption, Quantitative stool fat determination)

Type of test Stool

Normal findings

Fat: 5 g/24 hr
Retention coefficient: ≥95%

Test explanation and related physiology

This test is performed to confirm the diagnosis of steatorrhea. Steatorrhea occurs when the fat in the stool is high. It is suspected when the patient has large, greasy, and foul-smelling stools. Determining an abnormally high fecal fat content confirms the diagnosis. Short-gut syndrome and any condition that may cause malabsorption (e.g., sprue, Crohn's disease, Whipple's disease) or maldigestion (e.g., bile duct obstruction, pancreatic duct obstruction secondary to tumor or gallstones) are also associated with increased fecal fat. Children with cystic fibrosis may have steatorrhea. Mucous plugs obstruct their pancreatic ducts; thus the pancreatic enzymes (amylase, lipase, trypsin, and chymotrypsin) cannot be mixed with the food to assist with fat digestion.

The fecal fat test measures the fat content in the stool. The total output of fecal fat per 24 hours in a 3-day stool collection provides the most reliable measurement.

Interfering factors

- ✘ Drugs that may alter test results include enemas and laxatives, especially mineral oil.
- ✘ Drugs that may *decrease* levels of fecal fat include Metamucil and barium.

Procedure and patient care

Before

- Explain the procedure to the patient.
- Give the patient instructions regarding the appropriate diet (a diet diary may be requested by the laboratory):
  1. For adults, usually 100 g of fat per day is suggested for 3 days before and throughout the collection period.
  2. Children, and especially infants, cannot ingest 100 g of fat. Therefore a *fat retention coefficient* is determined by

measuring the difference between ingested fat and fecal fat and then expressing that difference (the amount of fat retained) as a percentage of the ingested fat:

$$\frac{\text{Ingested fat} - \text{Fecal fat}}{\text{Ingested fat}} \times 100\% = \text{Fat coefficient}$$

- Note that the fat retention coefficient in normal children and adults is 95% or greater. A low value indicates steatorrhea.
- Instruct the patient to defecate in a dry, clean container.
- Occasionally, a tongue blade is required to transfer the stool to the specimen container.
- Tell the patient not to urinate in the stool container.
- Inform the patient that even diarrheal stools should be collected.
- Instruct the patient that toilet paper should not be placed in the stool container.
- Tell the patient not to take any laxatives or enemas during this test because they will interfere with intestinal motility and alter test results.

During
- Collect each stool specimen and send immediately to the laboratory during the 24- to 72-hour testing period. Label each specimen and include the time and date of collection.
- If the specimen is collected at home, give the patient a large stool container to keep in the freezer.

After
- Inform the patient that a normal diet can be resumed.

Abnormal findings

▲   **Increased levels**
   Cystic fibrosis
   Malabsorption secondary to sprue, celiac disease, Whipple's disease, Crohn's disease (regional enteritis), or radiation enteritis
   Maldigestion secondary to obstruction of the pancreatico-biliary tree (e.g., cancer, stricture, gallstones)
   Short-gut syndrome secondary to surgical resection, surgical bypass, or congenital anomaly

ferritin

Type of test Blood

Normal findings
Male: 12-300 ng/ml or 12-300 μg/L (SI units)
Female: 10-150 ng/ml or 10-150 μg/L (SI units)
Children
  Newborn: 25-200 ng/ml
  1 month: 200-600 ng/ml
  2-5 months: 50-200 ng/ml
  6 months-15 years: 7-142 ng/ml

Test explanation and related physiology
The serum ferritin study is a good indicator of available iron stores in the body. Ferritin, the major iron storage protein, is normally present in the serum in concentrations directly related to iron storage. In normal patients 1 ng/ml of serum ferritin corresponds to approximately 8 mg of stored iron. Ferritin levels rise with age in males and postmenopausal females. In premenopausal females, levels stay about the same. Decreases in ferritin levels indicate a decrease in iron storage associated with iron deficiency anemia. A ferritin level of below 10 ng/100 ml is diagnostic of iron deficiency anemia. The decrease in serum ferritin level often precedes other signs of iron deficiency such as decreased iron levels or changes in red blood cell size, chromasia, and number. Only when protein depletion is severe can ferritin be decreased by malnutrition. Pregnancy is also associated with decreased ferritin levels. Increased levels are a sign of iron excess, as seen in hemochromatosis, hemosiderosis, iron poisoning, or recent blood transfusions. Increased ferritin is also noted in patients with megaloblastic anemia, hemolytic anemia, and chronic hepatitis. Further, ferritin is factitiously elevated in patients with chronic disease states such as neoplasm, alcoholism, uremia, collagen diseases, or chronic liver diseases. Ferritin is also used in patients with chronic renal failure to monitor iron stores.

A limitation of this study is that ferritin levels also can act as an "acute phase" reactant protein and may be elevated in conditions not reflecting iron stores (e.g., acute inflammatory diseases, infections, metastatic cancer, lymphomas). Elevations in ferritin occur 1 to 2 days after onset of the acute illness and peak at 3 to 5 days. If iron deficiency were to coexist in patients with these diseases, it may not be recognized because the levels of ferritin would be factitiously elevated by the concurring disease.

When combined with the serum iron level and total iron-binding capacity (TIBC, see p. 502), this test is useful in differentiating and classifying anemias. For example, in patients with iron deficiency anemia, the ferritin, iron, and transferrin saturation levels are low, whereas the TIBC and transferrin levels are high.

Interfering factors

- Recent transfusions and recent ingestion of a meal containing a high iron content may cause elevated ferritin levels.
- Recent administration of a radionuclide can cause abnormal levels if testing is performed by radioimmunoassay.
- Hemolytic diseases may be associated with an artificially high iron content.
- Disorders of excessive iron storage (e.g., hemochromatosis, hemosiderosis) are associated with high ferritin levels.
- Menstruating women may have decreased ferritin levels.
- Drugs that may *increase* ferritin levels include iron preparations.

Procedure and patient care

Before

- Explain the procedure to the patient.
- Tell the patient that no fasting is required.

During

- Collect approximately 5 to 7 ml of venous blood in a red-top tube.

After

- Apply pressure to the venipuncture site.

Abnormal findings

▲ **Increased levels**
  Hemochromatosis
  Hemosiderosis
  Megaloblastic anemia
  Hemolytic anemia
  Alcoholic/inflammatory
    hepatocellular disease
  Inflammatory disease
  Advanced cancers
  Chronic illnesses (e.g.,
    leukemias, cirrhosis,
    chronic hepatitis)
  Collagen vascular diseases

▼ **Decreased levels**
  Severe protein deficiency
  Iron deficiency anemia
  Hemodialysis

F

notes

fetal biophysical profile (Biophysical profile, [BPP])

Type of test Ultrasound; fetal activity study

Normal findings Score of 8-10 points (if amniotic fluid volume is adequate)

Possible critical values Less than 4 may necessitate immediate delivery.

Test explanation and related physiology

The BPP is a method of evaluating fetal status during the antepartal period based on five variables originating within the fetus: fetal heart rate, fetal breathing movement, gross fetal movements, fetal muscle tone, and amniotic fluid volume. Fetal heart rate reactivity is measured by the nonstress test (see p. 405), and the other four parameters are measured by ultrasound scanning.

The major premise behind the BPP is that variable assessments of fetal biophysical activity are more reliable than an examination of a single parameter (such as fetal heart rate). Indications for this test include factors such as postdate pregnancy, maternal hypertension, diabetes mellitus, vaginal bleeding, maternal Rh sensitization, maternal history of stillbirth, and premature rupture of membranes. The BPP is probably more useful in identifying a fetus that is in jeopardy than in predicting future fetal well-being.

The five parameters are briefly described here. Each parameter is scored and contributes either a 2 or a 0 to the score. Therefore 10 is the perfect score, and 0 is the lowest score.

1. *Fetal heart rate reactivity.* This is measured and interpreted in the same way as the nonstress test (see p. 405). The fetal heart rate is considered reactive when there are movement-associated fetal heart rate accelerations of at least 15 beats/min above baseline and 15 seconds in duration over a 20-minute period. A score of 2 is given for reactivity, and a score of 0 indicates that the fetal heart rate is nonreactive.

2. *Fetal breathing movements.* This parameter is assessed based on the assumption that fetal breathing movements indicate fetal well-being and their absence may indicate hypoxemia. Fetal breathing becomes increasingly

regular in frequency and uniformity after the thirty-sixth week of gestation. To earn a score of 2, the fetus must have at least one episode of fetal breathing lasting at least 60 seconds within a 30-minute observation. Absence of this breathing pattern is scored a 0 on the BPP. It is important to note that several factors can alter fetal breathing movements. For example, fetal breathing movements increase during the second and third hours after maternal meals and also at night. Fetal breathing movements may decrease in conditions such as hypoxemia, hypoglycemia, nicotine use, and alcohol ingestion.

3. *Fetal body movements.* Fetal activity is a reflection of neurologic integrity and function. The presence of at least three discrete episodes of fetal movements within a 30-minute observation period is given a score of 2. A score of 0 is given with two or fewer fetal movements in this time period. It is important to note that fetal activity is greatest 1 to 3 hours after the mother has consumed a meal. For this reason, it is often suggested that this test be arranged in relation to mealtime.

4. *Fetal tone.* In the uterus the fetus is normally in a position of flexion. However, the fetus also stretches, rolls, and moves in the uterus. The arms, legs, trunk, and head may be flexed and extended. A score of 2 is earned when there is at least one episode of active extension with return to flexion. An example of this would be the opening and closing of the hand. A score of 0 is given for slow extension with a return to only partial flexion; fetal movement not followed by return to flexion; limbs or spine in extension; and an open fetal hand.

5. *Amniotic fluid volume.* Amniotic fluid volume has been demonstrated to be an effective method of predicting fetal distress. Oligohydramnios (too little amniotic fluid) has been associated with fetal anomalies, uterine growth retardation, and postterm pregnancy. A score of 2 is given for this parameter when there is at least one pocket of amniotic fluid that measures 1 cm in two perpendicular planes. A score of 0 indicates either that fluid is absent in most areas of the uterine cavity or that the largest pocket measures 1 cm or less in the vertical axis.

A score of 8 or 10 with a normal amount of amniotic fluid indicates a healthy fetus. A score of 8 with oligohydramnios or a score of 4 to 6 is equivocal. An equivocal test result is interpreted as possibly abnormal. Some clinicians would recommend repeating the test within 24 hours. However, others may advocate extending testing after any equivocal or abnormal test result. A score of 0 or 2 is abnormal and indicates the need for assessment of immediate delivery.

Although the BPP is fairly new, it has already been modified. Some physicians omit the nonstress test if the ultrasound parameters are normal. Some physicians have added placental grading as a sixth parameter.

Doppler ultrasound evaluations of the placenta and the *umbilical artery velocity* can recognize alterations in umbilical artery flow and direction that may indicate fetal stress or illness.

Interfering factors

- Central nervous system stimulants such as catecholamine can increase BPP activities.
- Occasionally no movement is noted. If no eye movement or respiratory movement is noted, the fetus may be sleeping.

Procedure and patient care

Before

- Explain the procedure to the patient.
- Inform the patient that no fasting is required.

During

- Fetal heart rate reactivity is measured and interpreted from a nonstress test (see p. 405).
- Fetal breathing movements, fetal body movements, fetal tone, and amniotic fluid volume are determined by ultrasound imaging (see obstetric ultrasonography, p. 623)

After

- If the test results are abnormal or equivocal, support the patient in the next phase of the fetal evaluation process.

Abnormal findings

Fetal asphyxia
Congenital anomalies
Oligohydramnios
Intrauterine growth retardation
Postterm pregnancy
Fetal stress
Fetal death

fetal contraction stress test (CST, Oxytocin challenge test [OCT])

Type of test Electrodiagnostic

Normal findings Negative

Test explanation and related physiology

CST is used to evaluate the viability of a fetus. It documents the function of the placenta in its ability to supply adequate blood supply to the fetus.

The CST, frequently called the *oxytocin challenge test* (OCT), is a relatively noninvasive test of fetoplacental adequacy used in the assessment of high-risk pregnancy. For this study a temporary stress in the form of uterine contractions is applied to the fetus after the IV administration of oxytocin. The reaction of the fetus to the contractions is assessed by an external fetal heart monitor. Uterine contractions cause transient impediment of placental blood flow. If the placental reserve is adequate, the maternal-fetal oxygen transfer is not significantly compromised during the contractions, and the fetal heart rate (FHR) remains normal (a *negative* test). The fetoplacental unit can then be considered adequate for the next 7 days.

If the placental reserve is inadequate, the fetus does not receive enough oxygen during the contraction. This results in intrauterine hypoxia and late deceleration of the FHR. The test is considered to be *positive* if consistent, persistent, late decelerations of the FHR occur with two or more uterine contractions. False-positive results caused by uterine hyperstimulation can occur in 10% to 30% of patients. Thus positive test results warrant a complete review of other studies (e.g., amniocentesis) before the pregnancy is terminated by delivery.

The test is considered to be *unsatisfactory* if the results cannot be interpreted (e.g., because of hyperstimulation of the uterus, excessive movement of the mother, or deceleration of unknown meaning). In the case of unsatisfactory results, other means of management should be considered.

Two advantages of the CST are that it can be done at any time and that its results are available shortly afterward. Although this test can be performed reliably at 32 weeks of gestation, it usually is done after 34 weeks. CST can induce labor, and a fetus at 34 weeks is more likely to survive an unexpectedly induced delivery than a fetus at 32 weeks. Nonstress testing (see p. 405) of the fetus is the preferred test in almost every instance and can be performed more safely at 32 weeks; it can then be followed 2 weeks later by CST if necessary. The CST may be performed weekly until delivery terminates pregnancy.

A new noninvasive method of performing the CST is called the *breast stimulation or nipple stimulation technique*. Stimulation of the nipple causes nerve impulses to the hypothalamus that trigger the release of oxytocin into the mother's bloodstream. This causes uterine contractions and may eliminate the need for IV administration of oxytocin. Uterine contractions are usually satisfactory after 15 minutes of nipple stimulation (gentle twisting of the nipples). Advantages of this technique include the ease of performing the test; shorter duration of the study; and elimination of the need to start, monitor, and stop IV infusions.

Contraindications

- Patient pregnant with multiple fetuses because the myometrium is under greater tension and is more likely to be stimulated to premature labor
- Patient with a prematurely ruptured membrane, because labor may be stimulated by the CST
- Patient with placenta previa, because vaginal delivery may be induced
- Patient with abruptio placentae, because the placenta may separate from the uterus as a result of the oxytocin-induced uterine contractions
- Patient with a previous hysterotomy, because the strong uterine contractions may cause uterine rupture
- Patient with a previous vertical or classic cesarean section, because the strong uterine contractions may cause uterine rupture (The test can be performed, however, if it is carefully monitored and controlled.)
- Patient with pregnancy of less than 32 weeks, because early delivery may be induced by the procedure

Potential complications

- Premature labor

Interfering factors

- Hypotension may cause false-positive results.

Procedure and patient care

Before

- Explain the procedure to the patient.
- Obtain informed consent for the procedure.
- Teach the patient breathing and relaxation techniques.
- Record the patient's blood pressure and FHR before the test as baseline values.
- If the CST is performed on an elective basis, the patient may be kept NPO in case labor occurs.

F

During

- Note the following procedural steps:
  1. After the patient empties her bladder, place her in a semi-Fowler's position and tilted slightly to one side to avoid vena caval compression by the enlarged uterus.
  2. Check her blood pressure every 10 minutes to avoid hypotension, which may cause diminished placental blood flow and a false-positive test result.
  3. Place an external fetal monitor over the patient's abdomen to record the fetal heart tones. Attach an external tokodynamometer to the abdomen at the fundal region to monitor uterine contractions.
  4. Record the output of the fetal heart tones and uterine contractions on a two-channel strip recorder.
  5. Monitor baseline FHR and uterine activity for 20 minutes.
  6. If uterine contractions are detected during this pretest period, withhold oxytocin and monitor the response of the fetal heart tone to spontaneous uterine contractions.
  7. If no spontaneous uterine contractions occur, administer oxytocin (Pitocin) by IV infusion pump.
  8. Increase the rate of oxytocin infusion until the patient is having moderate contractions; then record the FHR pattern.
  9. After the oxytocin infusion is discontinued, continue FHR monitoring for another 30 minutes until the uterine activity has returned to its preoxytocin state. The body metabolizes oxytocin in approximately 20 to 25 minutes.
- Note that the CST is performed safely on an outpatient basis in the labor and delivery unit, where qualified nurses and necessary equipment are available. The test is performed by a nurse with a physician available.

- Note that, if sufficient contractions do not result from the *nipple stimulation technique*, the standard CST procedure is followed.
- Note that the duration of this study is approximately 2 hours.
- Tell the patient that the discomfort associated with the CST may consist of mild labor contractions. Usually, breathing exercises are sufficient to control any discomfort. Administer analgesics if needed.

After

- Monitor the patient's blood pressure and FHR.
- Discontinue the IV line and assess the site for bleeding.

Abnormal finding

Fetoplacental inadequacy

notes

fetal nonstress test (Nonstress test, NST, Fetal activity determination)

Type of test Electrodiagnostic

Normal findings "Reactive" fetus (heart rate acceleration associated with fetal movement)

Test explanation and related physiology

NST is a method of evaluating the viability of a fetus. It documents the function of the placenta in its ability to supply adequate blood to the fetus. The NST can be used to evaluate any high-risk pregnancy in which fetal well-being may be threatened.

The NST is a noninvasive study that monitors acceleration of the fetal heart rate (FHR) in response to fetal movement. This FHR acceleration reflects the integrity of the central nervous system and fetal well-being. Fetal activity may be spontaneous, induced by uterine contraction, or induced by external manipulation. Oxytocin stimulation is not used. Fetal response is characterized as "reactive" or "nonreactive." The NST indicates a *reactive fetus* when, with fetal movement, two or more FHR accelerations are detected, each of which must be at least 15 beats/min for 15 seconds or more within any 10-minute period. The test is 99% reliable in indicating fetal viability and negates the need for the contraction stress test (CST, see p. 401). If the test detects a *nonreactive fetus* (i.e., no FHR acceleration with fetal movement) within 40 minutes, the patient is a candidate for the CST. A 40-minute test period is used because this is the average duration of the sleep-wake cycle of the fetus. The cycle may vary considerably, however.

The NST is useful in screening high-risk pregnancies and in selecting patients who may require the CST. An NST is now routinely performed before the CST to avoid the complications associated with oxytocin administration. No complications are associated with the NST.

Procedure and patient care

Before

- Explain the procedure to the patient.
- Encourage verbalization of the patient's fears. The necessity for the study usually raises realistic fears in the expectant mother.

- If the patient is hungry, instruct her to eat before the NST is begun. Fetal activity is enhanced with a high maternal serum glucose level.

During

- After the patient empties her bladder, place her in Sims' position.
- Place an external fetal monitor on the patient's abdomen to record the FHR. The mother can indicate fetal movement by pressing a button on the fetal monitor whenever she feels the fetus move. FHR and fetal movement are concomitantly recorded on a two-channel strip graph.
- Observe the fetal monitor for FHR accelerations associated with fetal movement.
- If the fetus is quiet for 20 minutes, stimulate fetal activity by external methods such as rubbing or compressing the mother's abdomen, ringing a bell near the abdomen, or placing a pan on the abdomen and hitting the pan.
- Note that a nurse performs the NST in approximately 20 to 40 minutes in the physician's office or a hospital unit.
- Tell the patient that no discomfort is associated with NST.

After

- If the results detect a nonreactive fetus, inform the patient that she is a candidate for the CST.

Abnormal findings

Fetal stress
Fetal death

notes

fetal scalp blood pH

Type of test Blood

Normal findings
pH: 7.25-7.35
O_2 saturation: 30% to 50%
P_{O_2}: 18-22 mm Hg
P_{CO_2}: 40-50 mm Hg
Base excess: 0 to −10 mEq/L

Test explanation and related physiology

Measurement of fetal scalp blood pH provides valuable information on fetal acid-base status. This screening test is useful clinically for diagnosing fetal distress.

Although the oxygen partial pressure (P_{O_2}), carbon dioxide partial pressure (P_{CO_2}), and bicarbonate ion concentration can be measured with the fetal scalp blood sample, the pH is the most useful clinically. The pH normally ranges from 7.25 to 7.35 during labor; a mild decline within the normal range is noted with contractions and as labor progresses.

Fetal hypoxia causes anaerobic glycolysis, resulting in excess production of lactic acid. This causes an increase in hydrogen ion concentration (acidosis) and a decrease in pH. Acidosis reflects the effect of hypoxia on cellular metabolism. A high correlation exists between low pH levels and low Apgar scores.

Contraindications

- Patients with premature membrane rupture
- Patients with active cervical infection (e.g., gonorrhea)

Potential complications

- Continued bleeding from the puncture site
- Hematoma
- Ecchymosis
- Infection

Procedure and patient care

Before

- Explain the procedure to the patient.
- Obtain informed consent for this procedure.
- Tell the patient that no fasting or sedation is required.

During

- Note the following procedural steps:
  1. Amnioscopy is performed with the mother in the lithotomy position.
  2. The cervix is dilated, and the endoscope (amnioscope) is introduced into the cervical canal.
  3. The fetal scalp is cleansed with an antiseptic and dried with a sterile cotton ball.
  4. A small amount of petroleum jelly is applied to the fetal scalp to cause droplets of fetal blood to bead.
  5. After the skin on the scalp is pierced with a small metal blade, beaded droplets of blood are collected in long, heparinized capillary tubes.
  6. The tube is sealed with wax and placed on ice to retard cellular respiration, which can alter the pH.
  7. The physician performing the procedure applies firm pressure to the puncture site to retard bleeding.
  8. Scalp blood sampling can be repeated as necessary.
- Note that this study is performed by a physician in approximately 10 to 15 minutes.
- Tell the patient that she may be uncomfortable during the cervical dilation.

After

- Inform the patient that she may have vaginal discomfort and menstrual-type cramping.

After delivery

- Assess the newborn and identify and document the puncture site(s).
- Cleanse the fetal scalp puncture site with an antiseptic solution and apply an antibiotic ointment.

Abnormal finding

Fetal distress

notes

fetoscopy

Type of test   Endoscopy

Normal findings   No fetal distress

Test explanation and related physiology

Fetoscopy is an endoscopic procedure that allows direct visualization of the fetus via the insertion of a tiny, telescope-like instrument through the abdominal wall and into the uterine cavity (Figure 18). Direct visualization may lead to diagnosis of a severe malformation such as a neural tube defect. During the procedure fetal blood samples to detect congenital blood disorders (e.g., hemophilia, sickle cell anemia) can be drawn from a blood vessel in the umbilical cord for biochemical analysis. Fetal skin biopsies also can be done to detect primary skin disorders.

Fetoscopy is performed at approximately 18 weeks of gestation. At this time the vessels of the placental surface are of adequate size, and the fetal parts are readily identifiable. A therapeutic abortion would not be as hazardous at this time as it would be if it were done later in the pregnancy. An ultrasound is usually performed the day after the procedure to confirm the adequacy of the amniotic fluid and fetal viability.

Potential complications

- Spontaneous abortion
- Premature delivery
- Amniotic fluid leak
- Intrauterine fetal death
- Amnionitis

Procedure and patient care

Before

- Explain the procedure to the patient.
- Obtain informed consent.
- Assess the fetal heart rate before the test to serve as a baseline value.
- Administer meperidine (Demerol) if ordered before the test because it crosses the placenta and quiets the fetus. This prevents excessive fetal movement, which would make the procedure more difficult.

Figure 18 Fetoscopy for fetal blood sampling.

During
- Note the following procedural steps:
  1. The woman is placed in the supine position on an examining table.
  2. The abdominal wall is anesthetized locally.
  3. Ultrasonography is performed to locate the fetus and the placenta.
  4. The endoscope is inserted.
  5. Biopsies and blood samples may be obtained.
- Note that this procedure is performed by a physician in 1 to 2 hours.

- Tell the patient that the only discomfort associated with this study is the injection of the local anesthetic.

After

- Assess the FHR and compare with the baseline value to detect any side effects related to the procedure.
- Monitor the mother and fetus carefully for alterations in blood pressure, pulse, uterine activity, and fetal activity; vaginal bleeding; and loss of amniotic fluid.
- Administer RhoGAM to mothers who are Rh negative unless the fetal blood is found to be Rh negative.
- Note that a repeat ultrasound is usually performed the day after the procedure to confirm the adequacy of the amniotic fluid and fetal viability.
- Instruct the mother to avoid strenuous activity for 1 to 2 weeks following the procedure and to report any pain, bleeding, amniotic fluid loss, or fever.
- At times, if ordered, administer antibiotics prophylactically after the test to prevent amnionitis.

Abnormal findings

Developmental defects (e.g., neural tube defects)
Congenital blood disorders (e.g., hemophilia, sickle cell anemia)
Primary skin disorders

notes

fibrin degradation products (FDPs, Fibrin split products [FSPs], Fibrin breakdown products)

Type of test Blood

Normal findings <10 μg/ml or dilution <1:20

Possible critical values >40 μg/ml

Test explanation and related physiology

Measurement of FDPs provides a direct indication of the activity of the fibrinolytic system. The fibrinolytic system is an important part of the balance that exists in the body between clot formation and clot dissolution. Clot formation stimulates the activation of three major activators of the fibrinolytic system. These in turn act on plasminogen, which had previously been absorbed into the clot, to form plasmin. Plasmin degenerates the fibrin polymer of the clot into fragments called FDPs (X, D, E, and Y). If present in increased quantities, they can have an anticoagulant effect.

When present in large amounts, FDPs indicate increased fibrinolysis, as occurs in disseminated intravascular coagulation (DIC) and other secondary fibrinolytic disorders. This test is one of the DIC screening tests. FDPs are also present in thrombotic states such as venous thrombosis. The thrombosis stimulates the activation of the fibrinolytic system. Other diseases can potentially cause activation of the fibrinolytic system and elevate FDP levels. These may include extensive malignancy, tissue necrosis, and gram-negative sepsis. For example, thrombolytic therapy used in myocardial infarction is associated with increased FDPs. Streptokinase or urokinase stimulates the conversion of plasminogen to plasmin. The plasmin splits the fibrinogen polymer into FDPs, as discussed earlier.

Interfering factors

- Traumatic venipunctures may alter test results.
- ✗ Drugs that may cause *increased* levels include barbiturates, heparin, streptokinase, and urokinase.

Procedure and patient care

Before
- Explain the procedure to the patient.
- Tell the patient that no fasting is required.

During
- Draw the sample before initiating heparin therapy.
- Collect a venous blood sample (usually only 2 ml) in a small, blue-top tube or in the colored tube designated by the laboratory.
- Avoid excessive agitation of the blood sample.
- Note that it is best to place the blood on ice and take it immediately to the hematology laboratory.
- List on the laboratory slip any drugs that may cause elevated levels.

After
- Apply pressure to the venipuncture site.

Abnormal findings

▲   **Increased levels**
Disseminated intravascular coagulation
Heart/vascular surgery
Thromboembolic states

notes

fibrinogen (Factor I, Quantitative fibrinogen)

Type of test Blood

Normal finding

Adult: 200-400 mg/dl or 2-4 g/L (SI units)
Newborn: 125-300 mg/dl

Possible critical values <100 mg/dl

Test explanation and related physiology

Fibrinogen is essential to the blood clotting mechanism. It is part of the "common pathway" in the coagulation system. Fibrinogen is converted to fibrin by action of thrombin during the coagulation process. (See discussion of coagulating factors, p. 248.) Fibrinogen, which is produced by the liver, is also an acute-phase protein reactant. It rises sharply during instances of tissue inflammation or necrosis. High levels also may be a useful predictor for increased risk of coronary artery or cerebrovascular disease. Reduced levels can be seen in patients with liver disease, malnourished states, and consumptive coagulopathies (e.g., disseminated intravascular coagulation). Large-volume blood transfusions are also associated with low levels because banked blood does not contain fibrinogen. Reduced levels of fibrinogen will cause a prolonged protime and partial thromboplastin time.

Interfering factors

- Blood transfusions within the past month may affect test results.
- Fibrinolysins can attack fibrinogen and reduce the serum levels.
- ☛ Drugs that may cause *increased* levels include estrogens and oral contraceptives.
- ☛ Drugs that may cause *decreased* levels include anabolic steroids, androgens, asparaginase, phenobarbital, streptokinase, urokinase, and valproic acid.

Procedure and patient care

Before

- Explain the procedure to the patient.
- Tell the patient that no fasting is required.

During

- Collect one tube of venous blood in a blue-top tube.

After

- Apply pressure to the venipuncture site.

Abnormal findings

▲ **Increased levels**

Acute inflammatory reactions (e.g., rheumatoid arthritis, glomerulonephritis)

Trauma

Acute infection such as pneumonia

Coronary heart disease

Cigarette smoking

Pregnancy

▼ **Decreased levels**

Liver disease (e.g., hepatitis, cirrhosis)

Consumptive coagulopathy

Fibrinolysins

Congenital afibrinogenemia

Advanced carcinoma

Malnutrition

Large-volume blood transfusion

notes

folic acid (Folate)

Type of test Blood

Normal findings 5-20 µg/ml or 14-34 mmol/L (SI units)

Test explanation and related physiology

Folic acid, one of the B vitamins, is necessary for normal function of red and white blood cells (RBCs, WBCs) and for the adequate synthesis of certain purines and pyrimidines, which are precursors for deoxyribonucleic acid (DNA). As with vitamin B_{12} (see p. 741), folate depends on normal function of the intestinal mucosa.

Folic acid blood levels are performed to evaluate hemolytic disorders and to detect anemia caused by folic acid deficiency (in which the RBCs are abnormally large, causing a megaloblastic anemia). These RBCs have a shortened life span and impaired oxygen-carrying capacity.

The main causes of folic acid deficiency include dietary deficiency, malabsorption syndrome, pregnancy, and certain anticonvulsant drugs. Decreased folic acid levels are seen in patients with folic acid deficiency anemia (megaloblastic anemia), hemolytic anemia, malnutrition, malabsorption syndrome, malignancy, liver disease, sprue, and celiac disease. Some drugs (e.g., anticonvulsants, antimalarials, alcohol, aminopterin, and methotrexate) are folic acid antagonists and interfere with nucleic acid synthesis.

Elevated levels of folic acid may be seen in patients with pernicious anemia. The folic acid test may be done in conjunction with tests for vitamin B_{12} levels (see p. 741). This test for folate is often done in the workup for alcoholic patients to assess the patient's nutritional status. One must be depleted of folate for at least 5 months before megaloblastic anemia occurs.

Interfering factors

- ☛ Drugs that may cause *decreased* folic acid levels include alcohol, aminopterin, aminosalicylic acid (PAS), ampicillin, antimalarials, chloramphenicol, erythromycin, estrogens, methotrexate, oral contraceptives, penicillin, phenobarbital, phenytoin, and tetracyclines.
- Because radioimmunoassay is the method of choice for folic

acid determination, radionuclide administration should be avoided for at least 24 hours.

Procedure and patient care

Before

- Explain the procedure to the patient.
- Tell the patient that usually no fasting is required. (However, some laboratories prefer an 8-hour fast.)
- Instruct the patient not to consume alcoholic beverages before the test.
- Draw the specimen before starting folate therapy.

During

- Collect approximately 7 to 10 ml of venous blood in a red-top tube.
- Avoid hemolysis.
- Indicate on the laboratory slip any medications that may affect test results.

After

- Apply pressure to the venipuncture site.
- Transport the blood immediately to the laboratory after collection.

Abnormal findings

▲ **Increased levels**
Pernicious anemia
Vegetarianism
Recent massive blood
   transfusion

▼ **Decreased levels**
Folic acid deficiency
   anemia
Hemolytic anemia
Malnutrition
Malabsorption syndrome
   (e.g., sprue, celiac
   disease)
Malignancy
Liver disease
Pregnancy
Alcoholism
Anorexia nervosa
Chronic renal disease

gallbladder nuclear scanning (Hepatobiliary scintigraphy, Hepatobiliary imaging, Biliary tract radionuclide scan, Cholescintigraphy, DISIDA scanning, HIDA scanning, IDA gallbladder scanning)

Type of test Nuclear scan

Normal findings Gallbladder, common bile duct, and duodenum visualize within 60 minutes after radionuclide injection. (This confirms patency of the cystic and common bile ducts.)

Test explanation and related physiology

Through the use of iminodiacetic acid analogs (IDAs) labeled with technetium-99m (^{99m}Tc), the biliary tract can be evaluated in a safe, accurate, and noninvasive manner. These radionuclide compounds are extracted by the liver and excreted into the bile. Gamma rays emitted from the bile are detected by a scintillator, and a realistic image of the biliary tree is apparent.

Failure to visualize the gallbladder 60 to 120 minutes after injection of the radionuclide dye is virtually diagnostic of an obstruction of the cystic duct (acute cholecystitis). Delayed filling of the gallbladder is associated with chronic or acalculus cholecystitis. The identification of the radionuclide in the biliary tree, but not in the bowel, is diagnostic of common bile duct obstruction.

With cholescintigraphy, gallbladder function can be numerically determined by calculating the capability of the gallbladder to eject its contents. It is believed that an ejection fraction below 35% indicates chronic cholecystitis or functional obstruction of the cystic duct.

Occasionally morphine sulfate is given intravenously during nuclear scanning. The morphine causes increased ampullary contraction. Not only can this reproduce the patient's symptoms of biliary colic, but it also serves to force the bile containing the radionuclide into the gallbladder, shortening the expected time of visualization of the gallbladder. If no radionuclide is seen in the gallbladder with the use of morphine within 15 to 30 minutes, the diagnosis of acute cholecystitis is nearly certain.

Contraindications

- Pregnancy, because of the risk of fetal damage

Interfering factors

- If the patient has not eaten for more than 24 hours, the radionuclide may not fill the gallbladder. This would produce a false-positive result.

Procedure and patient care

Before

- Explain the procedure to the patient.
- Assure the patient that he or she will not be exposed to large amounts of radioactivity.
- Instruct the patient to fast for at least 2 hours before the test. This fasting is preferable but not mandatory.

During

- Note the following procedural steps:
  1. After IV administration of a ^{99m}Tc-labeled IDA analog (e.g., DISIDA, PIPIDA, HIDA), the right upper quadrant of the abdomen is scanned.
  2. Serial images are obtained over 1 hour.
  3. Subsequent images can be obtained at 15- to 30-minute intervals.
  4. If the gallbladder, common bile duct, or duodenum is not visualized within 60 minutes after injection, delayed images are obtained up to 4 hours later.
  5. When an *ejection fraction* is to be determined, the patient is given a fatty meal or cholecystokinin to evaluate emptying of the gallbladder. The gallbladder is continually scanned to measure the percentage of isotope ejected.
- Note that a radiologist performs this study in 1 to 4 hours in the nuclear medicine department.
- Tell the patient that the only discomfort associated with this procedure is the IV injection of radionuclide.

After

- Obtain a meal for the patient if indicated.

Abnormal findings

Acute cholecystitis
Chronic cholecystitis
Acalculus cholecystitis
Common bile duct obstruction secondary to gallstones, tumor, or stricture
Cystic duct syndrome

gallium scan

Type of test Nuclear scan

Normal findings

Diffuse, low level of gallium uptake, especially in the liver and
spleen

No increased gallium uptake within the body

Test explanation and related physiology

A gallium scan of the total body is usually performed 24, 48,
and 72 hours after an IV injection of radioactive gallium.
Gallium is a radionuclide that is concentrated by areas of
inflammation and infection, abscesses, and benign and malignant
tumors. However, not all types of tumors will concentrate
gallium. Lymphomas are particularly gallium avid. Other tumors
that can be detected by a gallium scan include sarcomas,
hepatomas, and carcinomas of the gastrointestinal tract, kidney,
uterus, stomach, and testicle.

This test is useful in detecting metastatic tumor, especially
lymphoma, even when other diagnostic imaging tests are
normal. The gallium scan also is useful in demonstrating a source
of infection in patients with a fever of unknown origin. Gallium
can be used to identify noninfectious inflammation within the
body in patients who have an elevated sedimentation rate.
Unfortunately this test is not specific enough to differentiate
among tumor, infection, inflammation, or abscess.

Contraindications

- Pregnancy, because of the risk of fetal damage

Procedure and patient care

Before

- Explain the procedure to the patient.
- Usually, administer a cathartic or enema to the patient to
  minimize increased gallium uptake within the bowel.

During

- Note the following procedural steps:
  1. The unsedated patient is injected with gallium.
  2. A total-body scan may be performed 4 to 6 hours later by
     slowly passing a radionuclide detector over the body.

3. Additional scans are usually taken 24, 48, and 72 hours later.
4. During the scanning process the patient is positioned in the supine, prone, and lateral positions.

- Note that a nuclear medicine technologist performs each scan in approximately 30 to 60 minutes. Repeated scanning is required. Repeated injections are not necessary.
- Inform the patient that test results are interpreted by a physician trained in nuclear medicine and are usually available 72 hours after the injection.

After

- Assure the patient that only tracer doses of radioisotopes have been used and that no precautions against radioactive exposure to others are necessary.

Abnormal findings

Tumor
Noninfectious inflammation
Infection
Abscess

notes

gamma-glutamyl transpeptidase (GGTP, γ-GTP, gamma-glutamyl transferase [GGT])

Type of test Blood

Normal findings
Male and female over age 45: 8-38 U/L
Female under age 45: 5-27 U/L
Elderly: slightly higher than adult level
Child: similar to adult level
Newborn: 5 times higher than adult level

Test explanation and related physiology
The enzyme GGTP participates in the transfer of amino acids and peptides across the cellular membrane and possibly participates in glutathione metabolism. Highest concentrations of this enzyme are found in the liver and biliary tract. Lesser concentration are found in the kidney, spleen, heart, intestine, brain, and prostate gland. This test is used to detect liver cell dysfunction, and it very accurately indicates even the slightest degree of cholestasis. This is the most sensitive liver enzyme in detecting biliary obstruction, cholangitis, or cholecystitis. As with leucine aminopeptidase and 5-nucleotidase, the elevation of GGTP generally parallels that of alkaline phosphatase; however, GGTP is more sensitive. Also, as with 5-nucleotidase and leucine aminopeptidase, GGTP is not increased in bone diseases as is alkaline phosphatase. A normal GGTP level with an elevated alkaline phosphatase level implies skeletal disease. Elevated GGTP and alkaline phosphatase levels imply hepatobiliary disease. GGTP is also not elevated in childhood or pregnancy.

Another important clinical aspect of GGTP is that it can detect chronic alcohol ingestion. Therefore it is very useful in the screening and evaluation of alcoholic patients. GGTP is elevated in approximately 75% of patients who chronically drink alcohol.

Why this enzyme is elevated after an acute myocardial infarction is not clear. It may represent the associated hepatic insult (if elevation occurs in the first 7 days) or the proliferation of capillary endothelial cells in the granulation tissue that replaces the infarcted myocardium. The elevation usually occurs 1 to 2 weeks after infarction.

Interfering factors
- Values may be decreased in late pregnancy.
- Drugs that may cause *increased* GGTP levels include alcohol, phenytoin (Dilantin), and phenobarbital.
- Drugs that may cause *decreased* levels include clofibrate and oral contraceptives.

Procedure and patient care

Before
- Explain the procedure to the patient.
- Tell the patient that an 8-hour fast is recommended. Only water is permitted.

During
- Collect approximately 7 to 10 ml of venous blood in a red-top tube.
- Indicate on the laboratory slip any medications the patient is taking that may affect test results.

After
- Apply pressure to the venipuncture site. Patients with liver dysfunction often have prolonged clotting times.

Abnormal findings

▲ **Increased levels**
   Hepatitis
   Cirrhosis
   Hepatic necrosis
   Hepatic tumor or metastasis
   Hepatotoxic drugs
   Cholestasis
   Jaundice
   Myocardial infarction
   Alcohol ingestion
   Pancreatitis
   Cancer of the pancreas
   Epstein Barr (infectious mononucleosis)
   Cytomegalovirus infections
   Reye's syndrome

gastrin

Type of test Blood

Normal findings

<200 pg/ml or <200 ng/L (SI units)
Levels are higher in elderly patients.

Test explanation and related physiology

Gastrin is a hormone produced by the G cells located in the distal part of the stomach (antrum). Gastrin is a potent stimulator of gastric acid. In normal gastric physiology an alkaline environment (created by food or antacids) stimulates the release of gastrin. Gastrin then stimulates the parietal cells of the stomach to secrete gastric acid. The pH environment in the stomach is thereby reduced. By negative feedback this low-pH environment suppresses further gastrin secretion.

Zollinger-Ellison (ZE) syndrome (gastrin-producing pancreatic tumor) and G-cell hyperplasia (overfunctioning of G cells in the distal stomach) are associated with high serum gastrin levels. Patients with these tumors have aggressive peptic ulcer disease. Unlike the patient with routine peptic ulcers, the patient with ZE syndrome or G-cell hyperplasia has a high incidence of complicated and recurrent peptic ulcers. It is important to identify this latter group of patients to institute more appropriate, aggressive medical and surgical therapy. The serum gastrin level is normal in the patient with routine peptic ulcer and greatly elevated in patients with ZE syndrome or G-cell hyperplasia.

However, it is important to note that patients who are taking antacid peptic ulcer medicines, have had peptic ulcer surgery, or have atrophic gastritis will have a high serum gastrin level. However, levels usually are not as high as in patients with ZE syndrome or G-cell hyperplasia.

Not all patients with ZE syndrome exhibit increased levels of serum gastrin. Some may have "top" normal gastrin levels, which makes these patients difficult to differentiate from patients with routine peptic ulcer disease. ZE syndrome or G-cell hyperplasia can be diagnosed in these "top" normal patients by *gastrin stimulation tests* using calcium or secretin. Patients with these diseases have greatly increased serum gastrin levels associated with the infusion of these drugs.

Interfering factors

- Peptic ulcer surgery.
  This creates a persistent alkaline environment, which is the strongest stimulant to gastrin.
- Ingestion of high-protein food can result in an increase in serum gastrin two to five times the normal level.
- Patients with diabetes who take insulin may have falsely elevated levels.
- Drugs that may *increase* serum gastrin levels include antacids, H_2-blocking agents (e.g., Tagamet, Zantac), and hydrogen pump inhibitors (e.g., Prilosec).
- Drugs that may *decrease* levels include anticholinergics and tricyclic antidepressants.

Procedure and patient care

Before

- Explain the procedure to the patient.
- Usually instruct the patient to fast for 12 hours. Water is permitted.
- Tell the patient to avoid alcohol for at least 24 hours.

During

- Collect approximately 5 to 7 ml of venous blood in a red-top tube.
- For the *calcium infusion test*, administer calcium gluconate intravenously for 3 hours. A preinfusion serum gastrin level is then compared with specimens taken every 30 minutes for 4 hours.
- For the *secretin test*, administer secretin intravenously. Preinjection and postinjection serum gastrin levels are taken at 15-minute intervals for 1 hour after injection.

After

- Apply pressure to the venipuncture site.

G

Abnormal findings

▲ **Increased levels**
   ZE syndrome
   G-cell hyperplasia
   Pernicious anemia
   Atrophic gastritis
   Gastric carcinoma
   Chronic renal failure
   Pyloric obstruction or gastric outlet obstruction
   Retained antrum after gastric surgery

notes

gastroesophageal reflux scan (GE reflux scan, Aspiration scan)

Type of test Nuclear scan

Normal findings No evidence of gastroesophageal reflux

Test explanation and related physiology

GE reflux scans are used to evaluate patients with symptoms of heartburn, regurgitation, vomiting, and dysphagia. They are also used to evaluate the medical or surgical treatment of patients with GE reflux. Finally, *aspiration scans* may be used to detect aspiration of gastric contents into the lungs.

Contraindications

- Patients who cannot tolerate abdominal compression
- Patients who are pregnant or lactating

Procedure and patient care

Before

- Explain the procedure to the patient.
- Assure the patient that no pain is associated with this test.
- Instruct the patient to eat a full meal just before the study.

During

- Note the following procedural steps:

GE reflux scan
  1. The patient is placed in the supine position and asked to swallow a tracer cocktail (e.g., orange juice, diluted hydrochloric acid, and technetium-99m-labeled colloid).
  2. Images are taken of the patient over the esophageal area.
  3. The patient is asked to assume other positions to determine whether GE reflux occurs and, if so, in what position.
  4. A large abdominal binder that contains an air-inflatable cuff is placed on the patient's abdomen. This is insufflated to increase abdominal pressure.
  5. Images are again taken over the esophageal area to determine if any GE reflux occurs.

Aspiration scans
  1. These scans may be performed by adding a radionuclide to the patient's evening meal and keeping the patient in the supine position until the next morning.

2. Images are made over the lung fields to detect esophago-tracheal aspiration of the tracer.

- In infants being evaluated for chalasia, note that the tracer is added to the feeding or formula. Nuclear tracer films are then taken over the next hour, with delayed films as needed.

- Note that this procedure is performed in the nuclear medicine department in approximately 30 minutes.

- Remind the patient that no discomfort is associated with this test.

After

- Assure the patient that he or she has ingested only a small dose of nuclear material. No radiation precautions need to be taken against the patient or his or her bodily secretions.

Abnormal findings

Gastroesophageal reflux
Pulmonary aspiration

notes

gastrointestinal bleeding scan (Abdominal scintigraphy, GI scintigraphy)

Type of test Nuclear scan

Normal findings No collection of radionuclide in GI tract

Test explanation and related physiology

The GI bleeding scan is a test used to localize the site of bleeding in patients who are having active GI hemorrhage. The scan also can be used in patients who have suspected intraabdominal (nongastrointestinal) hemorrhage from an unknown source. Localization of the source of GI or other bleeding can be quite difficult. When surgery is required under these circumstances, it is difficult, cumbersome, and prolonged. The surgeon may have extreme difficulty finding the source of bleeding. The bleeding scan helps localize the bleeding for the surgeon.

Arteriography has limitations in its evaluation of GI bleeding. Arteriography can determine the site of bleeding only if the rate of bleeding exceeds 0.5 ml/min for detection. The GI bleeding scan has several advantages over arteriography. It can detect bleeding if the rate is greater than 0.05 ml/min. Also, with the use of Tc-labeled red blood cells, delayed films (as long as 24 hours) can be obtained indicating the site of an intermittent or extremely slow intestinal bleed.

A GI scintigram is much more sensitive in locating the area of GI bleeding; however, it is not very specific in pinpointing the site or cause of bleeding. Usually, when positive, it cannot localize the exact source of bleeding any more accurately than to indicate the affected quadrant of the abdomen (e.g., right upper, left lower). This test is usually performed by injecting sulfur colloid labeled with technetium-99m (^{99m}Tc) or ^{99m}Tc-labeled red blood cells (RBCs) into the patient. If the patient is bleeding at a rate in excess of 0.05 ml/min, pooling of the radionuclide will ultimately be detected in the abnormal segment of the intestine. Few false-positive results occur. Again, it is important to recognize that the test only localizes the bleeding; it does not indicate the exact pathologic condition causing the bleeding. With this test result, if surgery is required, the surgeon is directed to the abnormal area and hopefully can detect and resect the pathologic bleeding source.

It is important to realize that this test can take at least 1 to 4 hours to obtain useful information. Unstable patients should not leave the intensive care environment for that long a period of time. Further, the unstable patient may need to go to surgery in minutes, and several hours may not be available to determine the region of active bleeding.

Contraindications

- Patients who are pregnant or lactating
- Medically unstable patients whose stay in the nuclear medicine department may be risky

Interfering factors

- Barium within the GI tract may mask a small source of bleeding.

Procedure and patient care

Before

- Explain the procedure to the patient.
- Assess the patient's vital signs to ensure that they are stable for the patient's transfer to and from the nuclear medicine department.
- Accompany the patient to the nuclear medicine department if vital signs are unstable.
- Assure the patient that only a small amount of nuclear material will be administered.
- Instruct the patient to notify the nuclear medicine technologist if he or she has a bowel movement during the test. Blood in the GI tract can act as a cathartic.
- Inform the patient that no pretest preparation is required.
- Inform the nuclear medicine technologist to notify the nurse of all bloody bowel movements that occur while the patient is in the nuclear medicine department.

During

- Note the following procedural steps:
  1. Ten millicuries of freshly prepared ^{99m}Tc-labeled sulfur colloid is administered intravenously to the patient. If ^{99m}Tc-labeled RBCs are to be used, 3 to 5 ml of the patient's own blood is combined with the ^{99m}Tc and reinjected into the patient.
  2. Immediately after administration of the radionuclide, the patient is placed under a scintillation camera.
  3. Multiple images of the abdomen are obtained at short

intervals (5 to 15 minutes). Scintigrams are recorded on Polaroid or x-ray film.

4. Detection of radionuclide in the abdomen indicates the site of bleeding. If no bleeding sites are noted in the first hour, the scan is repeated at hourly intervals for as long as 24 hours.

- Note that areas of the bowel hidden by the liver or spleen may not be adequately evaluated by this procedure. Also, the rectum cannot be easily evaluated, because other pelvic structures (e.g., the bladder) obstruct the view. If the initial study is negative and subsequent films give evidence of active bleeding, a repeat scan may be performed.
- Note that this test is usually performed in approximately 20 to 30 minutes by a technologist in the nuclear medicine department.
- Tell the patient that the only discomfort associated with this study is the injection of the radioisotope.

After

- Reevaluate the patient's vital signs on return to the nursing unit.
- Assure the patient that only tracer doses of radioisotopes have been used and that no precautions against radioactive exposure to others are necessary.

Abnormal findings

Ulcer
Tumor
Angiodysplasia
Polyps
Diverticulosis
Inflammatory bowel disease
Aortoduodenal fistula

notes

glucagon

Type of test Blood

Normal findings 30-210 pg/ml or 30-210 ng/L (SI units)

Test explanation and related physiology

Glucagon is a hormone secreted by the alpha cells of the pancreatic islets of Langerhans. It is secreted in response to hypoglycemia and increases the blood glucose. As serum glucose levels rise in the blood, glucagon is inhibited by a negative feedback mechanism.

Elevated glucagon levels may indicate the diagnosis of a *glucagonoma* (i.e., an alpha islet cell neoplasm). Glucagon deficiency occurs with extensive pancreatic resection or with burned out pancreatitis. Arginine is a potent stimulator of glucagon. If the glucagon levels fail to rise even with arginine infusion, the diagnosis of glucagon deficiency as a result of pancreatic insufficiency is confirmed.

In the insulin-dependent patient with diabetes, glucagon stimulation caused by hypoglycemia does not occur. To differentiate the causes of glucagon insufficiency (between pancreatic insufficiency and diabetes), *arginine stimulation* is performed. The patient with diabetes will have an exaggerated elevation of glucagon with arginine. In pancreatic insufficiency glucagon is not stimulated with arginine. Further, in patients with diabetes, hypoglycemia fails to stimulate glucagon release as would occur in a nondiabetic person.

Because glucagon is thought to be metabolized by the kidneys, renal failure is associated with high glucagon and, as a result, high glucose levels. When rejection of a transplanted kidney occurs, one of the first signs of rejection may be increased serum glucagon levels.

Interfering factors

- Test results may be invalidated if a patient has undergone a radioactive scan within the previous 48 hours.
- Levels may be elevated after prolonged fasting or moderate to severe exercise.
- Drugs that may cause *increased* levels include some amino acids (e.g., arginine), danazol, glucocorticoids, gastrin, insulin, and nifedipine.

☛ Drugs that may cause *decreased* levels include atenolol, propranolol, and secretin.

Procedure and patient care

Before
- Explain the procedure to the patient.
- Tell the patient that fasting is necessary for 10 to 12 hours
before the test. Only water is permitted.

During
- Collect a venous blood sample in a lavender-top tube.

After
- Apply pressure to the venipuncture site.
- Place the specimen on ice and send it immediately to the
laboratory.

Abnormal findings

▲ **Increased levels**
  Familial hypergluca-
      gonemia
  Glucagonoma
  Diabetes mellitus
  Chronic renal failure
  Severe stress including
      infection, burns, surgery,
      and acute hypoglycemia
  Acromegaly
  Hyperlipidemia
  Acute pancreatitis
  Pheochromocytoma

▼ **Decreased levels**
  Idiopathic glucagon
      deficiency
  Cystic fibrosis
  Chronic pancreatitis
  Postpancreatectomy
  Cancer of the pancreas

notes

glucose, blood (Blood sugar, Fasting blood sugar [FBS])

Type of test Blood

Normal findings

Cord: 45-96 mg/dl or 2.5-5.3 mmol/L (SI units)
Premature infant: 20-60 mg/dl or 1.1-3.3 mmol/L
Neonate: 30-60 mg/dl or 1.7-3.3 mmol/L
Infant: 40-90 mg/dl or 2.2-5.0 mmol/L
Child <2 years: 60-100 mg/dl or 3.3-5.5 mmol/L
Child >2 years to adult: 70-105 mg/dl or 3.9-5.8 mmol/L
Elderly: increase in normal range after age 50 years

Possible critical values

Adult male: <50 and >400 mg/dl
Adult female: <40 and >400 mg/dl
Infant: <40 mg/dl
Newborn: <30 and >300 mg/dl

Test explanation and related physiology

Through an elaborate feedback mechanism, glucose levels are controlled by insulin and glucagon. In the fasting state glucose levels are low. In response, glucagon is secreted. Glucagon causes glucose levels to rise.

After eating, glucose levels are elevated. Insulin is secreted. Insulin drives glucose into the cells to be metabolized to glycogen, amino acids, and fatty acids. Blood glucose levels diminish. Many other hormones such as adrenocorticosteroids, adrenocorticotropic hormone, epinephrine, and thyroxine can also affect glucose metabolism.

Serum glucose levels must be evaluated according to the time of day they are performed. For example, a glucose level of 135 mg/dl may be abnormal if the patient is in the fasting state, but this level would be within normal limits if the patient had eaten a meal within the last hour.

In general, true glucose elevations indicate diabetes mellitus; however, one must be aware of many other possible causes of hyperglycemia. Similarly, hypoglycemia has many causes. The most common cause is inadvertent insulin overdose in patients with brittle diabetes. If diabetes is suspected by elevated fasting blood levels, glycosylated hemoglobin (p. 449) or glucose tolerance tests (p. 444) can be performed.

Glucose determinations must be performed frequently in new patients with diabetes to monitor closely the insulin dosage to be administered. Finger stick blood glucose determinations are often performed before meals and at bedtime. Results are compared with a sliding-scale insulin chart ordered by the physician to provide coverage with SQ regular insulin.

Interfering factors

- Many forms of stress (e.g., general anesthesia, cerebrovascular accident, myocardial infarction) can cause increased serum glucose levels.
- Most IV fluids contain dextrose, which is quickly converted to glucose. Therefore most patients receiving IV fluids will have increased glucose levels.
- Many pregnant women experience some degree of glucose intolerance. If significant, it is called gestational diabetes.
- Drugs that may cause *increased* levels include antidepressants (tricyclics), beta-adrenergic blocking agents, corticosteroids, dextrose IV infusion, dextrothyroxine, diazoxide, diuretics, epinephrine, estrogens, glucagon, isoniazid, lithium, phenothiazines, phenytoin, salicylates (acute toxicity), and triamterene.
- Drugs that may cause *decreased* levels include acetaminophen, alcohol, anabolic steroids, clofibrate, disopyramide, gemfibrozil, insulin, monoamine oxidase inhibitors, pentamidine, propranolol, tolazamide, and tolbutamide.

Procedure and patient care

Before

- Explain the procedure to the patient.
- For FBS, keep the patient fasting at least 8 hours. Water is permitted.
- To prevent starvation, which may artificially raise the glucose levels, the patient should not fast longer than 16 hours.
- Withhold insulin or oral hypoglycemics until after blood is obtained.

During

- Collect approximately 7 ml of venous blood in a red- or gray-top tube.
- Glucose levels can also be evaluated by performing a finger stick and using either a visually read or a reflectance meter. The advantage of the *visually read* test is that it does not

require an expensive machine. However, the patient must be able to visually interpret the color of the reagent strip. Using *reflectance meters* (e.g., Glucometer, Accu Check bG, Stat Tek) improves the accuracy of the blood glucose determination. However, this method is more complex because it requires machine calibration and control testing.

After

- Apply pressure to the venipuncture site.
- Be certain that the patient receives a meal after fasting blood work.

Abnormal findings

▲ **Increased levels (hyperglycemia)**

Diabetes mellitus
Acute stress response
Cushing's syndrome
Pheochromocytoma
Chronic renal failure
Glucagonoma
Acute pancreatitis
Diuretic therapy
Corticosteroid therapy
Acromegaly

▼ **Decreased levels (hypoglycemia)**

Insulinoma
Hypothyroidism
Hypopituitarism
Addison's disease
Extensive liver disease
Insulin overdose
Starvation

notes

glucose, postprandial (2-hour postprandial glucose [2-hour PPG], 2-hour postprandial blood sugar, 1-hour glucose screen for gestational diabetes mellitus)

Type of test Blood

Normal findings

2-hour PPG
0-50 years: <140 mg/dl or <7.8 mmol/L (SI units)
50-60 years: <150 mg/dl
60 years and older: <160 mg/dl

1-hour glucose screen for gestational diabetes
<140 mg/dl

Test explanation and related physiology

For this study a meal acts as a glucose challenge to the body's metabolism. Normally insulin is secreted immediately after a meal in response to the elevated blood glucose level, causing the level to return to the premeal range within 2 hours. In patients with diabetes, the glucose level usually is still elevated 2 hours after the meal. The PPG is an easily performed screening test for diabetes mellitus. If the results are >140 mg/dl and <200 mg/dl, a glucose tolerance test (see p. 444) may be performed to confirm the diagnosis. If the 2-hour PPG is >200 mg/dl, the diagnosis of diabetes mellitus is confirmed.

The *1-hour glucose screen* is used to detect gestational diabetes mellitus (GDM). GDM affects 3% to 8% of pregnant women, with up to half of these women developing overt diabetes later in life. The detection and treatment of GDM may reduce the risk for several adverse perinatal outcomes (such as excessive fetal growth and birth trauma, fetal death, or neonatal morbidity).

Screening for GDM is performed with a 50-g oral glucose load, followed by a glucose level determination 1 hour later. Screening is done between weeks 24 and 28 of gestation. However, patients with risk factors, such as a previous history of GDM, may benefit from earlier screening. Patients whose serum glucose level equals or exceeds 140 mg/dl should be evaluated by a 3-hour glucose tolerance test (GTT) (see p. 444).

Interfering factors

- Stress can increase glucose levels.
- If the patient is not able to eat the entire test meal or vomits some or all of the meal, levels will be falsely decreased.

Procedure and patient care

Before

- For the *2-hour PPG*, instruct the patient to eat the entire meal (with at least 75 g of carbohydrates) and then not to eat anything else until the blood is drawn.
- For the *1-hour glucose screen for GDM*, give the fasting or nonfasting patient a 50-g oral glucose load.
- Instruct the patient not to smoke during the testing. Smoking may increase glucose levels.
- Inform the patient that he or she should rest during the 1- or 2-hour interval.

During

- Collect approximately 7 ml of blood in a red- or gray-top tube 1 or 2 hours after the patient has eaten the test meal.

After

- Apply pressure to the venipuncture site.

Abnormal findings

▲ **Increased levels**
  Diabetes mellitus
  Gestational diabetes
    mellitus
  Malnutrition
  Hyperthyroidism
  Acute stress response
  Cushing's syndrome
  Pheochromocytoma
  Chronic renal failure
  Glucagonoma
  Diuretic therapy
  Corticosteroid therapy
  Acromegaly
  Extensive liver disease

▼ **Decreased levels**
  Insulinoma
  Hypothyroidism
  Hypopituitarism
  Addison's disease
  Insulin overdose
  Malabsorption or mal-
    digestion

notes

glucose, urine (Urine sugar, Urine glucose)

Type of test Urine

Normal findings

Random specimen: Negative
24-hour specimen: <0.5 g/day or <2.78 mmol/day (SI units)

Test explanation and related physiology

A qualitative glucose test is usually part of a routine urinalysis. This screening test for the presence of glucose within the urine may indicate the likelihood of diabetes mellitus or other causes of glucose intolerance (see glucose, p. 434). This diagnosis must be confirmed by other tests (e.g., glucose tolerance test). Urine glucose tests are also used to monitor the effectiveness of diabetes therapy; however, this is largely supplanted today by finger stick determinations of blood glucose levels.

Glucose is filtered from the blood by the glomeruli of the kidney. Normally, all of the glucose is resorbed in the proximal renal tubules. When the blood glucose level exceeds the capability of the renal threshold to resorb the glucose (normally, around 180 mg/dl), it begins to spill over into the urine (glycosuria). As the blood glucose level increases further, greater amounts of glucose are spilled into the urine.

Glucosuria is not always abnormal. It may occur immediately after eating a high-carbohydrate meal. It can also occur in patients receiving dextrose-containing IV fluids. In patients who do not have diabetes, glucosuria can occur with a normal serum glucose level when kidney diseases affect the renal tubule. The renal threshold for glucose becomes abnormally low, and glucosuria occurs.

Interfering factors

- Any substance that can reduce the copper in Clinitest can produce positive results. This may include other sugars such as galactose, fructose, or lactose.
- Drugs that may cause false-positive tests with Clinitest but not with Clinistix or Tes-Tape include acetylsalicylic acid, aminosalicylic acid, ascorbic acid, cephalothin, chloral hydrate, nitrofurantoin, streptomycin, and sulfonamides.
- Drugs that may cause false-negative tests include ascorbic

acid (Clinistix, Tes-Tape), levodopa (Clinistix), and phenazopyridine (Clinistix, Tes-Tape).

▼ Drugs that may cause *increased* urine glucose levels include aminosalicylic acid, cephalosporins, chloral hydrate, chloramphenicol, dextrothyroxine, diazoxide, diuretics (loop and thiazide), estrogens, glucose infusions, isoniazid, levodopa, lithium, nafcillin, nalidixic acid, and nicotinic acid (large doses).

Procedure and patient care

Before

- Explain the procedure to the patient.
- Read the directions on the bottle or container of the reagent strips.
- Check the expiration date on the bottle before use.
- Inform the patient that urine tests for glucose may be performed at specified times during the day, generally before meals and at bedtime, and that test results may be used to determine insulin requirements.

During

- Because accuracy is necessary, collect a "fresh" urine specimen. The stagnant urine that has been in the bladder for several hours will not accurately reflect the serum glucose level at testing.
- Preferably, obtain a *double-voided specimen*:
  1. Collect a urine specimen 30 to 40 minutes before the time the urine specimen is actually needed.
  2. Discard this first specimen.
  3. Give the patient a glass of water to drink.
  4. At the required time obtain a second specimen, which is tested for glucose.
- Inform the patient that testing for glucose can be performed easily using enzyme tests such as Clinistix, Diastix, or Tes-Tape.
- Remember that urine glucose also can be determined using the Clinitest method (a copper-reducing approach).
- If a 24-hour specimen is required, refrigerate the urine during the collection period.

After

- Record the urine glucose results on the patient's chart.

Abnormal findings

▲ **Increased levels**

Diabetes mellitus

Pregnancy

Renal glycosuria

Hereditary defects in metabolism of other reducing substance (e.g., galactose, fructose, pentose)

Nephrotoxic chemicals (e.g., carbon monoxide, mercury, lead)

notes

G

glucose-6-phosphate dehydrogenase (G-6-PD screen)

Type of test Blood

Normal findings Negative (screening test) or 8-8.6 U/g of hemoglobin

Test explanation and related physiology

Glucose-6-phosphate dehydrogenase (G-6-PD) is an enzyme used in glucose metabolism. In the red blood cell a G-6-PD deficiency causes precipitation of hemoglobin and cellular membrane changes. This may result in hemolysis of variable severity. This disease is a sex-linked trait carried on the X chromosome. Affected males inherit this abnormal gene from their mothers, who are usually asymptomatic. In these males the disease consequence is most severe. Heterozygous women have variable expressions of the disease, from no symptoms to moderate symptoms if under a significant degree of stimulation.

In patients with G-6-PD deficiency, oxidizing drugs such as antimalarials, sulfa, aspirin, phenacetin, antipyretics, quinidine, sulfonamides, thiazide diuretics, tolbutamide (Orinase) and others can cause red blood cell destruction and hemolysis. Hemolysis may start as early as the first day and usually by the fourth day. Infections or acidosis can also precipitate a hemolytic process in these patients. Certain foods (e.g., fava beans) are oxidizing and therefore are harmful to the G-6-PD-deficient patient. This test is used to diagnose G-6-PD deficiency in suspected individuals.

Interfering factors

- With the dye reduction and glutathione screening testing, reticulocytosis (often associated with a hemolytic episode) may be associated with false high levels of G-6-PD.

Procedure and patient care

Before
- Explain the procedure to the patient.
- Tell the patient that no fasting is required.

During
- Collect approximately 5 ml of venous blood in a lavender- or green-top tube.
- Avoid hemolysis.

After

- Apply pressure to the venipuncture site.
- If the test indicates a G-6-PD deficiency, give the patient a list of drugs that may precipitate hemolysis. Instruct patients with the Mediterranean type of this disease not to eat fava beans. Teach patients to read labels on any over-the-counter drugs for the presence of agents (e.g., aspirin, phenacetin) that may cause hemolytic anemia.

Abnormal findings

▲ **Increased levels**

Pernicious anemia
Megaloblastic anemia
Chronic blood loss
Myocardial infarction
Hepatic coma
Hyperthyroidism

▼ **Decreased levels**

G-6-PD deficiency
Hemolytic anemia
Unusual nonspherocytic anemias

G

notes

glucose tolerance test (GTT, Oral glucose tolerance test [OGTT])

Type of test Blood; urine

Normal findings

Serum test

Fasting: 70-115 mg/dl or <6.4 mmol/L (SI units)
30 minutes: <200 mg/dl or <11.1 mmol/L
1 hour: <200 mg/dl or <11.1 mmol/L
2 hours: <140 mg/dl or <7.8 mmol/L
3 hours: 70-115 mg/dl or <6.4 mmol/L
4 hours: 70-115 mg/dl or <6.4 mmol/L

Urine test

Negative

Test explanation and related physiology

A normal fasting blood glucose, but a GTT peak and 2 hour value of greater than 200 mg/100 ml on more than one occasion is one of the National Diabetes Data Group (NDDG)'s criteria for the diagnosis of DM. The GTT is used when diabetes is suspected (retinopathy, neuropathy, diabetic-type renal diseases). It is also suggested for the following:

Patients with a family history of diabetes
Patients who are massively obese
Patients with a history of recurrent infections
Patients with delayed healing of wounds (especially on the lower legs or feet)
Women who have a history of delivering large babies, still-births, or neonatal births
Patients who have transient glycosuria or hyperglycemia during pregnancy, following myocardial infarction, surgery or stress

In the GTT the patient's ability to tolerate a standard oral glucose load is evaluated by obtaining serum and urine specimens for glucose level determinations before glucose administration and then at 30 minutes, 1 hour, 2 hours, 3 hours, and sometimes 4 hours afterwards. Normally there is a rapid insulin response to the ingestion of a large oral glucose load. This response peaks in 30 to 60 minutes and returns to normal in about 3 hours. Patients with an appropriate insulin response are able to tolerate the glucose load quite easily, with only a minimal

Figure 19 Glucose tolerance test curve for a diabetic patient and a prediabetic patient.

and transient rise in serum glucose levels within 1 to 2 hours after ingestion. In normal patients glucose does not spill over into the urine.

Patients with diabetes will not be able to tolerate this load. As a result, their serum glucose levels will be greatly elevated from 1 to 5 hours (Figure 19). Also, glucose can be detected in their urine. It is important to note that intestinal absorption may vary among individuals. For this reason, some centers prefer the glucose load to be administered intravenously.

The American Diabetes Association recommends that pregnant women who have not previously had an abnormal GTT should be tested at the 24th and 28th week of gestation with a 50-g dose of glucose. A glucose level of >140 mg/100 ml suggests that the women should be retested with a nonpregnant GTT 6 weeks or more after delivery.

Glucose intolerance also may exist in patients with oversecretion of hormones that have an ancillary affect on glucose, such as in patients with Cushing's syndrome, pheochromocytoma, acromegaly, aldosteronism, or hyperthyroidism. Patients with chronic renal failure, acute pancreatitis, myxedema, type IV lipoproteinemia, infection, or cirrhosis, can also have an abnormal GTT. Certain drugs mentioned in following paragraphs can also cause abnormal GTT results.

The GTT is also used to evaluate patients with reactive

hypoglycemia. This may occur as late as 5 hours after the initial glucose load.

Contraindications

- Patients with serious concurrent infections or endocrine disorders, because glucose intolerance will be observed even though these patients may not have diabetes

Potential complications

- Dizziness, tremors, anxiety, sweating, euphoria, or fainting during testing
  If these symptoms occur, a blood specimen is obtained. If the glucose level is too high, the test may need to be stopped and insulin administered.

Interfering factors

- Smoking during the testing period stimulates glucose because of the nicotine.
- Stress (e.g., from surgery, infection) can increase glucose levels.
- Exercise during the testing can affect glucose levels.
- Fasting or reduced caloric intake before GTT can cause glucose intolerance.
- Drugs that may cause glucose intolerance include antihypertensives, antiinflammatory drugs, aspirin, beta-blockers, furosemide, nicotine, oral contraceptives, psychiatric drugs, steroids, and thiazide diuretics.

Procedure and patient care

Before

- Explain the procedure to the patient.
- Educate the patient about the importance of having adequate food intake with adequate carbohydrates (150 g) for at least 3 days before the test.
- Instruct the patient to fast for 12 hours before the test.
- Instruct the patient to discontinue drugs (including tobacco) that could interfere with the test results
- Give the patient written instructions explaining the pretest dietary requirement.
- Obtain the patient's weight to determine the appropriate glucose loading dose (especially in children).

During

- Obtain fasting blood and urine specimens.
- Administer the oral glucose solution, usually a 75- to 100-g carbohydrate load.
- Give pediatric patients a carbohydrate load of 1.75 g/kg body weight, up to a maximum of 75 g.
- Instruct the patient to ingest the entire glucose load.
- Tell the patient that he or she cannot eat anything until the test is completed. However, encourage the patient to drink water. No other liquids should be taken.
- Inform the patient that tobacco, coffee, and tea are not allowed because they cause physiologic stimulation.
- Collect approximately 5 ml of venous blood in a gray-top tube at 30 minutes and at hourly periods. Apply pressure or a pressure dressing to the sites.
- Collect urine specimens at hourly periods.
- Mark on the tubes the time that the specimens are collected.
- Assess the patient for reactions such as dizziness, sweating, weakness, and giddiness. (These are usually transient.)
- For the IV-GTT, administer the glucose load intravenously over 3 to 4 minutes.
- Indicate on the laboratory slip any drugs that may affect test results.

After

- Send all specimens promptly to the laboratory.
- Allow the patient to eat and drink normally.
- Administer insulin or oral hypoglycemics if ordered.
- Apply pressure to the venipuncture site.

G

Abnormal findings

Diabetes mellitus
Acute stress response
Cushing's syndrome
Pheochromocytoma
Chronic renal failure
Glucagonoma
Acute pancreatitis
Diuretic therapy
Corticosteroid therapy
Acromegaly
Myxedema
Somogyi response to hypoglycemia
Post gastrectomy

notes

glycosylated hemoglobin (GHb, GHB, Glycohemoglobin, Hemoglobin [Hb] A$_{1c}$, Diabetic control index)

Type of test Blood

Normal findings Vary with laboratory method used

Adult/elderly: 4% to 8%
Child: usually <7%
Good diabetic control: 7%
Fair diabetic control: 10%
Poor diabetic control: 13% to 20%

G

Test explanation and related physiology

This test is used to monitor diabetes treatment. It measures the amount of hemoglobin A$_{1c}$ (HbA$_{1c}$) in the blood and provides an accurate long-term index of the patient's average blood glucose level. In adults about 98% of the hemoglobin in the red blood cells (RBCs) is hemoglobin A. About 7% of hemoglobin A consists of a type of hemoglobin (HbA$_1$) that can combine strongly with glucose in a process called "glycosylation." Once glycosylation occurs, it is not easily reversible.

The amount of glycosylated hemoglobin (glycohemoglobin [GHb]) depends on the amount of glucose available in the bloodstream over the RBCs' 120-day life span. Therefore determination of the GHb value reflects the average blood sugar level for the 100- to 120-day period before the test. The more glucose the RBC was exposed to, the greater the GHb percentage. One important advantage of this test is that the sample can be drawn at any time because it is not affected by short-term variations (e.g., food intake, exercise, stress, hypoglycemic agents, patient cooperation).

The GHb test is particularly beneficial for the following:

1. Evaluating the success and patient compliance of diabetic treatment
2. Comparing and contrasting the success of past and new forms of diabetic therapy
3. Determining the duration of hyperglycemia in patients with newly diagnosed diabetes
4. Providing a sensitive estimate of glucose imbalance in patients with mild diabetes
5. Individualizing diabetic control regimens

6. Providing a feeling of reward for many patients when the test shows achievement of good diabetic control
7. Evaluating the diabetic patient whose glucose levels change significantly day to day (brittle diabetic)
8. Differentiating short-term hyperglycemia in patients who do not have diabetes (e.g., recent stress or myocardial infarction) from those who have diabetes (where the glucose has been persistently elevated).

Interfering factors

- Hemoglobinopathies can affect results because the quantity of hemoglobin A (and, as a result, HbA_1) varies considerably in these diseases.
- Falsely elevated values occur when the RBC life span is lengthened because the hemoglobin A_1 has a longer period available for glycosylation.

Procedure and patient care

Before

- Explain the procedure to the patient.
- Tell the patient that fasting is not indicated.

During

- Collect approximately 5 ml of venous blood in a gray- or lavender-top tube.

After

- Apply pressure to the venipuncture site.

Abnormal findings

▲ **Increased levels**
Newly diagnosed diabetic
  patient
Poorly controlled diabetic
  patient
Nondiabetic hyperglyce-
  mia (e.g., acute stress
  response, Cushing's
  syndrome, pheochro-
  mocytoma, glucagonoma,
  corticosteroid therapy,
  or acromegaly)
Splenectomized patients
Pregnancy

▼ **Decreased levels**
Hemolytic anemia
Chronic blood loss
Chronic renal failure

notes

growth hormone (GH, Human growth hormone [HGH], Somatotropin hormone [SH])

Type of test Blood

Normal findings
Men: <5 ng/ml or <5 μg/L (SI units)
Women: <10 ng/ml or <10 μg/L
Children: 0-10 ng/ml or 0-10 μg/L
Newborn: 10-40 ng/ml or 10-40 μg/L

Test explanation and related physiology

This test is used to identify growth hormone deficiency in adolescents who have short stature, delayed sexual maturity, or other growth deficiencies. It is also used to document the diagnosis of GH excess in gigantic or acromegalic patients. Finally, it is often used as a screening test for pituitary hypofunction.

GH, or somatotropin, is secreted by the acidophil cells in the anterior pituitary gland and plays a central role in modulating growth from birth until the end of puberty. GH exerts its affects on many tissues through a group of peptides called somatomedins. The most common tested somatomedin is somatomedin-C, which is produced by the liver and has its major effect on cartilage.

If GH secretion is insufficient during childhood, limited growth and dwarfism may result. Also, a delay in sexual maturity may be a result in adolescents with reduced GH levels. Conversely, overproduction of GH during childhood results in gigantism, with the person reaching nearly 7 to 8 feet in height. An excess of GH during adulthood (after closure of long bone end plates) results in acromegaly, which is characterized by an increase in bone thickness and width but no increase in height.

GH tests are also used to confirm hypopituitarism or hyperpituitarism.

Normal GH levels overlap significantly with deficient levels. Low GH levels may indicate deficiency or may be normal for certain individuals at certain times of the day. To negate time variables in GH testing, GH can be drawn 1 to 1½ hours after deep sleep has occurred. Levels increase during sleep. Also, strenuous exercise can be performed for 30 minutes in an effort to stimulate GH production.

To negate the common variations in GH secretion, screening for *insulin-like growth factor* (IGF-1) or *somatomedin C* (see p. 780) provides a more accurate reflection of the mean plasma concentration of growth hormone. These proteins are not affected by the time of day or food intake as is GH. A GH stimulation test (see p. 455) can be performed to evaluate the body's ability to produce growth hormone.

Interfering factors

- Random measurements of growth hormone are not adequate determinants of GH deficiency, because hormone secretion is episodic.
- A radioactive scan performed within the week before the test may affect test results because levels are determined by radioimmunoassay.
- GH secretion is increased by stress, exercise, and low blood glucose levels.
- Drugs that may cause *increased* levels include amphetamines, arginine, dopamine, estrogens, glucagon, histamine, insulin, levodopa, methyldopa, and nicotinic acid.
- Drugs that may cause *decreased* levels include corticosteroids and phenothiazines.

Procedure and patient care

Before

- Explain the procedure to the patient.
- The patient should not be emotionally or physically stressed because this can increase GH levels.
- It is preferred that the patients be fasting and well rested. Water is permitted.

During

- Collect one red-top tube of venous blood.
- Because approximately two thirds of the total production of GH occurs during sleep, GH secretion also can be measured during hospitalization by obtaining blood samples while the patient is sleeping.

After

- Indicate the patient's fasting status and the time the blood is collected on the laboratory slip. Include the patient's recent activity (e.g., sleeping, walking, eating).
- Send the blood to the laboratory immediately after collection because the half-life of GH is only 20 to 25 minutes.

Abnormal findings

▲ **Increased levels**

Gigantism
Acromegaly
Diabetes mellitus
Anorexia nervosa
Stress
Major surgery
Hypoglycemia
Starvation
Deep-sleep state
Exercise

▼ **Decreased levels**

Pituitary insufficiency
Dwarfism
Hyperglycemia
Failure to thrive
Growth hormone deficiency

notes

growth hormone stimulation test (GH provocation test, Insulin tolerance test [ITT], Arginine test)

Type of test Blood

Normal findings Growth hormone levels >10 ng/ml or 10 μg/L (SI units)

Test explanation and related physiology

Because growth hormone (GH) (see p. 452) secretion is episodic, a random measurement of plasma GH is not adequate to make the diagnosis of GH deficiency. To diagnose GH deficiency, GH stimulation tests are needed. One of the most reliable GH simulators is insulin-induced hypoglycemia, in which the blood glucose declines to less than 40 mg/dl. Other GH stimulants include vigorous exercise and drugs (such as arginine, glucagon, levodopa, and clonidine).

Usually a *double-stimulated test* is performed using an arginine infusion followed by insulin-induced hypoglycemia. A GH concentration over 10 μg/L after stimulation effectively excludes the diagnosis of GH deficiency.

Contraindications

- Patients with epilepsy
- Patients with cerebrovascular disease
- Patients with myocardial infarction
- Patients with low basal plasma cortisol levels

Potential complications

- Hypoglycemia may be so significant and severe as to cause ketosis, acidosis, and shock. With close observation this is unlikely.

Interfering factors

- A radioactive scan performed within 1 week before the test may affect test results.

Procedure and patient care

Before

- Explain the procedure very carefully to the patient and, if appropriate, to the parents.
- Instruct the patient to remain NPO after midnight on the morning of the test. Water is permitted.

During

- Note the following procedural steps:
  1. A heparin lock IV line is inserted for the administration of medications and the withdrawal of frequent blood samples.
  2. Baseline blood levels are obtained for GH, glucose, and cortisol.
  3. Venous samples for GH are obtained at 0, 60, and 90 minutes after injection of arginine and/or insulin.
  4. Blood glucose levels are monitored at 15- to 30-minute intervals with the glucometer. The blood sugar should drop to less than 40 mg/dl for effective measurement of GH reserve.
- Monitor the patient for signs of hypoglycemia, postural hypotension, somnolence, diaphoresis, and nervousness. Ice chips are often given during the test for patient comfort.
- This procedure is usually performed by a nurse with a physician in proximity.
- This test takes approximately 2 hours to perform.
- Tell the patient that the minor discomfort associated with this test results from the insertion of the IV line and the hypoglycemic response induced by the insulin injection.
- GH also can be stimulated by vigorous exercise. This entails running or stair-climbing for 20 minutes. Blood samples of GH are obtained at 0, 20, and 40 minutes.

After

- Observe the venipuncture site for bleeding.
- Inform the patient and family that results may not be available for approximately 7 days. Many laboratories only run GH tests once per week.
- Give the patient cookies and punch or an IV glucose infusion.
- Send the blood to the laboratory immediately after collection, because the half-life of GH is only 20 to 25 minutes.

Abnormal findings

GH deficiency
Pituitary deficiency

Ham's test (Acid serum test for paroxysmal nocturnal hemoglobinuria [PNH])

Type of test Blood

Normal findings 10% to 50% hemolysis of red blood cells

Test explanation and related physiology

Ham's test is used to diagnose paroxysmal nocturnal hemoglobinuria (PNH). PNH is an acquired bone marrow stem cell defect. It affects the white blood cells (WBCs), red blood cells (RBCs), and platelets. Patients with this defect have evidence of hemolysis. When the WBCs, RBCs, and platelets are affected, the patient can develop aplastic anemia.

In patients with PNH, intravascular hemolysis of RBCs intermittently occurs during sleep. The RBCs of patients with PNH are more likely to lyse in an acid pH than are the RBCs of normal patients. This fact is the basis for the Ham's test. Ham's test is performed by incubating the suspected patient's RBCs with fresh autologous or compatible homologous serum adjusted to a pH of 6.5 using dilute hydrochloric acid. A positive test occurs when 10% to 80% hemolysis of RBCs is observed.

Contraindications

- Patients with recent blood transfusions

Procedure and patient care

Before

- Explain the procedure to the patient.
- Tell the patient that no fasting is required.

During

- Collect approximately 5 to 7 ml of venous blood in a lavender-top tube.
- Indicate if the patient has had a recent blood transfusion.

After

- Apply pressure or a pressure dressing to the venipuncture site.

Abnormal findings

▲ **Increased levels**
PNH
Type II congenital dyserythropoietic anemia

notes

haptoglobin

Type of test Blood

Normal findings
Adult: 100-150 mg/dl or 16-31 μmol/L (SI units)
Newborn: 0-10 mg/dl

Possible critical values <40 mg/dl

Test explanation and related physiology

The serum haptoglobin test is used to detect intravascular destruction (lysis) of red blood cells (RBCs), also called hemolysis. Haptoglobins are glycoproteins produced by the liver. These haptoglobins are powerful, free hemoglobin-binding proteins. In hemolytic anemias associated with the hemolysis of RBCs, the released hemoglobin is quickly bound to haptoglobin, and the new complex is quickly catabolized. This results in a diminished amount of free haptoglobin in the serum; this decrease cannot be quickly compensated for by normal liver production. As a result, the patient demonstrates a transient, reduced level of haptoglobin in the serum.

Haptoglobins are also decreased in patients with primary liver disease not associated with hemolytic anemias. This occurs because the diseased liver is unable to produce these glycoproteins. Hematoma can reduce haptoglobin levels by the absorption of hemoglobin into the blood and binding with haptoglobin.

Elevated haptoglobin concentrations are found in many inflammatory diseases and therefore can be used as a nonspecific "acute-phase" protein in much the same way as a sedimentation rate test (see p. 369). That is, levels of haptoglobin increase with severe infection, inflammation, tissue destruction, acute myocardial infarction, burns, and some cancers.

Interfering factors

- Ongoing infection can cause falsely elevated test results.
- ✗ Drugs that may cause *increased* haptoglobin levels include androgens and steroids.
- ✗ Drugs that may cause *decreased* levels include chlorpromazine, diphenhydramine, indomethacin, isoniazid, nitrofurantoin, oral contraceptives, quinidine, and streptomycin.

Procedure and patient care

Before
- Explain the procedure to the patient.
- Tell the patient that no fasting is required.

During
- Collect at least 2 ml of venous blood in a red-top tube.
- Avoid hemolysis, which may alter test results.

After Apply pressure to the venipuncture site.

Abnormal findings

▲ **Increased levels**
Collagen disease
Infection
Tissue destruction
Biliary obstruction
Nephritis
Pyelonephritis
Ulcerative colitis
Peptic ulcer
Myocardial infarction
Acute rheumatic disease
Neoplasia

▼ **Decreased levels**
Hemolytic anemia
Transfusion reactions
Prostatic heart valves
Systemic lupus erythematosus
Primary liver disease not associated with hemolytic anemia
Erythroblastosis fetalis
Hematoma
Tissue hemorrhage
Chronic liver disease

notes

Helicobacter Pylori antibodies test (*Campylobacter pylori*, Anti–*Helicobacter pylori* immunoglobulin G [IgG] antibody, Campylobacter-like organism [CLO] test)

Type of test Blood, microscopic examination of antral or duodenal biopsy specimen, breath test

Normal findings Not present

Test explanation and related physiology

Helicobacter pylori, a bacteria that can be found in the mucus overlying the gastric mucosa and on the mucosal cells that line the stomach, has been recognized as a risk factor for gastric diseases such as duodenal ulcers, gastritis, and gastric carcinoma.

There are several methods of detecting the presence of this organism. It can be cultured from a specimen of mucus obtained through a gastroscope (see p. 375). The organism can also be detected on a gastric mucosal biopsy.

Newer methods that are more easily performed and more accurate are available to detect this organism. Immunoassays to serum antibodies to *H. pylori* have been developed and are very accurate in detecting the presence of the organism. The IgG anti-*H. pylori* antibody is most commonly used. It becomes elevated 2 months after infection and stays elevated for over a year after treatment. The IgA anti-*H. pylori* antibody, like IgG, becomes elevated 2 months after infection but decreases 3 to 4 weeks after treatment. The IgM anti-*H. pylori* antibody is the first to become elevated (about 3 to 4 weeks) and is not detected after 2 to 3 months after treatment. These antibody titers are fast becoming the "gold standard" for *H. pylori* detection.

There is also a *breath test* available for the detection of *H. pylori*. The breath test depends on the ability of *H. pylori* to break down urea into carbon dioxide and ammonia via its enzyme, urease. A dose of radioactive ^{14}C or nonradioactive ^{13}C urea is given by mouth. The isotopic CO_2 concentration is determined by breath collection.

Interfering factors

- *H. pylori* can be transmitted by endoscopy procedures.

Procedure and patient care

Before

- Explain the procedure to the patient.
- Tell the patient that no fasting is required for the blood test.
- If a biopsy or culture will be obtained by endoscopy, see discussion of esophagogastroduodenoscopy (EGD) (p. 375).

During

- Collect a venous blood sample according to the protocol of the laboratory performing the test.
- A gastric or duodenal biopsy can be obtained by endoscopy. Keep the specimen moist by the addition of approximately 5 ml of sterile saline.
- For the *breath test*, a dose of radioactive ^{14}C or nonradioactive ^{13}C urea is given by mouth.

After

- Apply pressure to the venipuncture site.
- If endoscopy was used to obtain a culture, see procedure for EGD (p. 375). The specimen should be transported to the laboratory within 30 minutes after collection.

Abnormal findings

▲ **Increased levels**
    Acute and chronic gastritis
    Duodenal ulcer
    Gastric ulcer
    Gastric carcinoma

notes

hematocrit (Hct, Packed red blood cell volume, Packed cell volume [PCV])

Type of test Blood

Normal findings

Male: 42%-52% or 0.42-0.52 volume fraction (SI units)
Female: 37%-47% or 0.37-0.47 volume fraction (SI units)
Pregnant female: >33%
Elderly: values may be slightly decreased
Children (%)
  Newborn: 44 to 64
  2-8 wks: 39-59
  2-6 mos: 35-50
  6 mos-1 year: 29-43
  1-6 years: 30-40
  6-18 years: 32-44

Possible critical values <15% or >60%

Test explanation and related physiology

The Hct is a measure of the percentage of the total blood volume that is made up by the red blood cells (RBCs). The height of the RBC column is measured after centrifugation. It is compared to the height of the column of the total whole blood. The ratio of the height of the RBC column compared to the original total blood column is multiplied by 100%. This is the Hct value. It is routinely performed as part of a complete blood count. The Hct closely reflects the hemoglobin (Hgb) and RBC values. The Hct in percentage points usually is approximately three times the Hgb concentration in grams per deciliter when RBCs are of normal size and contain normal amounts of Hgb.

Abnormal values indicate the same pathologic states as abnormal RBC counts and Hgb concentrations (see pp. 708 and 465). Decreased levels indicate anemia (reduced number of RBCs). Increased levels can indicate erythrocytosis.

Like other RBC values, the Hct can be altered by many factors such as hydration status and RBC morphology.

Interfering factors

- Abnormalities in RBC size may alter Hct values.
- Extremely elevated white blood cell counts may affect values.
- Hemodilution and dehydration may affect the Hct level.

- Pregnancy usually causes slightly decreased values because of hemodilution.
- Living in high altitudes causes increased values.
- Values may not be reliable immediately after hemorrhage.
- Drugs that may cause *decreased* levels include chloramphenicol and penicillin.

Procedure and patient care

Before
- Tell the patient that no fasting is required.

During
- Collect approximately 5 to 7 ml of venous blood in a lavender-top tube; however, only 0.5 ml is required when using capillary tubes.
- Avoid hemolysis.

After
- Apply pressure to the venipuncture site.

Abnormal findings

▲ Increased levels
   Congenital heart disease
   Polycythemia vera
   Severe dehydration
   Erythrocytosis
   Severe diarrhea
   Eclampsia
   Burns
   Dehydration
   Chronic obstructive
      pulmonary disease

▼ Decreased levels
   Anemia
   Hyperthyroidism
   Cirrhosis
   Hemolytic reaction
   Hemorrhage
   Dietary deficiency
   Bone marrow failure
   Normal pregnancy
   Rheumatoid arthritis
   Multiple myeloma
   Malnutrition
   Leukemia
   Hemoglobinopathy

notes

hemoglobin (Hb, Hgb)

Type of test Blood

Normal findings
Male: 14-18 g/dl or 8.7-11.2 mmol/L (SI units)
Female: 12-16 g/dl or 7.4-9.9 mmol/L
Pregnant female: >11 g/dl
Elderly: values are slightly decreased
Children
   Newborn: 14-24 g/dl
   0-2 wks: 12-20 g/dl
   2-6 mos: 10-17 g/dl
   6 mos-1 year: 9.5-14 g/dl
   1-6 years: 9.5-14 g/dl
   6-18 years: 10-15.5 g/dl

Possible critical values <5.0 g/dl or >20 g/dl

Test explanation and related physiology
The Hgb concentration is a measure of the total amount of Hgb in the peripheral blood, which reflects the number of red blood cells (RBCs) in the blood. The test is normally performed as part of a complete blood count.

The hematocrit (Hct) in percentage points usually is approximately three times the Hgb concentration in grams per deciliter when RBCs are of normal size and contain normal amounts of Hgb. Abnormal values indicate the same pathologic states as abnormal RBC counts and Hct concentrations (see pp. 708 and 463). Decreased levels indicate anemia (reduced number of RBCs). Increased levels can indicate erythrocytosis. In addition, however, changes in plasma volume are more accurately reflected by the Hgb concentration. Slight decreases in the values of Hgb and the hematocrit during pregnancy reflect both the expanded blood volume due to a chronic state of overhydration and an increased number of RBCs. Hemoglobinopathies such as sickle cell disease and Hgb C disease are also associated with reduced hemoglobin levels.

Interfering factors
- Slight Hgb decreases normally occur during pregnancy because of the expanded blood volume.

- Living in high-altitude areas causes high Hgb values.
- Drugs that may cause *increased* levels include gentamicin and methyldopa (Aldomet).
- Drugs that may cause *decreased* levels include antibiotics, antineoplastic drugs, aspirin, indomethacin (Indocin), rifampin, and sulfonamides.

Procedure and patient care

Before

- Explain the procedure to the patient.
- Tell the patient that no fasting is required.

During

- Collect approximately 5 to 7 ml of venous blood in a lavender-top tube.
- Avoid hemolysis.
- List on the laboratory slip any drugs that may affect test results.

After

- Apply pressure to the venipuncture site.

Abnormal findings

▲ **Increased levels**

Congenital heart disease
Polycythemia vera
Hemoconcentration of
  the blood
Chronic obstructive
  pulmonary disease
Congestive heart failure
High altitudes
Severe burns
Dehydration

▼ **Decreased levels**

Anemia
Severe hemorrhage
Hemolysis
Hemoglobinopathies
Cancer
Nutritional deficiency
Lymphoma
Systemic lupus erythema-
  tosus
Sarcoidosis
Kidney disease
Chronic hemorrhage
Splenomegaly
Sickle cell anemia
Neoplasia

hemoglobin electrophoresis (Hgb electrophoresis)

Type of test Blood

Normal findings

Adult/elderly

Hgb A_1: 95% to 98%

Hgb A_2: 2% to 3%

Hgb F: 0.8% to 2%

Hgb S: 0%

Hgb C: 0%

Children: Hgb F

Newborn: 50% to 80%

6 months: 8%

>6 months: 1% to 2%

Test explanation and related physiology

Hgb electrophoresis is a test that identifies abnormal forms of Hgb (hemoglobinopathies). Although many different Hgb variations have been described, the more common types are A_1, A_2, F, S, and C. Each major Hgb type is electrically charged to varying degrees. When the hemoglobin from lysed RBCs is placed on electrophoresis paper and placed in an electromagnetic field, the Hgb variants migrate at different rates and therefore spread apart from each other. The migrations of the various forms of Hgb make up a series of bands on the paper. Therefore the bands correspond to the various forms of hemoglobin present. The pattern of bands is compared to normal and other well known abnormal patterns. Further, each band can be quantitated as a percentage of the total Hgb, indicating the severity of any recognized abnormality.

The form *Hgb A_1* constitutes the major component of Hgb in the normal red blood cell (RBC). *Hgb A_2* is only a minor component (2% to 3%) of the normal Hgb total. *Hgb F* is the major hemoglobin component in the fetus but normally exists in only minimal quantities in the normal adult. Levels of Hgb F greater than 2% in patients over 3 years of age are considered abnormal. Hgb F is able to transport oxygen when only small amounts of oxygen are available (as in fetal life). In patients requiring compensation for prolonged chronic hypoxia (as in congenital cardiac abnormalities), Hgb F may be found in increased levels to assist in the transport of the available oxygen.

Hgb S and *Hgb C* are abnormal forms of Hgb that occur predominantly in American blacks. The Hgb contents of some common hemoglobinopathies, as determined by electrophoresis, are indicated in Table 12.

Interfering factor

- Blood transfusions within the previous 12 weeks may alter test results.

Procedure and patient care

Before

- Explain the procedure to the patient.
- Tell the patient that no fasting is required.

During

- Collect approximately 7 ml of venous blood in a lavender-top tube.

After

- Apply pressure to the venipuncture site.

Abnormal findings

Sickle cell disease
Sickle cell trait
Hemoglobin C disease
Hemoglobin H disease
Thalassemia major
Thalassemia minor

notes

TABLE 12 Hemoglobin contents of some common hemoglobinopathies

			Percentage range			
	Hgb A1	Hgb A2	Hgb F	Hgb S	Hgb H	Hgb C
Sickle cell disease	0	2	2	80-100	0	0
Sickle cell trait	60-80	2-3	2	20-40	0	0
Hemoglobin C disease	0	2-3	2	0	0	90-100
Hemoglobin H disease	65-90	2-3	0	0	5-30	0
Thalassemia major	5-20	2-3	65-100	0	0	0
Thalassemia minor	50-85	4-6	1-3	0	0	0

hepatitis virus studies (Hepatitis-associated antigen [HAA], Australian antigen)

Type of test Blood

Normal findings Negative

Test explanation and related physiology

Hepatitis is an inflammation of the liver caused by viruses, alcohol ingestion, drugs, toxins, or overwhelming bacterial sepsis. The three common viruses now recognized as causing disease are hepatitis A, hepatitis B, and hepatitis non-A/non-B (also called hepatitis C) viruses. Hepatitis D and E viruses are much less common in the United States. The various types of hepatitis cannot be differentiated on the basis of their clinical presentation.

Hepatitis A virus (HAV) was originally called *infectious hepatitis*. It has a short incubation period and is highly contagious. During active infection HAV is excreted in the stool and transmitted via the oral-fecal contamination of food and drink. About half of those tested in the United States have had this form of hepatitis. Two types of antibodies to HAV can be detected.

The first type of antibody to HAV is immunoglobulin (Ig) M antibody (HAV-Ab/IgM), which appears approximately 3 to 4 weeks after exposure and returns to normal in approximately 8 weeks.

The second type of antibody is IgG (HAV-Ab/IgG). The IgG antibody can remain detectable for more than 10 years after the infection. If the IgM antibody is elevated in the absence of the IgG antibody, acute hepatitis is suspected. If, however, IgG is elevated in the absence of IgM elevation, this indicates the convalescent or chronic stage of HAV viral infection.

Hepatitis B virus (HBV) is commonly known as *serum hepatitis*. HBV is most frequently transmitted by blood transfusion; however, it also can be contracted via exposure to other body fluids. Besides the acute phase of hepatitis B, carrier and chronic states of this disease have been recognized.

HBV, also called the *Dane particle*, is made up of an inner core surrounded by an outer capsule. The outer capsule contains the hepatitis B surface antigen (HBsAg), formerly called Australian antigen. The inner core contains HBV core antigen (HBcAg).

TABLE 13 Hepatitis testing

Hepatitis test	Appears/disappears	Clinical significance
HBsAg	2-6 weeks/1-3 months	Active infection, carrier state
HBsAb	2-6 weeks/life	Convalescent, denotes immunity to HBV
HBcAb	2 weeks/3-6 months	Past infection, chronic hepatitis
HBeAg	3-5 days/2-4 weeks	Acute infection, denotes infectivity
HBeAb	1-4 weeks/4-6 years	Convalescent, denotes decreased infectivity

The hepatitis B e-antigen (HBeAg) is also found within the core. Antibodies to these antigens are called HBsAb, HBcAb, and HBeAb. The tests used to detect these antigens and antibodies include (Table 13):

1. *Hepatitis B surface antigen (HBsAg)*. This is the most fre-quently and easily performed test for hepatitis B, and this is the first test to become abnormal. HBsAg rises before the onset of clinical symptoms, peaks during the first week of symptoms, and returns to normal by the time jaun-dice subsides. HBsAg generally indicates active infection by HBV. If the level of this antigen persists in the blood, the patient is considered to be a carrier.

2. *Hepatitis B surface antibody (HBsAb)*. This antibody appears approximately 4 weeks after the disappear-ance of the surface antigen and signifies the end of the acute infection phase. HBsAb also signifies immu-nity to subsequent infection. Concentrated forms of this agent constitute the hyperimmunoglobulin given to patients who have come in contact with HBV-infected patients (e.g., contact by an inadvertent needle prick from a needle previously used on a patient with HBV infec-tion). HBsAb is the antibody that denotes immunity after administration of hepatitis B vaccine.

3. *Hepatitis B core antigen (HBcAg)*. No tests are currently available to detect this antigen.

4. *Hepatitis B core antibody (HBcAb)*. This antibody appears approximately 1 month after infection with HBsAg and declines (although it remains elevated) over several years. HBcAb is also present in patients with chronic hepatitis. The HBcAb level is elevated during the time lag between the disappearance of HBsAg and the appearance of HBsAb. This interval is called the "core window". During the core window, HBcAb is the only detectable marker of a recent hepatitis infection.

5. *Hepatitis B e-antigen (HBeAg)*. This antigen is generally not used for diagnostic purposes but rather as an index of infectivity. The presence of HBeAg correlates with early and active disease, as well as with high infectivity in acute HBV infection. The persistent presence of HBeAg in the blood predicts the development of chronic HBV infection.

6. *Hepatitis B e-antibody (HBeAb)*. This antibody indicates that an acute phase of HBV infection is over, or almost over, and that the chance of infectivity is greatly reduced.

Non-A, non-B hepatitis (NANB), also called *hepatitis C (HCV)*, is transmitted in a manner similar to that of HBV. The incubation period is 2 to 12 weeks after exposure. An HCV viral titer to detect HCV IgG antibodies is now available to detect these infections; however, no vaccine protection exists against this form of hepatitis.

Hepatitis D virus (HDV) is known to cause "delta hepatitis". The HDV antigen can be detected by immunoassay within a few days after infection. The IgM and total antibodies to HDV are detected early in the disease also. A persistent elevation of these antibodies indicates a chronic or carrier state.

Hepatitis E virus (HEV) was initially included in the NANB virus group but was isolated several years ago. No antigen or antibody tests are currently widely available and accurate for the serologic testing.

Procedure and patient care

Before

- Tell the patient that no fasting is required.

During

- Collect approximately 5 to 7 ml of venous blood in a red-top tube.
- Note that most of the testing for hepatitis is done by radioim-

munoassay. Usually a hepatitis profile that includes several HBV antigens and antibodies is performed.

After

- Apply pressure to the venipuncture site.
- Handle the specimen as if it were capable of transmitting hepatitis.
- Immediately discard the needle in the appropriate receptacle.
- Send the specimen promptly to the laboratory.

Abnormal findings

▲   **Increased levels**

Hepatitis A

Hepatitis B

Non-A, non-B hepatitis

Chronic carrier state, hepatitis B

Chronic hepatitis B

notes

herpes simplex (Herpesvirus type 2, Herpes simplex virus type 2 [HSV 2], Herpes genitalis)

Type of test Blood; microscopic

Normal findings

No virus present
No HSV antigens or antibodies present

Test explanation and related physiology

Herpes simplex virus can be classified either as type 1 or as type 2. *Type 1* (HSV 1) is primarily responsible for oral lesions (blisters on the lips called "cold sores") or even corneal lesions. *Type 2* (HSV 2) is a sexually transmitted viral infection of the urogenital tract. Vesicular lesions may occur on the penis, scrotum, vulva, perineum, perianal region, vagina, or cervix.

Because most infants become infected if they pass through a birth canal containing HSV, determining its presence at delivery is necessary. Congenital infections may result in problems such as microcephaly, chorioretinitis, and mental retardation in the newborn. Disseminated neonatal herpesvirus infections carry a high incidence of infant mortality. A vaginal delivery is possible if no virus is present, and birth by cesarean section is needed if HSV is present. Viral testing can be performed on males or females to determine the risk of sexual transmission.

Culture is still the gold standard for HSV detection and can identify HSV in 90% of infected patients. Serologic tests are more easily and conveniently available for detection of HSV 1 and HSV 2 antigen. Unfortunately the accuracy is not great. Only about 85% of patients who are culture positive have positive serologies. The advantage of antigen tests is that results can be available in a day. Serologic tests for antibodies are cumbersome because they require repeated blood tests during the acute and convalescent phases of an acute viral outbreak (about 2 weeks apart). A fourfold rise in titer is expected to diagnose acute initial herpes infection. Recurrent infections are far less likely to demonstrate titer elevations. Furthermore, perhaps more than 50% of people in the United States have positive herpes antibodies.

Procedure and patient care

Before

- Explain the procedure to the patient.
- Tell the female patient to refrain from douching and tub bathing before the cervical culture is performed.
- Obtain the urethral specimen from the male patient before voiding.
- Blood can be diagnostic in either sex.

During

- Obtain cultures as follows:

Urethral culture

1. A culture is taken by inserting a sterile swab gently into the anterior urethra or genital skin lesion of the male patient.
2. It is advisable to place the male patient in the supine position to prevent falling if vasovagal syncope occurs during introduction of the cotton swab or wire loop into the urethra.
3. The patient is observed for hypotension, bradycardia, pallor, sweating, nausea, and weakness.

Cervical culture

1. The female patient is placed in the lithotomy position, and a vaginal speculum is inserted.
2. Cervical mucus is removed with a cotton ball.
3. A sterile cotton-tipped swab is inserted into the endocervical canal and moved from side to side to obtain the culture. If a genital lesion is present, swabs from that area will be more sensitive in indicating infection.

- For pregnant women with herpes genitalis, note that the cervix is cultured weekly for the herpesvirus, beginning 4 to 6 weeks before the due date. Vaginal delivery is possible if the following criteria are met:
  1. The two most recent cultures are negative.
  2. The woman is not experiencing any symptoms.
  3. No lesions are visible on inspection of the vagina and vulva.
  4. Throughout pregnancy the woman has not had more than one positive culture, during which she was symptom free.

Blood for serology

- Obtain 5 to 7 ml of blood in a red-top tube.

After
- Inform the patient how to obtain the test results.

Abnormal finding

Herpesvirus infection

notes

holter monitoring (Ambulatory monitoring, Ambulatory electrocardiography, Event recorder)

Type of test Electrodiagnostic

Normal findings Normal sinus rhythm

Test explanation and related physiology

Holter monitoring is a continuous recording of the electrical activity of the heart. This can be performed for periods up to 72 hours. With this technique an electrocardiogram (ECG) is recorded continuously on magnetic tape during unrestricted activity, rest, and sleep. The Holter monitor is equipped with a clock that permits accurate time monitoring on the ECG tape. The patient is asked to carry a diary and record daily activities, as well as any cardiac symptoms that may develop during the period of monitoring.

Most units in present use are equipped with an "event marker." This is a button the patient can push when symptoms such as chest pain, syncope, or palpitations are experienced. This type of monitor is referred to as an *event recorder*.

The Holter monitor is used primarily to identify suspected cardiac rhythm disturbances and to correlate these disturbances with symptoms such as dizziness, syncope, palpitations, or chest pain. The monitor is also used to assess pacemaker function and the effectiveness of antiarrhythmic medications.

After completion of the determined time period, usually 24 to 72 hours, the Holter monitor is removed from the patient, and the record tape is played back at high speeds. The ECG tracing is usually interpreted by computer, which can detect any significant abnormal waveform patterns that occurred during the testing.

Contraindications

- Patients who are unable to cooperate with maintaining the lead placement from the monitor to the body
- Patients who are unable to maintain an accurate diary of significant activities or events

Interfering factor

- Interruption in the electrode contact with the skin

Procedure and patient care

Before

- Explain the procedure to the patient.
- Instruct the patient about care of the Holter monitor.
- Inform the patient about the necessity of ensuring good contact between the electrodes and the skin.
- Teach the patient how to maintain an accurate diary. Stress the need to record significant symptoms.
- Instruct the patient to note in the diary if any interruption in Holter monitoring occurs.
- Assure the patient that the electrical flow is coming from the patient and that he or she will not experience any electrical stimulation from the machine.
- Instruct the patient not to bathe during the period of cardiac monitoring.
- Tell the patient to minimize the use of electrical devices (e.g., electric toothbrushes, shavers), which may cause artificial changes in the ECG tracing.

During

- Prepare the sites for electrode placement with alcohol. (This is usually done in the cardiology department by a technologist.)
- Place the gel and electrodes at the appropriate sites. Usually the chest and abdomen are the most appropriate locations for limb-lead electrode placement. The precordial leads also may be placed.
- Usually do not use the extremities for electrode placement to minimize alterations in tracing that occur with normal physical activity.
- Encourage the patient to call if he or she has any difficulties.

After

- Gently remove the tape and other paraphernalia securing the electrodes.
- Wipe the patient clean of electrode gel.
- Inform the patient that the Holter monitoring interpretation will be available in a few days.

Abnormal findings

Cardiac arrhythmia (dysrhythmia)
Ischemic changes

human lymphocyte antigen B27 (HLA-B27 antigen)

Type of test Blood

Normal findings Negative

Test explanation and related physiology

The HLA antigens exist on the surface of white blood cells and on the surface of all nucleated cells in other tissues. These antigens can be detected most easily on the cell surface of lymphocytes. The presence or absence of these antigens is determined genetically. Each gene controls the presence or absence of HLA A, B, C, or D. Because HLA antigens are genetically determined, they are useful in paternity investigations.

The HLA system of antigens has been used to indicate tissue compatibility with tissue transplantation. If the HLA antigens of the donor are not compatible with the recipient, the recipient will make antibodies to those antigens and accelerate rejection. Transplant survival of the tissue is increased if HLA matching is compatible. In contrast, prior HLA sensitization causes antibodies to form in the blood recipient, which will shorten the survival of blood cells (red blood cells or platelets) when transfused.

The HLA system has also been used to assist in the diagnosis of certain other diseases, as they are often associated with these diseases. For example, HLA B27 is present in 80% of patients with Reiter's syndrome. When a patient presents with recurrent and multiple arthritic complaints, the presence of HLA B27 supports the diagnosis of Reiter's syndrome. HLA-B27 is found in 5% to 7% of normal patients. Other HLA-disease associations are mentioned in "Abnormal findings."

Procedure and patient care

Before

- Tell the patient that no fasting or special preparation is required.

During

- Collect at least 10 ml of venous blood in a heparinized solution.

After

- Apply pressure to the venipuncture site.

Abnormal findings

▲ **Increased levels (HLA antigens present)**
   Ankylosing spondylitis
   Reiter's syndrome
   Yersinia enterocolitica arthritis
   Anterior uveitis
   Graves disease
   Celiac disease/gluten enteropathy
   Chronic active hepatitis
   Multiple sclerosis
   Myasthenia gravis
   Dermatitis herpetiformis
   Psoriasis
   Juvenile diabetes
   Hemochromatosis
   Rheumatoid arthritis

notes

human T-cell lymphotrophic (HTLV) I/II antibody

Type of test Blood

Normal findings Negative

Test explanation and related physiology

Several forms of HTLV, a human retrovirus, affect humans. HTLV-I is associated with adult T-cell leukemia/lymphoma. HTLV-II is associated with adult hairy-cell leukemia and neurologic disorders such as tropical spastic paraparesis. Humans can be infected with these viruses, however, and not develop any malignancy or diseases.

The human immunodeficiency viruses (HIVs), which are known to be the cause of acquired immunodeficiency syndrome (AIDS), are also retroviruses; however, HTLV infection is not associated with AIDS. HTLV transmission is similar, however, to HIV transmission (e.g., body fluid contamination, intravenous drug use, sexual contact, breastfeeding).

Procedure and patient care

Before

- Explain the procedure to the patient.
- Tell the patient that no fasting is required.

During

- Collect approximately 7 ml of venous blood in a red-top tube.

After

- Apply pressure to the venipuncture site.

Abnormal findings

Acute HTLV infection
Adult T-cell leukemia
Hairy-cell leukemia
Tropical spastic paraparesis

17-hydroxycorticosteroids (17-OCHS)

Type of test Urine (24-hour)

Normal findings

Male

<8 years: <1.5 mg/24 hr
<12 years: <4.5 mg/24 hr
Adult: 4.5-10 mg/24 hr
Elderly: values lower than for adult

Female

<8 years: <1.5 mg/24 hr
<12 years: <4.5 mg/24 hr
Adult: 2.5-10 mg/24 hr
Elderly: values lower than for adult

Test explanation and related physiology

Elevated levels of 17-OCHS are seen in patients with hyperfunctioning of the adrenal gland (Cushing syndrome), whether this condition is caused by a pituitary or adrenal tumor, bilateral adrenal hyperplasia, or ectopic tumors producing adrenocorticotropic hormone (ACTH). Low levels of 17-OCHS are seen in patients who have a hypofunctioning adrenal gland (Addison's disease) as a result of destruction of the adrenals (by hemorrhage, infarction, metastatic tumor, or autoimmunity), surgical removal of an adrenal gland, congenital enzyme deficiency, hypopituitarism, or adrenal suppression after prolonged exogenous steroid ingestion.

Testing the urine for this hormone metabolite is only an indirect measure of adrenal function. Urine and plasma levels of cortisol (see p. 283) provide a much more accurate measurement of adrenal function. Because the excretion of cortisol metabolites follows a diurnal variation, a 24-hour collection is necessary.

Interfering factors

- Emotional and physical stress (e.g., infection) and licorice ingestion may cause increased adrenal activity.
- Drugs that may cause *increased* 17-OCHS levels include acetazolamide, chloral hydrate, chlorpromazine, colchicine,

erythromycin, meprobamate, paraldehyde, quinidine, quinine, and spironolactone.
- ✗ Drugs that may cause *decreased* levels include estrogens, oral contraceptives, phenothiazines, and reserpine.

Procedure and patient care

Before
- Explain the procedure to the patient.
- Note that drugs are usually withheld several days before the urine collection. Check with the physician and laboratory for specific guidelines.
- Assess the patient for signs of stress and report these to the physician.

During
- Do not administer to the patient any drugs that may interfere with test results.
- Begin the 24-hour urine collection after the patient urinates. Discard this urine and note this as the start time of the test.
- Collect all urine passed by the patient during the next 24 hours.
- Post the hours for the urine collection in a prominent spot.
- Note that it is not necessary to measure each urine specimen.
- Tell the patient to void before defecating so that the urine is not contaminated by feces.
- Inform the patient that toilet paper should not be placed in the collection container.
- Encourage the patient to drink fluids during the 24 hours, unless this is contraindicated for medical purposes.
- Collect the last specimen as close as possible to the end of the 24-hour collection. Add this to the container.
- Keep the urine specimen refrigerated or on ice during the entire collection.

After
- Send the urine to the chemistry laboratory as soon as the test is completed.
- List on the laboratory slip any medications the patient may be taking that can affect test results.

H

Abnormal findings

▲ **Increased levels**
Cushing's disease
Ectopic ACTH-producing
  tumors
Stress
Adrenal adenoma or
  carcinoma
Hyperthyroidism
Obesity

▼ **Decreased levels**
Adrenal hyperplasia (adre-
  nogenital syndrome)
Addison's disease
Adrenal suppression from
  steroid therapy
Hypopituitarism
Hypothyroidism

notes

5-hydroxyindoleacetic acid (5-HIAA)

Type of test Urine (24-hour)

Normal findings
2-6 mg/24 hr or 10.4-31.2 μmol/day (SI units)
Female levels lower than male levels

Test explanation and related physiology
Quantitative analysis of urine levels of 5-HIAA is used to detect and follow the clinical course of patients with carcinoid tumors. Carcinoid tumors are serotonin-secreting tumors that may grow in the appendix, intestine, lung, or any tissue derived from the neuroectoderm. These tumors contain *argentaffin-staining (enteroendocrine)* cells, which produce serotonin and other powerful neurohormones that are metabolized by the liver to 5-HIAA and excreted in the urine. These powerful neurohormones are responsible for the clinical presentation of carcinoid syndrome (bronchospasm, flushing, diarrhea). This test is used not only to identify patients with carcinoid tumor but also to reevaluate those with known tumor by using serial levels of urinary 5-HIAA. Rising levels of 5-HIAA indicate progression of tumor; falling levels of 5-HIAA indicate a therapeutic response of the tumor to antineoplastic therapy.

Interfering factors
- Bananas, plantain, pineapple, kiwi fruit, walnuts, plums, pecans, and avocados can factitiously elevate 5-HIAA levels.
- Drugs that may cause *increased* 5-HIAA levels include acetanilid, acetophenetidin (phenacetin), glyceryl guaiacolate (guaifenesin [Robitussin]), methocarbamol, acetaminophen, and reserpine.
- Drugs that may cause *decreased* levels include chlorpromazine, ethyl alcohol, heparin, imipramine (Tofranil), isoniazid (INH), levodopa, MAO inhibitors, methenamine, methyldopa (Aldomet), phenothiazines, promethazine (Phenergan), aspirin, and tricyclic antidepressants.

Procedure and patient care

Before
- Explain the procedure to the patient.
- Instruct the patient to refrain from eating foods containing

serotonin (e.g., plums, pineapples, bananas, eggplant, tomatoes, avocados, walnuts) for several days (usually 3) before and during testing.

During

- To begin the 24-hour urine collection, discard the patient's initial specimen and start the timing at that point.
- Collect all urine passed during the next 24 hours.
- Show the patient where to store the urine specimen.
- Keep the specimen on ice or in a refrigerator during the 24-hour collection. A preservative is needed to keep the specimen at an appropriate pH.
- Post the hours for urine collection in a noticeable place to prevent accidental discarding of the specimen.
- Instruct the patient to void before defecating so that urine is not contaminated by stool.
- Tell the patient not to put toilet paper in the urine container.
- Collect the last specimen as close as possible to the end of the 24-hour collection. Add this urine to the container.

After

- Send the urine specimen to the laboratory promptly.
- List on the laboratory slip any medications that may affect the test results.

Abnormal findings

▲ **Increased levels**
   Carcinoid tumors
   Noncarcinoid illness
   Cystic fibrosis
   Intestinal malabsorption

▼ **Decreased levels**
   Depression
   Migraine headaches

notes

hysterosalpingography (Uterotubography, Uterosalpingography, Hysterogram)

Type of test X-ray with contrast dye

Normal findings

Patent fallopian tubes
No defects in uterine cavity

Test explanation and related physiology

In hysterosalpingography the uterine cavity and fallopian tubes are visualized radiographically after the injection of contrast material through the cervix. Uterine tumors, intrauterine adhesions, and developmental anomalies can be seen. Tubal obstruction caused by internal scarring, tumor, or kinking also can be detected. A possible therapeutic effect of this test is that passage of dye through the tubes may clear mucous plugs, straighten kinked tubes, or break up adhesions. This test also may be used to document adequacy of surgical tubal ligation.

Contraindications

- Patients with infections of the vagina, cervix, or fallopian tubes, because there is risk of extending the infection
- Patients with suspected pregnancy, because contrast material might induce abortion

Potential complications

- Infection of the endometrium (endometritis)
- Infection of the fallopian tubes (salpingitis)
- Uterine perforation
- Allergic reaction to iodinated dye or shellfish
- This rarely occurs because the dye is not administered intravenously.

Procedure and patient care

Before

- Determine pregnancy status of the patient.
- Administer sedatives (e.g., diazepam [Valium]) or antispasmodics, if ordered, before the test.
- Tell the patient that no food or fluid restrictions are needed.

During

- Note the following procedural steps:
  1. After voiding, the patient is placed on the fluoroscopy table in the lithotomy position.
  2. With a speculum in the vagina, contrast material is injected through the cervix. The dye fills the entire upper genital tract (uterus and tubes).
  3. Fluoroscopy is performed, and x-ray films are taken.
- Note that this procedure is performed by a physician in approximately 15 to 30 minutes.
- Tell the patient that she may feel occasional, transient menstrual-type cramping and that she may have shoulder pain caused by subphrenic irritation from the dye as it leaks into the peritoneal cavity.

After

- Inform the patient that a vaginal discharge (sometimes bloody) may be present for 1 to 2 days after the test.
- Instruct the patient as to signs and symptoms of infection (e.g., fever, increased pulse rate, pain).

Abnormal findings

Uterine tumor (e.g., leiomyoma, cancer)
Developmental anomaly (e.g., uterus bicornis) of the uterus
Intrauterine adhesions
Uterine fistula
Obstruction, kinking, or twisting of the fallopian tubes
Extrauterine pregnancy
Tumor of the fallopian tubes

notes

hysteroscopy

Type of test Endoscopy

Normal findings Normal structure and function of the uterus

Test explanation and related physiology

Hysteroscopy is an endoscopic procedure that provides direct visualization of the uterine cavity by inserting a hysteroscope (a thin, telescope-like instrument) through the vagina and cervix and into the uterus. Hysteroscopy can be used to identify the cause of abnormal uterine bleeding, infertility, and repeated miscarriages. It is also used to identify, evaluate, and perform biopsies of uterine adhesions (Asherman syndrome), polyps, cancer, fibroids, and displaced intrauterine devices (IUDs).

In addition to diagnosing and evaluating uterine problems, hysteroscopy can also correct uterine problems. For example, uterine adhesions and small fibroids can be removed through the hysteroscope, thus avoiding open abdominal surgery. Hysteroscopy can also be used to perform endometrial ablation, which destroys the uterine lining to treat some cases of heavy dysfunctional uterine bleeding.

Contraindications

- Patients with pelvic inflammatory disease
- Patients with vaginal discharge

Potential complications

- Uterine perforation
- Infection

Procedure and patient care

Before

- Explain the procedure to the patient.
- Obtain informed consent for this procedure.
- Assess the pregnancy status of the patient.
- Instruct the patient to be NPO for at least 8 hours before the test.

During

- Note the following procedural steps:
  1. Hysteroscopy may be performed in the operating room or the doctor's office. Local, regional, general, or no anesthe-

sia may be used. (The type of anesthesia depends on other procedures that may be done at the same time.)

2. The patient is placed in the lithotomy position. The vaginal area is cleansed with an antiseptic solution.
3. The cervix may be dilated before this procedure.
4. The hysteroscope is inserted through the vagina and cervix and into the uterus.
5. A liquid or gas is released through the hysteroscope to expand the uterus for better visualization.
6. If minor surgery is to be performed, small instruments will be inserted through the hysteroscope.
7. For more detailed or complicated procedures, a laparoscope may be used (see p. 518) to concurrently view the outside of the uterus.

- Note that hysteroscopy is performed by a physician in approximately 30 minutes.

After

- Tell the patient that it is normal to have slight vaginal bleeding and cramps for a day or two after the procedure.
- Inform the patient that signs of fever, severe abdominal pain, or heavy vaginal discharge or bleeding should be reported to her physician.

Abnormal findings

Endometrial cancer, polyps or hyperplasia
Uterine fibroids
Asherman syndrome
Septate uterus
Displaced IUD

notes

immunoglobulin electrophoresis (Gamma globulin electrophoresis)

Type of test Blood

Normal findings

IgG (mg/dl)
Adults: 565-1765
Children: 250-1600
IgA (mg/dl)
Adults: 85-385
Children: 1-350
IgM (mg/dl)
Adult: 55-375
Children: 20-200
IgD and IgE: minimal

Test explanation and related physiology

Proteins within the blood are made up of albumin and globulin. Several types of globulin exist, one of which is gamma globulin. Antibodies are made up of gamma globulin protein and are called *immunoglobulins*. There are many classes of immunoglobulins (antibodies). *Immunoglobulin G (IgG)* constitutes approximately 75% of the serum immunoglobulins; therefore it constitutes the majority of circulating blood antibodies. *IgA* constitutes approximately 15% of the immunoglobulins within the body and is present primarily in secretions of the respiratory and gastrointestinal tract, in saliva, in colostrum and in tears. IgA is also present to a smaller degree in the blood. *IgM* is an immunoglobulin primarily responsible for ABO blood grouping and rheumatoid factor; it is also involved in the immunologic reaction to many other infections (e.g., hepatitis, gram-negative sepsis). IgM does not cross the placenta so that an elevation of IgM in the newborn indicates in utero infection such as rubella, CMV, or STS. *IgE* often mediates an allergic response and is measured to detect allergic diseases. *IgD*, which constitutes the smallest part of the immunoglobulins, is rarely evaluated or detected.

Serum immunoelectrophoresis is used to detect and monitor the course of diseases, including hypersensitivity diseases, immune deficiencies, autoimmune diseases, chronic infections, multiple myeloma, chronic viral infections, and intrauterine fetal infections. For this test the serum is placed on a slide containing agar gel, and an electric current is passed through this gel. Immunoglobulins are separated out and electrophoresed according to the quantity and difference in electrical charge. Specific antisera are placed alongside the slide to identify the specific type of immunoglobulin present.

Interfering factors

▼ Drugs that may cause *increased* immunoglobulin levels include therapeutic gamma globulin, hydralazine, isoniazid (INH), phenytoin (Dilantin), procainamide, and tetanus toxoid and antitoxin.

Procedure and patient care

Before

- Explain the procedure to the patient.
- Tell the patient that no fasting or special preparation is required.

During

- Collect 7 to 10 ml of venous blood in a red-top tube.
- Indicate on the laboratory slip if the patient has received any vaccinations or immunizations within the past 6 months. Also, list any drugs that may affect test results.

After

- Apply pressure to the venipuncture site.

Abnormal findings

▲ **Increased IgA levels**
Chronic liver diseases
(e.g., primary biliary cirrhosis)
Chronic infections
Inflammatory bowel disease

▼ **Decreased IgA levels**
Ataxia/telangiectasia
Congenital isolated deficiency
Hypoproteinemia (e.g., nephrotic syndrome or protein-losing enteropathies)
Immunosuppressive drugs (e.g., steroids, dextran)

▲ **Increased IgG levels**
Chronic granulomatous infections (e.g., tuberculosis, Wegener's granulomatosis, sarcoidosis)
Hyper immunization reactions
Chronic liver disease
Multiple myeloma (monoclonal IgG type)
Autoimmune diseases (e.g., rheumatoid arthritis, Sjögren's disease and SLE)
IUD devices

▼ **Decreased IgG levels**
Wiskott-Aldrich syndrome
Agammaglobulinemia
AIDS
Hypoproteinemia (e.g., Nephrotic syndrome or Protein-losing enteropathies)
Drug immunosuppression (e.g., steroids, dextran)
Non-IgG multiple myeloma
Leukemia

▲ **Increased IgM levels**
Waldenström's macroglobulinemia
Chronic infections (e.g., hepatitis, mononucleosis, sarcoidosis)
Autoimmune diseases (e.g., SLE or rheumatoid arthritis)
Acute infections
Chronic liver disorders (e.g., biliary cirrhosis)

▼ **Decreased IgM levels**
Agammaglobulinemia
Acquired immunodeficiency syndrome
Hypoproteinemia (e.g., nephrotic syndrome or protein-losing enteropathies)
Drug immunosuppression (e.g., steroids, dextran)
IgG or IgA multiple myeloma
Leukemia

▲ **Increased IgE levels**
Allergy reactions (e.g., hayfever, asthma, eczema, or anaphylaxis)
Allergic infections such as aspergillosis or parasites

▼ **Decreased IgE levels**
Agammaglobulinemia

insulin antibody test (Anti-insulin antibody)

Type of test Blood

Normal findings No antibody detected for bovine or porcine insulin

Test explanation and related physiology

Insulin antibodies appear in nearly all patients with diabetes treated with exogenous (human, bovine, or porcine) insulin. These antibodies develop from impurities in animal insulin or from antigenic stimulation of the insulin molecule. With the increased use of human insulin, the frequency of anti-insulin antibodies has significantly decreased. Insulin antibodies may also be produced in patients who have never received exogenous insulin. These autoantibodies are present in nearly 50% of children at the time of diagnosis of juvenile diabetes.

Anti-insulin antibodies reduce the amount of insulin available for glucose metabolism and may contribute to insulin resistance. These insulin antibodies are diagnostic of factitious hypoglycemia from surreptitious administration of insulin.

Interfering factor

- Radioactive scans within 7 days before the test may interfere with the test result.

Procedure and patient care

Before

- Tell the patient that no fasting is required.

During

- Collect a venous blood sample in a red-top tube.

After

- Apply pressure to the venipuncture site.

Abnormal findings

▲ **Increased levels**
Insulin resistance
Allergies to insulin
Factitious hypoglycemia

insulin assay

Type of test Blood

Normal findings
5-24 μU/ml or 36-179 pmol/L (SI units)
Newborn: 3-20 μU/ml

Possible critical values >30 mU/ml

Test explanation and related physiology

Insulin assay is used to diagnose insulinoma (tumor of the islets of Langerhans). It is also used in the evaluation of patients with fasting hypoglycemia.

Some investigators believe that measuring the ratio of the blood sugar and insulin on the same specimen obtained during the oral glucose tolerance test (GTT, see p. 444) is more reliable than measuring insulin levels alone. Combined with the oral GTT, the insulin assay can show characteristic curves. For example, patients with juvenile diabetes have low fasting insulin levels and display flat GTT insulin curves because of little or no increase in insulin levels. Patients who have mild cases of diabetes have normal fasting insulin levels and display GTT curves with a delayed rise.

When combined with a fasting blood sugar, insulin assay is very accurate in detecting insulinoma. After the patient fasts 12 to 14 hours, the insulin/glucose ratio should be less than 0.3. Patients with insulinoma have ratios greater than this. To increase the sensitivity and specificity of these combined tests for insulinoma, Turner and others have proposed the "amended" insulin/glucose ratios using variable mathematic "fudge" factors:

$$\frac{\text{serum insulin level} \times 100}{\text{serum glucose} - 30 \text{ mg/100 ml}}$$

A Turner amended ratio of over 50 suggests insulinoma.

Interfering factors

- Anti-insulin antibodies can interfere with insulin radioimmunoassay.
- Food intake and obesity may cause increased insulin levels.
- Recent administration of radioisotopes may affect test results.

✴ Drugs that may cause *increased* insulin levels include corticosteroids, levodopa, and oral contraceptives.

Procedure and patient care

Before
- Explain the procedure to the patient.
- Keep the patient NPO for 8 hours.

During
- Collect approximately 5 ml of venous blood in a red-top tube and pack it in ice.
- Avoid hemolysis.
- If the serum insulin level will be measured during the GTT, collect the blood sample before oral ingestion of the glucose load and often at designated intervals after glucose ingestion.

After
- Apply pressure to the venipuncture site.
- Transport the specimen immediately to the laboratory.

Abnormal findings

▲ **Increased levels**
Insulinoma
Cushing's syndrome
Acromegaly
Obesity
Fructose or galactose
    intolerance

▼ **Decreased levels**
Diabetes
Hypopituitarism

notes

intravenous pyelography (IVP, Excretory urography [EUG], Intravenous urography [IUG, IVU])

Type of test X-ray with contrast dye

Normal findings

Normal size, shape, and position of the kidneys, renal pelvis, ureters, and bladder

Normal kidney excretory function as evidenced by the length of time for passage of contrast material through the kidneys

Test explanation and related physiology

IVP is an x-ray study that uses radiopaque contrast material to visualize the kidneys, renal pelvis, ureters, and bladder. It is indicated on patients with:

Pain compatible with urinary stones

Blood in the urine

Proposed pelvic surgery to locate the ureters

Trauma to the urinary system

Urinary outlet obstruction

A suspected kidney tumor

Dye is injected intravenously, filtered out at the kidney by the glomeruli, and then passed through the renal tubules. X-ray films taken at set intervals over the next 30 minutes will show passage of the dye material through the kidneys and ureters and into the bladder.

If the artery leading to one of the kidneys is blocked, the dye cannot enter that part of the renal system, and that kidney or part thereof will not be visualized. If the artery is partially blocked, the length of time required for the appearance of the contrast material will be prolonged.

With primary glomerular disease (e.g., glomerulonephritis), the glomerular filtrate is reduced, which causes a reduction in the quantity of dye filtered. Therefore it requires more time for enough dye to enter the kidney filtrate and allow for renal opacification. As a result, kidney visualization is delayed. This indicates an estimate of renal function.

Defects in dye filling of the kidney can indicate renal tumors or cysts. Often intrinsic tumors, stones, extrinsic tumors, and scarring can partially or completely obstruct the flow of dye through the collecting system (pelvis, ureters, bladder). If the obstruction has been of sufficient duration, the collecting system proximal to the obstruction will be dilated (hydronephrosis). Retroperitoneal and pelvic tumors, aneurysms, and enlarged lymph nodes also can produce extrinsic compression and distortions of the opacified collecting system.

IVP is also used to assess the effect of trauma on the urinary system. Renal hematomas distort the renal contour. Renal artery laceration is suggested by nonopacification of one kidney. Laceration of the kidneys, pelvis, ureters, or bladder often causes urine leaks, which are identified by dye extravasation from the urinary system.

Further, IVP is used to assess a patient for congenital absence or malposition of the kidneys. Horseshoe kidneys (connection of the two kidneys), double ureters, and pelvic kidneys are typical congenital abnormalities.

Nephrotomography provides radiographic visualization of the kidney using tomographic technique following the IV injection of a radiopaque dye. Tomography permits examination of a single layer or plane of the organ that would otherwise be obscured by the surrounding structures.

Contraindications

- Patients who are allergic to shellfish or iodinated dyes
- Patients who are severely dehydrated, because this can cause renal shutdown and failure
  Geriatric patients are particularly vulnerable
- Patients with renal insufficiency, as evidenced by a blood urea nitrogen value greater than 40 mg/dl, because the iodinated nephrotoxic dye can worsen kidney function
- Patients with multiple myeloma, because the iodinated nephrotoxic dye can worsen renal function
- Patients who are pregnant, because of radiation exposure to the fetus

Potential complications

- Allergy to iodine dye
- Infiltration of contrast dye
- Renal failure
  This occurs most often in elderly patients who are chronically dehydrated before the dye injection.
- Hypoglycemia or acidosis may occur in patients who are taking Glucophage and receive iodine dye.

Interfering factors

- Fecal material, gas, or barium in the bowel may obscure visualization of the renal system.
- Abnormal renal function studies may prevent adequate visualization of the urinary tract.
- Retained barium from previous studies may obscure visualization. Studies using barium (e.g., barium enema) should be scheduled after an IVP.

Procedure and patient care

Before

- Explain the procedure to the patient. Inform the patient that several x-ray films will be taken over 30 minutes.
- Obtain informed consent if required by the institution.
- Check the patient for allergies to iodinated dye and shellfish.
- Give the patient a laxative (e.g., castor oil) or a cathartic, as ordered, the evening before the test.
- Inform the patient of the required food and fluid restrictions. Some institutions prefer abstinence from solid foods for 8 hours before testing. Some allow a clear-liquid breakfast on the test day.
- Ensure adequate hydration for the patient (IV or oral) before and after the test to avoid dye-induced renal failure.
- Note that pediatric patients will have decreased fasting times, as ordered on an individual basis.
- Note that elderly and debilitated patients should have fasting times indicated specifically for them.
- Note that patients receiving high rates of IV fluids may have infusion rates decreased for several hours before the study to increase the concentration of the dye within the urinary system.
- Assess the patient's blood urea nitrogen and creatinine levels. Abnormal renal function could deteriorate as a result of the dye injection.
- Schedule any barium studies after completion of the IVP.
- Give the patient an enema or suppository on the morning of the study, if ordered.

During

- Note the following procedural steps:
  1. The patient is taken to the radiology department and placed in the supine position.
  2. A plain film of the abdomen (KUB) is taken to ensure

that no residual stool obscures visualization of the renal system. This also screens for calculi in the renal collecting system.

3. Skin testing for iodine allergy is often done.
4. A peripheral IV line is started (if not in place), and a contrast dye (e.g., Hypaque, Renografin) is given.
5. X-ray films are taken at specific times, usually at 1, 5, 10, 15, 20, and 30 minutes, and sometimes longer, to follow the course of the dye from the cortex of the kidney to the bladder.
6. Tomography may be performed to identify a mass.
7. The patient is taken to the bathroom and asked to void.
8. A postvoiding film is taken to visualize the empty bladder.

- Note that occasionally it is necessary to partially occlude the ureters temporarily to obtain a better film of the collecting system in the upper part of the ureters. This is done by compressing the abdomen with an inflatable rubber tube, which is wrapped tightly around the abdomen slightly below the umbilicus.
- Note that this test is performed by a radiologist in approximately 45 minutes.
- Inform the patient that the dye injection often causes a transitory flushing of the face, a feeling of warmth, a salty taste in the mouth, or even transient nausea. Initial IV needle placement and lying on a hard x-ray table are the only other discomforts associated with IVP.

After

- Assess the patient's urinary output. A decreased output may be an indication of renal failure.
- See p. xviii for appropriate interventions concerning the care for patients with iodine allergy.
- Encourage the patient to drink fluids to counteract fluid depletion caused by the test preparation.
- Evaluate elderly and debilitated patients for weakness because of the combination of fasting and catharsis necessary for test preparation. Instruct these patients to ambulate only with assistance.
- Maintain the patient on adequate oral or IV hydration for several hours after the IVP.

🏠 Home care responsibilities

- After this test, patients must be encouraged to drink a lot of fluids to reestablish their normal state of hydration.
- Instructions to patients regarding urinary output are crucial. A decreased urine output may by an indication of impending renal failure.

Abnormal findings

Pyelonephritis
Glomerulonephritis
Kidney tumor (benign or malignant)
Renal hematoma
Renal laceration
Cyst or polycystic disease of the kidney
Congenital abnormality of the urologic tract
Renal or ureteral calculi
Trauma to the kidneys, ureters, or bladder
Tumor of the collecting system
Hydronephrosis
Extrinsic compression of the collecting system (e.g., caused by tumor, aneurysm)
Bladder tumor
Prostate enlargement (male)

notes

iron level and total iron-binding capacity (Fe and TIBC, Transferrin saturation, Transferrin)

Type of test Blood

Normal findings

Iron: 13-31 μmol/L (SI units)
  Males: 65-175 μg/dl
  Females: 50-170 μg/dl
  Newborn: 100-250 μg/dl
  Child: 50-120 μg/dl
TIBC:
  250-420 μg/dl or 45-73 μmol/L (SI units)
Transferrin:
  Adult male: 215-365 mg/dl
  Adult female: 250-380 mg/dl
  Newborn: 130-275 mg/dl
  Child: 203-360 mg/dl
Transferrin saturation:
  Males: 20% to 50%
  Females: 15%-50%

Test explanation and related physiology

Serum iron

Abnormal levels of iron are characteristic of many diseases, including iron deficiency anemia and hemochromatosis. Seventy percent of the iron in the body is found in the hemoglobin of the red blood cells (RBCs). The other 30% is stored iron in the form of *ferritin* (see p. 395) and hemosiderin. Iron is supplied by the diet. Iron is bound to a globulin protein called *transferrin*. The serum iron determination is a measurement of the quantity of iron bound to transferrin.

Iron deficiency anemia is a result of reduced serum iron. Iron deficiency anemia has many causes, including the following:

1. Insufficient iron intake
2. Inadequate gut absorption
3. Increased requirements (as in growing children and late pregnancy)
4. Loss of blood (as in menstruation, bleeding peptic ulcer, and colon neoplasm).

Iron deficiency results in a decreased production of hemoglobin, which in turn results in a small, pale (microcytic, hypochromic) RBC. A decreased serum iron level, elevated TIBC, and low transferrin saturation (TS) value are characteristic of iron deficiency anemia.

Iron overload or poisoning is called hemochromatosis or hemosiderosis. Excess iron is usually deposited in the brain, liver, and heart and causes severe dysfunction of these organs. Massive blood transfusions also may cause elevated serum iron levels, although only transiently. Transfusions should be avoided before serum iron level blood specimens are obtained in the evaluation of anemia. Because serum iron levels may vary significantly during the day, the blood specimen should be drawn in the morning, especially when the results are used to monitor iron replacement therapy.

Total iron binding capacity and transferrin

TIBC is a measurement of all proteins available for binding mobile iron. *Transferrin* represents the largest quantity of iron binding proteins. Therefore TIBC is an indirect yet accurate measurement of transferrin. Ferritin is not included in TIBC because it binds only stored iron. TIBC is increased in 70% of patients with iron deficiency.

Transferrin is a *negative* acute phase reactant protein. That is, in various acute inflammatory reactions, transferrin levels diminish. Transferrin also is diminished in the face of chronic illnesses such as malignancy, collagen vascular diseases, or liver diseases. Hypoproteinemia is also associated with reduced transferrin levels. Pregnancy and estrogen therapy are associated with increased transferrin levels.

TIBC varies minimally according to iron intake. The TIBC is more of a reflection of liver function (transferrin is produced by the liver) and nutrition than of iron metabolism. Transferrin values often are used to monitor the course of patients receiving hyperalimentation.

Total iron binding capacity and transferrin saturation

The percentage of transferrin and other mobile iron binding proteins saturated with iron is calculated by dividing the serum iron level by the TIBC:

$$\text{TS (\%)} = \frac{\text{Serum iron level}}{\text{TIBC}} \times 100\%$$

The normal value for TS is 20% to 50%. TS is decreased to

below 15% in patients with iron deficiency anemia. It is increased in patients with hemolytic, sideroblastic, or megaloblastic anemias. TS is also increased in patients with iron overload or poisoning. Increased intake or absorption of iron (as in hemochromatosis) leads to elevated iron levels. In such cases the TIBC is unchanged; as a result, the percentage of transferrin saturation is very high.

Chronic illness (e.g., infections, neoplasia, cirrhosis) is characterized by a low serum iron level, decreased TIBC, and normal TS. Pregnancy is marked by high levels of protein, including transferrin. Because iron requirements are high, it is not unusual to find low serum iron levels, high TIBC, and a low percentage of TS in late pregnancy.

Contraindication

- Patients with hemolytic diseases, because they may have an artificially high iron content

Interfering factors

- Recent blood transfusions may affect test results.
- Recent ingestion of a meal containing high iron content may affect test results.
- Hemolytic diseases may be associated with an artificially high iron content.
- Drugs that may cause *increased* iron levels include chloramphenicol, dextran, estrogens, ethanol, iron preparations, methyldopa, and oral contraceptives.
- Drugs that may cause *decreased* iron levels include adrenocorticotropic hormone (ACTH), cholestyramine, chloramphenicol, colchicine, deferoxamine, methicillin, and testosterone.
- Drugs that may cause *increased* TIBC levels include fluorides and oral contraceptives.
- Drugs that may cause *decreased* TIBC levels include ACTH and chloramphenicol.

Procedure and patient care

Before

- Keep the patient fasting for 12 hours before the blood test. Water is permitted.

During

- Collect approximately 5 to 7 ml of venous blood in a red-top tube. The specimen should always be obtained using a 20-gauge or larger needle.

- Avoid hemolysis, because the iron contained in the RBC will pour out into the serum and cause artificially high iron levels.
- Indicate on the laboratory slip any drugs that may affect test results.

After

- Apply pressure to the venipuncture site.

Abnormal findings

▲ **Increased serum iron levels**
  Hemosiderosis
  Hemochromatosis
  Hemolytic anemia
  Hepatitis
  Hepatic necrosis
  Lead toxicity
  Iron poisoning
  Massive transfusion
  Lead toxicity

▼ **Decreased serum iron levels**
  Insufficient dietary iron
  Chronic blood loss
  Inadequate absorption of iron
  Pregnancy (late)
  Iron deficiency anemia
  Neoplasia
  Chronic gastrointestinal blood loss
  Chronic hematuria
  Chronic heavy physiologic or pathologic menstruation

▲ **Increased TIBC levels**
  Oral contraceptives
  Pregnancy (late)
  Polycythemia vera
  Iron deficiency anemia

▼ **Decreased TIBC levels**
  Hypoproteinemia
  Inflammatory diseases
  Cirrhosis
  Hemolytic anemia
  Pernicious anemia
  Sickle cell anemia

notes

17-ketosteroids (17-KS)

Type of test   Urine (24-hour)

Normal findings
Male: 7-25 mg/24 hr or 24-88 μmol/day (SI units)
Female: 4-15 mg/24 hr or 14-52 μmol/day (SI units)
Elderly: values decrease with age
Child
   Under 12 years: <5 mg/24 hr
   12-15 years: 5-12 mg/24 hr

Test explanation and related physiology
17-KS are metabolites of the testosterone and nontestosterone androgenic sex hormones that are secreted from the adrenal cortex and the testes. The principal 17-ketosteroid is dehydro-epiandrosterone (DHEA). In men approximately one third of the hormone metabolites come from testosterone that is made in the testes, and two thirds come from nontestosterone androgens made in the adrenal cortex; in women and children, almost all the 17 KS are metabolites from nontestosterone androgenic hormones derived from the adrenal cortex. Therefore this test is very useful in diagnosing adrenocortical dysfunction. It is important to note that 17 KS are not metabolites of cortisol and do not reflect levels of cortisol production. Elevated 17-KS levels are frequently seen in patients with congenital adrenal hyperplasia and androgenic tumors of the adrenal glands. In these diseases excess steroid synthesis is of the "noncortisol" androgenic sterols. These diseases frequently cause virilization syndromes. Low levels of 17-KS have little clinical significance.

Interfering factors
- ✘ Drugs that may cause *increased* 17-KS levels include antibiotics, chloramphenicol, chlorpromazine, dexamethasone, meprobamate, phenothiazines, quinidine, secobarbital, and spironolactone (Aldactone).
- ✘ Drugs that may cause *decreased* levels include estrogen, oral contraceptives, probenecid, promazine, reserpine, salicylates (prolonged use), and thiazide diuretics.

Procedure and patient care

Before

- Explain the procedure to the patient.
- Withhold all drugs (with physician approval) for several days beforehand.
- Assess the patient for signs of stress and report these to the physician.

During

- Begin the 24-hour urine collection after the patient urinates; discard this specimen.
- Collect all urine passed by the patient during the next 24 hours.
- Post the hours for the urine collection in a prominent spot.
- Remember that it is not necessary to measure each urine specimen.
- Tell the patient to void before defecating so that the urine is not contaminated by feces.
- Inform the patient that toilet paper should not be placed in the collection container.
- Encourage the patient to drink fluids during the 24 hours, unless this is contraindicated for medical purposes.
- Remember that the urine collection needs a preservative.
- Refrigerate the urine throughout the collection.
- Collect the last specimen as close as possible to the end of the 24-hour period. Add this to the urine collection.

After

- Indicate on the laboratory slip the start and end times of the specimen collection.
- List on the laboratory slip any medications that may affect test results.
- Send the specimen to the laboratory as soon as the test is completed.

K

Abnormal findings

▲ **Increased levels**
Congenital adrenal hyper-
plasia
Pregnancy
Adrenocorticotropic
hormone administration
Cushing syndrome
Testosterone- or estrogen-
secreting tumors of the
adrenals, ovaries, or
testes
Severe stress or infection
Hyperpituitarism
Ovarian neoplasia
Stein-Leventhal syndrome

▼ **Decreased levels**
Addison's disease
Hypogonadism
(Klinefelter syndrome)
Hypopituitarism
Myxedema
Severe debilitating disease
Nephrosis
Gout
Castration
Thyrotoxicosis
Severe stress or infection
Chronic illnesses

notes

kidney, ureter, and bladder x-ray study (KUB, Flat plate of the abdomen, Plain film of the abdomen, Scout film)

Type of test   X-ray

Normal findings

No evidence of calculi
Normal gastrointestinal (GI) gas pattern

Test explanation and related physiology

The KUB is a *flat plate*, or simple x-ray film, of the abdomen. It is often referred to as a *plain film*, or *scout film*, of the abdomen. The KUB is similar to the supine view on an *obstruction series* (see p. 590) and can be performed to demonstrate the size, shape, location, and malformations of the kidneys and bladder. The KUB can also be used to identify calculi in these organs and in the ureters. This is often one of the first studies done to diagnose other intraabdominal diseases such as intestinal obstruction, soft tissue masses, and a ruptured viscus. The KUB is useful in detecting abnormal accumulations of gas within the GI tract and finding ascites. This study involves no contrast medium and poses no risk to the patient.

Contraindication

- Patients who are pregnant

Interfering factor

- Retained barium from previous studies can obscure visualization.

Procedure and patient care

Before

- Explain the procedure to the patient.
- Tell the patient that no fasting or sedation is required.
- Schedule this study before any barium studies.
- Ensure that the male patient has a lead sheet over his testicles to prevent their irradiation.
- Note that the female ovaries cannot be shielded because of their proximity to the kidneys, ureters, and bladder.

K

During

- Note that in the radiology department the patient is placed in the supine position with the arms extended overhead. X-ray films are taken of the patient's abdomen.
- Note that the KUB is performed by a radiologic technologist in a few minutes and is interpreted by a radiologist.
- Inform the patient that results are available in approximately 1 hour.
- Tell the patient that no discomfort is associated with this study.

After

- Schedule intravenous pyelography or GI studies after completion of the KUB.

Abnormal findings

Calculi
Abnormal accumulation of bowel gas
Ascites
Soft tissue masses
Ruptured viscus
Congenital anomalies in the location, size and number of
  kidneys
Organomegaly
Bladder distention

notes

lactate dehydrogenase Lactic dehydrogenase (LDH)

Type of test Blood

Normal findings

Adult/elderly: 45-90 U/L (30° C), 115-225 IU/L, or 0.4-1.7 μmol/L (SI units)

Isoenzymes
    Adult/elderly:
        LDH-1: 17% to 27%
        LDH-2: 27% to 37%
        LDH-3: 18% to 25%
        LDH-4: 3% to 8%
        LDH-5: 0% to 5%
Child: 60-170 U/L (30° C)
Infant: 100-250 U/L
Newborn: 160-450 U/L

Test explanation and related physiology

LDH is found in the cells of many body tissues, especially the heart, liver, red blood cells, kidneys, skeletal muscle, brain, and lungs. Because LDH is widely distributed through the body, the total LDH level is not a specific indicator of any one disease affecting any one organ. When disease or injury affects the cells that contain LDH, the cells lyse, and LDH is spilled into the bloodstream, where it is identified in higher than normal levels. The LDH is a measure of total LDH. There are actually five separate fractions (isoenzymes) that make up the total LDH. Each tissue contains a predominance of one or more LDH enzymes.

In general, isoenzyme LDH-1 comes mainly from the heart; LDH-2 comes primarily from the reticuloendothelial system; LDH-3 comes from the lungs and other tissues; LDH-4 comes from the kidney, placenta, and pancreas; and LDH-5 comes mainly from the liver and striated muscle. In normal persons LDH-2 makes up the greatest percentage of total LDH.

With myocardial injury, the serum LDH level rises within 24 to 48 hours after a myocardial infarction (MI), peaks in 2 to 3 days, and returns to normal in approximately 5 to 10 days. This makes the serum LDH level especially useful for a delayed diagnosis of patients with MI (e.g., in which the patient reports having had severe chest pain 4 days earlier). In healthy individuals the LDH 2 fraction is greater than the LDH 1 fraction. Therefore the normal LDH 1 to LDH 2 ratio is less than one. The reversal of the normal ratio (i.e., the ratio is greater than 1) is referred to as a "flipped LDH." In an acute MI the flipped LDH ratio usually appears in 12 to 24 hours and is present within 48 hours in approximately 80% of patients. In the patient with chest pain caused by angina only, the LDH will probably not be elevated.

LDH is also measured in other body fluids. Elevated urine levels of total LDH indicates neoplasm or injury to the urologic system. When the LDH in an effusion (pleural, cardiac or peritoneal) is >60% of the serum total LDH (i.e., effusion LDH/serum LDH ratio is greater than 0.6), the effusion is said to be an *exudate* and not a transudate.

Interfering factors

- Strenuous exercise may cause an elevation of total LDH and specifically LDH 1, 2, and 5
- Hemolysis of blood will cause false-positive LDH levels.
- Drugs that may cause *increased* LDH levels include alcohol, anesthetics, aspirin, clofibrate, fluorides, mithramycin, narcotics, and procainamide.
- Drugs that may cause *decreased* levels include ascorbic acid.

Procedure and patient care

Before

- Explain the procedure to the patient.
- Tell the patient that no fasting is required.
- Inform the patient if he or she will be receiving frequent venipuncture for the evaluation of an MI.

During

- Collect approximately 7 to 10 ml of venous blood in a red-top tube.
- Because many diseases cause an increased LDH level, identify disease conditions on the laboratory slip.
- Record the data and time when blood was drawn on the laboratory slip for an accurate evaluation of the temporal pattern of enzyme elevations.

After

- Apply pressure to the venipuncture site.

Abnormal findings

▲ **Increased values**

Myocardial infarction

Pulmonary disease (e.g., embolism, infarction, pneumonia, congestive heart failure)

Hepatic disease (e.g., hepatitis, active cirrhosis, neoplasm)

Red blood cell disease (e.g., hemolytic or megaloblastic anemia or red blood cell destruction from prosthetic heart valves)

Skeletal muscle disease and injury (e.g., muscular dystrophy, recent very strenuous exercises, or muscular trauma)

Renal parenchymal disease (e.g., infarction, glomerulonephritis, acute tubular necrosis, kidney transplantation rejection)

Intestinal ischemia and infarction

Testicular tumors (seminoma or dysgerminomas)

Lymphoma and other reticuloendothelial system tumors

Advanced solid tumor malignancies

Pancreatitis

Diffuse disease or injury (e.g., heat stroke, collagen disease, shock, hypotension)

notes

lactic acid (Lactate)

Type of test Blood

Normal findings
Venous blood: 0.5 to 2.2 mmol/L
Arterial blood: 0.9 to 1.7 mmol/L

Test explanation and related physiology

Under conditions of normal oxygen availability to tissues, glucose is metabolized to CO_2 and H_2O for energy. When oxygen to the tissues is diminished, anaerobic metabolism of glucose occurs, and lactate (lactic acid) is formed instead of CO_2 and H_2O. To compound the problem of lactic acid buildup, when the liver is hypoxic, it fails to clear the lactic acid. Lactic acid levels accumulate, causing lactic acidosis (LA). Therefore blood lactate is a fairly sensitive and reliable indicator of tissue hypoxia. The hypoxia may be caused by local tissue hypoxia (e.g., mesenteric ischemia, extremity ischemia) or generalized tissue hypoxia such as exists in shock. Lactic acid blood levels are used to document the presence of tissue hypoxia, determine the degree of hypoxia, and monitor the effect of therapy. Type I LA is caused by diseases that increase lactate but are not hypoxic related, such as glycogen storage diseases, liver diseases, or drugs. LA caused by hypoxia is classified as type II. Shock, convulsions, and extremity ischemia are the most common causes of type II LA. Type III LA is idiopathic and is most commonly seen in nonketotic patients with diabetes. The pathophysiology of lactic acid accumulation in type III is not known.

Interfering factors
- The prolonged use of a tourniquet or clenching of hands increases lactate levels.
- � Drugs that *increase* levels include cyanide, ethanol, aspirin, phenformin, and nalidixic acid

Procedure and patient care

Before
- Explain the procedure to the patient.
- Tell the patient that no fasting is required.

During
- Instruct the patient to avoid making a fist before and while blood is being withdrawn.
- Avoid the use of a tourniquet if possible.
- Collect approximately 7 ml of venous blood or 4 to 7 ml of arterial blood in a red-top tube

After
- Apply pressure to the venipuncture site.

Abnormal findings

▲   **Increased levels**
   Shock
   Tissue ischemia
   Carbon monoxide poisoning
   Severe liver disease
   Genetic errors of metabolism
   Diabetes mellitus (nonketotic)

notes

lactose tolerance test

Type of test Blood

Normal findings

Blood: Adult/elderly: rise in plasma glucose levels >20 mg/dl.
No abdominal cramps or diarrhea.
Breath: <50 ppm hydrogen increase over baseline.

Test explanation and related physiology

This test is performed to detect lactose intolerance. Lactose is a disaccharide typically found in dairy products. Because lactose-intolerant patients have an absence of lactase, lactose digestion will not occur. Thus the small bowel is flooded with a high lactose load. Bacterial metabolism of the lactose occurs within the intestine. This creates a strong cathartic effect. Symptoms of lactose intolerance include abdominal cramping, flatus, abdominal bloating, and diarrhea.

Although all adults have some degree of lactase reduction, severe lactose intolerance can occur in patients with inflammatory bowel disease, short-gut syndrome, and other malabsorption syndromes. Lactase deficiency can be congenital and become apparent in the newborn. These infants present with vomiting, diarrhea, malabsorption, and failure to thrive.

In the test the patient is provided a lactose load. If lactase is not present in sufficient quantities, lactose is not metabolized to glucose and galactose. Plasma levels of glucose do not rise as expected. Therefore lower-than-expected serum glucose levels suggest intestinal lactase deficiency. Patients who have malabsorption without lactase deficiency will also fail to elevate the blood glucose levels. They also fail to have a glucose rise with an oral glucose load.

There is also a breath test part to this test in which the exhaled air is analyzed for hydrogen content. The hydrogen content is directly proportional to the amount of lactose not broken down and absorbed.

Interfering factors

- Enterogenous steatorrhea
- Strenuous exercise
- Smoking, which may increase blood glucose levels

- Patients with diabetes may have glucose levels that exceed 20 mg/dl despite lactase insufficiency.

Procedure and patient care

Before

- Explain the procedure to the patient. Inform the patient that four blood samples will be needed.
- Instruct the patient to fast 8 hours before testing.
- Instruct the patient to avoid strenuous exercise for 8 hours before testing. This may factitiously affect the blood glucose level.
- Inform the patient that smoking is prohibited before testing. This may falsely increase the blood glucose level.

During

- Obtain 5 to 7 ml of venous blood in a gray-top tube from the fasting patient.
- Provide a specified dose of lactose for the patient. Usually dilute 100 g of lactose with 200 ml of water for ingestion in adults.
- Note that pediatric doses of lactose are based on weight.
- Collect three more blood samples at 30, 60, and 120 minutes after the ingestion of lactose.
- Tell the patient that the only discomfort is the venipuncture; however, patients with lactase deficiency will have the symptoms previously described.
- If the breath test is being done, the exhaled air is evaluated for hydrogen content at 30, 60, and 120 minutes after the ingestion of lactose.

After

- Apply pressure to the venipuncture site.
- Note that patients with abnormal test results may receive a monosaccharide tolerance test (e.g., glucose or galactose tolerance test).

Abnormal findings

▼ **Decreased levels**

Lactase insufficiency

Enterogenous diarrhea

laparoscopy (Pelvic endoscopy, Gynecologic video laparoscopy)

Type of test Endoscopy

Normal findings Normal-appearing abdominal and pelvic organs

Test explanation and related physiology

Laparoscopy is used to directly visualize the abdominal and pelvic organs when pathology is suspected. It is used to evaluate patients with:

Acute abdominal/pelvic pain
Chronic abdominal/pelvic pain
Suspected advanced cancer
Abdominal mass of uncertain etiology

During laparoscopy the abdominal organs can be visualized by inserting a scope through the abdominal wall and into the peritoneum (Figure 20). Usually a television camera is applied to the scope, and the view of the scope is seen on color monitors. This is particularly helpful in diagnosing abdominal and pelvic adhesions, tumors and cysts affecting any abdominal organ, and tubal and uterine causes of infertility. Endometriosis, ectopic

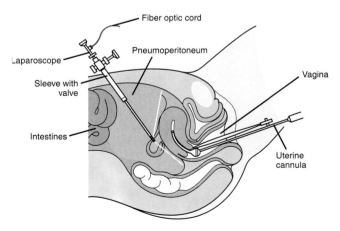

Figure 20 Laparoscopy directed to the pelvis.

pregnancy, ruptured ovarian cyst, and salpingitis can be detected during an evaluation for pelvic pain. This procedure is also used to stage cancers and determine their resectability. Surgical procedures (e.g., cholecystectomy, appendectomy, hernia repair, tubal ligation, oophorectomy, hiatal hernia repair, and bowel resection) can be performed with the laparoscope. Laparoscopy affords many advantages to the patient in comparison with an open laparotomy, including reduced pain, length of stay, and time off from work.

Contraindications

- Patients who have had multiple surgical procedures, because adhesions may have formed between the viscera and the abdominal wall
- Patients with suspected intraabdominal hemorrhage, because visualization through the scope is obscured by the blood

Potential complications

- Perforation of the bowel, with spilling of intestinal contents into the peritoneum
- Hemorrhage

Interfering factors

- Adhesions or extreme obesity may obstruct the field of vision.

Procedure and patient care

Before

- Explain the procedure to the patient.
- Ensure that an informed consent for this procedure is obtained. Because of the possibility of intraabdominal injury, an open laparotomy may be required. Be sure the patient is aware of that.
- If enemas are ordered to clear the bowel, assist the patient as needed and record the results.
- Because the procedure is usually performed with the patient under general anesthesia, follow routine general anesthesia precautions.
- Shave and prepare the patient's abdomen as ordered.
- Keep the patient NPO after midnight on the day of the test. IV fluids may be given.
- Instruct the patient to void before going to the operating room because a distended bladder can be easily penetrated.

During

- After general anesthesia is induced, a catheter and nasogastric tube are inserted to minimize the risk of penetrating a distended stomach or bladder with the initial needle placement.
- Note the following procedural steps:
  1. Laparoscopy is performed in the operating room. The patient is initially placed in the supine position. Other positions may be assumed to maximize visibility.
  2. After the abdominal skin is cleansed, a blunt-tipped (Verres) needle is inserted through a small incision in the periumbilical area and into the peritoneal cavity. Alternatively, a slightly larger incision is placed in the skin, and the abdominal wall is separated under direct vision. The peritoneal cavity is entered directly. Adhesions can be lysed under direct vision.
  3. The peritoneal cavity is filled with approximately 3 to 4 L of carbon dioxide to separate the abdominal wall from the intraabdominal viscera, enhancing visualization of pelvic and abdominal structures.
  4. A laparoscope is inserted through a trocar to examine the abdomen (Figure 20). Other trocars can be placed as conduits for other instrumentation.
  5. After the desired procedure is completed, the laparoscope is removed, and the carbon dioxide is allowed to escape.
  6. The incision(s) is closed with a few skin stitches and covered with an adhesive bandage.
- Note that laparoscopy is performed by a surgeon.
- Inform the patient who will be under general anesthesia that she will feel no discomfort. Most patients will have mild incisional pain later, however, and also may complain of shoulder or subcostal discomfort from pneumoperitoneum.

After

- Assess the patient frequently for signs of bleeding (increased pulse rate, decreased blood pressure), perforated viscus (abdominal tenderness, guarding, decreased bowel sounds). Report any significant findings to the physician.
- If patients have shoulder or subcostal discomfort from pneumoperitoneum, assure them that this usually lasts only 24 hours. Minor analgesics usually relieve this discomfort.
- If a surgical procedure has been performed laparoscopically, provide appropriate specific postsurgical care.

Abnormal findings

Abdominal adhesions
Ovarian tumor or cyst
Endometriosis
Ectopic pregnancy
Pelvic inflammatory disease
Uterine fibroids
Abscess or Infection
Cancer
Ascites
Portal hypertension
Other abdominal pathology

notes

L

Legionnaires' disease antibody test

Type of test Blood

Normal findings No *Legionella* antibody titer

Test explanation and related physiology

Legionnaires' disease was originally described as a fulminating pneumonia caused by *Legionella pneumophila*, a tiny gram-negative rod-shaped bacterium. This organism can also cause an influenza type of illness called *Pontiac fever*.

The diagnosis of Legionnaires' disease can be made by culturing this organism from suspected infected fluids such as blood, sputum, lung tissue or pleural fluid. Sputum for this test is best obtained by transtracheal aspiration or from bronchial washings. However, growth of this organism in culture is difficult. A negative culture does not mean that the patient does not have Legionnaires' disease. Another method of diagnosis is by directly identifying the organism in a microscopic smear of infected fluid with the use of direct fluorescent antibody methods. If positive, this allows for a rapid diagnosis of *Legionella*. However, this is difficult also because the concentration of the bacteria may not be high enough to see the bacterium in the specimen.

The most common and easiest method for diagnosis is detection of the antibody directed against the Legionnaires' bacterium in the patient's blood. A presumptive diagnosis of Legionnaires' disease can be made in a symptomatic person when a single antibody titer is 1:256 or greater. A fourfold rise in titer to at least 1:128 between the acute (1-week) and the convalescent (3-week) phase convalescent titer is diagnostic.

Procedure and patient care

Before

- Tell the patient that no fasting is required.

During

- For blood: Collect approximately 5 to 7 ml of blood in a red-top tube.
- For culture: Obtain sputum as indicated in sputum culture, p. 784.

After
- Apply pressure to the venipuncture site.

Abnormal finding

▲ **Increased levels**
  Legionnaires' disease

notes

L

leucine aminopeptidase (LAP)

Type of test Blood; urine (24-hour)

Normal findings
Blood
  Male: 80-200 U/ml
  Female: 75-185 U/ml
Urine: 2-18 U/24 hr

Test explanation and related physiology

LAP is an intracellular enzyme that exists in the hepatobiliary system and to a much smaller degree in the pancreas and small intestine. When disease or injury affects these organs, the cells lyse, and LAP is spilled out into the bloodstream. LAP is mainly used in diagnosing liver disorders and in the differential diagnosis of increased levels of alkaline phosphatase (ALP, see p. 35). LAP levels tend to parallel ALP levels in hepatic disease. LAP is a sensitive indicator of cholestasis; however, unlike ALP, LAP remains normal in bone disease. LAP can be detected in both the blood and the urine. Patients with elevated serum LAP levels will always show elevations in urine levels. When the urine LAP level is elevated, however, the blood level may have already returned to normal.

This enzyme was originally thought to be elevated during pregnancy and to be an indication of the viability of the fetal-placental unit. However, it has been found that the enzyme found in pregnancy is immunochemically different than LAP.

Interfering factors

- Pregnancy may cause increased values.
- ☛ Drugs that may cause *increased* LAP levels include estrogens and progesterones.

Procedure and patient care

Before
- Explain the procedure to the patient.
- Tell the patient that no fasting is required.

During
- Collect approximately 7 to 10 ml of venous blood in a red-top tube.

- If a urine sample is needed, follow the procedure for a 24-hour urine collection (see p. 381).
- Indicate on the laboratory slip any medications the patient is taking that may affect test results.

After

- Apply pressure to the venipuncture site. Patients with liver dysfunction often have prolonged clotting times.

Abnormal findings

▲ **Increased levels**

Hepatitis
Cirrhosis
Hepatic necrosis
Hepatic ischemia
Hepatic tumor
Hepatotoxic drugs
Cholestasis
Gallstones

L

notes

lipase

Type of test Blood

Normal findings 0-110 units/L or 0-417 U/L (SI units) (values are method dependent)

Test explanation and related physiology

The most common cause of an elevated serum lipase level is acute pancreatitis. Lipase is an enzyme secreted by the pancreas into the duodenum to break down triglycerides into fatty acids. As with amylase (see p. 49), lipase appears in the bloodstream following damage to or disease affecting the pancreatic acinar cells.

Because lipase was thought to be produced only in the pancreas, elevated serum levels were considered to be specific to pathologic pancreatic conditions. It is now apparent that other conditions can be associated with elevated lipase levels. Lipase is excreted through the kidneys. Therefore elevated lipase levels are often found in patients with renal failure. Intestinal infarction or obstruction also can be associated with lipase elevation. However, the lipase elevations in nonpancreatic diseases are less than 3 times the upper limit of normal, as compared with pancreatitis, where they are often 5 to 10 times normal values. Still other conditions such as cholangitis, mumps, cholecystitis, or peptic ulcer are more rarely associated with elevated lipase levels.

In acute pancreatitis elevated lipase levels usually parallel serum amylase levels. The lipase levels usually rise a little later than amylase (24 to 48 hours after the onset of pancreatitis) and remain elevated for 5 to 7 days. Because lipase peaks later and remain elevated longer than serum amylase, it is more useful in the diagnosis of acute pancreatitis later in the course of the disease. Lipase levels are less useful in more chronic pancreatic diseases (e.g., chronic pancreatitis, pancreatic carcinoma).

Interfering factors

- Drugs that may cause *increased* lipase levels include bethanechol, cholinergics, codeine, indomethacin, meperidine, methacholine, and morphine.
- Drugs that may cause *decreased* levels include calcium ions.

Procedure and patient care

Before
- Explain the procedure to the patient.
- Instruct the patient to remain NPO, except for water, for 8 to 12 hours before the test.

During
- Collect 5 to 7 ml of venous blood in a red-top tube.
- Indicate on the laboratory slip drugs that may affect test results.

After
- Apply pressure to the venipuncture site.

Abnormal findings

Acute pancreatitis
Chronic relapsing pancreatitis
Pancreatic cancer
Pancreatic pseudocyst
Acute cholecystitis
Cholangitis
Extrahepatic duct obstruction
Renal failure
Bowel obstruction or infarction
Salivary gland inflammation or tumor
Peptic ulcer disease

notes

---

lipoproteins (High-density lipoprotein [HDL], Low-density lipoprotein [LDL], Very low–density lipoprotein [VLDL])

Type of test Blood

Normal findings
HDL
   Male: >45 mg/dl or >0.75 mmol/L (SI units)
   Female: >55 mg/dl or >0.91 mmol/L (SI units)
LDL: 60-180 mg/dl or <3.37 mmol/L (SI units)
VLDL: 25% to 50%

Test explanation and related physiology
Lipoproteins are considered to be an accurate predictor of coronary heart disease (CHD). As part of the "lipid profile," these tests are performed to indicate persons at risk for developing heart disease and to monitor therapy if abnormalities are found.

Lipoproteins are proteins in the blood whose main purpose is to transport cholesterol, triglycerides, and other insoluble fats. They are used as markers indicating the levels of lipids within the bloodstream. With the use of electrophoresis, these lipoproteins can be grouped into chylomicrons, which are primarily triglycerides; LDLs (beta-lipoproteins), which are primarily cholesterol; VLDLs (prebeta-lipoproteins), which are mainly triglycerides; and HDLs (alpha-lipoproteins), which are predominantly protein with small amount of cholesterol. The "lipid profile" usually includes total cholesterol, triglycerides, HDL, LDL, and VLDL.

HDLs are carriers of cholesterol. They are produced in the liver and to a smaller degree in the intestines. It is suspected that the purpose of HDLs is to remove the cholesterol from the peripheral tissues and to transport this to the liver for excretion. Also, HDLs may have a protective effect by preventing cellular uptake of cholesterol and lipids. These potential actions may be the source of the protective cardiovascular characteristics associated with HDLs ("good cholesterol") within the blood. Both HDL and total cholesterol are independent variables of risk of CHD. When combined in a ratio fashion, the accuracy of prediction is increased. The total cholesterol/HDL ratio should be at least 5:1, with 3:1 being ideal. See Table 7, p. 233.

LDLs are cholesterol rich. Cholesterol carried by LDLs can be deposited into the peripheral tissues and is associated with an increased risk of arteriosclerotic heart and vascular disease. Therefore high levels of LDL ("bad cholesterol") are atherogenic. The LDL level should be less than 160 mg/dl in persons with coronary artery disease and less than 180 mg/dl in those without disease. LDL is very difficult to isolate and measure. Therefore the LDL is most usually derived by the Friedwald formula. In this formula LDL is derived by subtracting the HDL plus one fifth of the triglycerides from the total cholesterol:

$$LDL = Total\ cholesterol - (HDL + Triglycerides/5)$$

There are other formulas for deriving LDL, which may account for different sets of normal values.

VLDLs, although carrying a small amount of cholesterol, are the predominant carriers of blood triglycerides. To a lesser degree, VLDLs are also associated with an increased risk of arteriosclerotic occlusive disease. The VLDL value is usually expressed as a percentage of total cholesterol. Levels in excess of 25% to 50% are associated with increased risk of coronary disease.

Interfering factors

- Smoking and alcohol ingestion decrease HDL levels.
- Binge eating can alter lipoprotein values.
- HDL values are age and sex dependent.
- HDL values, like cholesterol, tend to significantly decrease for as long as 3 months following myocardial infarction.
- HDL is elevated in hypothyroid patients and diminished in hyperthyroid patients.
- Drugs that may cause increased lipoprotein levels include aspirin, oral contraceptives, phenothiazines, steroids, and sulfonamides.

Procedure and patient care

Before

- Instruct the patient to fast for 12 to 14 hours before testing. Only water is permitted.
- Inform the patient that dietary indiscretion within the previous few weeks may influence lipoprotein levels.

During

- Collect 5 to 10 ml of venous blood in a red-top tube.
- Indicate on the laboratory slip any drugs that may affect test results.

After
- Apply pressure to the venipuncture site.
- Instruct patients with high lipoprotein levels regarding diet, exercise, and appropriate body weight.

Abnormal findings

▲ **Increased HDL levels**
Familial HDL lipoproteinemia
Excessive exercise

▼ **Decreased HDL levels**
Familial low HDL
Hepatocellular disease (e.g., hepatitis or cirrhosis)
Hypoproteinemia (e.g., nephrotic syndrome or malnutrition)

▲ **Increased LDL and VLDL**
Familiar LDL lipoproteinemia
Nephrotic syndrome
Glycogen storage diseases (e.g., von Gierke's disease)
Hypothyroidism
Alcohol consumption
Chronic liver disease (e.g., hepatitis or cirrhosis)
Hepatoma
Gammopathies (e.g., multiple myeloma)
Familial hypercholesterolemia type IIa
Cushing's syndrome
Apoprotein CII deficiency

▼ **Decreased LDL and VLDL**
Familial hypolipoproteinemia
Hypoproteinemia (e.g., malabsorption, severe burns, or malnutrition)
Hyperthyroidism

notes

liver biopsy

Type of test Microscopic examination of tissue

Normal findings Normal liver histology

Test explanation and related physiology

Liver biopsy is a safe, simple, and valuable method of diagnosing pathologic liver conditions. For this study a specially designed needle is inserted through the abdominal wall and into the liver. A piece of liver tissue is removed for microscopic examination. Percutaneous liver biopsy is used in the diagnosis of various liver disorders such as cirrhosis, hepatitis, drug reaction, granuloma, and tumor. Biopsy is indicated for the following:

1. Patients with unexplained hepatomegaly
2. Patients with persistently elevated liver enzymes
3. Patients with suspected primary or metastatic tumor, as determined by other studies
4. Patients with unexplained jaundice
5. Patients with suspected hepatitis
6. Patient with suspected infiltrative diseases (e.g., sarcoidosis, amyloidosis)

The biopsy may be performed by a "blind" stick or directed with the use of a computed tomography (CT) or magnetic resonance imaging (MRI) scan. Directed scans are used if there is a specific area of the liver that is suspicious and from which tissue must be obtained (e.g., a metastatic tumor). The "blind" stick is used if the liver is diffusely involved.

Contraindications

- Uncooperative patients who cannot remain still and hold their breath during sustained exhalation
- Patients with impaired hemostasis
- Patients with anemia who could not tolerate major blood loss associated with inadvertent puncture of an intrahepatic blood vessel
- Patients with infections in the right pleural space or right upper quadrant, because the biopsy may spread the infection
- Patients with obstructive jaundice
  In these patients, bile within the ducts is under pressure and may subsequently leak into the abdominal cavity after needle penetration.

- Patients with a hemangioma
  This is a very vascular tumor, and bleeding after a biopsy may be severe.

Potential complications

- Hemorrhage caused by inadvertent puncture of a blood vessel within the liver
- Chemical peritonitis caused by inadvertent puncture of a bile duct, with subsequent leakage of bile into the abdominal cavity
- Pneumothorax (collapsed lung) caused by improper placement of the biopsy needle into the adjacent chest cavity

Procedure and patient care

Before

- Explain the procedure to the patient. Many patients are apprehensive about it.
- Obtain an informed consent.
- Ensure that all coagulation tests are normal.
- Instruct the patient to keep NPO after midnight on the day of the test.
- Administer any sedative medications as ordered.

During

- Note the following procedural steps:
  1. The patient is placed in the supine or left lateral position.
  2. The skin area used for puncture is anesthetized locally.
  3. The patient is asked to exhale and hold the exhalation. This causes the liver to descend and reduces the possibility of a pneumothorax. Frequently the patient practices exhalation two or three times before insertion of the needle.
  4. During the patient's sustained exhalation, the physician rapidly introduces the biopsy needle into the liver and obtains liver tissue.
     a. Several types of needles are available.
     b. Occasionally the biopsy needle is inserted under CT guidance. This is especially useful when tissue from a specific area of the liver is needed.
  5. The needle is withdrawn from the liver.
- Note that this test is performed by a physician in approximately 15 minutes.
- Inform the patient that he or she may have minor discomfort during injection of the local anesthetic and needle insertion.

After

- Place the tissue sample into a specimen bottle containing for-malin and send it to the pathology department.
- Apply a small dressing over the needle insertion site.
- Place the patient on his or her right side for approximately 1 to 2 hours. In this position, the liver capsule is com-pressed against the chest wall, thereby decreasing the risk of hemorrhage or bile leak.
- Assess the patient's vital signs frequently for evidence of hem-orrhage (increased pulse, decreased blood pressure) and peri-tonitis (increased temperature).

Abnormal findings

Benign tumor
Malignant tumor (primary or metastatic)
Abscess
Cyst
Hepatitis
Infiltrative diseases (e.g., amyloidosis, hemochromatosis, cirrhosis)

L

notes

liver/spleen scanning (Liver scanning)

Type of test Nuclear scan

Normal findings Normal size, shape, and position of the liver and spleen

Test explanation and related physiology

This radionuclide procedure is used to outline and detect structural changes of the liver and spleen. A radionuclide, usually technetium sulfur-labeled albumin colloid, is administered intravenously. Later a gamma ray scintillator is placed over the right and left upper quadrants of the patient's abdomen. This records the distribution of the radioactive particles emitted from the liver and spleen. Images are obtained comparable to the gamma ray emission and are recorded on film.

Because the scan can only demonstrate filling defects greater than 2 cm in diameter, false-negative results may occur in patients with space-occupying lesions (e.g., tumors, cysts, granulomas, abscesses) smaller than 2 cm. The liver scan can detect tumors, cysts, granulomas, abscesses, and diffuse infiltrative processes affecting the liver (e.g., amyloidosis, sarcoidosis).

Single Photon Emitting Computed Tomography (SPECT) has significantly improved the quality and accuracy of liver scanning. With SPECT scanning, the radionuclide is injected, and the scintillator is placed to receive images from multiple angles (around the circumference of the patient). This greatly increases the accuracy of nuclear liver scanning. With the use of radioactive carbon, nitrogen, or oxygen, anatomic and biochemical changes can be visualized within the liver. This method of liver scanning is called PET scanning (p. 660).

This scan can also identify portal hypertension. Normally most of the radionuclide administered during a liver scan is taken up by the liver. If the liver-to-spleen ratio is reversed (i.e., the spleen takes up more of the radionuclide), reversal of hepatic blood flow exists as a result of portal hypertension.

Splenic hematoma, abscess, cyst, tumor, infarction, and infiltrate processes such as granulomas also can be detected.

Contraindications

- Patients who are pregnant or lactating, because of risk of damage to the fetus or infant.

Interfering factor

- Barium in the GI tract overlying the liver or spleen will produce defects on the scan that may be mistaken for masses.

Procedure and patient care

Before

- Explain the procedure to the patient.
- Tell the patient that no fasting or premedication is required.
- Assure the patient that he or she will not be exposed to large amounts of radiation, because only tracer doses of isotopes are used.

During

- Note the following procedural steps:
  1. The patient is taken to the nuclear medicine department, where the radionuclide is administered intravenously.
  2. Thirty minutes after injection, a gamma ray detector is placed over the right upper quadrant of the patient's abdomen.
  3. The patient is placed in supine, lateral, and prone positions so that all surfaces of the liver can be visualized.
  4. The radionuclide image is recorded on x-ray film.
- Note that this procedure is performed by a trained technologist in approximately 1 hour. A physician trained in nuclear medicine interprets the results.
- Tell the patient that the only discomfort associated with this procedure is the IV injection of the radionuclide.

After

- Because only tracer doses of radioisotopes are used, inform the patient that no precautions need to be taken by others against radiation exposure.

L

Abnormal findings

Primary or metastatic tumor of the liver or spleen
Abscess of the liver or spleen
Hematoma of the liver or spleen
Hepatic or splenic cyst
Hemangioma
Lacerations of the liver or spleen
Infiltrative processes (e.g., sarcoidosis, amyloidosis, tuberculosis, or granuloma of the liver or spleen)
Cirrhosis
Portal hypertension
Accessory spleen
Splenic infarction

notes

long-acting thyroid stimulator (LATS, Thyroid-stimulating immunoglobulin [TSIG])

Type of test Blood

Normal findings Negative

Test explanation and related physiology

The LATS antibody is an IgG immunoglobulin directed against the thyroid cell plasma membrane. LATS initially was thought to mimic the action of thyroid-stimulating hormone (TSH). It has recently been found to be a part of a group of IgG immunoglobulins directed against the thyroid cell membrane. These immunoglobulins are all associated with Graves' disease and in some cases of Hashimoto's thyroiditis. Their use is helpful in the evaluation of patients for whom the diagnosis of Grave's disease is complicated by borderline or conflicting data needed to support the diagnosis. Other components of this system include *thyroid-stimulating immunoglobulin (TSI)* and *TSH binding inhibiting immunoglobulin (TBII)*.

Like TSI and TBII, LATS can be found in 75% of the patients with Graves' disease. It also can be found in some patients with Hashimoto's thyroiditis and in some patients with hyperparathyroidism. LATS is found most frequently in patients with Graves' disease associated with exophthalmos and/or pretibial edema. Its effect on the thyroid is long lasting, and titers do not decrease until nearly 1 year after successful treatment of the thyroid disease. Because LATS crosses the placenta, it may be found in neonates whose mothers have Graves' disease.

Interfering factors

- Recent administration of radioactive iodine may affect test results.

Procedure and patient care

Before

- Explain the procedure to the patient.
- Tell the patient that no fasting or special preparation is required.

During
- Collect approximately 5 ml of venous blood in a red-top tube.
- Notify the laboratory if the patient has received radioactive iodine in the preceding 2 days.
- Handle the blood sample gently. Hemolysis may interfere with interpretation of test results.

After
- Apply pressure to the venipuncture site.

Abnormal findings

▲   **Increased levels**
    Hyperthyroidism
    Malignant exophthalmos
    Graves' disease

notes

lumbar puncture and cerebrospinal fluid examination (LP and CSF examination, Spinal tap, Spinal puncture, Cerebrospinal fluid analysis)

Type of test Fluid analysis

Normal findings

Pressure: less than 200 cm H_2O
Color: clear and colorless
Blood: none
Cells:
　RBC: 0
　WBC:
　　Total
　　　Neonate: 0-30 cells/μl
　　　1-5 years: 0-20 cells/μl
　　　6-18 years: 0-10 cells/μl
　　　Adult: 0-5 cells/μl
　　Differential
　　　Neutrophils: 0%-6%
　　　Lymphocytes: 40%-80%
　　　Monocytes: 15%-45%
Culture and sensitivity: no organisms present
Protein: 15-45 mg/dl CSF (up to 70 mg/dl in elderly adults and children)
Protein electrophoresis
　Prealbumin: 2%-7%
　Albumin: 56%-76%
　Alpha$_1$ globulin: 2%-7%
　Alpha$_2$ globulin: 4%-12%
　Beta globulin: 8% to 18%
　Gamma globulin: 3% to 12%
　Oligoclonal bands: none
　IgG: 0-4.5 mg/dl
Glucose: 50-75 mg/dl CSF or 60% to 70% of blood glucose level
Chloride: 700-750 mg/dl
Lactate dehydrogenase (LDH): <2-7.2 U/ml
Lactic acid: 10-25 mg/dl
Cytology: no malignant cells

L

Serology for syphilis: negative
Glutamine: 6-15 mg/dl

Test explanation and related physiology

By placing a needle in the subarachnoid space of the spinal column, one can measure the pressure of that space and obtain CSF for examination and diagnosis. Lumbar puncture may also be used therapeutically to inject therapeutic or diagnostic agents and to administer spinal anesthetics.

Examination of the CSF includes evaluation for the presence of blood, bacteria, and malignant cells, along with quantification of the amount of glucose and protein present. Color is noted, and various other tests such as a serologic test for syphilis (see p. 797) are performed.

Pressure

By attaching a sterile manometer to the needle used for LP, the pressure within the subarachnoid space can be measured. A pressure above 200 cm H_2O is considered abnormal and indicative of increased spinal pressure. Because the subarachnoid space surrounding the brain is freely connected to the subarachnoid space of the spinal cord, any increase in intracranial pressure will be directly reflected as an increase at the lumbar site. Tumors, infection, hydrocephalus, and intracranial bleeding can cause increased intracranial and spinal pressure. Intracranial pressure is related to the volume of CSF fluid. Also, because the cranial venous sinuses are connected to the jugular veins, obstruction of those veins or the superior vena cava increases intracranial pressure.

Pressures are routinely measured at the beginning and end of an LP. If there is a significant difference in these values, one must suspect a spinal cord obstruction (tumor). Large differences in opening and closing pressures are also seen in patients with hydrocephalus. One must be aware that children who are crying and holding their breath may have transient elevations of pressure that reduce as the child relaxes.

Color

Normal CSF is clear and colorless. Color differences can occur with hyperbilirubinemia, hypercarotenemia, melanoma, or elevated proteins. A cloudy appearance may indicate an increase in the white blood cell (WBC) count or protein. A red tinge to the CSF indicates the presence of blood.

Blood

Normally, CSF contains no blood. Blood may be present because of bleeding into the subarachnoid space or because the needle used in the LP has inadvertently penetrated a blood vessel on the way into the subarachnoid space. With a "traumatic puncture," the blood within the CSF will clot. No clotting occurs in a patient with subarachnoid hemorrhage. Also, with a traumatic tap, the fluid clears toward the end of the procedure as successive CSF samples are obtained. This clearing does not occur with a subarachnoid hemorrhage.

Cells

The number of red blood cells is merely an indication of the amount of blood present within the CSF. Except for a few lymphocytes, the presence of WBCs in the CSF is abnormal. The presence of polymorphonuclear leukocytes (neutrophils) is indicative of bacterial meningitis or cerebral abscess. When mononuclear leukocytes are present, viral or tubercular meningitis or encephalitis is suspected. Leukemia or other primary or metastatic malignant tumors may cause elevated WBCs. Pleocytosis is a term used to indicate turbidity of CSF caused by an increased number of cells within the fluid.

Culture and sensitivity

The organisms that cause meningitis or brain abscess can be cultured from the CSF. Organisms found also may include atypical bacteria, fungi, or *Mycobacterium tuberculosis*. A Gram stain (p. 784) of the CSF may give the clinician preliminary information about the causative infectious agent. This may allow appropriate antibiotic therapy to be initiated before the 24 to 72 hours necessary to complete the culture and sensitivity report.

Protein

Normally, very little protein is found in CSF because protein is a large molecule that does not cross the blood-brain barrier. Normally, the proportion of albumin to globulin is higher in CSF than in blood plasma (see p. 686) because albumin is smaller in size than globulin and therefore can pass more easily through the blood-brain barrier. Disease such as meningitis, encephalitis, or myelitis can alter the permeability of the blood-brain barrier, allowing protein to leak into the CSF. Furthermore, CNS tumors may produce and secrete protein into the CSF.

CSF protein electrophoresis is very important in the diagnosis of CNS diseases. Patients with multiple sclerosis, neurosyphilis, or other immunogenic degenerative central neurologic disease have elevated immunoglobulins in their CSF. The detection of *oligoclonal gamma globulin bands* is highly suggestive of inflammatory and autoimmune diseases of the central nervous system, especially multiple sclerosis (MS). Myelin-basic protein, a component of myelin (substance that surrounds normal nerve tissue) is elevated when demyelinating diseases such as MS or amyotrophic lateral sclerosis occur.

Glucose

The glucose level is decreased when the bacteria or cells within the CSF increase in number and catabolize the glucose. The cells may be inflammatory cells in response to infection or inflammation or cells that are shed by tumors. A blood sample for glucose (see p. 434) is usually drawn before the spinal tap is performed. A CSF glucose level less than 60% of the blood glucose may indicate meningitis or neoplasm.

Chloride

The chloride concentration in CSF may be decreased in patients with meningeal infections, tubercular meningitis, and conditions of low blood chloride levels. An increase in the chloride level in CSF is not neurologically significant; it correlates with the blood levels of chloride (see p. 230). CSF is not routinely evaluated for chloride; this test is done only if specifically requested.

Lactate dehydrogenase

Quantification of LDH (specifically fractions 4 and 5; see p. 511) is helpful in diagnosing bacterial meningitis. The source of LDH is the neutrophils that fight the invading bacteria. When the LDH level is elevated, infection or inflammation is suspected. The elevated WBC count associated with central nervous system (CNS) leukemia is also associated with elevated LDH levels. The nerve tissue in the CNS is also high in LDH (isoenzymes 1 and 2). Therefore disease directly affecting the brain or spinal cord (e.g., stroke) is associated with elevated LDH levels.

Lactic acid

Elevated levels indicate anaerobic metabolism associated with decreased oxygenation of the brain. CSF lactic acid is increased in both bacterial and fungal meningitis but not in viral meningitis.

Cytology

Examination of cells found in the CSF can determine if they are malignant. Tumors in the central nervous system may shed cells from their surface. These cells can float freely in CSF. Their presence suggests neoplasm as the cause of any neurologic symptoms.

Tumor markers

Increased levels of tumor markers such as carcinoembryonic antigen, alpha-fetoprotein, or human chorionic gonadotropin may indicate metastatic tumor.

Serology for syphilis

Latent syphilis is diagnosed by performing one of many presently available serologic tests on CSF. These include the Wasserman test, the Venereal Disease Research Laboratory test (see p. 797), and the fluorescent treponemal antibody (FTA) test (see p. 797). The FTA test is presently considered to be the most sensitive and specific. When test results are positive, the diagnosis of neurosyphilis is made, and appropriate antibiotic therapy is initiated.

Glutamine

Elevated glutamine levels are helpful in the detection and evaluation of hepatic encephalopathy and hepatic coma. The glutamine is made by increased levels of ammonia, which are commonly associated with liver failure. See serum ammonia (p. 41). Levels of glutamine are also often increased in patients with Reye's syndrome.

Contraindications

- Patients with increased intracranial pressure
  The LP may induce cerebral or cerebellar herniation through the foramen magnum.
- Patients who have severe degenerative vertebral joint disease
  It is very difficult to pass the needle through the degenerated arthritic interspinal space.
- Patients with infection near the LP site
  Meningitis can result from contamination of CSF with infected material.

Potential complications

- Persistent CSF leak, causing severe headache
- Puncture of subcutaneous blood vessel during this procedure
- Introduction of bacteria into CSF, causing suppurative meningitis

- Herniation of the brain through the tentorium cerebelli or herniation of the cerebellum through the foramen magnum In patients with increased intracranial pressure, the quick reduction of pressure in the spinal column by the LP may induce herniation of the brain, causing compression of the brain stem. This results in deterioration of the patient's neurologic status and death.
- Inadvertent puncture of the spinal cord caused by inappropriately high puncture of the spinal cord
- Puncture of the aorta or vena cava, causing serious retroperitoneal hemorrhage
- Transient back pain and pain or paresthesia in the legs

Procedure and patient care

Before

- Explain the procedure to the patient. Many patients have misconceptions regarding LP. Allay the patient's fears and allow time to verbalize concerns.
- Obtain informed consent if required by the institution.
- Perform a baseline neurologic assessment of the legs by assessing the patient's strengths, sensation, and movement.
- Tell the patient that no fasting or sedation is required.
- Instruct the patient to empty the bladder and bowels before the procedure.
- Explain to the patient that he or she must lie very still throughout this procedure. Movement may cause traumatic injury. Encourage the patient to relax and take deep, slow breaths with the mouth open.

During

- Note the following procedural steps:
  1. This study is a sterile procedure that can be easily performed at the bedside. The patient is usually placed in the lateral decubitus (fetal) position (Figure 21).
  2. The patient is instructed to clasp the hands on the knees to maintain this position. Someone usually helps the patient maintain this position. (A sitting position also may be used.)
  3. A local anesthetic is injected into the skin and subcutaneous tissues after the site has been aseptically cleaned.
  4. A spinal needle containing an inner obturator is placed through the skin and into the spinal canal.
  5. The subarachnoid space is entered.

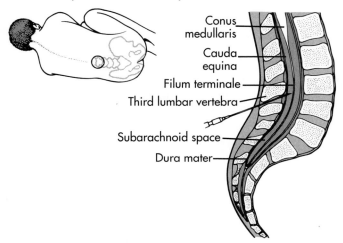

Figure 21 Patient position for lumbar puncture.

L

6. The insert (obturator) is removed, and CSF can be seen slowly dripping from the needle.
7. The needle is attached to a sterile manometer, and the pressure (opening pressure) is recorded.
8. Before the pressure reading is taken, the patient is asked to relax and straighten the legs to reduce the intraabdominal pressure, which causes an increase in CSF pressure.
9. Three sterile test tubes are filled with 5 to 10 ml of CSF.
10. The pressure (closing pressure) is measured.
- Note that, if blockage in CSF circulation in the spinal subarachnoid space is suspected, a *Queckenstedt-Stookey* test may be performed. For this test the jugular vein is occluded either manually by digital pressure or by a medium-sized blood pressure cuff inflated to approximately 20 mm Hg. Within 10 seconds after jugular occlusion, CSF pressure should increase from 15 to 40 cm H_2O and then promptly return to normal within 10 seconds after release of the pressure. A sluggish rise or fall of CSF pressure suggests partial blockage of CSF circulation. No rise after 10

seconds suggests a complete obstruction within the spinal canal.
- Note that this procedure is performed by a physician in approximately 20 minutes.
- Inform the patient that this procedure is described as uncomfortable or painful by most patients. Some patients complain of feeling pressure from the needle. Some patients complain of a shooting pain in their legs.

After
- Apply digital pressure and an adhesive dressing to the puncture site.
- Place the patient in the prone position with a pillow under the abdomen to increase the intraabdominal pressure, which will indirectly increase the pressure in the tissues surrounding the spinal cord. This retards continued CSF flow from the spinal canal.
- Encourage the patient to drink increased amounts of fluid with a straw to replace the CSF removed during the lumbar puncture. Drinking with a straw will enable the patient to keep the head flat.
- Usually keep the patient in a reclining position for up to 12 hours to avoid the discomfort of potential postpuncture spinal headache. Allow the patient to turn from side to side as long as the head is not raised.
- Label and number the specimen jars appropriately and deliver them immediately to the laboratory after the test. Refrigeration will alter test results. A delay between collection time and testing can invalidate results, especially cell counts.
- Assess the patient for numbness, tingling, and movement of the extremities; pain at the injection site; drainage of blood or CSF at the injection site; and the ability to void. Notify the physician of any unusual findings.

🏠 Home care responsibilities

- The patient should be kept flat in bed for up to 12 hours to avoid a postprocedure spinal headache.
- Encourage the patient to drink increased amounts of fluid to replace CSF removed during the LP.
- Instruct the patient to report any abnormalities, such as numbness and tingling in the legs, to the physician.

Abnormal findings

Brain neoplasm
Spinal cord neoplasm
Cerebral hemorrhage
Encephalitis
Myelitis
Tumor
Neurosyphilis
Degenerative brain disease
Autoimmune disorder
Hepatic encephalopathy
Coma
Meningitis
Encephalitis
Viral or tubercular meningitis
Cerebral abscess
Degenerative cord or brain disease
Multiple sclerosis
Acute demyelinating polyneuropathy
Subarachnoid bleeding
Reye syndrome
Metastatic tumor

notes

L

lung biopsy

Type of test Microscopic examination of tissue

Normal findings No evidence of pathology

Test explanation and related physiology

This invasive procedure is used to obtain a specimen of pulmonary tissue for a histologic examination by using either an open or a closed technique. The *open method* involves a limited thoracotomy. The *closed technique* includes methods such as transbronchial lung biopsy, transbronchial needle aspiration biopsy, transcatheter bronchial brushing, percutaneous needle biopsy, and video assisted thoracostomy (VAT).

Lung biopsy is indicated to determine the pathology of pulmonary parenchymal disease. Carcinomas, granulomas, infections, and sarcoidosis can be diagnosed with this procedure. The procedure is also useful in detecting environmental exposures, infections, or familial disease, which may lead to better prevention and treatment.

Contraindications

- Patients with bullae or cysts of the lung
- Patients with suspected vascular anomalies of the lung
- Patients with bleeding abnormalities
- Patients with pulmonary hypertension
- Patients with respiratory insufficiency

Potential complications

- Pneumothorax
- Pulmonary hemorrhage
- Empyema

Procedure and patient care

Before

- Explain the procedure to the patient.
- Ensure that informed and signed consent is obtained.
- Instruct the patient that fasting is usually ordered. The patient may be kept NPO after midnight on the day of the test.
- Administer the preprocedural medications 30 to 60 minutes before the test as ordered.

- Instruct the patient to remain still during the lung biopsy. Any movement or coughing could cause laceration of the lung by the biopsy needle.

During

- Note that the patient's position depends on the method used and that the histologic lung specimen may be obtained by several different methods:

Transbronchial lung biopsy

1. This technique is performed via flexible fiberoptic bronchoscopy, using cutting forceps.
2. Fluoroscopy is used to ensure proper opening and positioning of the forceps on the lesions.
3. Fluoroscopy also permits visualization of the "tug" of the lung as the specimen is removed.

Transbronchial needle aspiration

1. The needle is inserted through the bronchoscope and into the tumor or desired area, where aspiration is performed with the attached syringe.
2. The needle is retracted within its sheath, and the entire catheter is withdrawn from the fiberoptic scope.

Transbronchial brushing

1. A small brush is moved back and forth over the suspicious area in the bronchus or its branches.
2. The cells adhere to the brush, which is then removed and used to make microscopic slides.

Percutaneous needle biopsy

1. In this method for obtaining a closed specimen, the biopsy is obtained after using fluoroscopic x-ray or CT scan determination of the desired site.
2. The procedure is carried out by using a cutting needle or by aspiration with a spinal-type needle to obtain a specimen.

Open lung biopsy

1. The patient is taken to the operating room, and general anesthesia is provided.
2. The patient is placed in the supine or lateral position, and an incision is made into the chest wall.
3. After a piece of lung tissue is removed, the lung is sutured.
4. Chest tube drainage is used for approximately 24 hours after an open lung biopsy.

Thorascopic lung biopsy

1. The lung is collapsed with a double lumen endotracheal tube placed during induction of general anesthesia.
2. With the use of a thoracoscope (similar to a laparoscope [p. 518]), the lung is grasped, and a piece is cut off with the use of a cutting/stapling device. Large wedge lung resections can be obtained.
3. The scope and trocars are removed, and a small chest tube is left in place.
4. The tiny incisions are closed, and the procedure is completed.

- Note that this procedure is performed by a surgeon in less than 30 to 60 minutes.
- During the lung biopsy procedure, assess the patient carefully for signs of respiratory distress (e.g., shortness of breath, rapid pulse, cyanosis).
- Tell the patient that most patients describe this procedure as painful.

After

- Place biopsy specimens in appropriate containers for histologic and microbiologic examination.
- Observe the patient's vital signs frequently for signs of bleeding (increased pulse, decreased blood pressure) and shortness of breath.
- Assess the patient's breath sounds and report any decrease on the biopsy side.
- Obtain a chest x-ray film to check for complications (e.g., pneumothorax).
- Observe the patient for signs of pneumothorax (e.g., dyspnea, tachypnea, decrease in breath sounds, anxiety, restlessness).

Abnormal findings

Carcinoma

Granuloma

Exposure lung diseases (e.g., black lung, asbestosis)

Sarcoidosis

Infection

lung scan (Ventilation/perfusion scanning [VPS], Pulmonary scintiphotography, V/Q scan)

Type of test Nuclear scan

Normal findings Diffuse and homogeneous uptake of nuclear material by the lungs

Test explanation and related physiology

This nuclear medicine procedure is used to identify defects in blood *perfusion* of the lung in patients with suspected pulmonary embolism. Blood flow to the lungs is evaluated using a macroaggregated albumin (MAA) tagged with technetium (Tc), which is injected into the patient's peripheral vein. Because the diameter of the radionuclide aggregates is larger than that of the pulmonary capillaries, the aggregates become temporarily lodged in the pulmonary vasculature. A scintillator (gamma camera) detects the gamma rays from within the lung microvasculature. With the use of light conversion, a realistic image of the lung is obtained on film.

A homogeneous uptake of particles that fills the entire pulmonary vasculature conclusively rules out pulmonary embolism. If a defect in an otherwise smooth and diffusely homogeneous pattern is seen, a perfusion abnormality exists. This can indicate pulmonary embolism. Unfortunately, many other serious pulmonary parenchymal lesions (e.g., pneumonia, pleural fluid, emphysematous bullae) also cause a defect in pulmonary blood perfusion. Therefore, although the scan may be sensitive, it is not specific, because many different pathologic conditions can cause the same abnormal results.

The chest x-ray film aids in assessing the perfusion scan, because a defect on the perfusion scan seen in the same area as an abnormality on the chest x-ray film does not indicate pulmonary embolism. Rather, the defect may represent pneumonia, atelectasis, effusion, and so on. However, when a perfusion defect occurs in an area of the lung that is normal on a chest x-ray study, pulmonary embolus is likely.

Specificity of a perfusion scan also can be enhanced by performance of a *ventilation scan,* which detects parenchymal abnormalities in ventilation (e.g., pneumonia, pleural fluid, emphysematous bullae). The ventilation scan reflects the patency of the pulmonary airways, using krypton gas or

L

Tc-diethylenetriamine pentaacetic acid (DTPA) as an aerosol. When vascular obstruction (embolism) is present by perfusion scan, ventilation scans demonstrate a normal wash-in and wash-out of radioactivity from the embolized lung area. If parenchymal disease (e.g., pneumonia) is responsible for the perfusion abnormality, however, wash-in or wash-out will be abnormal. Therefore the "mismatch" of perfusion and ventilation findings is characteristic of embolic disorders, whereas the "match" is indicative of parenchymal disease. When ventilation and perfusion scan are performed synchronously, this is called a *ventilation/perfusion (V/Q) scan*. Most nuclear physicians read the lung scan as one of several categories: negative for PE, low probability of PE, high probability of PE, or positive for PE.

Contraindications

- Patients who are pregnant

Interfering factors

- Patients with known pulmonary parenchymal problems (e.g., pneumonia, emphysema, pleural effusion, tumors)
  These problems will give the picture of a perfusion defect and simulate pulmonary embolism.

Procedure and patient care

Before

- Explain the procedure to the patient.
- Obtain informed consent if required by the institution.
- Assure the patient that he or she will not be exposed to large amounts of radioactivity, because only tracer doses of isotopes are used.
- Although rarely done, if iodine-131 will be administered, give the patient 10 drops of Lugol's solution several hours before the test as a blocking agent for the thyroid gland. This will prevent iodine uptake by the thyroid gland.
- Tell the patient that no fasting is required.
- Note that a recent chest x-ray film should be available.
- Instruct the patient to remove jewelry around the chest area.

During

- Note the following procedural steps:
  1. The unsedated, nonfasting patient suspected of having a pulmonary embolism is taken to the nuclear medicine department.

Perfusion scan

2. The patient is given a peripheral IV injection of radionuclide-tagged MAA.

3. While the patient lies in the appropriate position, a gamma ray detector is passed over the patient and records radionuclide uptake on Polaroid or x-ray film.

4. The patient is placed in the supine, prone, and various lateral positions, which allows for anterior, posterior, lateral, and oblique views, respectively.

5. The results are interpreted by a physician trained in diagnostic nuclear medicine.

Ventilation scan

6. The patient breathes the tracer through a face mask with a mouthpiece.

7. Less patient cooperation is needed with a krypton tracer. Ventilation scans can even be performed on comatose patients using krypton. Krypton images can be obtained before, during, or after perfusion images.

8. In contrast, Tc-DTPA images are usually done before perfusion images and require patient cooperation with deep breathing and appropriate use of breathing equipment to prevent contamination.

- Note that this test is usually performed by a physician in approximately 30 minutes.
- Tell the patient that no discomfort is associated with this test other than the peripheral venipuncture.

After

- Inform the patient that no radiation precautions are necessary.

Abnormal findings

Pulmonary embolism
Pneumonia
Tuberculosis
Emphysema
Tumor
Asthma
Atelectasis
Bronchitis
Chronic obstructive pulmonary disease

luteinizing hormone assay (LH assay, Lutropin) and Follicle-stimulating hormone (FSH)

Type of test   Blood

Normal findings

	LH (IU/L)	FSH (IU/L)
Adult		
Male	1.24-7.8	1.42-15.4
Female		
Follicular phase	1.68-15	1.37-9.9
Ovulatory peak	21.9-56.6	6.17-17.2
Luteal phase	0.61-16.3	1.09-9.2
Postmenopause	14.2-52.3	19.3-100.6
Child (age 1-10 years)		
Male	0.04-3.6	0.3-4.6
Female	0.03-3.9	0.68-6.7

(Values may vary, depending on laboratory method.)

Test explanation and related physiology

LH and FSH are glycoproteins that are produced in the anterior pituitary gland. These two hormones then act on the ovary or testes. In the female FSH stimulates the development of follicles in the ovary. In the male FSH stimulates Sertoli cell development. In the female LH stimulates follicular production of estrogen, ovulation, and formation of a corpus luteum. In the male LH stimulates testosterone production from the Sertoli cells. In females the mid-cycle peak of FSH is necessary for follicle/ovum formation. LH also must peak about that same time to stimulate corpus luteal formation that could potentially support a embryo if fertilization were to occur.

Spot urines for LH have become very useful in the evaluation and treatment of infertility. Because LH is rapidly excreted into the urine, the plasma LH surge that precedes ovulation by 24 hours can be recognized quickly and easily. This is used to indicate the period when the women is most fertile. The best time to obtain a urine specimen is between 11 AM and 3 PM. Usually the woman begins to test her urine on the day following her menses and continues to do so daily. Home kits using a color change as an endpoint are now marketed to make this process even more convenient.

These hormones are used in the evaluation of infertility. Performing an LH assay is an easy way to determine if ovulation has occurred. An LH surge in blood levels indicates that ovulation has taken place. Daily samples of serum LH around the woman's midcycle can detect the LH surge, which is believed to occur on the day of maximal fertility.

These assays also determine whether a gonadal insufficiency is primary (problem with the ovary/testicle) or secondary (caused by pituitary insufficiency resulting in reduced levels of FSH and LH). Elevated levels of FSH and LH in patients with gonadal insufficiency indicate primary gonadal failure, as may be seen in women with polycystic ovaries or menopause. In secondary gonadal failure, LH and FSH levels are low as a result of pituitary failure or some other pituitary-hypothalamic pathology.

Interfering factors

- Recent use of radioisotopes may affect test results if the testing method is performed by radioimmunoassay.
- Human chorionic gonadotropin (HCG) and thyroid-stimulating hormone may interfere with some immunoassay methods. Therefore patients with HCG-producing tumors and hypothyroid patients should be expected to have falsely high LH levels.
- Drugs that may *increase* LH levels include anticonvulsants, clomiphene, naloxone, and spironolactone.
- Drugs that may *decrease* LH levels include estrogens, progesterones, testosterone, digoxin, oral contraceptives, and phenothiazines.

Procedure and patient care

Before
- Explain the procedure to the patient.
- Tell the patient that no food or fluid restrictions are needed.

During
- Collect approximately 7 to 10 ml of venous blood in a red-top tube.
- Note that the patient may also perform LH assays at home using a home urine test or a 24-hour urine test.
- Indicate the date of the last menstrual period on the laboratory slip. Note if the woman is postmenopausal.

After
- Apply pressure to the venipuncture site.

Abnormal findings

▲ **Increased levels**

Menopause
Ovarian dysgenesis
  (Turner's syndrome)
Testicular dysgenesis
  (Klinefelter syndrome)
Castration
Anorchia
Hypogonadism
Polycystic ovaries
Complete testicular femi-
  nization syndrome
Precocious puberty
Pituitary adenoma

▼ **Decreased levels**

Pituitary failure
Hypothalamic failure
Stress
Anorexia nervosa
Malnutrition

notes

Lyme disease test

Type of test Blood

Normal findings Negative (low titers of IgM and IgG antibodies)

Test explanation and related physiology

Lyme disease was first recognized in Lyme, Connecticut, in 1975. It is caused by a spirochete called *Borrelia burgdorferi*. The disease usually begins in the summer with a skin lesion called erythema chronicum migrans (ECM), which occurs at the site of a bite by a deer tick, usually *Ixodes dammini* or *pacificus*. Ticks are the best documented vectors of this spirochete, which is the causative agent for Lyme disease.

Cultures of ECM can isolate the spirochete in half of the cases. However, it is hard to culture and takes a long time to grow. Cultures of the blood or cerebrospinal fluid are even less helpful. Currently, serologic studies are the most sensitive and specific tests for the detection of Lyme disease. These tests determine titers of specific immunoglobulin M (IgM) and specific IgG antibodies to the *B. burgdorferi* spirochete. Levels of specific IgM antibody peak during the third to sixth week after disease onset and then gradually decline.

Titers of specific IgG antibodies are generally low during the first several weeks of illness, reach maximal levels 4 to 6 months later, usually after the patient has developed arthritis, and often remain elevated for years. A single titer of specific IgM antibody may suggest the diagnosis. Acute and convalescent sera can be tested to verify the diagnosis.

The Centers for Disease Control and Prevention (CDC) requires the following for the diagnosis to be made with certainty:

Isolation of *B. burgdorferi* from an infected tissue or specimen

Identification of IgM and IgG antibodies to *B. burgdorferi* in the blood or CSF

Acute and convalescent blood samples with significant positive antibody titers.

Interfering factors

- Previous infection with *B. burgdorferi* can cause positive serologic testing. These patients no longer have Lyme disease.

- Other spirochete diseases (syphilis or leptospirosis) can cause false-positive results.

Procedure and patient care

Before
- Explain the procedure to the patient.
- Tell the patient that no fasting or special preparation is required.

During
- Collect approximately 7 to 10 ml of venous blood in a red-top tube.

After
- Apply pressure to the venipuncture site.

Abnormal finding

Lyme disease

notes

lymphangiography (Lymphangiogram, Lymphography)

Type of test X-ray with contrast dye

Normal findings Normal-sized lymph nodes containing no filling defects

Test explanation and related physiology

The lymphatic system consists of lymph vessels and lymph nodes. Assessment of this system is important, because cancer lymphomas and Hodgkin's disease often spread via the lymphatic system. With the help of lymphangiography, the pathologic lymph nodes can be localized for surgical removal or for inclusion in radiation therapy ports.

Lymphangiography is especially useful in patients suspected of having lymphatic pathology (lymphoma or metastatic tumor). The test allows one to demonstrate the extent and level of lymphatic metastasis. The lymphangiogram is also useful in staging lymphoma patients and in evaluating the results of chemotherapy or radiation therapy. Because the contrast medium remains in the lymph nodes for 6 months to 1 year, repeat plain x-ray films may be done for continued follow-up of disease progression or response to treatment.

This test is also useful in the evaluation of patient with chronic leg swelling. Lack of flow of the dye into the pelvic lymphatic vessels indicates lymphatic vessel obstruction as the cause of the leg edema.

Contraindications

- Patients with an allergy to iodine dye or shellfish
- Patients with severe chronic lung diseases, cardiac disease, or advanced kidney or liver disease

Potential complications

- Lipoid (lipid) pneumonia
  This occurs if the contrast medium flows into the thoracic duct and causes micropulmonary emboli. These small emboli usually disappear after several weeks or months.
- Allergic reaction or allergy to iodine dye.

Procedure and patient care

Before

- Explain the procedure to the patient.
- Obtain informed consent if required by the institution.
- Tell the patient that no fasting or sedation is required.
- Inform the patient that, if a blue-colored dye is used, he or she may note a bluish tinge in the urine. Excessive infiltration or IV administration of the lymphatic stain may create a transient bluish tint to a part of or the entire skin surface.

During

- Note the following procedural steps:
    1. In the radiology department the patient is placed on an x-ray table in the supine position.
    2. A lymphatic stain is injected into the subcutaneous tissue between each of the first three toes in each foot to outline the lymphatic vessels. See Figure 22. (The stain can also be injected into the web of the skin between the fingers.)
    3. After the stain is taken up by the lymphatic vessels, they can be easily seen.
    4. A local anesthetic is injected.
    5. A small incision is made on the top of the foot (or hand).
    6. The lymphatic vessel is identified and cannulated to infuse the iodine contrast agent.
    7. The dye is slowly infused into the vessel. Usually a low-rate infusion pump is used. The patient must lie very still during the injection.
    8. The flow of iodine dye is followed by fluoroscopy.
    9. When the dye reaches the upper lumbar level, the flow of dye is discontinued.
    10. X-ray films are taken of the chest, abdomen, and pelvis to demonstrate the filling of the lymph nodes. Often the patient is asked to return in 24 hours to have additional x-ray studies done.
    11. On completion of the injection, the cannula is removed and the incision is sutured closed.
- See p. xviii for appropriate interventions concerning the care for patients with iodine allergy.
- Note that this procedure is performed by a radiologist in approximately 3 hours. Additional x-ray films are usually taken 24 to 48 hours later.

Figure 22 Lymphangiography. Note the small lymphatic vessels that become apparent after the injection of a lymphatic stain into the web space of the feet. (From Pagana KD, Pagana TJ: *Mosby's manual of diagnostic and laboratory tests,* St Louis, 1998, Mosby.)

- Inform the patient that discomfort may be felt when the blue stain is injected subcutaneously and the feet are locally anesthetized.

After

- Observe the injection and incision sites for evidence of cellulitis. If the patient will be returning home, instruct him or her to evaluate the site for redness, pain, and swelling.
- Inform the patient that the sutures should be removed 7 to 10 days after the test.

Abnormal findings

Hodgkin's disease
Metastatic tumor involving the lymph glands
Lymphoma

lymphocyte immunophenotyping (AIDS T-lymphocyte cell markers, CD4 marker, CD4/CD8 ratio, CD4 percentage)

Type of test Blood

Normal findings

Cells	Percent	No. of cells/μl
T cells	60-95	800-2500
T helper (CD4) cells	60-75	600-1500
T suppressor (CD8) cells	25-30	300-1000
B cells	4-25	100-450
Natural killer cells	4-30	75-500
CD4/CD8 ratio	>1	

Test explanation and related physiology

This test is used to detect the progressive depletion of CD4 T lymphocytes, which is associated with an increased likelihood of clinical complications from acquired immunodeficiency syndrome (AIDS). Test results can also indicate if an AIDS patient is at risk for developing opportunistic infections.

T lymphocytes are responsible for cellular immunity. CD4 helper cells and CD8 suppressor cells are examples of T lymphocytes. There are three related measurements of CD4 T lymphocytes. The first measurement is the *total CD4 cell count*. This is measured in whole blood and is the product of the white blood cell count, the lymphocyte differential count, and the percentage of lymphocytes that are CD4 T cells. The second measurement, the *CD4 percentage*, is a more accurate prognostic marker. It measures the percentage of CD4 lymphocytes in the whole blood sample by using immunophenotyping with flow cytometry. This procedure relies on detecting specific antigenic determinants on the surface of the CD4 lymphocyte by antigen-specific monoclonal antibodies labeled with a fluorescent dye. The third prognostic marker, which is also more reliable than the total CD4 count, is the *ratio of CD4 cells to CD8 (T-suppressor) cells*.

Of the three T-cell measurements, the total CD4 count is the most variable. The Multicenter AIDS Cohort Study suggests that the last two measurements are more accurate than the total CD4 count.

The pathogenesis of AIDS is largely attributed to a decrease in the T lymphocyte that bears the CD4 receptor. Progressive depletion of CD4 T lymphocytes is associated with an increased likelihood of clinical complications from AIDS. Therefore CD4 measurement is a prognostic marker that can indicate whether a patient infected with HIV is at risk for developing opportunistic infections. The measurement of CD4 cell levels is used for deciding the initiation of *Pneumocystis carinii* pneumonia prophylaxis and the use of antiviral therapy and for determining the prognosis of patients with human immunodeficiency virus (HIV) infection.

The dosage of immunosuppressive medications used after organ transplant is also monitored with the use of lymphocyte phenotyping. Lymphomas and other lymphoproliferative diseases are now classified and treated according to the predominant lymphocyte type identified. In some instances, prognosis of these diseases depends on lymphocyte phenotyping.

As the CD4 cell measurements decrease, the percentage of persons developing AIDS increases. Forty-eight percent of patients can be expected to develop AIDS within 6 months when their CD4 count is 100 cells/mm^3. It is recommended that antiviral therapy be started in patients whose CD4 count is less than 500 to 600 cells/mm^3. *Pneumocystis carinii* pneumonia prophylaxis should start when the CD4 count is less than 200 to 300 cells/mm^3.

CD4 prognostic markers also can be useful in guiding the approach to the patient's symptoms. Complaints such as cough and headache are common in most people; however, in patients infected with HIV, these symptoms often raise concerns about opportunistic infections. If the CD4 cell count exceeded 500 cells/mm^3 in the past 6 months, there is a very low probability that these symptoms result from opportunistic infections. Knowing this, the patient and physician can feel comfortable with routine care.

Contraindications

- Patients who are not emotionally prepared for the prognosis that the results may indicate

Interfering factors

- Diurnal variation
- A recent viral illness can decrease total T lymphocyte counts.
- Nicotine and very strenuous exercise have been shown to decrease lymphocyte counts.

- Steroids can *increase* lymphocyte counts.
- Immunosuppressive drugs will *decrease* lymphocyte counts.

Procedure and patient care

Before

- Explain the procedure to the patient.
- Tell the patient that no fasting or preparation is required.
- Maintain a nonjudgmental attitude toward the patient's sexual practices. Allow the patient ample time to express his or her concerns regarding the results.

During

- Record the time of day when the blood specimen is being obtained.
- Observe universal body and blood precautions. Wear gloves when handling blood products from all patients.
- Obtain 10 ml of blood in a large green-top tube (containing sodium heparin).
- Obtain 5 ml of blood in a small purple-top tube (containing ethylenediaminetetraacetic acid).
- Never recap needles. Dispose of needles and syringes required for obtaining the blood specimen in a puncture-proof container designed for this purpose.

After

- Keep the specimen at room temperature. Do not refrigerate.
- The specimen must be evaluated within 24 hours.
- Most specimens are sent to a central laboratory. Be sure to draw the blood immediately before the courier's departure to the central laboratory.
- Apply pressure to the venipuncture site.
- Instruct the patient to observe the venipuncture site for infection. Patients with AIDS are immunocompromised and susceptible to infection.
- Encourage the patient to discuss his or her concerns regarding the prognostic information that may be obtained by these results.

Abnormal findings

▲ **Increased counts**

Chronic lymphocytic
 leukemia
B cell lymphoma
T cell lymphoma

▼ **Decreased counts**

Organ transplant patients
HIV positive patients
Congenital
 immunodeficiency

notes

magnesium

Type of test Blood

Normal findings
Adults: 1.2-2 mEq/L
Child: 1.4-17 mEq/L
Newborn: 1.4-2 mEq/L

Possible critical values <0.5 mEq/L or >3 mEq/L

Test explanation and related physiology

Most of the magnesium found within the body exists intracellularly. About half is in the bone. Most of the magnesium is bound to an adenosine triphosphate (ATP) molecule and is important in phosphorylation of ATP (important as the main source of energy for the body). Therefore this electrolyte is critical in nearly all metabolic processes.

Most organ functions, including neuromuscular tissue, also depend on magnesium. It is especially important to monitor magnesium levels in cardiac patients. Low magnesium may increase cardiac irritability and aggravate cardiac arrhythmias. Hypermagnesemia retards neuromuscular conduction and is demonstrated as cardiac conduction slowing (widened PR and Q-T intervals with wide QRS).

As intracellular elements, potassium, magnesium, and calcium (in order of quantity) are intimately tied together in maintaining a neutral intracellular electrical charge. That is why it is hard to maintain a normal potassium level when a patient has low magnesium blood levels.

Magnesium deficiency occurs in patients who are malnourished. Toxemia of pregnancy is also believed to be associated with reduced magnesium levels. Symptoms of magnesium depletion are mostly neuromuscular (i.e., weakness, irritability, tetany, electrocardiographic changes, delirium, and convulsions).

Increased magnesium levels most commonly are associated with ingestion of magnesium-containing antacids. Because most of the serum magnesium is excreted by the kidney, chronic renal diseases cause elevated magnesium levels. Symptoms of increased Mg include lethargy, nausea and vomiting, and slurred speech.

Interfering factors

- Hemolysis should be avoided when collecting this specimen.
- Drugs that *increase* magnesium levels include thyroid medication, antacids, laxatives, calcium-containing medication, lithium, loop diuretics, and aminoglycosides antibiotics.
- Drugs that *decrease* magnesium levels include diuretics, some antibiotics, and insulin.

Procedure and patient care

Before

- Explain the procedure to patient.
- Tell the patient that no special diet or fasting is required.

During

- Collect approximately 5 to 7 ml of venous blood in a red- or green-top tube.
- Avoid hemolysis.
- Indicate on the laboratory slip any drugs that may affect test results.

After

- Apply pressure to the venipuncture site.

M

Abnormal findings

▲ **Increased levels**

Renal insufficiency
Uncontrolled diabetes
Addison's disease
Hypothyroidism
Ingestion of magnesium-
  containing antacids or
  salts

▼ **Decreased levels**

Malnutrition
Malabsorption
Hypoparathyroidism
Alcoholism
Chronic renal disease
Diabetic acidosis

notes

magnetic resonance imaging (MRI, Nuclear magnetic resonance [NMRI])

Type of test Magnetic field study

Normal findings No evidence of pathology

Test explanation and related physiology

MRI is a noninvasive diagnostic scanning technique that provides valuable information about the body's biochemistry by placing the patient in a magnetic field. MRI is based on how hydrogen atoms behave when they are placed in a magnetic field and then disturbed by radiofrequency signals. The unique feature about MRI is that is does not require exposure to ionizing radiation. MRI has several advantages over computed tomography (CT) scanning, including the following:

1. MRI provides better contrast between normal tissue and pathologic tissue.
2. Obscuring bone artifacts that occur in CT scanning do not occur in MRI scanning.
3. Because rapidly flowing blood appears dark, which results from its quick motion, many blood vessels appear as dark lumens. This provides a natural contrast to the blood vessels when using MRI.
4. Because spatial information depends only on how the magnetic fields are varied in space, it is possible to image the transverse, sagittal, and coronal planes directly with MRI.

Although the full usefulness of MRI is yet to be determined, it shows promise in the evaluation of the following areas:

1. Head and surrounding structures
2. Spinal cord and surrounding structures
3. Face and surrounding structures
4. Neck
5. Mediastinum
6. Heart and great vessels
7. Liver
8. Kidney
9. Prostate
10. Bone and joints
11. Breast
12. Extremities and soft tissues

An important advantage of MRI imaging is that serial studies can be performed on the patient without any risk. This is useful in assessing the response of cancer to radiotherapy and chemotherapy. A major disadvantage of MRI is that patient eligibility is reduced as compared with CT scanning. For example, examination of patients requiring cardiac monitoring or having metal implants, metal joint replacements, pins for open reduction of fractures, pacemakers, or cerebral aneurysm clips will result in MRI image degradation and may endanger the patient.

Contraindications

- Patients who are extremely obese (over 300 pounds)
- Patients who are pregnant, because the long-term effects of MRI are not known at this time
- Patients who are confused or agitated
- Patients who are claustrophobic
- Patients who are unstable and require continuous life-support equipment, because monitoring equipment cannot be used inside the scanner room
- Patients with implantable metal objects such as pacemakers, infusion pumps, aneurysm clips, inner ear implants, and metal fragments in one or both eyes, because the magnet may move the object within the body and may injure the patient

Interfering factor

- Movement during the scan may cause artifacts on MRI.

Procedure and patient care

Before

- Explain the procedure to the patient.
- Inform the patient that there is no exposure to radiation.
- Obtain informed consent if required by the institution.
- Tell the patient that he or she can drive without assistance after the procedure.
- Tell patients that they may read or talk to a child in the scanning room during the procedure, because no risk of radiation from the procedure exists.
- Assess the patient for any contraindications for testing (e.g., aneurysm clips).
- If possible, show the patient a picture of the scanning machine and encourage verbalization of anxieties. Some patients may experience claustrophobia. Antianxiety medications may be helpful for those with mild claustrophobia.

M

- Instruct the patient to remove all metal objects (e.g., dental bridges, jewelry, hair clips, belts, credit cards), because they will create artifacts on the scan. The magnetic field can damage watches and credit cards. Also, movement of metal objects within the magnetic field can be detrimental to anyone within the field.
- Inform the patient that he or she will be required to remain motionless during this study. Any movement can cause artifacts on the scan.
- Tell the patient that, during the procedure he or she may hear a thumping sound. Earplugs are available if the patient wishes to use them.
- Inform the patient that no fluid or food restrictions are necessary before MRI.
- For comfort, instruct the patient to empty his or her bladder before the test.

During

- Note the following:
  1. The patient lies on a platform that slides into a tube containing the doughnut-shaped magnet.
  2. The patient is instructed to lie very still during the procedure.
  3. During the scan, the patient can talk to and hear the staff via microphone or earphones placed in the scanner.
  4. A contrast medium called gadolinium (Magnevist) has been approved by the U.S. Food and Drug Administration. This is a paramagnetic enhancement agent that crosses the blood-brain barrier. It is especially useful for distinguishing edema from tumors. If this is to be administered, approximately 10 to 15 ml is injected in the vein. Imaging can begin shortly after the injection. No dietary restrictions are necessary before using this agent.
- Note that this procedure is performed by a qualified radiologic technologist in approximately 30 to 90 minutes.
- Tell the patient that the only discomfort associated with this procedure may be lying still on a hard surface and a possible tingling sensation in teeth containing metal fillings. Also, an injection may be needed for administration of Magnevist.

After

- Inform the patient that no special postprocedural care is needed.

Abnormal findings

Brain

Cerebral tumor
Cerebral infarction
Aneurysm
Arteriovenous malformation
Hemorrhage
Subdural hematoma
Multiple sclerosis

Other

Tumor (primary or metastatic)
Myocardial infarction
Atherosclerotic plaques
Aortic dissection
Aortic occlusion and stenosis
Abscess
Edema
Congenital heart disease
Dementia
Bone destructive lesion
Joint disorder
Degenerative vertebral disks

M

notes

mammography (Mammogram)

Type of test X-ray

Normal findings
Class I: Negative
Class II: Benign
Class III: Benign—short-term follow-up suggested
Class IV: Suspicious—further evaluation suggested
Class V: Cancer highly suspected

Test explanation and related physiology

Mammography is an x-ray examination of the breast used to identify cancers. In many cases, these cancers can be detected before they become palpable lesions.

Although mammography is not a substitute for breast biopsy, it is reliable and accurate when interpreted by a skilled radiologist. The accuracy of detection of breast cancer with mammography has been approximately 85%. Usually cancers that are not detected by mammography are in areas of the breast not well imaged by x-ray machine (the high axillary tail of the breast). Almost 35% of breast cancers are not palpable and are detected only by mammography. The combination of mammography and close physical examination provides the best approach to detect breast cancer at its earliest stage.

The American Cancer Society suggests that every women over the age of 40 years should have a mammogram yearly. The National Cancer Institutes (NCI) suggest that women in their 40s should have mammography every other year and annually after 50. However, the NCI suggests that women who are at increased risk for breast cancer should have them annually after 40.

Mammography also can detect other diseases of the breast. These include acute suppurative mastitis, abscess, fibrocystic changes, gross cysts, benign tumors (e.g., fibroadenoma), and intraglandular lymph nodes.

A women receives minimal radiation exposure during this mammography (about 0.5 rads per view). Most mammograms include two views of each breast. Females under the age of 25 years are most susceptible to the neoplastic effects of ionizing radiation. Therefore mammography is rarely performed in these women.

Mammography can also be used to locate a non-palpable mammographically identifiable lesion for biopsy. The most common method is called *preoperative mammogram localization* of the mammogram abnormality followed by open biopsy. Before surgery a wire is placed to lead the surgeon to the abnormality. Nonoperative *stereotactic biopsy* with needle or *mammotomy* probes is the newest and least invasive manner of obtaining tissue from a nonpalpable mammographic abnormality. With the use of stereotaxis, a computer guides a core biopsy needle or mammotome probe into the abnormality. When fired, the biopsy equipment is in the center of the lesion, and specimens are obtained for biopsy. No surgery or sutures are required.

Contraindications

- Patients who are pregnant, because of the risk of fetal damage
- Women under the age of 25 years

Interfering factors

- Talc powder can give the impression of calcification within the breast.
- Jewelry worn around the neck can preclude total visualization of the breast.
- Breast augmentation implants prevent total visualization of the breast.
- Previous breast surgery can alter or distort the mammogram findings.

Procedure and patient care

Before

- Explain the procedure to the patient.
- Inform the patient that some discomfort may be experienced during breast compression. This compression allows better visualization of the breast tissue. Assure the patient that the breast will not be harmed by the compression.
- Tell the patient that no fasting is required.
- Explain to the patient that a minimal radiation dose will be used during the test.
- Instruct the patient to disrobe above the waist and put on an x-ray gown.

During

- Note the following procedural steps:
  1. The patient is taken to the radiology department and seated in front of a mammogram machine.

M

2. One breast is placed on the x-ray plate.
3. The x-ray cone is brought down on the top of the breast to compress it gently between the broadened cone and the x-ray plate.
4. The x-ray film is exposed. This is the craniocaudal view.
5. The x-ray plate is turned about 45 degrees medially and placed on the inner aspect of the breast.
6. The broadened cone is brought in medially and again gently compresses the breast. This creates the medio-lateral view.
7. Occasionally other views such as *direct lateral* (90-degree) or *magnified spot views* are obtained to more clearly visualize an area of suspicion.

- Note that mammography is performed by a radiologic technologist in approximately 10 minutes. The x-ray films are interpreted by a radiologist. Tell the patient that very little discomfort is associated with mammography. Remind the patient that some pain may be caused by the pressure required to compress the breast tissue while the x-ray films are being taken. If the patient has very tender breasts, this may be painful.

After

- Take this opportunity to instruct the patient in breast self-examination.

Abnormal findings

Breast cancer
Benign tumor (e.g., fibroadenoma)
Breast cyst
Fibrocystic changes
Breast abscess
Suppurative mastitis

notes

Meckel's diverticulum nuclear scan

Type of test   Nuclear medicine

Normal findings   No increased uptake of radionuclide in the right lower quadrant of the abdomen

Test explanation and related physiology

Meckel's diverticulum is the most common congenital abnormality of the intestinal tract. It is a persistent remnant of the omphalomesenteric tract. The diverticulum usually occurs in the ileum, approximately 2 feet proximal to the ileocecal valve. Approximately 20% to 25% of Meckel's diverticulum is lined internally by ectopic gastric mucosa. This gastric mucosa can secrete acid and cause ulceration of the intestinal mucosa nearby. Bleeding, inflammation, and intussusception are other potential complications of this congenital abnormality. The majority of these complications occur by 2 years of age.

Both normal gastric mucosa within the stomach and ectopic gastric mucosa in Meckel's diverticulum concentrate ^{99m}Tc pertechnetate. When this radionuclide is injected intravenously, it is concentrated in the ectopic gastric mucosa of Meckel's diverticulum. One can then expect to see a hot spot in the right lower quadrant of the abdomen at about the same time as the normal stomach mucosa is visualized. This is a very sensitive and specific test for this congenital abnormality.

It is possible that Meckel's diverticulum is present but contains no ectopic gastric mucosa within. Usually these are not symptomatic. No concentration of radionuclide will occur within the diverticulum. This test is not helpful in these cases.

Other conditions can simulate a hot spot compatible with Merkel's diverticulum containing ectopic gastric mucosa. Usually these are associated with inflammatory processes within the abdomen (e.g., appendicitis or ectopic pregnancy).

Procedure and patient care

Before

- Explain the procedure to the patient.
- Advise the patient to refrain from eating or drinking anything for 6 to 12 hours before the examination.
- A histamine H2-receptor antagonist is usually given for 1 to 2 days before the scan. This blocks secretion of the radionu-

M

clide from the ectopic gastric mucosa and improves visualization of Meckel's diverticulum.

During

- The patient lies in a supine position, and a large-view nuclear detector camera is placed over the patient's abdomen to identify concentration of nuclear material after intravenous injection.
- Images are taken at 5-minute intervals for 1 hour.
- Patients may be asked to lie on their left side to minimize the excretion of the radionuclide from the normal stomach, flooding the intestine with radionuclide and precluding visualization of Meckel's diverticulum.
- Occasionally glucagon is provided to prolong intestinal transit time and avoid downstream contamination with the radionuclide.
- Occasionally gastrin is given to increase the uptake of the radionuclide by the ectopic gastric mucosa.
- There is no pain associated with this test.

After

- The patient is asked to void, and a repeat image is obtained. This is to ensure that Meckel's diverticulum has not been hidden by a distended bladder.
- Because only tracer doses of radioisotopes are used, inform the patient that no precautions need to be taken by others against radiation.

Abnormal findings

Meckel's diverticula

notes

mediastinoscopy

Type of test Endoscopy

Normal findings No abnormal mediastinal lymph node tissue

Test explanation and related physiology

Mediastinoscopy is a surgical procedure in which a mediastinoscope (a lighted instrument scope) is inserted through a small incision made at the suprasternal notch. The scope is passed into the superior mediastinum to inspect the mediastinal lymph nodes and to remove biopsy specimens. Because these lymph nodes receive lymphatic drainage from the lungs, their assessment can provide information on intrathoracic diseases such as carcinoma, granulomatous infections, and sarcoidosis. Therefore mediastinoscopy is used in establishing the diagnosis of various intrathoracic diseases.

This procedure is also used to "stage" patients with lung cancer and to assess whether they are surgical candidates. Evidence of metastasis is usually a contraindication to thoracotomy because the tumor is considered inoperable. Tumors occurring in the mediastinum (e.g., thymoma or lymphoma) can also be biopsied through the mediastinoscope.

Potential complication

- Puncture of the esophagus, trachea, or blood vessels

Procedure and patient care

Before

- Explain the procedure to the patient.
- Ensure that the physician has obtained the informed consent for this procedure.
- Check whether the patient's blood needs to be typed and crossmatched.
- Provide preoperative care as with any other surgical procedure.
- Keep the patient NPO after midnight on the day of the test.
- Administer preprocedural medication approximately 1 hour before the test as ordered.

During

- Note the following procedural steps:
  1. The patient is taken to the operating room for this surgical procedure.
  2. The patient is placed under general anesthesia.
  3. An incision is made in the suprasternal notch.
  4. The mediastinoscope is passed through this neck incision and into the superior mediastinum.
  5. The lymph nodes are biopsied.
  6. The scope is withdrawn, and the incision is sutured closed.
- Note that this procedure is performed by a surgeon in approximately 1 hour.
- Inform the patient that he or she is asleep during the procedure.

After

- Provide postoperative care as with any other surgical procedure.
- Assess for mediastinal crepitus on auscultation, which may indicate mediastinal air from pneumothorax or the bronchus or esophagus.
- Note that distended neck veins and pulsus paradoxus may indicate lack of cardiac filling due to a large mediastinal hematoma.

🏠 Home care responsibilities

- Assess for cough or shortness of breath, which may indicate a pneumothorax.
- Note that subcutaneous emphysema may indicate a pneumothorax.
- Observe for hypotension and tachycardia, which may indicate bleeding from the biopsy site or the great vessels.
- Evaluate for hoarseness, which may indicate injury to the recurrent laryngeal nerve.
- Assess for fever, chills, and sepsis, which may indicate mediastinitis from infection.

Abnormal findings

Lung cancer
Metastasis
Sarcoidosis
Thymoma
Tuberculosis
Hodgkin's disease
Lymphoma
Infection

notes

mononucleosis spot test (Mononuclear heterophil test, Heterophil antibody test, Monospot test)

Type of test Blood

Normal findings Negative (<1:28 titer)

Test explanation and related physiology

The mononucleosis test is performed to aid in the diagnosis of infectious mononucleosis (IM), a disease caused by the Epstein-Barr virus (EBV). Usually young adults are affected by mononucleosis. The clinical presentation is fever, pharyngitis, lymphadenopathy, and splenomegaly. Approximately 2 weeks after the onset of the disease, many patients are found to have immunoglobulin M (IgM) heterophil antibodies in their serum that react against warm red blood cells (RBCs). When these antibodies are present in serial dilutions of greater than 1:56, infectious mononucleosis can be strongly considered. However, false-positive results can occur in patients who have other diseases that cause elevation of heterophil antibodies. Examples include patients with lymphoma, systemic lupus erythematosus, Burkitt's lymphoma, leukemia, and some gastrointestinal cancers. Burkitt's lymphoma is strongly associated with EBV.

Several heterophil agglutination tests are available, but the most frequently performed is the rapid slide spot test for infectious mononucleosis (monospot test). Heterophil antibodies normally present in most individuals are produced in increased quantities in patients with IM. These antibodies strongly and readily agglutinate horse RBCs. The spot slide test is performed by adding the patient's serum to horse RBCs on a slide. If agglutination occurs, heterophil antibodies are present in the patient's serum, indicating an EBV virus infection. About 30% of the cases of IM are "heterophil antibody negative". When the diagnosis of IM is still suspected, a repeat monospot test or EBV serology is done (see p. 366).

Procedure and patient care

Before

- Explain the procedure to the patient.
- Tell the patient that no fasting or special preparation is required.

During

- Collect approximately 7 to 10 ml of venous blood in a red-top tube.

After

- Apply pressure to the venipuncture site.

Abnormal findings

Infectious mononucleosis
Chronic EBV infection
Chronic fatigue syndrome
Burkitt's lymphoma
Some forms of chronic hepatitis

notes

M

myelography (Myelogram)

Type of test X-ray with contrast dye

Normal findings Normal spinal canal

Test explanation and related physiology

By placing radiopaque dye (or air) into the subarachnoid space of the spinal canal, the contents of the canal can be radiographically outlined. Cord tumors, meningeal tumors, metastatic spinal tumors, herniated intravertebral disks, and arthritic bone spurs can be readily detected by this study. These lesions appear as canal narrowing or as varying degrees of obstruction to the flow of the dye column within the canal. The entire canal (from lumbar to cervical areas) can be examined. This test is indicated in patients with severe back pain or localized neurologic signs that suggest the canal as the location of these injuries. Because this test is usually performed by lumbar puncture (LP, see p. 539), all the potential complications of that procedure exist.

Different types of contrast material can be used for myelography. Pantopaque is most often used as the *oil-based medium*. An oil-based dye can cause meningeal irritation.

A *water-soluble* contrast material, metrizamide (Amipaque), is now frequently used for myelography. Metrizamide has two advantages over the oil-based medium. First, metrizamide does not need to be removed at the end of the procedure, because it is water soluble and will be completely resorbed. Second, metrizamide is less viscous than the iodine, oil-based dye and therefore permits better visualization of small areas (e.g., nerves, nerve roots, nerve sheaths). Metrizamide may precipitate seizure activity after the procedure. To prevent this, the patient should be well hydrated and should avoid medications that could decrease the seizure threshold. A water-soluble contrast agent, Omnipaque, has a significantly lower risk of central nervous system (CNS) toxicity than does metrizamide and is now more routinely used.

To avoid the side effects associated with radiopaque dyes, some neurosurgeons prefer to use *air-contrast* myelography. After air myelography, the patient is positioned with the head lower than the trunk to prevent air from gravitating to the cerebral space and causing headaches.

Contraindications

- Patients with multiple sclerosis, because exacerbation may be precipitated by myelography
- Patients with increased intracranial pressure, because LP may cause herniation of the brain
- Patients with infection near the LP site, because this may precipitate a bacterial meningitis
- Patients who are allergic to shellfish or iodinated dye

Potential complications

- Headache
- Meningitis
- Herniation of the brain
- Seizures
- Allergic reaction to iodinated dye.

Procedure and patient care

Before

- Explain the procedure to the patient.
- Ensure that the physician has obtained written and informed consent for this procedure.
- Assess the patient for allergies to iodinated contrast dye or shellfish.
- Ascertain whether the patient has recently taken phenothiazines, tricyclic antidepressants, CNS stimulants, or amphetamines if a water-soluble contrast (metrizamide) will be used. These medications should be avoided, because they could decrease the seizure threshold.
- Have the patient empty the bladder and bowel before myelography if possible.
- Explain to the patient that he or she must lie very still during the procedure.
- Note that food and fluid restrictions vary according to the type of dye used. Check with the radiology department for specific restrictions.
- Inform the patient that he or she will be tilted into an up-and-down position on the table so that the dye can properly fill the spinal canal and provide adequate visualization in the desired area.

During

- Note the following procedural steps:
  1. A lumbar puncture (see p. 544) is performed.

M

2. Fifteen ml of cerebrospinal fluid (CSF) is withdrawn, and 15 ml or more of radiopaque dye or air is injected into the spinal canal. Because the specific gravity of the dye is greater than that of the CSF, the direction of dye flow will depend on the tilt of the table and the patient's position.

3. With the needle in place, the patient is placed in the prone position on the tilt table with the head tilted down. A foot support and shoulder brace or harness will keep the patient from sliding.

4. The lights are turned off, and the column of dye is followed in a cephalad direction with fluoroscopy.

5. Representative x-ray films are taken.

6. Obstructions to the flow of the dye are evident, and the level of the lesion is easily detected.

7. After myelography is performed, the needle is removed, and a dressing is applied.

8. The patient is returned to the unit on a stretcher and is kept on bed rest.

- Note that this procedure is done by a radiologist in approximately 45 minutes.
- Keep in mind that patient response varies from mild discomfort to severe pain.

After

- Note that nursing interventions after the procedure depend on the type of contrast used.
- Usually place the patient on bed rest for several hours afterward as indicated. Position the patient as specifically ordered by the physician in consultation with the radiologist. The head position varies with the dye used. For example, the head is usually elevated after using oil-based and water-soluble contrast agents. After an air-contrast study, the head is positioned lower than the trunk.
- Observe the patient for signs and symptoms of meningeal irritation (e.g., fever, stiff neck, occipital headache, photophobia).
- Observe the patient for seizure activity if metrizamide dye was used.
- If metrizamide was used, do *not* administer medications (e.g., phenothiazines) that may precipitate seizure activity.
- Monitor the patient's vital signs and ability to void.

- Encourage the patient to drink fluids to enhance excretion of the dye and to hasten replacement of CSF.
- See p. xviii for appropriate interventions concerning the care for patients with iodine allergy.

🏠 **Home care responsibilities**

- After this test, safe positioning of the patient's head will be determined by the type of dye used in the procedure.
- Encourage the patient to drink fluids to enhance excretion of the dye and to replace CSF.
- Tell the patient to report any signs of meningeal irritation such as fever, stiff neck, occipital headache, photophobia.

Abnormal findings

Cord tumor
Meningeal tumor
Metastatic spinal tumor
Meningioma
Cervical ankylosing spondylosis
Arthritic lumbar stenosis
Herniated intravertebral disks
Arthritic bone spurs
Neurofibroma
Avulsion of nerve roots
Cysts
Astrocytoma

M

notes

myoglobin

Type of test Blood

Normal findings 0-85 ng/ml or 0-85 nmol/L (SI units)

Test explanation and related physiology

Myoglobin is an oxygen-binding protein found in cardiac and skeletal muscle. Measurement of myoglobin is an index of damage to the myocardium in myocardial infarction (MI) or reinfarction. Increased levels, which indicate cardiac muscle injury or death, occur in about 3 hours. Although this test is more sensitive than creatine phosphokinase isoenzymes (see p. 290), it is not as specific. Trauma, inflammation, or ischemic changes to the noncardiac skeletal muscles also can cause elevated levels of myoglobin. The benefit of myoglobin over CPK-MB (see p. 290) is that it may become elevated earlier in some patients. This may prove beneficial, since thrombolytic therapy is to be started within the first 6 hours after an MI.

As already indicated, disease or trauma of the skeletal muscle also causes elevations in myoglobin. With sudden and severe muscle injury, myoglobin levels can get very high. Myoglobin can also be measured in the urine. Because myoglobin is excreted in the urine and is nephrotoxic, urine levels must be monitored in these patients. The routine urine dipstick for hemoglobin will also react to screen for myoglobin.

Interfering factors

- Recent administration of radioactive substances may affect test results.
- Increased myoglobin levels can occur after IM injections.

Procedure and patient care

Before

- Explain the procedure to the patient.
- Tell the patient that no fasting is required.

During

- Collect approximately 5 ml of venous blood in a red-top tube.

After
- Apply pressure to the venipuncture site.

Abnormal findings

▲ **Increased levels**
   Myocardial infarction
   Skeletal muscle inflammation (myositis)
   Malignant hyperthermia
   Muscular dystrophy
   Skeletal muscle ischemia
   Skeletal muscle trauma
   Rhabdomyolysis

notes

M

5′-nucleotidase

Type of test Blood

Normal findings 0.0-1.6 U or 27-233 nmol/sec/L (SI units)

Test explanation and related physiology

5′-Nucleotidase is an enzyme specific to the liver. The 5′-nucleotidase level is elevated in patients with liver diseases, especially those associated with cholestasis. It provides information similar to alkaline phosphatase (ALP). However, ALP is not specific to the liver. Diseases of the bone, sepsis, pregnancy, and other diseases can cause ALP to be elevated. When doubt as to the cause of an elevated ALP exists, 5′-nucleotidase is recommended. If that enzyme is elevated along with the ALP, the source of the pathology is certainly in the liver. If the 5′-nucleotidase is normal in the face of an elevated ALP, the source of pathology is outside the liver (bone, kidney or spleen). Gamma-glutamyl transpeptidase (GGTP) (p. 442) is used similarly since it is also specific to the liver.

Interfering factors

✴ Drugs that may cause *increased* 5′-nucleotidase levels include hepatotoxic agents.

Procedure and patient care

Before
- Explain the procedure to the patient.
- Tell the patient that no fasting is required.

During
- Collect approximately 7 to 10 ml of venous blood in a red-top tube.
- Indicate on the laboratory slip any medication the patient may be taking to aid in the interpretation of test results.

After
- Apply pressure to the venipuncture site. Patients with liver dysfunction often have prolonged clotting times.

Abnormal findings

▲ **Increased levels**
  Bile duct obstruction
  Cholestasis
  Hepatitis
  Cirrhosis
  Hepatic necrosis
  Hepatic ischemia
  Hepatic tumor
  Hepatotoxic drugs

notes

N

obstruction series

Type of test X-ray

Normal findings
No evidence of bowel obstruction
No abnormal calcifications
No free air

Test explanation and related physiology

The obstruction series is a group of x-ray films performed on the abdomen of patients with suspected bowel obstruction, paralytic ileus, perforated viscus, abdominal abscess, kidney stones, appendicitis, or foreign body ingestion. This series of films usually consists of at least two x-ray studies. The first is an *erect abdominal* film that should include visualization of both diaphragms. The film is examined for evidence of free air under either diaphragm, which is pathognomonic for a perforated viscus. This view is also used to detect air-fluid levels within the intestine; the presence of an air-fluid level is compatible with bowel obstruction or paralytic ileus. Occasionally patients are too ill to stand erect. In this case, an x-ray film can be taken with the patient in the left lateral decubitus position. If free air is present, it will be seen between the liver and the right side of the abdominal wall. As with the erect-position film, air-fluid levels also can be detected.

The second view in the obstruction series is usually a *supine abdominal* x-ray study. This is very similar to the kidney, ureter, and bladder x-ray study (see p. 509). An abdominal abscess may be seen as a cluster of tiny bubbles within one localized area. A calcification within the course of the ureter could indicate a kidney ureteral stone. A small calcification in the right lower quadrant on the film of a patient complaining of pain in this quadrant may be an appendicolith. A gas-filled, distended bowel is compatible with bowel obstruction or paralytic ileus. The obstruction series can also be used to monitor the clinical course of patients with gastrointestinal (GI) disease. For example, repeated obstruction series on patients who have a partial small bowel obstruction or paralytic ileus can indicate worsening or improvement of the clinical situation.

Frequently a *cross-table lateral* view of the abdomen is included in an obstruction series to detect abdominal aorta calcification, which often occurs in older patients. The calcification represents the anterior wall of the aorta. If an aortic aneurysm exists, this calcification will be seen to protrude from the spine.

Finally, the *supine abdominal* x-ray study can be used as a "scout film" before performing GI or abdominal x-ray studies that use contrast, such as a barium enema (see p. 133) or intravenous pyelogram (see p. 497).

Contraindications

- Patients who are pregnant

Interfering factor

- Previous GI barium contrast study
  Although at times barium within the GI tract can preclude the identification of other important calcifications (e.g., kidney stones), barium can be helpful in outlining the GI anatomy.

Procedure and patient care

Before

- Explain the procedure to the patient.
- Ensure that all radiopaque clothing has been removed.
- Remind the patient that no GI contrast will be used.

During

- Although the procedure varies from facility to facility, note that usually a supine abdominal x-ray film, erect abdominal film, and perhaps a lower erect chest film are taken. Often a cross-table lateral x-ray film is also included.
- Note that the obstruction series is performed in minutes in the radiology department by a radiologic technologist; however, it can be performed at the bedside with a portable x-ray machine. A radiologist interprets the films.
- Tell the patient that no discomfort is associated with this study.

After

- Note that no special aftercare is needed.

Abnormal findings

Kidney stone
Bowel obstruction
Organomegaly
Presence of a foreign body
Bladder distention
Abdominal abscess
Perforated viscus
Abdominal aortic calcification
Appendicolithiasis
Paralytic ileus
Abdominal aortic aneurysm
Peritoneal effusion/ascites
Abnormal position of the kidneys
Soft tissue masses

notes

octreotide scan (Carcinoid nuclear scan, neuroendocrine nuclear scan)

Normal findings No evidence of increased uptake throughout the body

Test explanation and related physiology

Octreotide scans are used to identify and localize neuroendocrine primary and metastatic tumors. These scan are indicated on patients with known neuroendocrine tumors.

Most neuroendocrine tumors have a somatostatin receptor on the cellular membrane. Octreotide is an analog of somatostatin. When combined with a radiopharmaceutical (such as I^{123} or Indium-111 DTPA), the radiolabeled octreotide will attach to the somatostatin receptors of the neuroendocrine tumor cells. With the use of a scintillator camera, the uptake can be identified. This test is used to identify primary and metastatic neuroendocrine tumors. It is also used to monitor the course of the disease.

The use of **S**ingle **P**hoton **E**mission **C**omputed **T**omography (SPECT) imaging improves the sensitivity of this test. Many different types of hormone-producing tumors can be detected by this scan. Most notable include carcinoid, gastrinoma, insulinoma, glucagonoma, pheochromocytoma, and small-cell lung cancer. Other abnormalities can pick up octreotide. They would include granulomatous infections such as sarcoidosis or tuberculosis, rheumatoid arthritis, and nonhormonal cancers (breast, lymphoma, and non-small cell lung cancers).

Contraindication

- Patients who are pregnant or lactating, because of risk of damage to the fetus or infant.

Interfering factor

- Barium in the GI tract overlying the liver or spleen will produce defects on the scan that may be mistaken for masses.

Procedure and patient care

Before

- Explain the procedure to the patient.
- Tell the patient that no fasting or premedication is required.
- Assure the patient that he or she will not be exposed to

O

large amounts of radiation, because only tracer doses of isotopes are used.

- If an iodinated radionuclide is to be performed, ensure that
the patient does not have an allergy to iodine.
- If an iodinated dye is to be performed, administer 5 drops of
Lugol's solution (iodine) daily for 3 days. This will avoid
uptake of the radionuclide by the thyroid gland.
- If the patient has been receiving octreotide as a form of antineoplastic treatment, this must be discontinued for 2 weeks
before scanning.

During

- Note the following procedural steps:
  1. The patient is taken to the nuclear medicine department,
     where the radionuclide is administered intravenously.
  2. One hour after injection, a gamma ray detector/camera is
     successively placed over the entire body.
  3. The patient is placed in supine, lateral, and prone posi-
     tions so that all surfaces can be visualized.
  4. The radionuclide image is recorded on film. SPECT
     images may also be performed.
  5. Usually the patient is given a fatty meal 2 hours after oct-
     reotide injection to clear the radiopharmaceutical from
     the gallbladder.
  6. After 4 hours the patient is given a strong laxative to clear
     the octreotide from the bowel.
  7. Repeat scanning is again performed at 2, 4, 24, and 48
     hours after administration of the octreotide.
- Note that the imaging procedure is performed by a trained
technologist in approximately ½ hour. A physician trained
in nuclear medicine interprets the results.
- Inform the patient that the only discomfort associated with
this procedure is the IV injection of the radionuclide.

After

- Because only tracer doses of radioisotopes are used, inform
the patient that no precautions need to be taken by others
against radiation exposure.

Abnormal findings

Carcinoid tumors
Neuroendocrine tumors
Granulomatous infections such as sarcoidosis and tuberculosis

oculoplethysmography (OPG)

Type of test Manometric

Normal findings Normal and equal blood flow in both carotid arteries

Test explanation and related physiology

OPG is a noninvasive study used to indirectly measure blood flow in the ophthalmic artery. Because the ophthalmic artery is the first major branch of the internal carotid artery, its blood flow reflects the carotid blood flow and the alternative blood flow to the brain.

For this study, eye pressures are measured through suction cups placed on the eyes for the recording. OPG is indicated in patients who have symptoms of carotid occlusive disease (e.g., transient ischemic attacks, carotid bruits, neurologic symptoms [e.g., dizziness, fainting]). If indicated, this procedure may be followed by cerebral angiography. This test is often performed as a follow-up after carotid endarterectomy to prove patency of the carotid artery. Carotid Doppler flow studies (see p. 221) are more easily performed and therefore are now being used more frequently.

Contraindications

- Patients who have had eye surgery within the last 2 to 6 months
- Patients who have a lens implant
- Patients who have had retinal detachment
- Patients with cataracts
- Patients who are allergic to local anesthetics

Potential complications

- Conjunctival hemorrhage
- Corneal abrasions
  If corneal abrasions occur, the patient's eye is patched, and a lubricant (e.g., Dacriose solution) is applied
- Transient photophobia

Procedure and patient care

Before

- Explain the procedure to the patient.
- Instruct the patient to remove contact lenses if applicable.

- Inform patients with glaucoma to take their usual medications and eye drops.
- Tell the patient that no fasting or sedation is necessary.

During

- Note the following procedural steps:
  1. The patient is asked to lie on his or her back on a table or bed.
  2. Blood pressure in both arms is taken before the test.
  3. Electrocardiographic (ECG) electrodes are applied to the patient's extremities to detect abnormal cardiac rhythms.
  4. Anesthetic eye drops are instilled in both eyes to minimize discomfort.
  5. Small detectors are attached to the earlobes to detect blood flow to the ear through the external carotid artery.
  6. Tracings for both ears are taken and compared.
  7. Suction cups resembling contact lenses are applied directly to the eyeball.
  8. Tracings of the pulsations within each eye are recorded.
  9. A vacuum source is applied to the suction cup. This increased pressure causes the pulse in both eyes to disappear temporarily, because all blood flow to the eye is stopped.
  10. When the suction source is stopped, the blood flow returns to the eyes. Both pulses should return simultaneously.
  11. The time difference in the pulse rate from one eye to the other, one ear to the other, and one ear to the eye on the other side is measured in milliseconds. If internal carotid stenosis is present, blood flow to the eye will be delayed.
- Note that a trained technologist performs this test in approximately 20 to 30 minutes.
- Tell the patient that eyes usually burn slightly when the ophthalmic drops are applied.
- Inform the patient that, when suction is applied, he or she may feel a pulling sensation and vision may temporarily be lost.

After

- Inform the patient that the eye anesthesia usually wears off in approximately 30 minutes.
- Instruct the patient not to rub his or her eyes for at least 2 hours. If tears appear, the eye should be blotted dry.

- Inform the patient that contact lenses should not be inserted for at least 2 hours after OPG.
- Tell the patient that the eyes may appear bloodshot for several hours after the test. Artificial tears may be instilled to soothe any irritation in the eyes.
- Inform the patient to wear sunglasses if photophobia is present.

Abnormal finding

Carotid atherosclerotic stenosis

notes

O

oncoscint scan (Immunoscintigraphy)

Type of test Nuclear medicine

Normal findings No increased uptake of radionuclide in the body

Test explanation and related physiology

Immunoscintigraphy is a new procedure. At present, it is used to detect recurrent metastatic colorectal or ovarian cancer. The radionuclide indium chloride-111 is attached to a monoclonal antibody that is commonly on the cell surface of colorectal and ovarian cancer cells. When injected, this radionuclide-antibody conjugate attaches to the cancer cells. With the use of a gamma camera, whole-body images are obtained. Areas of increased uptake may represent tumor.

This scan is not 100% accurate and can be incorrectly negative up to 30% of the time. When positive, however, its accuracy meets or exceeds the accuracy of a computed tomography (CT) scan. It is very helpful in determining the source of a rising tumor marker (see CEA, p. 201, or CA-125, p. 186) in patients with an otherwise normal diagnostic evaluation. Also, it is very helpful in differentiating CT-recognized changes as being postsurgical or postradiation anatomic changes from recurrent cancer. The first two do not take up tracer; recurrent cancer does. One must be aware that uptake of the radionuclide normally occurs in the liver, spleen, and bowel.

Contraindications

- Nursing mothers

Procedure and patient care

Before

- Explain the procedure to the patient.
- Explain that no fasting is required before the test.
- Because the radionuclide can be concentrated in areas of degenerated joint disease, abdominal aortic aneurysms, abdominal inflammatory processes, or inflammatory bowel disease, a careful history should be obtained before scanning.

During

- The patient is injected with the radiolabeled monoclonal antibody.

- Initial images are obtained 48 to 72 hours after IV infusion.
- The patient is asked to lie on a padded table.
- A nuclear counter camera is placed over the anterior or posterior surface of the chest, abdomen, and pelvis. Approximately 10 minutes is required for each view.
- The patient may be asked to return the following day or the day after that for repeated images.
- Little or no discomfort is associated with this procedure.
- The procedure takes approximately 1 hour each day for at least 1 to 4 days.
- This procedure is performed in the nuclear medicine department.

After

- Because only tracer doses of radioisotopes are used, inform the patient that no precautions need to be taken by others against radiation exposure.

Abnormal findings

▲ **Increased uptake**
  Colorectal cancer
  Ovarian cancer

notes

O

osmolality, blood (Serum osmolality)

Type of test Blood

Normal findings
Adult/elderly: 285-295 mOsm/kg H_2O
Child: 275-290 mOsm/kg H_2O

Possible critical values
<265 mOsm/kg H_2O
>320 mOsm/kg H_2O

Test explanation and related physiology

Osmolality measures the concentration of dissolved particles in blood. As the amount of free water in the blood increases or the amount of particles decreases, osmolality decreases. As the amount of water in the blood decreases or the amount of particles increases, osmolality increases. Osmolality increases with dehydration and decreases with overhydration.

The serum osmolality test is useful in evaluating fluid and electrolyte imbalance. The test is very helpful in the evaluation of seizures, ascites, hydration status, acid-base balance, and suspected ADH abnormalities. Osmolality is also helpful in identifying the presence of organic acids, sugars, or ethanol. In these cases there is an "osmolal gap." This gap represents the difference between what the osmolality should be (based on calculations of serum sodium, glucose and BUN—the three most important solutes in the blood) and the osmolality as truly measured. If the "gap" is large, the presence of solutes such as organic acids (ketones), unusually high levels of glucose, or ethanol by-products is suspected.

Finally, osmolality also has an important role in evaluation of coma patients. Values of 385 mOsm/kg of water are associated with stupor in patients with hyperglycemia. When values of 400 to 420 are detected, grand mal seizures can occur. Values greater than 420 can be lethal. The simultaneous use of urine osmolality (p. 602) helps in the interpretation and evaluation of problems with osmolality.

Interfering factors

- Diseases such as cerebrovascular accident (stroke) or brain tumors may interfere with test results through inappropriate secretion of ADH.

Procedure and patient care

Before
- Explain the procedure to the patient.
- Tell the patient that no fasting is required.

During
- Collect approximately 5 to 10 ml of venous blood in a red-top tube.
- For pediatric patients, draw blood from a heel stick.

After
- Apply pressure to the venipuncture site.

Abnormal findings

▲ **Increased levels**
Hypernatremia
Dehydration
Hyperglycemia
Mannitol therapy
Azotemia
Uremia
Ingestion of ethanol, methanol, or ethylene glycol
Hyperosmolar nonketotic hyperglycemia
Diabetes insipidus
Hypercalcemia
Renal tubular necrosis
Severe pyelonephritis
Ketosis
Shock

▼ **Decreased levels**
Hyponatremia
Overhydration
Syndrome of inappropriate antidiuretic hormone secretion (SIADH)
Paraneoplastic syndromes associated with lung carcinoma

O

notes

osmolality, urine (Urine osmolality)

Type of test   Urine

Normal findings

12- to 14-hour fluid restriction: >850 mOsm/kg H_2O
   (SI units)
Random specimen: 50-1400 mOsm/kg H_2O, depending on
   fluid intake (SI units)

Possible critical values

<100 mOsm/kg H_2O in overhydration
>800 mOsm/kg H_2O in dehydration

Test explanation and related physiology

Osmolality is the measurement of the number of dissolved particles in a solution. It is a more exact measurement of urine concentration than specific gravity, because specific gravity depends on the number and precise nature of the particles in the urine. Specific gravity also requires correction for the presence of glucose or protein, as well as for temperature; in contrast, osmolality depends only on the number of particles of solute in a unit of solution. Osmolality also can be measured over a wider range than specific gravity and with greater accuracy.

Osmolality is used in the precise evaluation of the concentrating ability of the kidney. This test is also used to monitor fluid and electrolyte balance. Osmolality is valuable in the workup of patients with renal disease, the syndrome of inappropriate antidiuretic hormone (SIADH) secretion, and diabetes insipidus. Osmolality may be used as part of the urinalysis when the patient has glycosuria or proteinuria or has had tests that use radiopaque substances. In these situations, the urine "osmolar gap" is increased because of other organic osmolal particles. The "osmolar gap" is the sum of all the particles expected to be in the urine (electrolytes, urea, and glucose) compared to the actual measurement of the osmolality. Normally, the osmolar gap is 80 to 100 mOsm/kg/H_2O. The urine osmolality is more easily interpreted when the serum osmolality (p. 600) is simultaneously performed.

Procedure and patient care

Before

- Explain the procedure to the patient.
- Tell the patient that no special preparation is necessary for a random urine specimen.
- Inform the patient that preparation for a fasting urine specimen may require a high-protein diet for 3 days before the test. Instruct the patient to eat a dry supper the evening before the test and to drink no fluids until the test is completed the next morning.

During

- Collect a first-voided urine specimen for a random sample.
- For a fasting specimen, instruct the patient to empty the bladder at approximately 6 AM and to discard the urine. Collect the test urine at 8 AM.
- Indicate on the laboratory slip the patient's fasting status.

After

- Send the specimen to the laboratory.
- Provide food and fluids for the patient.

Abnormal findings

▲ Increased levels
Syndrome of inappropriate ADH secretion (SIADH)
Acidosis
Shock
Hypernatremia
Hepatic cirrhosis
Congestive heart failure
Addison's disease

▼ Decreased levels
Diabetes insipidus
Hypercalcemia
Excess fluid intake
Renal tubular necrosis
Aldosteronism
Hypokalemia
Severe pyelonephritis

notes

oximetry (Pulse oximetry, Ear oximetry, Oxygen saturation)

Type of test Photodiagnostic

Normal findings ≥95%

Possible critical values ≤75%

Test explanation and related physiology

Oximetry is a noninvasive method of monitoring arterial blood oxygen saturation (SaO_2). The SaO_2 is the ratio of oxygenated hemoglobin to the total amount of hemoglobin. The SaO_2 is expressed as a percentage; for example, a saturation of 95% indicates that 95% of the total hemoglobin attachments for oxygen have oxygen attached to them. The SaO_2 is an accurate approximation of oxygen saturation obtained from arterial blood gas study (see p. 104). By correlating the SaO_2 and the patient's physiologic status, a close estimate of the partial oxygen pressure (PO_2) can be obtained.

Oximetry is typically used for monitoring the patient's oxygenation status during the perioperative period (or any time of heavy sedation) and for patients receiving mechanical ventilation. This test is also frequently used in many clinical situations, such as pulmonary rehabilitation programs, stress testing, and sleep laboratories. Oximetry can be used to assess the body's response to various drugs such as theophylline, which causes bronchodilation, and methacholine, which evokes bronchospasm in people with asthma. This test is commonly used to titrate levels of oxygen on hospitalized patients.

Procedure and patient care

Before

- Explain the procedure to the patient.
- Tell the patient that no fasting is required.

During

- Rub the patient's earlobe, pinna (upper part of the ear), or fingertip to increase blood flow.
- Clip the monitoring probe or sensor to the ear or finger. The sensor warms and increases blood flow to the tissue. A beam of light passes through the tissue, and the sensor measures the amount of light the tissue absorbs (Figure 23).

Figure 23 Oximetry. The pulse oximeter passes a beam of light through the tissue. The amount of light absorbed by the oxygen-saturated hemoglobin is measured by the sensor.

- Note that this study is usually performed by a respiratory therapist or nurse at the patient's bedside in a few minutes.
- Tell the patient that no discomfort is associated with this study.

After

- Note that no special aftercare is needed.

Abnormal findings

▲ **Increased levels**
Increased inspired O_2
Hyperventilation

▼ **Decreased levels**
Inadequate O_2 in inspired air
Hypoxic lung diseases
Hypoxic cardiac diseases
Severe hypoventilation states

notes

Papanicolaou smear (Pap smear, Pap test, Cytologic test for cancer)

Type of test   Microscopic examination

Normal findings   No abnormal or atypical cells

Test explanation and related physiology

A Pap smear is taken to detect neoplastic cells in cervical and vaginal secretions. This test is based on the fact that normal cells and abnormal cervical and endometrial neoplastic cells are shed into the cervical and vaginal secretions. By examining these secretions microscopically, one can detect early cellular changes compatible with premalignant conditions or an existing malignant condition. The Pap smear is 95% accurate in detecting cervical carcinoma; however, its accuracy in detection of endometrial carcinoma is only approximately 40%. In the past, the cells were classified as Class 1 (indicating absence of atypical or abnormal cells) through Class 5 (cytologic findings conclusive of malignancy).

A general movement has occurred over the last 10 years to reclassify Pap smear reporting in terms of cervical intraepithelial neoplasia (CIN). This is a simple designation of the spectrum of intraepithelial dysplasia, which usually occurs before invasive cervical cancer. The subclasses of CIN are defined as follows:

CIN 1: mild and mild-to-moderate dysplasia
CIN 2: moderate and moderate-to-severe dysplasia
CIN 3: severe dysplasia and carcinoma in situ

Most recently, the Bethesda System for reporting cervical/vaginal cytologic diagnoses was developed and revised by the National Cancer Institute. This system includes evaluation of the following:

Adequacy of specimen
General categorization (optional)
Descriptive diagnosis
Epithelial cell abnormalities (squamous and glandular cells)

A Pap smear also may be performed to follow some abnormalities (e.g., infertility). An abnormal maturation index (MI) is characteristic of an estrogen-progesterone imbalance. The MI is calculated by determining the ratio of parabasal cervical cells to intermediate cells to superficial cells. The normal ovulating adult MI is 0/70/30. The MI is used more frequently for determination of menstrual status and ovarian function.

Pap smears should be part of the routine pelvic examination, which is usually performed once a year on women over 18 years of age (or even earlier when the patient is sexually active). Opinions differ regarding the necessity for annual Pap smears. The American Cancer Society recommends that a Pap smear be taken annually for two negative examinations, then repeated once every 3 years until age 65 in asymptomatic women. More frequent testing may be indicated for patients with venereal infections, those with a family history of cervical cancer, and those whose mothers had ingested diethylstilbestrol during their pregnancies.

Contraindications

- Patients presently having routine normal menses, because this can alter test interpretation.
- Patients with vaginal infections.
- Cellular changes that may be misinterpreted as dysplastic may transiently occur during these infections.

Interfering factors

- A delay in fixing a specimen allows the cells to dry, destroys effectiveness of the stain, and makes cytologic interpretation difficult.
- Using lubricating jelly on the speculum can alter the specimen.
- Douching and tub bathing may wash away cellular deposits and interfere with the test results.
- Menstrual flow may alter test results.
- Infections may interfere with hormonal cytology.
- Drugs such as digitalis and tetracycline may alter the test results by affecting the squamous epithelium.

Procedure and patient care

Before

- Explain the procedure to the patient.
- Instruct the patient not to douche or tub bathe during the 24 hours before the Pap smear. (Some physicians prefer that patients refrain from sexual intercourse for 24 to 48 hours before the test.)
- Instruct the patient to empty her bladder before the examination.

- Tell the patient that no fasting or sedation is required.

During

- Note the following procedural steps:
  1. The patient is placed in the lithotomy position.
  2. A vaginal speculum is inserted to expose the cervix.
  3. Material is collected from the cervical canal by rotating a moist, saline cotton swab or spatula within the cervical canal and in the squamocolumnar junction. See Figure 24.
  4. The cells are immediately wiped across a clean glass slide and fixed either by immersing the slide in equal parts of 95% alcohol and ether or by using a commercial spray (e.g., Aqua Net hair spray). The secretions must be fixed before drying, because drying will distort the cells and make interpretation difficult.
  5. The slide is labeled with the patient's name, age, and parity and with the date of her last menstrual period.
  6. The patient's medication history (e.g., oral contraceptives) and the reason for the examination should be written on the laboratory request form.
- Note that a Pap smear is obtained by a nurse or a physician in approximately 10 minutes.
- Tell the patient that no discomfort, except for insertion of the speculum, is associated with this procedure.

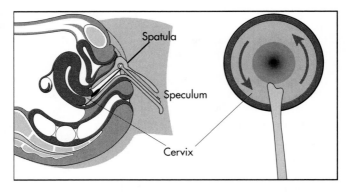

Figure 24 Papanicolaou (Pap) smear. **A,** The vaginal speculum is shown in position to allow direct visualization of the cervix. **B,** The cervix is scraped with bifid end of a wooden spatula. (From Pagana KD, Pagana TJ: *Mosby's manual of diagnostic and laboratory tests,* St Louis, 1998, Mosby.)

After
- Inform the patient that usually she will not be notified unless further evaluation is necessary.

Abnormal findings

Cancer
Infertility
Venereal disease
Reactive inflammatory changes
Fungal infection
Parasitic infection
Herpes infection

notes

paracentesis (Peritoneal fluid analysis, Abdominal paracentesis, Ascitic fluid cytology, Peritoneal tap)

Type of test Fluid analysis

Normal findings

Gross appearance: Clear, serous, light yellow, <50 ml
Red blood cells (RBCs): None
White blood cells (WBCs): <300/μl
Protein: <4.1 g/dl
Glucose: 70-100 mg/dl
Amylase: 138-404 U/L
Ammonia: <50 μg/dl
Alkaline phosphatase
    Adult male: 90-240 U/L
    Female <45 years: 76-196 U/L
    Female >45 years: 87-250 U/L
Lactate dehydrogenase (LDH): Similar to serum lactate dehydrogenase
Cytology: No malignant cells
Bacteria: None
Fungi: None
Carcinoembryonic antigen (CEA): Negative

Test explanation and related physiology

Paracentesis is an invasive procedure entailing the insertion of a needle or catheter into the peritoneal cavity (Figure 25) for removal of ascitic fluid for diagnostic and therapeutic purposes.

Diagnostically, paracentesis is performed to obtain and analyze fluid to determine the etiology of the peritoneal effusion. Peritoneal fluid is classified as to whether it is a transudate or exudate. This is an important differentiation and is very helpful in determining the etiology of the effusion. *Transudates* are most frequently caused by congestive heart failure, cirrhosis, nephrotic syndrome, myxedema, peritoneal dialysis, and hypoproteinemia. *Exudates* are most often found in infectious or neoplastic conditions. However, collagen vascular disease, gastrointestinal diseases, trauma, and drug hypersensitivity also may cause an exudative effusion.

Therapeutically this procedure is done to remove large amounts of fluid from the abdominal cavity. Usually these patients experience transient relief of symptoms (shortness of

Figure 25 Paracentesis. A catheter is placed through the skin and abdominal muscle wall, into the peritoneal cavity containing free fluid.

breath, distention, and early satiety) because of the fluid within the abdominal cavity.

The peritoneal fluid is usually evaluated for gross appearance, RBCs, WBCs, protein, glucose, amylase, ammonia, alkaline phosphatase, LDH, cytology, bacteria, fungi, and other tests such as CEA levels. Each is discussed separately. Urea and creatinine may be measured if there is a question that the fluid may represent urine from a perforated bladder.

Gross appearance

Transudative peritoneal fluid may be clear, serous, and light yellow, especially in patients with hepatic cirrhosis. Milk-colored peritoneal fluid may result from the escape of chyle from blocked abdominal or thoracic lymphatic ducts. Conditions that may cause lymphatic blockage include lymphoma, carcinoma, and tuberculosis involving the abdominal or thoracic lymph nodes. The triglyceride value in a chylous effusion exceeds 110 mg/dl.

Exudative fluid is cloudy or turbid fluid. Bloody fluid may be the result of a traumatic tap (the aspirating needle penetrates a blood vessel), intra-abdominal bleeding, tumor, or hemorrhagic pancreatitis. Bile-stained, green fluid may result from a ruptured gallbladder, acute pancreatitis, or perforated intestines.

Cell counts

Normally no RBCs should be present. The presence of RBCs may indicate neoplasms, tuberculosis, or intraabdominal bleeding. Increased WBC counts may be seen with peritonitis, cirrhosis, and tuberculosis. Usually these counts are performed manually using a simple hemacytometer.

Protein count

Total protein levels greater than 3 g/dl are characteristic of *exudates*, whereas *transudates* usually have a protein content of less than 3 g/dl. It is now thought that the *albumin gradient* between serum and ascitic fluid can differentiate better between the transudate and exudate nature of ascites than can the total protein content. This gradient is obtained by subtracting the ascitic albumin value from the serum albumin value. Values of 1.1 g/dl or more suggest a transudate, and values less than 1.1 g/dl suggest an exudate. The total protein ratio (fluid/serum) has been used to differentiate exudate from transudate. A total protein ratio of fluid to serum of greater than 0.5 is considered to be an exudate.

Glucose

Usually peritoneal glucose levels approximate serum glucose levels. Decreased levels may indicate tuberculous/bacterial peritonitis or peritoneal carcinomatosis.

Amylase

Increased amylase levels may be seen in patients with pancreatic trauma; pancreatic pseudocyst; acute pancreatitis; and intestinal necrosis, perforation, or strangulation. In these diseases the amylase level is usually >1.5 times higher than serum levels.

Ammonia

High ammonia levels occur in ruptured or strangulated intestines and also with a ruptured appendix or ulcer.

Alkaline phosphatase

Levels of alkaline phosphatase are greatly increased in infarcted or strangulated intestines.

Lactate dehydrogenase

A peritoneal fluid/serum LDH ratio of greater than 0.6 is typical of an exudate. An exudate is identified with a higher degree of accuracy if the peritoneal fluid/serum protein ratio is greater than 0.5 and the peritoneal fluid/serum LDH ratio is greater than 0.6.

Cytology

A cytologic study is performed to detect tumors. It can be difficult to differentiate malignancy from severe inflammatory mesothelial cells. Cytology examination of the fluid is improved by spinning down a large volume of fluid and examining the sediment. Large numbers of cells can be seen and compared to each other.

Bacteria

Usually the fluid is cultured, and the antibiotic sensitivities are determined. Gram stains are often performed.

Gram stain and bacteriologic culture

The presence of bacteria may indicate intraabdominal infection. Culture and Gram stains identify the organisms involved in the infection (see p. 784).

Fungi

Fungi may indicate infections with histoplasmosis, candidiasis, or coccidioidomycosis.

Carcinoembryonic antigen

Peritoneal fluid levels for CEA are associated with abdominal malignancy, usually arising from the gastrointestinal tract.

Contraindications

- Patients with coagulation abnormalities or bleeding tendencies
- Patients with only a small amount of fluid and extensive previous abdominal surgery

Potential complications

- Hypovolemia if a large volume of peritoneal fluid was removed
- Peritonitis

Procedure and patient care

Before

- Explain the procedure to the patient.
- Obtain informed consent for this procedure.
- Tell the patient that no fasting or sedation is necessary.
- Have the patient urinate or empty the bladder before the test. This will help to prevent accidental bladder trauma.
- Measure abdominal girth.
- Obtain the patient's weight.

- Obtain baseline vital signs.

During

- Note the following procedural steps:
  1. Position the person in a high Fowler's position in bed.
  2. Paracentesis is performed under strict sterile technique. A paracentesis tray usually contains all necessary supplies.
  3. The needle insertion site is aseptically cleansed and anesthetized locally.
  4. A scalpel may be used to make a stab wound in the skin to allow the cannula or needle to enter.
  5. A trocar, cannula, or needle is threaded through the incision.
  6. Tubing is attached to the cannula. The other end of the tubing is placed in the collection receptacle (usually a container with a pressurized vacuum).
- Note that this procedure is performed by a physician at the patient's bedside, in a procedure room, or in the physician's office in less than 30 minutes. Usually the volume removed is limited to about 4 L at any one time to avoid hypovolemia if the ascites is rapidly reaccumulated.
- Although local anesthetics eliminate pain at the insertion site, tell the patient that he or she will feel a pressure-like pain as the needle is inserted.

After

- All tests performed on peritoneal fluid should be performed immediately to avoid false results due to chemical or cellular deterioration.
- Place a small bandage over the needle site.
- Label the specimen with the patient's name, date, source of fluid, and diagnosis.
- Send the specimen promptly to the laboratory.
- Observe the puncture site for bleeding, continued drainage, or signs of inflammation.
- Measure the abdominal girth and weight of the patient; compare with baseline values.
- Monitor vital signs for evidence of hemodynamic changes. Watch for signs of hypotension if a large volume of fluid was removed.
- Write any recent antibiotic therapy on the laboratory requisition slip.
- Because of the high protein content of ascitic fluid, albumin infusions may be ordered after paracentesis to compensate

for protein loss. Monitor serum protein and electrolyte (especially sodium) levels.

- Occasionally ascitic fluid continues to leak out of the needle tract after removal of the needle. A suture can stop that. If unsuccessful, a collection bag should be applied to the skin to allow for measurement of the volume of fluid loss.

Abnormal findings

Exudate
Lymphoma
Carcinoma
Tuberculosis
Peritonitis
Pancreatitis
Ruptured viscus

Transudate
Hepatic cirrhosis
Portal hypertension
Nephrotic syndrome
Hypoproteinemia
Congestive heart failure
Abdominal trauma
Peritoneal bleeding

notes

P

parathyroid hormone (PTH, Parathormone)

Type of test Blood

Normal findings

Intact (whole): 10-65 pg/ml
N terminal: 8-24 pg/ml
C terminal: 50-330 pg/ml

Test explanation and related physiology

PTH is secreted by the parathyroid gland in response to hypocalcemia. This test is useful in establishing a diagnosis of hyperparathyroidism and distinguishing nonparathyroid from parathyroid causes of hypercalcemia. Increased PTH levels are seen in patients with hyperparathyroidism (primary, secondary or tertiary); in patients with nonparathyroid, ectopic PTH-producing tumors (pseudohyperparathyroidism); or as a normal compensatory response to hypocalcemia in patients with malabsorption or vitamin D deficiency.

It is important to measure serum calcium simultaneously with the measurement of PTH. Most laboratories have a PTH/calcium nomogram already made up, indicating what PTH level is considered normal for each calcium level.

Decreased PTH levels are seen in patients with hypoparathyroidism or as a compensatory response to hypercalcemia in patients with metastatic bone tumors, sarcoidosis, vitamin D intoxication, or milk-alkali syndrome. Of course, surgical ablation of the parathyroids is another cause of hypoparathyroidism.

Whole (intact) PTH is metabolized to several different fragments, including an N terminal, a midregion or midmolecule, and a C terminal. The intact PTH and all fragments generally provide accurate information concerning the level of PTH in the blood. The intact PTH is probably most often tested since it is most reliable.

Interfering factors

- Recent injection of radioisotopes may interfere with this test.
- Drugs that *increase* PTH include anticonvulsants, steroids, isoniazid, lithium, and rifampin.
- Drugs that *decrease* PTH include cimetidine and propranolol.

Procedure and patient care

Before
- Explain the procedure to the patient.
- Keep the patient NPO except for water after midnight on the day of the test.

During
- Obtain a morning blood specimen, because diurnal rhythm affects PTH levels. (Check with the laboratory if the patient works at night.)
- Collect 5 to 10 ml of venous blood in a red-top tube. Note that some laboratories require 15 ml of blood in an iced plastic syringe.
- Obtain a serum calcium level determination at the same time if ordered. The serum PTH and serum calcium levels are important in the differential diagnosis.

After
- Indicate the time the blood was drawn on the laboratory slip, because a diurnal rhythm affects test results.
- Apply pressure to the venipuncture site.

Abnormal findings

▲ Increased levels
Hyperparathyroidism
secondary to adenoma
or carcinoma of the
parathyroid gland
Non-PTH-producing
tumors (paraneoplastic
syndrome)
Lung carcinoma
Kidney carcinoma
Hypocalcemia
Chronic renal failure
Malabsorption syndrome
Vitamin D deficiency
Rickets
Osteomalacia
Congenital renal defect

▼ Decreased levels
Hypoparathyroidism
Hypercalcemia
Metastatic bone tumor
Sarcoidosis
Autoimmune destruction
of the parathyroid
glands
Vitamin D intoxication
Milk-alkali syndrome
Graves' disease
Hypomagnesemia
DiGeorge syndrome

P

partial thromboplastin time, activated (APTT, Partial thromboplastin time [PTT])

Type of test Blood

Normal findings

APTT: 30-40 seconds

PTT: 60-70 seconds

Patients receiving anticoagulant therapy: 1.5-2.5 times control
value in seconds

Possible critical values

APTT: >70 seconds

PTT: >100 seconds

Test explanation and related physiology

The PTT test is used to assess the intrinsic system and the
common pathway of clot formation. PTT evaluates factors I
(fibrinogen), II (prothrombin), V, VIII, IX, X, XI, and XII.
When any of these factors exists in inadequate quantities, as in
hemophilia A and B or consumptive coagulopathy, the PTT
is prolonged. Because factors II, IX, and X are vitamin
K-dependent factors, biliary obstruction, which precludes gastrointestinal absorption of fat and fat-soluble vitamins (e.g.,
vitamin K), can reduce their concentration and thus prolong the
PTT. Because coagulation factors are made in the liver, hepatocellular diseases will also prolong the PTT.

Heparin has been found to inactivate prothrombin (factor II)
and prevent the formation of thromboplastin. These actions
prolong the intrinsic clotting pathway for approximately 4 to
6 hours after each dose of heparin. Therefore heparin is capable
of providing therapeutic anticoagulation. The appropriate dose
of heparin can be monitored by the PTT. PTT test results are
given in seconds, along with a control value. The control value
may vary slightly from day to day because of the reagents used.

Recently activators have been added to the PTT test reagents
to shorten normal clotting time and provide a narrow normal
range. This shortened time is called the *activated* PTT (APTT).
The normal APTT is 30 to 40 seconds. Desired ranges
for therapeutic anticoagulation are 1.5 to 2.5 times normal (e.g.,
70 seconds). The APTT specimen should be drawn 30 to
60 minutes before the patient's next heparin dose is given. If the

APTT is less than 50 seconds, the patient may not be receiving therapeutic anticoagulation and needs more heparin. An APTT greater than 100 seconds indicates that too much heparin is being given; the risk of serious spontaneous bleeding exists when the APTT is this high. The effects of heparin can be reversed immediately by the administration of 1 mg of protamine sulfate for every 100 units of the heparin dose.

Heparin's effect, unlike that of warfarin, is immediate and short-lived. When a thromboembolic episode (e.g., pulmonary embolism, arterial embolism, thrombophlebitis) occurs, immediate and complete anticoagulation is most rapidly and safely achieved by heparin administration. This drug is often given during cardiac and vascular surgery to prevent intravascular clotting during clamping of the vessels. Often, small doses of heparin (5000 U subcutaneously every 12 hours) are given to prevent thromboembolism in high-risk patients. This dose alters the PTT very little, and the risk of spontaneous bleeding is minimal.

Interfering factors

☞ Drugs that may prolong PTT test values include antihistamines, ascorbic acid, chlorpromazine, heparin, and salicylates.

Procedure and patient care

Before

- Explain the procedure to the patient.
- If the patient is receiving heparin by intermittent injection, plan to draw the blood specimen for the APTT 30 minutes to 1 hour before the next dose of heparin.
- If the patient is receiving continuous heparin, draw the blood at any time.

During

- Collect 5 to 14 ml of venous blood in one or two blue-top tubes.

After

- Apply pressure to the venipuncture site. Remember, if the patient is receiving anticoagulants or has coagulopathies, the bleeding time will be increased.
- Assess the patient to detect possible bleeding. Check for blood in the urine and all other excretions and assess the patient for bruises, petechiae, and low back pain.

- If severe bleeding occurs, note that the anticoagulant effect of heparin can be reversed by parenteral administration of protamine sulfate.

Abnormal findings

▲ **Increased levels**

Acquired or congenital clotting factor deficiencies

Cirrhosis of the liver

Vitamin K deficiency

Leukemia

Disseminated intravascular coagulation

Heparin administration

Hypofibrinogenemia

Von Willebrand's disease

Hemophilia

▼ **Decreased levels**

Early stages of disseminated intravascular coagulation

Extensive cancer

notes

parvovirus B19 antibody

Type of test Blood

Normal findings Negative for IgM and IgG specific antibodies to parvovirus B19

Test explanation and related physiology

The parvovirus group includes several species-specific viruses of animals. The parvovirus B19 is known to be a human pathogen. Many of the severe manifestations of B19 viremia relate to the ability of the virus to infect and lyse red blood cell precursors in the bone marrow. The name B19 was derived from the code number of the human serum in which the virus was discovered.

Erythema infectiosum is the most common manifestation of B19 infection and occurs predominantly in children. This pathogen is also referred to as "fifth disease" because it was classified in the late nineteenth century as the fifth in a series of six exanthems of childhood. This infection is also sometimes referred to as "academy rash."

Recently, parvovirus B19 has been associated with a number of other clinical problems, including: joint inflammation, purpura, hydrops fetalis, and aplastic anemia.

Because of the recently discovered spectrum of disease caused by parvovirus B19, laboratory diagnosis has come into great demand. Serologic testing for parvovirus B19 specific IgM and IgG antibodies can be detected. Acute infections can be determined by B19-compatible symptoms and the presence of IgM antibodies that remain detectable up to a few months. Past infection or immunity is documented by IgG antibodies that persist indefinitely. Fetal infection may be recognized by hydrops fetalis and the presence of B19 DNA in amniotic fluid or fetal blood.

Procedure and patient care

Before

- Explain the procedure to the patient.
- Tell the patient that no fasting or special preparation is necessary.

During

- Collect a venous blood sample according to the laboratory protocol.

After

- Apply pressure to the venipuncture site.
- Inform the patient that it normally requires approximately 2 to 3 days to get test results.

Abnormal findings

▲ **Increased levels**

Erythema infectiosum (fifth disease)
Joint arthralgia and arthritis
Hydrops fetalis
Fetal loss
Transient aplastic anemia
Chronic anemia in immunodeficient patients
Bone marrow failure

notes

pelvic ultrasonography (Obstetric echography, Pregnant uterus ultrasonography, Pelvic ultrasonography in pregnancy, Obstetric ultrasonography, Vaginal ultrasound)

Type of test Ultrasound

Normal findings Normal fetal and placental size and position

Test explanation and related physiology

Ultrasound examination of the female patient is a harmless, noninvasive method of evaluating the female genital tract and fetus. In real-time ultrasound, high-frequency sound waves are emitted from the transducer and penetrate the structure (uterus, ovaries, parametria, placenta, fetus) to be studied. These sound waves are bounced back to a sensor within the transducer and by electronic conversion are arranged into a pictorial image of the desired organ.

It should be noted that pelvic ultrasonography can be performed with the transducer placed on the anterior abdomen (see Figure 1, p. 2) or in the vagina with a specially designed vaginal probe. The view obtained from both transducers complements the information gained from either one alone. Vaginal ultrasound adds significant accuracy in identifying paracervical, endometrial, and ovarian pathology that otherwise may not be detected with the anterior abdominal probe.

Pelvic ultrasonography may be useful in the *obstetric patient* to diagnose the following circumstances:

1. Making an early diagnosis of normal pregnancy and abnormal pregnancy (e.g., tubal pregnancy)
2. Identifying multiple pregnancies
3. Differentiating a tumor (e.g., hydatidiform mole) from a normal pregnancy
4. Determining the age of the fetus by the diameter of the head. This is often combined with computed tomography scan of the pelvis to compare measurements of the fetal head to the maternal pelvis. This is helpful in identifying cephalopelvic disproportion.
5. Measuring the rate of fetal growth
6. Identifying placental abnormalities such as abruptio placentae and placenta previa
7. Determining the position of the placenta (Ultrasound

P

localization of the placenta is done before amniocentesis.)

8. Making differential diagnoses of various uterine and ovarian enlargements (e.g., polyhydramnios, neoplasms, cysts, abscesses)
9. Determining fetal position
10. Ectopic pregnancy

Pelvic ultrasound is used in the *nonpregnant woman* to monitor the endometrium in patients who take tamoxifen and to aid in the diagnosis of:

1. Ovarian cyst
2. Ovarian tumor
3. Tubo-ovarian abscess
4. Uterine fibroids
5. Uterine cancer
6. Pelvic inflammatory disease (PID)
7. Thickened uterine endometrium (stripe) (caused by cancer, hyperplasia, etc.)

See rectal ultrasonography, p. 682.

Contraindications

- Patients with latex allergy
  Vaginal ultrasound requires placement of the probe in a latex condom-like sac. Patients with a latex allergy may react significantly to that contact.

Interfering factors

- Patients who have had recent gastrointestinal (GI) contrast studies, because barium creates severe distortion of reflective sound waves
- Patients with air-filled bowels, because gas does not transmit the sound waves well
- Failure to fill the bladder, which may make the image uninterpretable

Procedure and patient care

Before

- Explain the procedure to the patient.
- Assure the patient that this study has no known deleterious effect on maternal or fetal tissues, even when it is repeated several times.
- Give the patient three to four glasses (200 to 350 ml) of water or other liquid 1 hour before the examination, and instruct her *not* to void until after the procedure is com-

pleted. This will permit visualization of the bladder, which is used as a reference point in pelvic anatomy.

- No water is required if the ultrasound is to be done vaginally only.
- If a transabdominal ultrasound is required urgently and there is not time to fill the bladder by ingestion or administration of fluids, a bladder catheter is inserted, and the bladder is filled with water.
- Tell the patient that no fasting or sedation is required.

During

- Note the following procedural steps:
  1. The patient is taken to the ultrasound room and placed in the supine position on the examining table.
  2. The ultrasonographer, usually a radiologist, applies a greasy, conductive paste to the abdomen to enhance sound transmission and reception.
  3. A transducer is passed vertically and horizontally over the skin.
  4. If a vaginal probe is used, it is inserted via the vagina and angled to identify the various parts of the pelvis.
  5. Pictures are taken of the reflections.
  6. During the examination, fetal structures are pointed out to the mother.
- Note that this procedure is performed in approximately 20 minutes.
- Inform the patient that no discomfort is associated with this study, other than having a full bladder and the urge to void. Some patients may be uncomfortable lying on a hard x-ray table.

After

- Remove the lubricant from the patient's skin.
- Provide an opportunity for the patient to void.

P

Abnormal findings

Tubal pregnancy
Abdominal pregnancy
Hydatidiform mole
Intrauterine growth retardation
Multiple fetuses
Fetal death
Abruptio placentae
Abnormal fetal position (e.g., breech, transverse)
Placenta previa
Polyhydramnios
Neoplasm of the ovaries, uterus, or fallopian tubes
Cysts
Abscesses
Hydrocephalus of the fetus
Intrauterine device localization

notes

percutaneous transhepatic cholangiography
(PTC, PTHC)

Type of test X-ray with contrast dye

Normal findings Normal gallbladder and biliary ducts

Test explanation and related physiology

By passing a needle through the liver and into an intrahepatic bile duct, the biliary system can be directly injected with iodinated x-ray contrast dye. The intrahepatic and extrahepatic biliary ducts and occasionally the gallbladder can be visualized and studied for partial or total obstruction caused by gallstones, benign strictures, malignant tumors, congenital cysts, and anatomic variations. This is especially helpful in jaundiced patients. If the jaundice is found to result from extrahepatic obstruction, a catheter can be left in the bile duct and used for external drainage of bile. Furthermore, a stent can be placed across a stricture to decompress the biliary system internally.

Both PTC and endoscopic retrograde cholangiopancreatography (ERCP)(see p. 361) are the only methods available to visualize the biliary tree in jaundiced patients. ERCP is used more frequently because of its lower complication rate. But PTC is the only way to visualize the biliary tree after most gastric surgery. Occasionally (if the pancreatic duct and the common bile duct form a common channel), part or all of the pancreatic duct can be filled with dye from the same injection.

Contraindications

- Patients with evidence of mild cholangitis
  Dye injections increase biliary pressure and cause bacteremia, which may lead to septicemia and shock.
- Patients who cannot cooperate and remain still
- Patients with prolonged clotting times

Potential complications

- Allergic reaction to iodinated dye.
  This is rare because no iodine is being injected into the venous system.
- Peritonitis caused by bile extravasation from the liver after the needle has been removed
- Bleeding caused by inadvertent puncture of a large hepatic blood vessel

- Sepsis and cholangitis resulting from injection of the dye into an already infected and obstructed bowel duct
  The pressure of injection pushes the bacteria into the bloodstream, causing a bacteremia.

Interfering factor

- The presence of barium from a previous upper GI series or barium enema x-ray study may preclude visualization of the biliary tree.

Procedure and patient care

Before

- Explain the procedure to the patient.
- Obtain informed consent for this procedure.
- Type and crossmatch the patient's blood. The patient may bleed and require a transfusion or surgery.
- Check to make sure that the patient's coagulation studies are within the normal ranges.
- Keep the patient NPO after midnight on the day of the test. A laxative may be ordered.
- Premedicate the patient as indicated, usually with atropine and meperidine.

During

- Note the following procedural steps:
  1. The patient is placed in the supine position on an x-ray table in the radiology department.
  2. The abdominal wall or lower chest wall (over the liver) is anesthetized with lidocaine (Xylocaine).
  3. With the use of televised fluoroscopic monitoring, the needle is advanced through the skin and into the liver (Figure 26).
  4. When bile flows freely through the needle, radiographic dye is injected.
  5. X-ray films are taken immediately.
  6. If an obstruction is found, a catheter or stent is placed over a guide wire and left temporarily in the biliary tract to establish drainage and decompression of the biliary tract.
- Note that PTC is performed by a radiologist in approximately 1 hour, during which time the patient must lie still.
- Inform the patient that abdominal pain may be felt for several hours after the test. Occasionally the patient also may have

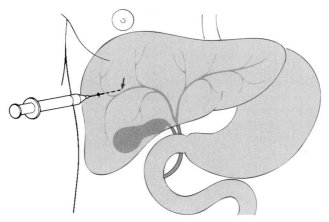

Figure 26 Percutaneous transhepatic cholangiography. A needle attached to a syringe is passed through the abdominal wall and into the liver. With continuous aspiration, a biliary branch is punctured. Through that needle, a wire is placed into the biliary tree. A catheter is then placed over the wire.

right shoulder-top pain because of diaphragmatic irritation of leaking bile or blood.

After
- Keep the patient on bed rest for several hours.
- If indicated, place a sandbag over the insertion site.
- Observe the patient for hemorrhage or bile leakage. A small amount of bleeding is usually present.
- Keep the patient NPO for a few hours after the test in the event he or she has any intraabdominal bleeding or bile extravasation that requires surgery.
- Repeatedly assess the patient's vital signs for evidence of hemorrhage.
- Assess the patient for signs of bacteremia or sepsis.
- If a catheter is left in the biliary tract, establish a sterile, closed drainage system.
- Withhold pain medications to avoid blunting the abdominal signs associated with hemorrhage or bile extravasation.

Abnormal findings

Tumors, strictures, or gallstones of the hepatic or common
  bile duct
Sclerosing cholangitis
Biliary sclerosis
Cysts of the common bile duct
Tumors, strictures, inflammation, or pseudocysts of the
  pancreatic duct
Anatomic biliary or pancreatic duct variations

notes

pericardiocentesis

Type of test Fluid analysis

Normal findings Minimal amount of clear, straw-colored fluid without evidence of any bacteria, blood, or malignant cells

Test explanation and related physiology

Pericardiocentesis, which involves the aspiration of fluid from the pericardial sac with a needle, may be performed for therapeutic and diagnostic purposes. Therapeutically, the test is performed to relieve cardiac tamponade by removing fluid and improving diastolic filling. Diagnostically, pericardiocentesis is performed to remove a sample of pericardial fluid for laboratory examination to determine the cause of the fluid. This is similar to the evaluation described for peritoneal and pleural fluid on p. 610 and p. 806, respectively.

Contraindications

- Patients who are uncooperative because of the risk of lacerations to the epicardium or coronary artery
- Patients with a bleeding disorder
  Inadvertent puncture of the myocardium may create uncontrollable bleeding into the pericardial sac, leading to tamponade.

Potential complications

- Laceration of the coronary artery or myocardium
- Needle-induced ventricular arrhythmias (dysrhythmias)
- Myocardial infarction
- Pneumothorax caused by inadvertent puncture of the lung
- Liver laceration caused by inadvertent puncture
- Pleural infection
- Vasovagal arrest

Procedure and patient care

Before

- Explain the procedure to the patient.
- Obtain informed consent for this procedure.
- Restrict fluid and food intake for at least 4 to 6 hours (if this is an elective procedure).

P

- Obtain IV access for infusion of fluids and cardiac medications if required.
- Administer pretest medication. Atropine is frequently given to prevent the vasovagal reflex of bradycardia and hypotension.

During

- Note the following procedural steps:
  1. The patient is placed in the supine position.
  2. An area in the fifth to sixth intercostal space at the left sternal margin (or subxyphoid) is prepared and draped.
  3. After skin anesthesia is performed, a large-bore, pericardiocentesis needle is placed on a 50-ml syringe and introduced into the pericardial sac (Figure 27).
  4. An electrocardiographic lead is often attached by a clip to

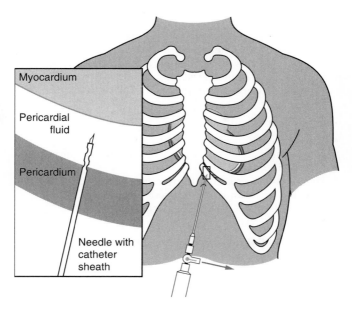

Figure 27 Pericardiocentesis procedure and aspiration of pericardial fluid. For recurrent cardiac tamponade and large pericardial effusion, the indwelling catheter may remain.

the needle to identify any ST-segment elevations, which may indicate penetration into the epicardium.

5. Pericardial fluid is aspirated and placed in multiple specimen containers.
6. Some patients who have recurring cardiac tamponade may require placement of an indwelling pericardial catheter for continuous draining for 1 to 3 days.
7. With certain types of pericarditis, medications (e.g., antibiotics, antineoplastic drugs, corticosteroids) may be instilled during pericardiocentesis.

- Note that a physician usually performs this procedure in the cardiac catheterization laboratory, operating room, or emergency room in approximately 10 to 20 minutes.
- Tell the patient that this procedure is associated with very little discomfort. Most patients feel pressure as the needle is inserted into the pericardial sac.

After

- Closely monitor the patient's vital signs. An increased temperature may indicate infection. Pericardial bleeding would be marked by hypotension or pulsus paradoxus (abnormal decrease in systolic blood pressure during inspiration).
- Label and number the specimen tubes that contain the pericardial fluid and deliver them to the appropriate laboratories for examination. Note the following possibilities:
  1. Usually the fluid is taken to the chemistry laboratory, where the color, turbidity, glucose, albumin, protein, and lactic dehydrogenase levels are obtained (see discussion of thoracentesis, p. 806).
  2. A tube of blood often goes to the hematology laboratory, where the quantities of red and white blood cells are recorded.
  3. The bacteriology laboratory performs routine cultures, Gram stains, fungal studies, acid-fast bacilli smears, and cultures.
  4. When malignancy is suspected, the fluid should be sent for cytology.
- Apply a sterile dressing to the catheter if one has been left for continuing pericardial drainage.
- Establish a closed system if continued pericardial drainage is required. This is usually performed via the straight drainage method.

P

- Note that to minimize infection, pericardial catheters, if used, are usually removed after 2 days, although there are exceptions. After the sutures are cut and the catheter is removed, apply a sterile dressing to the puncture site.

Abnormal findings

Pericarditis
Uremia
Hypoproteinemia
Congestive heart failure
Metastatic cancer
Blunt or penetrating cardiac trauma
Rupture of ventricular aneurysm

notes

phenylketonuria test (PKU test, Guthrie test, Phenylalanine screening)

Type of test Blood; urine

Normal findings
Blood: negative (<2 mg/dl) (Guthrie technique)
Urine: no green coloration

Possible critical values ≥4 mg/dl (Guthrie technique)

Test explanation and related physiology

An inherited disease, PKU is characterized by deficiency of the enzyme phenylalanine hydroxylase, which converts phenylalanine to tyrosine. Phenylalanine is an essential amino acid necessary for growth; however, any excess must be degraded by conversion to tyrosine. An infant with PKU lacks the ability to make this necessary conversion. Thus phenylalanine accumulates in the body and spills over into the urine. If the amount of phenylalanine is not restricted in infants with PKU, progressive mental retardation results. Dietary control must begin early to avoid brain damage; therefore diagnosis must be made early.

Routine screening of newborn infants for PKU is now mandatory in most of the United States. It is important to note that this test is not valid until the newborn has ingested an ample amount (for 2 or 3 days) of the amino acid phenylalanine, which is a constituent of both human and cow's milk. If the child is not eating well or does not weigh at least 5 lbs, the test should not be done because results may be invalid. The urine PKU test is normally done after 6 weeks of age if, for some reason, a blood test was not done in the hospital. If the tests are positive, a blood phenylalanine test should be performed.

Interfering factors

- Premature infants may have false-positive results because of delayed development of the liver enzymes.
- Ketonuria can produce an altered urine color reaction.
- Infants tested before 24 hours of age may have false-negative results.
- Feeding problems (e.g., vomiting) may cause false-negative results.
- ✍ Drugs that may influence screening results include antibiotics, aspirin, and salicylates.

Procedure and patient care

Before

- Inform the mother about the purpose of the test and the method of performance.
- Assess the infant's feeding patterns before performing the PKU test. An inadequate amount of protein ingested before performing the test can cause false-negative results.

During

- Place a few drops of blood from a heel stick on filter paper for the Guthrie test. This test is performed after the newborn has ingested an ample amount (for 2 to 3 days) of the amino acid phenylalanine.
- Indicate on the laboratory slip the present date and time, date and time of birth, and time of first milk-feeding.
- Note that urine tests also may be used to detect PKU in infants who are at least 6 weeks of age. These tests are usually done at the infant's first checkup:
  1. For the *diaper test*, drop 10% ferric chloride on a diaper that contains fresh urine. A green spot indicates probable PKU.
  2. For the *Phenistix* test, press a test stick against a diaper containing urine or dip the stick in the urine. A green color reaction indicates probable PKU.

After

- If test results are positive, inform the mother that dietary control must begin immediately to prevent brain damage in the infant. This is done by substituting Lofenalac for milk. Later, strained foods low in protein are added to the infant's diet. The dietary treatment is monitored by blood and urine testing.
- Instruct women with PKU who wish to have children to begin a low-phenylalanine diet before conception and continue throughout the pregnancy. The risk of producing a mentally retarded infant is very high if the mother remains on a general diet.

Abnormal findings

PKU
Low-birth weight infants
Galactosemia
Hepatic encephalopathy

phosphate (P, PO₄, inorganic phosphorus)

Type of test Blood

Normal findings

Adult: 3-4.5 mg/dl or 0.97-1.45 mmol/L (SI units)
Elderly: values slightly lower than adult
Child: 4.5-6.5 mg/dl or 1.45-2.1 mmol/L (SI units)
Newborn: 4.3-9.3 mg/dl or 1.4-3 mmol/L (SI units)

Possible critical values <1 mg/dl

Test explanation and related physiology

Phosphorus in the body is in the form of a phosphate. Phosphorus and phosphate will be used interchangeably throughout this and other discussions. Most of the phosphate in the body is a part of organic compounds. Only a small part in of total body phosphate is inorganic phosphate (i.e., not part of another organic compound). It is the *inorganic* phosphate that is measured when one requests a "phosphate," "phosphorus," "inorganic phosphorus," or "inorganic phosphate". Most of the body's inorganic phosphorus is combined with calcium within the skeleton; however, approximately 15% of the phosphorus exists in the blood as a phosphate salt.

Dietary phosphorus is absorbed in the small bowel. The absorption is very efficient, and only rarely is hypophosphatemia caused by gastrointestinal malabsorption. Phosphorus levels are determined by calcium metabolism, parathormone (parathyroid hormone [PTH]), renal excretion, and to a lesser degree, by intestinal absorption. Because an inverse relationship exists between calcium and phosphorus, a decrease of one mineral results in an increase in the other. The regulation of phosphate by PTH is such that PTH tends to decrease phosphate resorption in the kidney. PTH and vitamin D, however, tend to stimulate phosphate absorption weakly within the gut.

Interfering factors

- Laxatives or enemas containing sodium phosphate can increase phosphorus levels.
- Recent carbohydrate ingestion, including IV glucose administration, causes decreased phosphorus levels because phosphorus enters the cell with glucose.

- ☛ Drugs that may cause *increased* levels include methicillin and vitamin D (excessive).
- ☛ Drugs that may cause *decreased* levels include antacids and mannitol.

Procedure and patient care

Before

- Keep the patient NPO after midnight on the day of the test.
- If indicated, discontinue IV fluids with glucose for several hours before the test.

During

- Collect approximately 5 to 10 ml of venous blood in a red-top tube.
- Avoid hemolysis. Handle the tube carefully.
- Use a heel stick to draw blood from infants.

After

- Take the specimen to the laboratory immediately.
- Indicate on the laboratory slip the time the blood was obtained. Apply pressure to the venipuncture site.

Abnormal findings

▲ **Increased levels (hyperphosphatemia)**

Renal failure
Increased dietary or IV intake of phosphorus
Acromegaly
Hypoparathyroidism
Bone metastasis
Sarcoidosis
Hypocalcemia
Liver disease
Renal failure
Acidosis
Rhabdomyolysis
Advanced lymphoma or myeloma
Hemolytic anemia

▼ **Decreased levels (hypophosphatemia)**

Inadequate dietary ingestion of phosphorus
Chronic antacid ingestion
Hyperparathyroidism
Hypercalcemia
Chronic alcoholism
Vitamin D deficiency
Diabetic acidosis
Hyperinsulinism
Rickets (childhood)
Osteomalacia (adult)
Malnutrition
Alkalosis
Sepsis

plasminogen (Fibrinolysin)

Type of test Blood

Normal findings 2.5-4.5 mmol/ml or 6.1 ± 2.3 Committee on Thrombolytic Agents (CTA) units

Test explanation and related physiology

This test is used to diagnose suspected plasminogen deficiency in patients who present with multiple thromboembolic episodes. Plasminogen is a protein involved in the fibrinolytic process of intravascular blood clot dissolution (see Figure 11, p. 251). Plasminogen is converted to plasmin by proteolytic cleavage. This reaction can be catalyzed by urokinase, streptokinase, or tissue plasminogen activator (t-PA). Plasmin can destroy fibrin and dissolve clots. This fibrinolytic system is a normal part of the balance between coagulation and fibrinolysis.

Plasminogen levels are occasionally measured during fibrinolytic therapy (for coronary and peripheral arterial occlusion) and are diminished with full fibrinolysis. Decreased levels of plasminogen are also found in hyperfibrinolytic states (e.g., disseminated intravascular coagulation [DIC], primary fibrinolysis). Because plasminogen is made in the liver, patients with cirrhosis or other severe liver diseases can be expected to have decreased levels. There are rare cases of hereditary deficiencies of this protein. Pregnancy and, especially, eclampsia are associated with increased levels of plasminogen. Inflammatory conditions may have mild elevations of plasminogens, which are "acute phase reactant" proteins.

Procedure and patient care

Before
- Explain the procedure to the patient.
- Tell the patient that no fasting is required.

During
- Collect a venous blood sample in a blue-top tube containing sodium citrate.
- Avoid excessive agitation of the blood sample.

After

- Apply pressure to the venipuncture site, especially if the patient is suspected of having a hyperfibrinolytic process (e.g., DIC).

Abnormal findings

▲ **Increased levels**

Pregnancy

▼ **Decreased levels**

Hyperfibrinolytic state (e.g., DIC, fibrinolysis)

Primary liver disease

Syndrome associated with hypercoagulation (e.g., venous and arterial clotting)

Rare congenital deficiencies

Malnutrition

notes

platelet aggregation test

Type of test Blood

Normal findings Depend on the platelet agonist used

Test explanation and related physiology

Platelet aggregation is an important part of hemostasis. Surrounding an area of acute blood vessel endothelial injury is a clump of platelets. Normal platelets adhere to this area of injury, and through a series of chemical reactions, they attract other platelets to the area. This is platelet aggregation, the first step of hemostasis. After this step, the normal coagulation factor waterfall occurs (see Figure 11, p. 251). Certain diseases that affect either platelet number or function can inhibit platelet aggregation and thereby prolong bleeding times. Congenital syndromes, uremia, myeloproliferative disorders, and drugs are associated with abnormal platelet aggregation. If blood is passed through a heart-lung or dialysis pump, platelet injury can occur and aggregation can be reduced.

Platelet aggregation is measured by determining the turbidity of platelet-rich plasma in which platelet aggregation has been stimulated in vitro. Turbidity is then measured within an aggregometer, and a curve indicating light transmission per unit of time is plotted. Normal curves have been identified for each platelet aggregation stimulant that is used.

Interfering factors

- Factors that may cause increased levels include blood storage temperature, hyperbilirubinemia, hemoglobinemia, hyperlipidemia, and platelet count.
- Drugs that may cause *decreased* levels include aspirin, antibiotics, sodium warfarin (Coumadin), and heparin.

Procedure and patient care

Before

- Explain the procedure to the patient.
- Tell the patient that no fasting is required.

During

- Collect 5 to 7 ml of venous blood in a blue-top tube.
- If the patient is receiving any drugs that may interfere with

platelet aggregation or has any diseases such as jaundice, hyperlipidemia, or hemolysis, this should be listed on the laboratory request slip.

After

- Apply pressure to the venipuncture site.
- Remember that abnormalities in platelet aggregation can prolong bleeding time, and a significant hematoma at the venipuncture site may occur.

Abnormal findings

Prolonged platelet aggregation
Various congenital disorders (e.g., Wiskott-Aldrich syndrome, Bernard-Soulier syndrome, glycogen storage)
Connective tissue disorder (e.g., lupus erythematosus)
Recent cardiopulmonary or dialysis bypass
Various myeloproliferative diseases
Primary protein disease
von Willebrand's disease
Uremia

notes

platelet antibody detection (Antiplatelet antibody detection)

Type of test Blood

Normal findings No antiplatelet antibodies identified

Test explanation and related physiology

Immune-mediated destruction of platelets may be caused either by autoantibodies directed against antigens located on the same person's platelets or by alloantibodies that develop after exposure to transfused platelets received from a donor. These antibodies are usually directed to an antigen on the platelet membrane such as human lymphocyte antigen (HLA) (see p. 479) or platelet-specific antigens such as PLA1, PLA2.

Antibodies directed to platelets cause early destruction of the platelets and subsequent thrombocytopenia. Immunologic thrombocytopenia includes the following:

Idiopathic thrombocytopenia purpura (ITP)
Platelet-associated IgG antibodies are detected in 90% of these patients.

Posttransfusion purpura
This is a rare syndrome characterized by the sudden onset of severe thrombocytopenia a few hours to a few days after transfusion of red blood cells or platelets. This is usually associated with an antibody to ABO, HLA, or PLA antigens on the RBC.

Maternal-fetal platelet antigen incompatibility (neonatal thrombocytopenia)
This occurs when the fetal platelet contains a PLA1 antigen that is absent in the mother. Neonatal thrombocytopenia can also occur if the mother has ITP autoantibodies that are passed through the placenta and destroy the fetal platelets also.

Drug-induced thrombocytopenia
This is usually caused by platelet-associated IgG antibodies. These antibodies are the result of a hypersensitivity to certain drugs. A host of drugs are known to induce autoimmune-mediated thrombocytopenia. They are *cimetidine*, analgesics (salicylates, acetaminophen), antibiotics (cephalosporins, penicillin, *sulfonamides*), *quinidine*-like drugs, hypnotics (phenobarbital), oral hypoglycemic agents

P

(e.g., chlorpropamide), heavy metals (e.g., gold, organic arsenicals), diuretics (e.g., chlorothiazide), and others (e.g., digoxin, propylthiouracil, Antabuse, *heparin*). The medications in italics are the most common offenders.

Interfering factor
- Blood transfusion may cause the development of isoantibodies to HLA antigens on the platelets or red blood cells.

Procedure and patient care

Before
- Tell the patient that no fasting is required.

During
- Collect 10 to 30 ml of blood in a red-top tube. The amount of blood required depends on the initial platelet count.

After
- Apply pressure to the venipuncture site.
- Assure adequate hemostasis in all patients who are suspected to have thrombocytopenia.

Abnormal findings
Idiopathic thrombocytopenia purpura
Neonatal thrombocytopenia
Posttransfusion purpura
Drug-induced thrombocytopenia
Paroxysmal hemoglobinuria

notes

platelet count (Thrombocyte count)

Type of test Blood

Normal findings

Adult/elderly: 150,000-400,000/mm³ or 150 to 400 × 10⁹/L (SI units)

Premature infant: 100,000-300,000/mm³

Newborn: 150,000-300,000/mm³

Infant: 200,000-475,000 mm³

Child: 150,000-400,000/mm³

Possible critical values   <50,000 or >1 million/mm³

Test explanation and related physiology

The platelet count is an actual count of the number of platelets (thrombocytes) per cubic milliliter of blood. It is performed on all patients who develop petechiae (small hemorrhages in the skin), spontaneous bleeding, or increasingly heavy menses, or it is used to monitor the course of the disease or therapy for thrombocytopenia or bone marrow failure.

Platelet activity is essential to blood clotting. Counts of 150,000 to 400,000/mm³ are considered normal. Counts less than 100,000/mm³ are considered to indicate *thrombocytopenia*; *thrombocytosis* is said to exist when counts are greater than 400,000/mm³. *Thrombocythemia* is a term used to indicate a platelet count in excess of 1 million/mm³. The most common associative disease with spontaneous thrombocytosis is malignancy (leukemia, lymphoma, or solid tumors, such as colon). Thrombocytosis may also occur with polycythemia vera and postsplenectomy syndromes.

Spontaneous hemorrhage may occur with thrombocytopenia. If thrombocytopenia is severe, the platelets are often hand counted. Spontaneous bleeding is a serious danger when platelet counts fall below 20,000/mm³. Petechiae and ecchymosis also occur at that level of thrombocytopenia. With counts above 40,000/mm³, spontaneous bleeding rarely occurs, but prolonged bleeding from trauma or surgery may occur at this level. Causes of thrombocytopenia (decreased number of platelets) include the following:

1. Reduced production of platelets (secondary to bone marrow failure or infiltration of fibrosis, tumor, etc.)

P

2. Sequestration of platelets (secondary to hypersplenism)
3. Accelerated destruction of platelets (secondary to antibodies [see antiplatelet antibodies p. 643], infections, drugs, prosthetic heart valves)
4. Consumption of platelets (secondary to disseminated intravascular coagulation)
5. Platelet loss from hemorrhage
6. Dilution, with large volume, of blood transfusions that contain very few, if any, platelets

Interfering factors

- Living in high altitudes may cause increased platelet levels.
- Because platelets can clump together, automated counting is subject to at least a 10% to 15% error.
- Strenuous exercise may cause increased levels.
- Decreased levels may be seen before menstruation.
- Drugs that may cause *increased* levels include oral contraceptives.
- Drugs that may cause *decreased* levels include acetaminophen, aspirin, chemotherapeutic agents, chloramphenicol, colchicine, H_2-blocking agents (cimetidine, Zantac), hydralazine, indomethacin, isoniazid (INH), quinidine, streptomycin, sulfonamides, thiazide diuretics, and tolbutamide (Orinase).

Procedure and patient care

Before

- Tell the patient that no fasting is required.

During

- Collect approximately 5 to 7 ml of peripheral venous blood in a lavender-top tube.
- List on the laboratory slip any drugs or other factors that may affect test results.

After

- Apply pressure to the venipuncture site.
- If the results indicate that the patient has a serious platelet deficiency:
  1. Observe the patient for signs and symptoms of bleeding.
  2. Check for blood in the urine and all excretions.
  3. Assess the patient for bruises, petechiae, bleeding from the gums, epistaxis, and low back pain.

4. Reassess all venipuncture sites for signs of hematoma formation.

Abnormal findings

▲ **Increased levels (thrombocytosis)**

Malignant disorder
Polycythemia vera
Postsplenectomy syndrome
Rheumatoid arthritis
Iron deficiency anemia

▼ **Decreased levels (thrombocytopenia)**

Hypersplenism
Hemorrhage
Immune thrombocytopenia
Leukemia and other myelofibrosis disorders
Thrombotic thrombocytopenia
Inherited thrombocytopenia disorders (e.g., Wiskott-Aldrich, Bernard Soulier, or Zieve syndromes)
Disseminated intravascular coagulation
Systemic lupus erythematosus
Pernicious anemia
Hemolytic anemia
Cancer chemotherapy
Infection

P

notes

platelet volume, mean (Mean platelet volume [MPV])

Type of test Blood

Normal findings 25 μm in diameter

Test explanation and related physiology

The MPV is a measure of the volume of a large number of platelets determined by an automated analyzer. MPV is to platelets as mean corpuscular volume (see p. 711) is to the red blood cell.

The MPV varies with total platelet production. In cases of thrombocytopenia, despite a normal reactive bone marrow (e.g., hypersplenism), the normal bone marrow releases immature platelets to attempt to maintain a normal platelet count. These immature platelets are larger, and the MPV is elevated. When bone marrow production of platelets is inadequate, the platelets that are released are small. This will be reflected as a low MPV; in this way the MPV is very useful in the differential diagnosis of thrombocytopenic disorders.

Interfering factors

- Blood collection tubes with ethylenediaminetetraacetic acid can create a variation of as much as 25% in the size of the platelets.

Procedure and patient care

Before

- Explain the procedure to the patient.
- Tell the patient that no fasting is required.

During

- Collect 5 to 7 ml of venous blood in a lavender-top tube.

After

- Apply pressure to the venipuncture site.
- If the patient is known to have a low platelet count:
  1. Observe the patient for signs and symptoms of bleeding.
  2. Check for blood in the urine and all excretions.
  3. Assess the patient for bruises, petechiae, bleeding of the gums, epistaxis, and low back pain.

Abnormal findings

▲ **Increased levels**
Valvular heart disease
Immune thrombo-
cytopenia
Massive hemorrhage
B_{12}/folate deficiency
Myelogenous leukemia

▼ **Decreased levels**
Aplastic anemia
Chemotherapy-induced
myelosuppression
Wiskott-Aldrich syndrome

notes

P

plethysmography, arterial

Type of test Manometric

Normal findings

<20 mm Hg difference in systolic blood pressure of the lower extremity compared with the upper extremity

Normal pulse wave amplitude showing a steep upswing, an acute narrow peak, and a more gentle downslope containing a dicrotic notch (normal arterial pulse wave)

Test explanation and related physiology

Plethysmography is usually performed to rule out occlusive disease of the lower extremities; however, it also can identify arteriosclerotic disease in the upper extremity. This test does require one normal extremity against which the other extremities may be compared.

Arterial plethysmography is performed by applying three blood pressure cuffs to the proximal, middle, and distal parts of the extremity. These are then attached to a pulse volume recorder (plethysmograph), and each pulse wave can be displayed. A reduction in amplitude of a pulse wave in any of the three cuffs indicates arterial occlusion immediately proximal to the area where the decreased amplitude is noted. Also, measurements of arterial pressures are performed at each cuff site. A difference in pressure greater than 20 mm Hg indicates a degree of arterial occlusion in the extremity. A positive result is reliable evidence of arteriosclerotic peripheral vascular occlusion. However, a negative result does not definitely exclude this diagnosis, because extensive vascular collateralization can compensate for even a complete arterial occlusion.

Although it is not as accurate as arteriography (see p. 113), plethysmography is performed without serious complications and can be done for seriously ill patients who cannot be transported to the arteriography laboratory.

Interfering factors

- Arterial occlusion proximal to the extremity
- Cigarette smoking, because nicotine can cause transient arterial constriction

Procedure and patient care

Before

- Explain the procedure to the patient.
- Tell the patient that no fasting is required.
- Inform the patient that this test is painless.
- Tell the patient that he or she must lie still during the testing procedure.
- Remove all clothing from the patient's extremities.
- Instruct the patient to avoid smoking for at least 30 minutes before the test. Nicotine creates constriction of the peripheral arteries and alters the test results.

During

- Note the following procedural steps:
  1. The patient is placed in the semirecumbent position.
  2. The cuffs are applied to the extremities and then inflated to 65 mm Hg to increase their sensitivity to pulse waves.
  3. The pulse waves are recorded on the plethysmographic paper.
  4. The amplitudes and form of the pulse wave of each cuff are measured and compared. A marked reduction in wave amplitude indicates arterial occlusive disease.
- Note that this test usually is performed in the noninvasive vascular laboratory or at the patient's bedside by a noninvasive vascular technologist in approximately 30 minutes.
- Inform the patient that results are usually interpreted by a physician and are available in a few hours.
- Remind the patient that no discomfort is associated with this test.

After

- Encourage the patient to verbalize any concerns regarding the test results.

Abnormal findings

Arterial occlusive disease
Arterial trauma
Small vessel diabetic changes
Vascular diseases (e.g., Raynaud's phenomenon)
Arterial embolization

P

plethysmography, venous (Cuff pressure test)

Type of test Manometric

Normal findings Patent venous system without evidence of thrombosis or occlusion

Test explanation and related physiology

Plethysmography measures changes in the volume of an extremity. Usually this test is performed on a leg to exclude deep-vein thrombosis. During this test, blood pressure cuffs are placed on the proximal, middle, and distal parts of the extremity and attached to a pulse volume recorder. The leg volume can then be recorded as a baseline value. The venous system is occluded by inflating the most proximal cuff (*occlusion cuff*); the most distal cuff (*recording cuff*) should record a sudden increase in venous volume. When the occlusion cuff is released, the venous volume of the leg should return to preocclusion baseline levels. In patients with venous obstruction, no initial increase in leg volume is recorded. Because venous outflow is obstructed, the venous volume of the leg will not dissipate quickly.

The results of venous plethysmography are less accurate than those of venography (see p. 888); however, no complications are associated with this noninvasive study. Plethysmography can be performed easily and quickly on any patient with suspected venous disease. Furthermore, with the use of portable plethysmography, this test can be performed at the bedside for extremely ill patients.

Doppler flow studies are now being performed to identify deep-vein thrombosis, but Doppler flow studies are less accurate in evaluating the venous system below the knee.

Interfering factor

- Venous occlusion more proximal to the site of the occlusion cuff

Procedure and patient care

Before

- Explain the procedure to the patient.
- Tell the patient that no fasting is required.
- Assure the patient that no discomfort is associated with the study.

- Instruct the patient to lie still during the testing.
- Remove all clothing from the patient's extremity to be tested.

During

- Note the following procedural steps:
  1. A large, inflatable occlusion cuff is placed on the proximal part of the extremity, usually a leg.
  2. A second, smaller plethysmographic monitor or recording cuff is placed more distal on the leg. A third cuff may be placed in between the proximal and distal cuffs.
  3. The second cuff is inflated to 10 mm Hg to facilitate recognition of small changes in the leg's venous volume.
  4. The effects of respiration on the leg's venous volume are evaluated. If no significant changes occur with respiration, venous occlusion can be suspected.
  5. The occlusion cuff is inflated to 50 mm Hg. The monitor cuff should demonstrate a rise in venous volume, displayed on the pulse-monitor recorder.
  6. After the highest volume is recorded in the monitor cuff, the occlusion cuff is rapidly deflated. The leg should return to its preocclusion volume within 1 second. If return to preocclusion baseline values is delayed for a long period, venous thrombosis is suspected.
  7. Often this test is performed concomitantly with Doppler ultrasound of the venous system (see p. 329).
- Note that this test is usually performed in the noninvasive vascular laboratory or at the patient's bedside by a noninvasive vascular technologist in approximately 30 minutes.
- Remind the patient that no discomfort is associated with this test.

After

- Note that no special aftercare is needed.

Abnormal findings

Partial venous obstruction
Total venous obstruction

notes

pleural biopsy

Type of test Microscopic examination of tissue

Normal findings No evidence of pathology

Test explanation and related physiology

This test is indicated when the pleural fluid obtained by thoracentesis (see p. 806) is exudative fluid, which suggests infection, neoplasm, or tuberculosis. The pleural biopsy is indicated to distinguish among these disease processes. It is also performed when a plain chest x-ray indicates a pleural-based tumor, reaction, or thickening.

Pleural biopsy is the removal of pleural tissue for histologic examination. It is usually performed by a percutaneous needle biopsy. It also can be performed via thoracoscopy, which is done by inserting a laparoscope into the pleural space for inspection and biopsy of the pleura. Pleural tissue also may be obtained by an *open pleural biopsy*, which involves a limited thoracotomy and requires general anesthesia. For this procedure, a small intercostal incision is made, and the biopsy of the pleura is done under direct observation. The advantage of these open procedures is that a larger piece of pleura can be obtained.

Contraindications

- Patients with prolonged bleeding or clotting times

Potential complications

- Bleeding or injury to the lung
- Pneumothorax

Procedure and patient care

Before

- Explain the procedure to the patient.
- Obtain informed consent for this procedure.
- Tell the patient that no fasting or sedation is required.
- Instruct the patient to remain very still during the procedure.
- Any movement may cause inadvertent needle damage.

During

- Note the following procedural steps for percutaneous needle biopsy:
  1. This procedure is usually performed with the patient in

a sitting position with his or her shoulders and arms elevated and supported by a padded overbed table.

2. After the presence of the fluid has been determined by the thoracentesis technique, the skin overlying the biopsy site is anesthetized and pierced with a scalpel blade.

3. A needle is inserted with a cannula until fluid is removed (some fluid is left in the pleural space after the thoracentesis to make the biopsy easier).

4. The inner needle is removed, and a blunt-tipped, hooked biopsy trocar attached to a three-way stopcock is inserted into the cannula.

5. The patient is instructed to expire all air and then perform the Valsalva maneuver to prevent air from entering the pleural space.

6. The cannula and biopsy trocar are withdrawn while the hook catches the parietal wall and takes a specimen with its cutting edge.

7. Usually three biopsy specimens are taken from different sites at the same session.

8. The specimens are placed in a fixative solution and sent to the laboratory immediately.

9. After the specimens are taken, additional parietal fluid can be removed.

- Note that this procedure is performed by a physician at the patient's bedside, in a special procedure room, or in the physician's office in approximately 30 minutes.

- Because of the local anesthetic, tell the patient that little discomfort is associated with this procedure.

After

- Apply an adhesive bandage to the biopsy site.
- Note that a chest x-ray film is usually taken to detect the potential complication of pneumothorax.
- Observe the patient for signs of respiratory distress (e.g., shortness of breath, diminished breath sounds) on the side of the biopsy.
- Observe the patient's vital signs frequently for evidence of bleeding (increased pulse, decreased blood pressure).
- Ensure that the biopsy specimen is sent immediately to the laboratory.

🏠 **Home care responsibilities**

- Instruct the patient to report any signs of shortness of breath.
- Note any signs of bleeding, such as decreasing blood pressure or increasing pulse.

Abnormal findings

Neoplasm
Tuberculosis

notes

porphyrins and porphobilinogens

Type of test Urine (fresh and 24-hour)

Normal findings

	Male (μg/24 hrs)	Female (μg/24 hrs)
Total porphyrins	8-149	3-78
Uroporphyrin	4-46	3-22
Coproporphyrin	<96	<60

Porphobilinogens: 0-2 mg/24 hr or 0-8.8 μmol/day (SI units)

Test explanation and related physiology

This test is a quantitative measurement of porphyrins and porphobilinogen. Along with measurement of aminolevulinic acid, the various forms of porphyria can be identified.

Porphyria is a group on genetic disorders associated with enzyme deficiencies involved with porphyrin synthesis. Porphyrins (e.g., uroporphyrin and coproporphyrin) and porphobilinogens are important building blocks in the synthesis of heme. Heme in incorporated into hemoglobin within the erythroid cells. Porphyrias are classified according to the location of the accumulation of the porphyrin precursors. In most forms of porphyria, increased levels of porphyrins and porphobilinogen are found in the urine. Heavy metal (lead) intoxication is also associated with increased porphyrins in the urine.

This test is a quantitative analysis of urinary porphyrins and porphobilinogens. If porphyrins are present, the urine may be colored amber-red or burgundy; the urine may turn even darker after standing in the light. Urine tests for porphyrins are not as accurate as plasma measurements and pattern identification for the various forms of porphyria. However, the urine tests are an accurate screening for porphyria, especially the intermittent variety. Although the test can also be done on a fresh stool specimen, random and 24 hour urine collections are more accurate.

Interfering factors

☛ Drugs that may alter test results include aminosalicylic acid (PAS), barbiturates, chloral hydrate, chlorpropamide (Diabinese), ethyl alcohol, griseofulvin, morphine, oral contraceptives, phenazopyridine (Pyridium), procaine, and sulfonamides.

Procedure and patient care

Before
- Explain the procedure to the patient.
- Tell the patient that no fasting is required.

During

Porphobilinogens
- Collect a freshly voided urine specimen.
- Protect the specimen from light.
- For both porphobilinogens and porphyrins, indicate on the laboratory slip any drugs that may affect test results.

Porphyrins
- Instruct the patient to begin a 24-hour urine collection after voiding. Discard the initial specimen and start the 24-hour timing at that point.
- Collect all the urine passed during the next 24 hours.
- Instruct the patient to avoid alcohol during the collection period.
- Show the patient where to store the urine container.
- Keep the specimen on ice or refrigerated during the 24 hours.
- Keep the urine in a light-resistant specimen bottle with a preservative to prevent degradation of the light-sensitive porphyrin.
- Indicate the starting time on the urine container and the laboratory slip.
- Post the times for urine collection in a prominent place to prevent accidental discarding of the specimen.
- Instruct the patient to void before defecating so that urine is not contaminated by feces.
- Remind the patient not to put toilet paper in the collection container.
- Encourage the patient to drink fluids during the 24 hours unless contraindicated for medical purposes.
- Collect the last specimen as close as possible to the end of the 24-hour period. Add this urine to the collection.

After
- Transport the urine specimens promptly to the laboratory.

Abnormal findings

▲   **Increased levels**
    Porphyrias
    Liver disease
    Lead poisoning
    Pellagra

notes

positron emission tomography (PET)

Type of test Nuclear scan, x-ray

Normal findings Normal patterns of tissue metabolism

Test explanation and related physiology

PET is a unique technique that combines the early biochemical assessment of pathology achieved by nuclear medicine with the precise localization achieved by computerized tomography (CT). PET is able to penetrate the body's metabolism by recording tracers of nuclear annihilations in body tissue. The selected tracers are chemically designed to measure body processes (e.g., blood flow and volume, protein metabolism).

A chemical compound with the desired biologic activity is labeled with a radioactive isotope that decays by emitting a positron (or positive electron). The positron combines with an electron, and the two are mutually annihilated with emission of two gamma rays. The gamma rays penetrate the surrounding tissue and are recorded outside the body by a circular array of detectors. Because the gamma rays travel in almost exactly opposite directions, their source can be established with a high degree of accuracy. A computer reconstructs the spatial distribution of the radioactivity for a selected plane within the patient and displays the resulting image on a cathode ray screen. PET provides noninvasive regional assessment of many biochemical processes essential to the functioning of the organ being studied.

The technology of PET is now well developed, and both its capabilities and limitations are being increasingly understood. Many PET studies are being carried out with results that cannot be obtained by other techniques. These include:

1. Determination of regional metabolism in the heart and brain (e.g., radioactive glucose used to map biochemical activity in the brain)
2. Studies of tissue permeability
3. Measurement of the size of infarcts in the heart from a coronary occlusion
4. Investigation into the physiology of psychosis
5. Assessment of the effects of drugs on diseased or malfunctioning tissues
6. Possibility of measuring the effects of cancer treatment by

changes in malignant tissues and by biochemical reactions in surrounding normal tissues

Interfering factors

- Recent use (within 24 hours) of caffeine, alcohol, or tobacco may affect test results.
- Excessive anxiety may affect brain function evaluation.
- Drugs that may influence results include tranquilizers and sedatives.

Procedure and patient care

Before

- Explain the procedure to the patient. Because many patients have not heard of this study, they are often anxious and require emotional support.
- Obtain informed consent if required by the institution.
- Inform the patient that he or she may have two IV lines inserted, one for infusion of the radioisotope and the other for serial blood samples.
- Inform the patient that he or she does not need to restrict food or fluids on the day of the test; however, the patient should refrain from alcohol, caffeine, and tobacco for 24 hours.
- Instruct patients with diabetes to take their pretest dose of insulin at a meal 3 to 4 hours before the test.
- Tell the patient that no sedatives or tranquilizers should be taken because he or she may need to perform certain mental activities during the test.
- Tell the patient to empty the bladder before the test for comfort.

During

- Note the following procedural steps:
  1. The patient is positioned in a comfortable, reclining chair.
  2. Two IV lines are inserted.
  3. The radioactive material can be infused through an IV line or inhaled as a radioactive gas.
  4. The gamma rays that penetrate the tissues are recorded outside the body by a circular array of detectors and are displayed by a computer.
  5. If the brain is being scanned, the patient may be asked to perform different cognitive activities (e.g., reciting the

Pledge of Allegiance) to measure changes in brain activity during reasoning or remembering.

6. Extraneous auditory and visual stimuli are minimized by a blindfold and ear plugs.

- Note that this procedure is performed by a physician or trained technologist in approximately 60 to 90 minutes.
- Tell the patient that the only discomfort associated with this study is insertion of the two IV lines.

After

- Instruct the patient to change position slowly from lying to standing to avoid postural hypotension.
- Encourage the patient to drink fluids and urinate frequently to aid removal of the radioisotope from the bladder.

Abnormal findings

Myocardial infarction
Cerebrovascular accident (stroke)
Epilepsy
Parkinson's disease
Dementia
Alzheimer's disease
Schizophrenia
Coronary artery disease
Pulmonary edema
Pneumonia
Brain tumor
Breast tumor
Huntington's disease

notes

potassium, blood (K⁺)

Type of test Blood

Normal findings

Adults/elderly: 3.5-5 mEq/L or 3.5-5 mmol/L (SI units)
Child: 3.4-4.7 mEq/L
Infant: 4.1-5.3 mEq/L
Newborn: 3.9-5.9 mEq/L

Possible critical values

Adult: <2.5 or >6.5 mEq/L
Newborn: <2.5 or >8 mEq/L

Test explanation and related physiology

Potassium is the major cation within the cell. The intracellular potassium concentration is approximately 150 mEq/L, whereas the normal serum potassium concentration is approximately 4 mEq/L. Because the serum concentration of potassium is so small, minor changes in concentration have significant consequences. K is excreted by the kidneys. There is no resorption of K from the kidneys. Therefore, if K is not adequately supplied in the diet (or by IV administration in the patient who is unable to eat), serum K levels can drop rapidly.

Serum potassium concentration depends on many factors, including the following:

1. *Aldosterone* (and, to a lesser extent, the glucocorticosteroids). This hormone tends to increase renal losses of potassium.
2. *Sodium resorption*. As sodium is resorbed, potassium is lost.
3. *Acid-base balance*. Alkalotic states tend to lower serum potassium levels by causing a shift of potassium into the cell. Acidotic states tend to raise serum potassium levels by reversing that shift.

Symptoms of *hyperkalemia* include irritability, nausea, vomiting, intestinal colic, and diarrhea. The electrocardiogram may demonstrate peaked T waves, a widened QRS complex, and depressed ST segment. Signs of *hypokalemia* are related to a decrease in contractility of smooth, skeletal, and cardiac muscles, which results in weakness, paralysis, hyporeflexia, ileus, increased cardiac sensitivity to digoxin, cardiac arrhythmias, flattened T

P

waves, and prominent U waves. This electrolyte has profound effects on the heart rate and contractility. The potassium level should be carefully followed in patients with uremia, Addison's disease, vomiting and diarrhea, and steroid therapy and in patients taking potassium-depleting diuretics. K must be closely monitored in patients taking digitalis-like drugs because cardiac arrhythmias may be induced by hypokalemia and digoxin.

Interfering factors

- Movement of the forearm with a tourniquet in place may increase potassium levels.
- Hemolysis of blood during venipuncture causes increased levels.
- Drugs that may cause *increased* potassium levels include aminocaproic acid, antibiotics, antineoplastic drugs, captopril, epinephrine, heparin, histamine, isoniazid (INH), lithium, mannitol, potassium-sparing diuretics, potassium supplements, and succinylcholine.
- Drugs that may cause *decreased* levels include acetazolamide, aminosalicylic acid (PAS), amphotericin B, carbenicillin, cisplatin, diuretics (potassium wasting), glucose infusions, insulin, laxatives, lithium carbonate, penicillin G sodium (high doses), phenothiazines, salicylates (aspirin), and sodium polystyrene sulfonate (Kayexalate).

Procedure and patient care

Before

- Explain the procedure to the patient.
- Tell the patient that no special diet or fasting is required.

During

- Instruct the patient to avoid opening and closing the hand after a tourniquet is applied.
- Collect approximately 5 to 7 ml of venous blood in a red- or green-top tube.
- Avoid hemolysis.
- Indicate on the laboratory slip any drugs that may affect test results.

After

- Apply pressure to the venipuncture site.
- Evaluate the patient with increased or decreased potassium levels for cardiac arrhythmias.

- Monitor for hypokalemia in patients taking digoxin and diuretics.
- If indicated, administer resin exchanges (e.g., Kayexalate enema) to correct hyperkalemia.

Abnormal findings

▲ **Increased levels (hyperkalemia)**

Excessive dietary intake
Excessive IV intake
Acute or chronic renal failure
Hypoaldosteronism
Aldosterone-inhibiting diuretics
Crush injury to tissues
Hemolysis
Transfusion of hemolyzed blood
Infection
Acidosis
Dehydration

▼ **Decreased levels (hypokalemia)**

Deficient dietary intake
Deficient IV intake
Burns
Gastrointestinal disorders (e.g., diarrhea, vomiting)
Diuretics
Hyperaldosteronism
Cushing's syndrome
Renal tubular acidosis
Licorice ingestion
Insulin administration
Glucose administration
Ascites
Renal artery stenosis
Cystic fibrosis
Trauma
Surgery

P

notes

potassium, urine (K$^+$)

Type of test Urine (24-hour)

Normal findings

25-120 mEq/L/day or 25-120 mmol/day (SI units)
Values vary greatly with diet

Test explanation and related physiology

Potassium is the major cation within the cell (see p. 663. Potassium can be measured in both a spot and a 24-hour urine collection.

The urine potassium concentration depends on many factors. Aldosterone and, to a lesser extent, glucocorticosteroids tend to increase the renal losses of potassium. Acid-base balance is dependent on potassium excretion to a small degree. In alkalotic states, H$^+$ ions can be resorbed in exchange for K$^+$ ions. The kidneys cannot resorb potassium. Therefore the intake of potassium is balanced by kidney excretion through the urine.

Interfering factors

- Dietary intake affects potassium levels.
- Excessive intake of licorice may cause increased levels of potassium in the urine.
- Drugs that may cause *increased* levels include diuretics, glucocorticoids, and salicylates.

Procedure and patient care

Before
- Explain the procedure to the patient.
- Tell the patient that no special diet is required.

During
- Instruct the patient to begin the 24-hour urine collection after voiding.
- Discard the initial specimen and start the 24-hour timing at that point.
- Collect all urine passed during the next 24 hours.
- Show the patient where to store the urine container.
- Keep the specimen on ice or refrigerated during the entire 24 hours.

- Indicate the starting time on the urine container and the laboratory slip.
- Post the hours for urine collection in a noticeable place to prevent accidental discarding of the specimen.
- Instruct the patient to void before defecating so that the urine is not contaminated by feces.
- Remind the patient not to put toilet paper in the collection container.
- Encourage the patient to drink fluids during the 24 hours.
- Instruct the patient to collect the last specimen as close as possible to the end of the 24-hour collection. Add this urine to the container.

After

- Transport the urine specimen promptly to the laboratory.

Abnormal findings

▲ **Increased levels**
    Chronic renal failure
    Renal tubular acidosis
    Cushing's syndrome
    Hyperaldosteronism
    Excessive intake of licorice
    Alkalosis
    Diuretic therapy

▼ **Decreased levels**
    Dehydration
    Addison's disease
    Malnutrition
    Vomiting
    Diarrhea
    Malabsorption
    Acute renal failure

notes

P

prealbumin (PAB, Thyroxine-binding prealbumin [TBPA], Thyretin, Transthyretin)

Type of test Blood; urine (24-hour); cerebrospinal fluid (CSF) analysis

Normal findings

Serum

Adult/elderly: 15-36 mg/dl or 150-360 mg/L (SI units)
Child
    Cord: 13 mg/dl or 130 mg/L (SI units)
    1 year: 10 mg/dl or 100 mg/L
    2-36 months: 16-28 mg/dl or 160-280 mg/L

Urine (24-hour)

0.017-0.047 mg/day

Cerebrospinal fluid

Approximately 2% of total CSF protein

Possible critical values Serum prealbumin levels <10.7 mg/dl indicate severe nutritional deficiency.

Test explanation and related physiology

Prealbumin is one of the major plasma proteins. Because prealbumin can bind thyroxine, it is also called *thyroxine-binding prealbumin* (TBA). However, prealbumin is secondary to thyroxine-binding globulin in the transportation of triiodothyronine (T_3) and thyroxine (T_4). Prealbumin also plays a role in the transport and metabolism of vitamin A.

Since prealbumin levels in serum fluctuate more rapidly in response to alterations in synthetic rate than do those of other serum proteins, clinical interest in the quantification of serum prealbumin has centered on its usefulness as a marker of nutritional status. Its half-life of 1.9 days is much less than the 21-day half-life of albumin (see p. 686). Because prealbumin has a short half-life, it is a sensitive indicator of any change affecting protein synthesis and catabolism. Because of this, prealbumin is frequently ordered to monitor the effectiveness of total parenteral nutrition (TPN).

Prealbumin is significantly reduced in hepatobiliary disease because of impaired synthesis. Prealbumin is also a negative acute-phase reactant protein; serum levels decrease in inflammation, malignancy, and protein-wasting diseases of the intestines or kidneys. Since zinc is required for synthesis of prealbumin, low levels occur with a zinc deficiency. Increased levels of prealbumin occur in Hodgkin's disease and during chronic kidney disease.

Interfering factors

- Coexistent inflammation may make test result interpretation impossible.
- Drugs that may cause *increased* levels include anabolic steroids, androgens, and prednisolone.
- Drugs that may cause *decreased* levels include amiodarone, estrogens, and oral contraceptives.

Procedure and patient care

Before

- Explain the procedure to the patient.
- Tell the patient that no food or fluid restrictions are needed.
- If the patient is going to collect a 24-hour urine specimen, provide a collection bottle.

During

- Collect a venous blood sample in a red-top tube.

After

- Apply pressure to the venipuncture site.
- Transport the 24-hour urine specimen promptly to the laboratory.
- Inform the patient how and when to obtain the results of this study.

Abnormal findings

▲ **Increased levels**
  Some cases of nephrotic
    syndrome
  Hodgkin's disease
  Chronic kidney disease
  Pregnancy

▼ **Decreased levels**
  Malnutrition
  Liver damage
  Burns
  Salicylate poisoning
  Inflammation

pregnancy tests (Human chorionic gonadotropin [HCG])

Type of test   Blood; urine

Normal findings

Qualitative: negative; positive in pregnancy
Quantitative
  Whole HCG

Gestation (wk)	Whole HCG (mIU/ml)
<1	5-50
2	50-500
3	100-10,000
4	1,000-30,000
5	3,500-115,000
6-8	12,000-270,000
12	15,000-220,000
Males and nonpregnant females	<5

B subunit: normal values depend on the method and test used

Test explanation and related physiology

All pregnancy tests are based on the detection of HCG, which is secreted by the placental trophoblast after the ovum is fertilized. HCG will appear in the blood and urine of pregnant women as early as 10 days after conception. In the first few weeks of pregnancy, HCG markedly rises, and serum levels are higher than urine levels. After about a month, HCG is about the same in either specimen.

HCG is made up of alpha and beta subunits. The alpha subunit is the same for all the glycoprotein hormones. The beta subunit is specific for HCG.

It is important to know that all these pregnancy studies demonstrate the presence of HCG. Methods of pregnancy testing fall into three categories: immunologic, radioimmunologic, and radioreceptor assays. Biologic (animal) tests have been used since the 1920s. They are primarily of historical interest today and are not discussed here.

Immunologic tests (agglutination inhibition test [AIT]) (blood and urine)

Immunologic tests are performed using commercially prepared antibodies against the whole HCG molecule and can be completed within 2 minutes or 2 hours, depending on the method used. Previous immunologic tests had a high false-positive rate and were usually not positive until about 28 days after the last menses. However, immunologic testing for the beta subunit of HCG greatly improved accuracy and shortened the time for positive testing (18 days). Now, with the development of monoclonal antibodies, immunoassays can identify very small levels of HCG, and pregnancy can be detected 3 to 7 days after conception. Several immunologic tests are now commercially available for testing by the public. In these tests the patient's urine is tested, and its color is compared to a standard containing a known small amount of HCG. If the color matches that standard, pregnancy is present. These tests take from 5 to 120 minutes to perform.

Radioimmunoassay (RIA) (serum)

The RIA is a highly sensitive and reliable blood test for the detection of the beta unit of HCG. This study requires a blood sample; however, RIA also may be performed with a urine test. The test can be done in 1 to 5 hours. This test is so sensitive that pregnancy can be diagnosed before the first missed menstrual period.

Radioreceptor assay (RRA) (serum)

The RRA for serum HCG is highly sensitive and accurate. This test can be performed in 1 hour. The major advantage of this study is its reliable diagnosis of early gestation in patients requesting an early termination of pregnancy and in cases in which infertile couples are anxious to confirm pregnancy. This study is 90% to 95% accurate 6 to 8 days after conception. Even the minute amounts of HCG secreted in an ectopic pregnancy can be measured. This test is also used in looking for early spontaneous abortion in patients who have difficulties maintaining early pregnancy.

• • •

Normally HCG is not present in nonpregnant women. In a very small number of women (<5%), HCG exists in minute levels. The presence of HCG does not necessarily indicate a normal pregnancy. Ectopic pregnancy, hydatidiform mole of the uterus, and choriocarcinoma of the uterus can all produce HCG. Germ cell tumors (choriocarcinoma and embryonal cell cancers) of the testes or ovaries can produce HCG in men and nonpregnant women, respectively. Primary liver cell cancers (hepatoma) can also make HCG. In tumors HCG is used as a valuable tumor marker that can be used to monitor and identify tumor activity.

Interfering factors

- Tests performed too early in the pregnancy, before a significant HCG level exists, may cause false-negative results.
- Hematuria and proteinuria in the urine may cause false-positive results.
- Hemolysis of blood may interfere with test results.
- Urine pregnancy tests can very according to the dilution of the urine. HCH levels may not be detectable on a dilute urine but may be quite detectable on a concentrated urine.
- Drugs that may cause false-negative urine results include diuretics (by causing diluted urine) and promethazine.
- Drugs that may cause false-positive results include anticonvulsants, antiparkinsonian drugs, hypnotics, and tranquilizers (especially promazine and its derivatives).

Procedure and patient care

Before
- Explain the procedure to the patient.
- If a urine specimen will be collected, give the patient a urine container the evening before so that she can provide a first-voided morning specimen. This specimen generally contains the greatest concentration of HCG.

During
- Collect the first-voided urine specimen for urine testing.
- Collect approximately 7 to 10 ml of venous blood in a red-top tube for serum testing. Avoid hemolysis.

After
- Apply pressure to the venipuncture site.
- Emphasize to the patient the importance of antepartal health care.

Abnormal findings

▲ **Increased levels**
Pregnancy
Ectopic pregnancy
Hydatidiform mole of the uterus
Choriocarcinoma of the uterus, testes, or ovaries
Tumor

▼ **Decreased levels**
Threatened abortion
Incomplete abortion
Dead fetus

pregnanediol

Type of test   Urine (24-hour)

Normal findings
<9 years: <0.1 mg/day
10-15 years: 0.1-1.2 mg/day
Adult male: 0-1.9 mg/day
Adult female
   Follicular phase: <2.6 mg/day
   Luteal: 2.6-10.6 mg/day
Pregnancy
   First trimester: 10-35 mg/day
   Second trimester: 35-70 mg/day
   Third trimester: 70-100 mg/day

Test explanation and related physiology

Urinary pregnanediol is measured to evaluate progesterone production by the ovaries and placenta. The main effect of progesterone is on the endometrium. It initiates the endometrial secretory phase in anticipation of implantation of a fertilized ovum. Normally progesterone is secreted by the ovarian corpus luteum following ovulation. Both serum progesterone levels and the urine concentration of progesterone metabolites (pregnanediol and others) are significantly increased during the later half of an ovulatory cycle. Pregnanediol is the most easily measured metabolite of progesterone.

Because pregnanediol levels rise rapidly after ovulation, this study is useful in documenting whether ovulation has occurred and, if so, its exact time. During pregnancy pregnanediol levels normally rise because of the placental production of progesterone. Repeated assays can be used to monitor the status of the placenta in women who are having difficulty becoming pregnant or maintaining a pregnancy. It is also used to monitor "high risk" pregnancies.

Hormone assays for urinary pregnanediol are primarily used today to monitor progesterone supplementation in patients with an inadequate luteal phase. Urinary assays may be supplemented by plasma assays (progesterone assay, see p. 676), which are quicker and more accurate.

Interfering factors

- �308 Drugs that may cause *increased* levels include adrenocortico-tropic hormone.
- �308 Drugs that may cause *decreased* levels include oral contraceptives and progesterones.

Procedure and patient care

Before

- Explain the procedure to the patient.
- Tell the patient that usually no special diet is required.
- Inform the patient that no sedation or fasting is necessary.

During

- Instruct the patient to begin the 24-hour urine collection. Discard the initial specimen and start the 24-hour timing at that point.
- Collect all urine passed for the next 24 hours.
- Show the patient where to store the urine collection.
- Keep the specimen on ice or refrigerated during the 24 hours. Check with the laboratory to see if a preservative is needed.
- Indicate the starting time on the urine container and the laboratory slip.
- Post the hours for urine collection in a noticeable place to prevent accidental discarding of the specimen.
- Instruct the patient to void before defecating so that the urine is not contaminated by feces.
- Remind the patient not to put toilet paper in the collection container.
- Encourage the patient to drink fluids during the 24 hours.
- Instruct the patient to collect the last specimen as close as possible to the end of the 24-hour collection. Add this urine to the container.

After

- Record on the laboratory slip the date of the last menstrual period or the week of gestation during pregnancy.

Abnormal findings

▲ **Increased levels**
Ovulation
Pregnancy
Luteal cysts of ovary
Arrhenoblastoma of ovary
Hyperadrenocorticalism
Choriocarcinoma of ovary
Adrenocortical hyperplasia

▼ **Decreased levels**
Threatened abortion
Fetal death
Toxemia of pregnancy
Amenorrhea
Ovarian hypofunction
Placental failure
Preeclampsia
Ovarian neoplasm
Breast neoplasm

notes

P

progesterone assay

Type of test Blood

Normal findings (extraction/radioimmunoassay)

<9 years: <20 ng/dl
10-15 years: 20 ng/dl
Adult male: 10-50 ng/dl
Adult female
   Follicular phase: <50 ng/dl
   Luteal: 300-2,500 ng/dl
   Postmenopausal: <40 ng/dl
Pregnancy
   First trimester: 725-4,400 ng/dl
   Second trimester: 1,950-8,250 ng/dl
   Third trimester: 6,500-22,900 ng/dl

Test explanation and related physiology

The major effect of progesterone is to induce the development of the secretory phase of the endometrium in anticipation of implantation of a fertilized ovum. Normally, progesterone is secreted by the ovarian corpus luteum following ovulation. Serum progesterone level is significantly increased during the later half of the ovulatory cycle. Normally, blood samples drawn at days 8 and 21 of the menstrual cycle show a large increase in progesterone levels in the latter specimen, indicating that ovulation has occurred. Therefore this study is useful in documenting whether ovulation has occurred and, if so, its exact time. This is very useful information for a women who has difficulty becoming pregnant. A series of measurements can help define the day of ovulation.

In pregnancy progesterone is produced by the corpus luteum for the first few weeks. After that, the placenta begins to make progesterone. Progesterone levels should progressively rise during pregnancy because of the placental production. Repeated assays can be used to monitor the status of the placenta in cases of "high-risk" pregnancy. Progesterone assay is also used today to monitor progesterone supplementation in patients with an inadequate luteal phase to maintain an early pregnancy.

Interfering factors

- Recent use of radioisotopes may affect test results.
- Hemolysis caused by rough handling of the sample may affect test results.
- Drugs that may interfere with test results include estrogen and progesterone.

Procedure and patient care

Before

- Explain the procedure to the patient.
- Tell the patient that no fasting is required.

During

- Collect approximately 5 to 7 ml of venous blood in a red-top tube.
- Indicate the date of the last menstrual period on the laboratory slip.

After

- Apply pressure to the venipuncture site.

Abnormal findings

▲ **Increased levels**

   Ovulation
   Pregnancy
   Luteal cysts of ovary
   Hyperadrenocorticalism
   Adrenocortical hyperplasia
   Choriocarcinoma of ovary
   Molar pregnancy

▼ **Decreased levels**

   Preeclampsia
   Toxemia of pregnancy
   Threatened abortion
   Placental failure
   Fetal death
   Ovarian neoplasm
   Amenorrhea
   Ovarian hypofunction

notes

progesterone receptor assay (PR assay, PRA, PgR)

Type of test Tumor-specimen analysis

Normal values

Negative: <10 fmol/g of tissue
Positive: >10 fmol/g of tissue

Test explanation and related physiology

The PR assay is used in determining the prognosis and treatment of breast cancer and, to a lesser degree, other cancers. These assays help to determine whether a tumor is likely to respond to endocrine medical or surgical therapy. The test is done on breast cancer specimens when a primary or recurrent cancer is identified; it is usually done in conjunction with estrogen receptor (ER) assay (see p. 383) to increase the predictability of a tumor response to hormone therapy. PR levels tend to be higher in the breast cancer of postmenopausal women. PR-positive tumors are suspected to be associated with a better prognosis than PR-negative tumors. Tumor response rates to medical or surgical hormonal manipulation are potentiated if the ER assay is positive. Response rates are as follows:

ER positive, PR positive 75%
ER negative, PR positive 45%
ER positive, PR negative 35%
ER negative, PR negative 15

In the past, 1 g of the breast cancer specimen has been sent to a centralized laboratory, where the PR protein is quantified in the cytoplasm or nucleus of breast cancer cells. A newer method, however, provides more accurate information on paraffin-embedded tissue using immunohistochemical staining for PR proteins.

Other tumors (such as ovarian, melanoma, uterine, or pancreatic) are occasionally studied for ER and PR assay. This is mostly done within clinical trials. To date, hormonal therapy has not been very successful with these tumors.

Interfering factors

- Exogenous hormone use
- Use of hormones such as progesterone or estrogen may cause false-negative results.

Procedure and patient care

Before

- Prepare the patient for breast biopsy per routine protocol.
- Record the menstrual status of the patient.
- Record any exogenous hormone the patient may have used during the last 2 months.
- Instruct the patient to discontinue exogenous hormones before breast biopsy.

During

- The surgeon obtains tissue.
- The specimen is place on ice and sent to the laboratory immediately.
- In the pathology department, part of the specimen is used for routine histology. A smaller part is sent to a central laboratory for PR analysis.
- Results are usually available in 2 weeks.

After

- Provide routine postoperative care.

Abnormal findings

▲ **Increased levels**
  Hormonally dependent cancer

notes

P

prolactin levels (PRLs)

Type of test   Blood

Normal findings

Adult male: 0-20 ng/ml
Adult female: 0-20 ng/ml
Pregnant female: 20-400 ng/ml

Test explanation and related physiology

Prolactin is a hormone secreted by the anterior pituitary gland (adenohypophysis). In females prolactin promotes lactation. Its role in males is not clear. During sleep, prolactin levels increase twofold to threefold, to circulating levels equaling those of pregnant women. With breast stimulation, pregnancy, nursing, stress, or exercise, a surge of this hormone occurs. It is elevated in patients with prolactin-secreting pituitary acidophilic or chromophobic adenomas. To a lesser extent, moderately high prolactin levels have been observed in women with secondary amenorrhea (i.e., postpubertal) and galactorrhea. Paraneoplastic tumors (e.g., lung cancer) may cause ectopic secretion of prolactin as well. In general, very high prolactin levels are more likely to be caused by pituitary adenoma than other causes.

The prolactin level is helpful for monitoring the disease activity of pituitary adenomas. Several *prolactin stimulation tests* (with TRH or chlorpromazine) and *prolactin suppression tests* (with levodopa) have been designed to help differentiate pituitary adenoma from some of the other causes of prolactin overproduction.

Interfering factors

- Stress from illness, trauma, surgery or even the fear of a blood test can elevate prolactin levels. In cases in which the patient is fearful of venipuncture, it is best to place a heparin lock and withdraw the blood specimen 2 hours later.
- Drugs that may cause *increased* values include phenothiazines, oral contraceptives, reserpine, opiates, verapamil, histamine antagonists, monoamine oxidase inhibitors, estrogens, and antihistamines.
- Drugs that may cause *decreased* values are ergot alkaloid derivatives, clonidine, levodopa, and dopamine.

Procedure and patient care

Before

- Explain the procedure to the patient.
- Tell the patient no fasting or special preparation is required.
- Inform the patient that this blood sample should be drawn in the morning.
- Record the use of any medication that may affect results.

During

- Obtain 5 to 7 ml of venous blood in a red-top tube.
- Transfer the specimen to the laboratory as soon as possible. If a delay occurs, the specimen should be placed on ice.

After

- Apply pressure to the venipuncture site.

Abnormal findings

▲ **Increased levels**

Galactorrhea
Amenorrhea
Prolactin-secreting pituitary tumor
Infiltrative diseases of the hypothalamus and pituitary stalk (e.g., granuloma, sarcoidosis)
Hypothyroidism
Renal failure
Anorexia nervosa
Perineoplastic ectopic production of prolactin
Metastatic cancer to the pituitary gland
Polycystic ovary syndrome
Stress such as anorexia nervosa, surgery, strenuous exercise, trauma, or severe illness
Empty sella syndrome

▼ **Decreased levels**

Pituitary apoplexy
Pituitary destruction from tumor (craniopharyngioma)

P

prostate/rectal sonogram (Ultrasound prostate)

Type of test Ultrasound

Normal findings Normal size, contour, and consistency of the prostate gland

Test explanation and related physiology

Rectal ultrasound of the prostate is a very valuable tool in the early diagnosis of prostate cancer. When combined with rectal digital examination and prostate-specific antigen (see p. 684), very small prostate cancers can be identified. Prostate/rectal sonography is also helpful in evaluating the seminal vessels and other perirectal tissue. Ultrasound is very helpful in guiding the direction of a prostate biopsy and can be extremely helpful in quantitating the volume of prostate cancer. When radiation therapy implantation is required for treatment, ultrasound is used to map the exact location of the prostate cancer. Rectal ultrasound is very helpful in staging rectal cancers as well. The depth of transmural involvement and presence of extrarectal extension can be accurately assessed.

Real-time ultrasonography requires the emission of high-frequency sound waves from a special transducer placed in the rectum. The sound waves are bounced back to the transducer and electronically converted into a pictorial image.

Contraindications

- Patients with latex allergy
  Rectal ultrasound requires placement of the probe in a latex condom-like sac. Patients with a latex allergy may react significantly to that contact.

Interfering factor

- Stool within the rectum

Procedure and patient care

Before

- Explain the procedure to the patient.
- Instruct the patient that a small-volume rectal enema is required approximately 1 hour before the ultrasound examination.

During

- The patient is placed in the left lateral decubitus position.
- A digital rectal examination may be performed to assess the prostate gland or rectal tumor.
- A draped and lubricated ultrasound probe is placed within the rectum.
- Scans are performed in various spatial planes.

After

- Provide the patient with tissue material to cleanse the perianal area.

Abnormal findings

Prostate cancer
Benign prostatic hypertrophy
Prostatitis
Seminal vesicle tumor
Prostate abscess
Perirectal abscess
Intrarectal or perirectal tumor

notes

P

prostate-specific antigen (PSA)

Type of test Blood

Normal findings <4 ng/ml

Test explanation and related physiology

PSA is a glycoprotein (part carbohydrate, part protein) normally found in the cytoplasm of prostatic epithelial cells. This antigen can be detected in all males; however, its level is greatly increased in patients with prostatic cancer. The higher the levels, the greater the tumor burden. Furthermore, the PSA assay is a sensitive test for monitoring response to therapy. Successful surgery, radiation, or hormone therapy is associated with a marked reduction in the PSA blood level. Subsequent significant elevation in PSA indicates the recurrence of prostatic cancer.

Prostate-specific antigen is more sensitive and specific than other prostatic tumor markers such as prostatic acid phosphatase (PAP, see p. 7). Also, PSA is more accurate than PAP in monitoring response and recurrence of tumor after therapy.

PSA (and PAP) levels also may be minimally elevated in patients with benign prostatic hypertrophy (BPH) and prostatitis. PSA levels greater than 10 ng/ml indicate a high probability for prostate cancer. Lower values may be compatible with BPH or early prostate cancer. Several formulas have been created to partially correct for BPH, which normally occurs in elderly men (e.g., predicted PSA = 0.12 × gland volume [in cubic centimeters] as determined by ultrasound). PSA levels have been age adjusted by some investigators. Levels above those predicted by age or size of gland would be compatible with cancer. Another way to tell whether moderate elevations in PSA levels are caused by cancer or BPH is to repeat the PSA level at 3- to 6-month intervals. A rising trend would indicate cancer. PSA has been recommended for routine use in screening men over 50 years of age. When combined with direct digital rectal examination, it can detect 90% of prostate cancers.

Interfering factors

Rectal examinations, known to falsely elevate PAP levels, may also minimally elevate PSA levels. To avoid this problem, the PSA specimen should be drawn before rectal examination of the prostate or several hours afterwards.

Prostatic manipulation by biopsy or transurethral resection of the prostate (TURP) may elevate the PSA levels. The blood test should be done before the surgery or 6 weeks afterwards.

Procedure and patient care

Before

- Explain the procedure to the patient.
- Tell the patient that no fasting is required.

During

- Collect approximately 5 ml of blood in a red-top tube.

After

- Apply pressure to the venipuncture site.

Abnormal findings

▲ **Increased levels**

Prostate cancer
Benign prostatic hypertrophy
Prostatitis

notes

P

protein, blood (Albumin, blood; Serum albumin; Serum globulin; Total protein, protein electrophoresis)

Type of test Blood

Normal findings

Adult/elderly
  Total protein: 6.4-8.3 g/dl or 64-83 g/L (SI units)
  Albumin: 3.5-5 g/dl or 35-50 g/L (SI units)
  Globulin: 2.3-3.4 g/dl
    Alpha$_1$ globulin: 0.1-0.3 g/dl or 1-3 g/L (SI units)
    Alpha$_2$ globulin: 0.6-1 g/dl or 6-10 g/L (SI units)
    Beta globulin: 0.7-1.1 g/dl or 7-11 g/L (SI units)
Children
  Total protein
    Premature infant: 4.2-7.6 g/dl
    Newborn: 4.6-7.4 g/dl
    Infant: 6-6.7 g/dl
    Child: 6.2-8 g/dl
  Albumin
    Premature infant: 3-4.2 g/dl
    Newborn: 3.5-5.4 g/dl
    Infant: 4.4-5.4 g/dl
    Child: 4-5.9 g/dl

Test explanation and related physiology

Proteins are constituents of muscle, enzymes, hormones, transport vehicles, hemoglobin, and several other key functional and structural entities within the body. They are the most significant component contributing to the osmotic pressure within the vascular space. This osmotic pressure keeps fluid within the vascular space, minimizing extravasation of fluid.

Albumin and globulin constitute most of the protein within the body and are measured in the total protein. *Albumin* is a protein that is formed within the liver. It makes up approximately 60% of the total protein. The major effect of albumin within the blood is to maintain colloidal osmotic pressure. Furthermore, albumin transports important blood constituents such as drugs, hormones, and enzymes. Albumin is synthesized within the liver and is therefore a measure of hepatic function. When disease affects the liver cell, the hepatocyte loses its ability to synthesize albumin. The serum albumin level is greatly decreased. Because the half-life of albumin is 12 to 18 days, however, severe impairment of hepatic albumin synthesis may not be recognized until after that period.

Globulins are the key building block of antibodies. Their role in maintaining osmotic pressure is far less than that of albumin. Alpha$_1$ globulins are mostly alpha$_1$ antitrypsin. Some transporting proteins such as thyroid and cortisol-binding globulin also contribute to this electrophoretic zone. Alpha$_2$ globulins include serum haptoglobins (bind hemoglobin during hemolysis), ceruloplasmin (carrier for copper), prothrombin, and cholinesterase (an enzyme used in the catabolism of acetylcholine). Beta globulins include lipoproteins, transferrin, plasminogen, and complement proteins; beta$_2$ globulins include fibrinogen. Gamma globulins are the immune globulins (antibodies) (see p. 491). To a lesser degree, globulins also act as transport vehicles.

Serum albumin and globulin are measures of nutrition. Malnourished patients, especially after surgery, have a greatly decreased level of serum proteins. Burn patients and patients who have protein-losing enteropathies and uropathies have low levels of protein, despite normal synthesis. Pregnancy, especially the third trimester, is usually associated with reduced total proteins.

In some diseases albumin is selectively diminished, and globulins are normal or increased to maintain a normal total protein level. For example, in collagen vascular diseases (e.g., lupus erythematosus), capillary permeability is increased. Albumin, a molecule much smaller than globulin, is selectively lost into the extravascular space. Another group of diseases similarly associated with low albumin, high globulin, and normal total protein levels is chronic liver diseases. In these diseases the liver cannot produce albumin, but globulin is adequately made in the reticuloendothelial system. In both these types of diseases, the albumin level is low, but the total protein level is normal because of increased globulin levels. These changes, however, can be detected if one measures the albumin/globulin ratio. Normally this ratio exceeds 1.0. The diseases just described that selectively affect albumin levels are associated with lesser ratios. Increased total protein levels, particularly the globulin fraction, occur with multiple myeloma and other gammopathies. It is important to note that the albumin fraction of the total protein can be factitiously elevated in dehydrated patients.

Serum protein electrophoresis can separate the various components of blood protein into bands or zones according to their electrical charge. Several well-established electrophoretic patterns have been identified and can be associated with specific diseases (Table 14).

TABLE 14 Protein electrophoresis patterns in specific diseases

Pattern	Electrophoresis	Disease
Acute reaction	↓ Albumin ↑ Alpha$_2$ globulin	Acute infections, tissue necrosis, burns, surgery, stress, myocardial infarction
Chronic inflammatory	sl. ↓ Albumin sl. ↑ Gamma globulin $\overline{N}$ Alpha$_2$ globulin	Chronic infection, granulomatous diseases, cirrhosis, rheumatoid-collagen diseases
Nephrotic syndrome	↓↓ Albumin ↑↑ Alpha$_2$ globulin $\overline{N}$ ↑ Beta globulin	Nephrotic syndrome
Far-advanced cirrhosis	↓ Albumin ↑ Gamma globulin Incorporation of beta and gamma peaks	Far-advanced cirrhosis
Polyclonal gamma globulin elevation	↑↑ Gamma globulin with a broad peak	Cirrhosis, chronic infection, sarcoidosis, tuberculosis, endocarditis, rheumatoid-collagen disease
Hypogamma-globulinemia	↓ Gamma globulin with normal other globulin levels	Light-chain multiple myeloma
Monoclonal gammopathy	Thin spikes in gamma globulin	Myeloma, macroglobulinemia, gammopathies

↓, Decreased; ↑, increased; sl. ↓, slightly decreased; sl. ↑, slightly increased; $\overline{N}$, normal; ↓↓, greatly decreased; ↑↑, greatly increased.

Interfering factors

- Prolonged application of a tourniquet can increase both fractions of total proteins.
- Sampling of peripheral venous blood proximal to an IV administration site can result in an inaccurately low protein level. Likewise, massive IV infusion of crystalloid fluid can result in acute hypoproteinemia.
- Drugs that may cause *increased* protein levels include anabolic steroids, androgens, corticosteroids, dextran, growth hormone, insulin, phenazopyridine, and progesterone.
- Drugs that may cause *decreased* protein levels include ammonium ions, estrogens, hepatotoxic drugs, and oral contraceptives.

Procedure and patient care

Before
- Explain the procedure to the patient.
- Tell the patient that no fasting is usually required.

During
- Collect approximately 5 to 7 ml of blood in a red-top tube.

After
- Apply pressure to the venipuncture site. Patients with liver dysfunction often have prolonged clotting times.

Abnormal findings

▲ **Increased albumin levels**
Dehydration

▼ **Decreased albumin levels**
Malnutrition
Pregnancy
Liver disease
Protein-losing enteropathies
Protein-losing nephropathies
Third-space losses
Overhydration
Increased capillary permeability
Inflammatory disease
Familial idiopathic dysproteinemia

▲ **Increased alpha₁ globulin levels**

Inflammatory disease

▼ **Decreased alpha₁ globulin levels**

Juvenile pulmonary emphysema

▲ **Increased alpha₂ globulin levels**

Nephrotic syndrome
Inflammatory disease

▼ **Decreased alpha₂ globulin levels**

Hemolysis
Wilson's disease
Hyperthyroidism
Severe liver dysfunction

▲ **Increased beta globulin levels**

Hypercholesterolemia
Iron deficiency anemia

▼ **Decreased beta globulin levels**

Malnutrition

▲ **Increased gamma globulin levels (see p. 493 for specific gamma immunoglobulin specifics)**

Multiple myeloma
Waldenström's macro-globulinemia
Chronic inflammatory disease
Malignancy
Hyperimmunization
Acute and chronic infection

▼ **Decreased gamma globulin levels**

Genetic immune disorders
Secondary immune deficiency

notes

prothrombin time (PT, Pro-time, International normalized ratio [INR])

Type of test Blood

Normal findings

11.0-12.5 seconds; 85% to 100%
Full anticoagulant therapy: 1.5-2 times control value; 20%
    to 30%

Possible critical values

>20 seconds
Full anticoagulant therapy: >3 times control value

Test explanation and related physiology

The PT is used to evaluate the adequacy of the extrinsic system and common pathway in the clotting mechanism. The PT measures the clotting ability of factors I (fibrinogen), II (prothrombin), V, VII, and X. When these clotting factors exist in deficient quantities, the PT is prolonged. Many diseases and drugs are associated with decreased levels of these factors. These include the following:

1. *Hepatocellular liver disease* (e.g., cirrhosis, hepatitis, neoplastic invasive processes)

    Factors I, II, V, VII, IX, and X are produced in the liver. With severe hepatocellular dysfunction, synthesis of these factors will not occur, and serum concentration of these factors will be decreased. Even a small decrease in factor VII will result in marked prolongation of the PT.

2. *Obstructive biliary disease* (e.g., bile duct obstruction secondary to tumor or gallstones or intrahepatic cholestasis secondary to sepsis or drugs)

    As a result of the biliary obstruction, the bile necessary for fat absorption fails to enter the gut, and fat malabsorption results. Vitamins A, D, E, and K are fat soluble and also are not absorbed. Because the synthesis of factors II, VII, IX, and X depends on vitamin K, these factors will not be adequately produced, and serum concentrations will fall. Factor VII is the first to decrease and will result in prolongation of PT.

    Parenchymal (hepatocellular) liver disease can be differentiated from obstructive biliary disease by determina-

P

tion of the patient's response to parenteral vitamin K administration. If the PT returns to normal after 1 to 3 days of vitamin K administration (10 mg IM twice a day), one can safely assume that the patient has obstructive biliary disease that is causing vitamin K malabsorption. If, on the other hand, the PT does not return to normal with the vitamin K injections, one can assume that severe hepatocellular disease exists and that the liver cells are incapable of synthesizing the clotting factors, no matter how much vitamin K is available.

3. *Coumarin ingestion*

   The coumarin derivatives dicumarol and warfarin (Coumadin, Panwarfin) are used to prevent coagulation in patients with thromboembolic disease (e.g., pulmonary embolism, thrombophlebitis, arterial embolism). These drugs interfere with the production of vitamin K-dependent clotting factors, which results in a prolongation of PT, as already described. The adequacy of coumarin therapy can be monitored by following the patient's PT. Appropriate coumarin therapy for full anticoagulation should prolong the PT by 1.5 to 2 times the control value (or 20% to 30% of the normal value if percentages are used).

• • •

PT test results are usually given in seconds, along with a control value. The control value usually varies somewhat from day to day because the reagents used may vary. The patient's PT should be approximately equal to the control value. Some laboratories report PT values as percentages of normal activity, because the patient's results are compared with a curve representing normal clotting time. Normally the patient's PT is 85% to 100%.

To have uniform PT results for physicians in different parts of the country and the world, the World Health Organization has recommended that PT results now include the use of the *international normalized ratio (INR)* value. The reported INR results are independent of the reagents or methods used because the standard method of obtaining therapeutic anticoagulation by keeping PT ratios of 1.5 to 2 times the control value in certain clinical indications would be converted to a figure that takes the sensitivity of the thromboplastin used as reagent and the type of instrument into account. These international sensitivity indices are different for various thromboplastins and according to whether mechanical or photo-optical methods and instruments are used. Many hospitals are now reporting PT times in both absolute and INR numbers. Therapeutic INR is usually considered to be 2 to 3.5 in most institutions, depending on the clinical situation.

Interfering factors

- Alcohol intake can increase PT levels.
- A high-fat diet may decrease PT levels.
- ✘ Drugs that may cause *increased* levels include allopurinol, aminosalicylic acid, barbiturates, beta-lactam antibiotics, chloral hydrate, cephalothins, chloramphenicol, chlorpromazine (Thorazine), cholestyramine, cimetidine, clofibrate, colestipol, ethyl alcohol, glucagon, heparin, methyldopa (Aldomet), neomycin, oral anticoagulants, propylthiouracil, quinidine, quinine, salicylates, and sulfonamides.
- ✘ Drugs that may cause *decreased* levels include anabolic steroids, barbiturates, chloral hydrate, digitalis, diphenhydramine (Benadryl), estrogens, griseofulvin, oral contraceptives, and vitamin K.

Procedure and patient care

Before

- Explain the procedure to the patient.
- Tell the patient that no fasting is required.
- If the patient is receiving warfarin, obtain the blood specimen before the patient is given the daily dose of warfarin. The daily dose may be increased, decreased, or kept the same, depending on the PT test results for that day.

During

- Collect approximately 5 to 7 ml of venous blood in a blue-top tube.
- List on the laboratory slip any drugs that may affect test results.

After

- Apply pressure to the venipuncture site. Remember, hemostasis will be delayed if the patient is taking warfarin or if the patient has any coagulopathies.
- If the PT is greatly prolonged, evaluate the patient for bleeding tendencies (i.e., check for blood in the urine and all

P

excretions and assess the patient for bruises, petechiae, and low back pain.

- If severe bleeding occurs, the anticoagulant effect of warfarin can be reversed by the slow parenteral administration of vitamin K (phytonadione).
- Because of drug interactions, instruct the patient not to take any medication unless specifically ordered by the physician.

🏠 Home care responsibilities

- Patients taking warfarin will be regulated by PT and INR values.
- Teach these patients to evaluate themselves for bleeding tendencies. Patients should assess themselves for bruises, petechiae, low back pain, and bleeding gums. Blood may be detected in the urine and stool.
- Because of many drug interactions, instruct patients on warfarin therapy not to take any other medications unless approved by their physician.

Abnormal findings

▲ **Increased levels**

Cirrhosis
Hepatitis
Vitamin K deficiency
Salicylate intoxication
Bile duct obstruction
Coumarin ingestion
Disseminated intravascular coagulation
Massive blood transfusion
Hereditary factor deficiency

notes

pulmonary angiography (Pulmonary arteriography, Bronchial angiography)

Type of test X-ray with contrast dye

Normal findings Normal pulmonary vasculature

Test explanation and related physiology

Through an injection of a radiographic contrast material into the pulmonary arteries, pulmonary angiography permits visualization of the pulmonary vasculature. Angiography is used to detect pulmonary embolism and a variety of congenital and acquired lesions of the pulmonary vessels.

When pulmonary embolism is suspected, lung scanning should be performed first. If the lung scan is normal, pulmonary embolism is ruled out. If the scan is equivocal, however, the diagnosis of pulmonary embolism is questionable, because pathologic parenchymal processes (e.g., emphysema, pneumonia) also may cause abnormalities on the lung scan. Definitive diagnosis for pulmonary embolism may require pulmonary angiography. This may be especially important in patients with peptic ulcers for whom anticoagulant treatment for pulmonary embolism may be associated with significant risks. Also, in rare instances, pulmonary embolectomy rather than anticoagulation is considered critical for patient survival. In these cases the angiographic location of the clot is important.

Bronchial angiography is now being done in some facilities to identify bleeding sites in the lungs. For this procedure, catheters are placed transarterially into the orifice of bronchial arteries. Radiopaque material is then injected, and the arteries are visualized. If a bleeding site is identified, the site can be injected with a sclerosing agent to prevent further bleeding.

Contraindications

- Patients with allergies to shellfish or iodinated dye
- Patients who are pregnant
- Patients with bleeding disorders

Potential complications

- Allergic reaction to iodinated dye
  Hypoglycemia or acidosis may occur in patients who are taking Glucophage and receive iodine dye.

P

- Cardiac arrhythmia
  Premature ventricular contractions during right-sided heart catheterization may lead to ventricular tachycardia and ventricular fibrillation.

Procedure and patient care

Before

- Explain the procedure to the patient.
- Ensure that written and informed consent for this procedure is obtained.
- Inform the patient that a warm flush will be felt when the dye is injected.
- Check the patient for allergies to iodinated dyes and shellfish.
- Determine if the patient has ventricular arrhythmias (dysrhythmias).
- Keep the patient NPO after midnight on the day of the test.
- Administer preprocedural medications as ordered. Atropine is given to decrease secretions. Meperidine is used for sedation and relaxation.

During

- Note the following procedural steps:
  1. The patient is placed on an x-ray table in the supine position.
  2. Electrocardiographic electrodes are attached for cardiac monitoring.
  3. The catheter is placed into the femoral vein and passed into the inferior vena cava.
  4. With fluoroscopic visualization, the catheter is advanced to the right atrium and the right ventricle.
  5. The catheter is manipulated into the main pulmonary artery, where the dye is injected.
  6. X-ray films of the chest are immediately taken in timed sequence. This allows all vessels visualized by the injection to be photographed. If filling defects are seen in the contrast-filled vessels, pulmonary emboli are present.
  7. If *bronchial angiography* is performed, the femoral artery is cannulated instead of the vein. The rest of the procedure is similar to that in preceding paragraphs.
- Note that this test is performed by a physician in approximately 1 hour.
- During injection of dye, remind the patient that he or

she will feel a burning sensation and flush throughout
the body.

After

- Observe the catheter insertion site for inflammation, hemorrhage, and hematoma.
- Assess the patient's vital signs for evidence of bleeding
  (decreased blood pressure, increased pulse).
- Apply cold compresses to the puncture site if needed to
  reduce swelling or discomfort.
- Inform the patient that coughing may occur after this study.
- Educate the patient regarding the need for bed rest for
  12 to 24 hours after the test.

Abnormal findings

Pulmonary embolism
Congenital and acquired lesions of the pulmonary vessels
  (e.g., pulmonary hypertension)
Tumor

notes

P

pulmonary function tests (PFTs)

Type of test Airflow assessment

Normal findings Vary with the patient's age, sex, height, and weight

Test explanation and related physiology

PFTs are performed to detect abnormalities in respiratory function and to determine the extent of any pulmonary abnormality. The main reasons for pulmonary function tests include the following:

1. Preoperative evaluation of the lungs and pulmonary reserve. When planned thoracic surgery will result in loss of functional pulmonary tissue, as in lobectomy (removal of part of a lung) or pneumonectomy (removal of an entire lung), a significant risk of pulmonary failure exists if preoperative pulmonary function is already severely compromised by other diseases such as chronic obstructive pulmonary disease (COPD).

2. Evaluation of response to bronchodilator therapy. Some patients with COPD have a spastic component to their obstructive disease that may respond to long-term use of bronchodilators. Pulmonary function studies performed before and after the use of bronchodilators will identify that group of patients.

3. Differentiation between restrictive and obstructive forms of chronic pulmonary disease. *Restrictive* defects (e.g., pulmonary fibrosis, tumors, chest-wall trauma) occur when ventilation is disturbed by a limitation in chest expansion. Inspiration is primarily affected. *Obstructive* defects (e.g., emphysema, bronchitis, asthma) occur when ventilation is disturbed by an increase in airway resistance. Expiration is primarily affected.

4. Determination of the diffusing capacity of the lungs (D_L). Rates are based on the difference in concentration of gases in inspired and expired air.

5. Performance of inhalation tests in patients with inhalation allergies.

PFTs routinely include spirometry, measurement of air flow rates, and calculation of lung volumes and capacities. Exercise pulmonary stress testing can also be performed to provide data concerning the patient pulmonary reserve.

Spirometry is performed first. On the basis of age, height, weight, race, and sex, normal values for the volumes and flow rates can be predicted. If the actual values are greater than 80% of predicted values, the person is considered normal. Spirometry provides information about obstruction or restriction of air flow. If airflow rates are significantly diminished (<60% of normal), spirometry can be repeated after bronchodilators are administered by nebulizer. If airflow rates are improved by 20%, the chronic use of bronchodilators may be recommended to the patient. Measurement of lung capacities (combination of two or more lung volumes) can be performed.

Gas exchange studies measure the diffusing capacity of the lung (D_L) (i.e., the amount of gas exchanged across the alveolar-capillary membrane per minute). Arterial blood gases (see p. 104) are also a part of pulmonary function studies as the information obtained is used in calculations of lung function data.

PFTs routinely include determination of the following:

Forced vital capacity. FVC is the amount of air that can be forcefully expelled from a maximally inflated lung position. This volume is decreased below the expected value in obstructive and restrictive pulmonary diseases.

Forced expiratory volume in 1 second. FEV_1 is the volume of air expelled during the first second of the FVC. In patients with obstructive disease, airways are narrowed and resistance to flow is high. Therefore not as much air can be expelled in 1 second, and FEV_1 will be reduced below the predicted value. In restrictive lung disease, FEV_1 is decreased not because of airway resistance but because the amount of air originally inhaled is less. One should therefore measure the FEV_1/FVC ratio. A normal value of 80% is found in patients with restrictive lung disease. In obstructive lung disease this ratio is considerably less than 80%. The FEV_1 measurement will reliably improve with bronchodilator therapy if a spastic component to an obstructive disease exists.

Maximal midexpiratory flow. MMEF is the maximal rate of airflow through the pulmonary tree during forced expiration. This is also called *forced midexpiratory flow.* This test is independent of the patient's effort or cooperation. MMEF is reduced below expected values in obstructive diseases and normal in restrictive diseases.

P

Maximal volume ventilation. MVV, formerly called *maximal breathing capacity*, is the maximal volume of air that the patient can breathe in and out during 1 minute. MVV is decreased below the expected value in both restrictive and obstructive pulmonary disease.

A comprehensive pulmonary function study also may include evaluation of the following lung volumes and lung capacities, many of which are illustrated in Figure 28:

Tidal volume. TV or V_T is the volume of air inspired and expired with each normal respiration.

Inspiratory reserve volume. IRV is the maximal volume of air that can be inspired from the end of a normal inspiration. It represents forced inspiration over and beyond the tidal volume.

Expiratory reserve volume. ERV is the maximal volume of air that can be exhaled after a normal expiration.

Residual volume. RV is the volume of air remaining in the lungs following forced expiration.

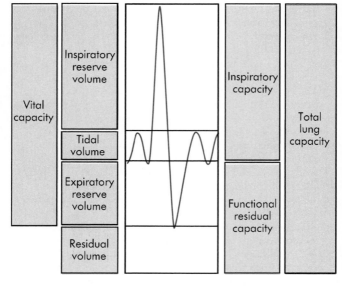

Figure 28 Relationship of lung volumes and capacities.

Inspiratory capacity. IC is the maximal amount of air that can be inspired after a normal expiration (IC = TV + IRV).

Functional residual volume. FRV is the amount of air left in the lungs after a normal expiration (FRV = ERV + RV).

Vital capacity. VC is the maximal amount of air that can be expired after a maximal inspiration (VC = TV + IRV + ERV).

Total lung capacity. TLC is the volume to which the lungs can be expanded with the greatest inspiratory effort (TLC = TV + IRV + ERV + RV).

Minute volume. MV, sometimes called *minute ventilation*, is the volume of air inhaled and exhaled per minute.

Dead space. Dead space is the part of the tidal volume that does not participate in alveolar gas exchange. This would include the air within the trachea.

Forced expiratory flow$_{200-1200}$. FEF$_{200-1200}$ is the airflow rate of expired air between 200 ml and 1200 ml during the FVC. This is the portion of the airflow curve that is most affected by airway obstruction.

Forced expiratory flow$_{25-75}$. FEF$_{25-75}$ is the airflow rate of expired air between 25% and 75% of the flow during the FVC. This is the part of the airflow curve that is most affected by airway obstruction.

Peak inspiratory flow rate. PIFR is the flow rate of inspired air during maximum inspiration. This is used to indicate large (trachea and bronchi) airway disease.

Contraindications

- Patients who are in pain because of the inability to cooperate by deep inspiration and expiration
- Patients who are unable to cooperate because of age or mental incapability

Procedure and patient care

Before

- Explain the test to the patient.
- Inform the patient that cooperation is necessary to obtain accurate results.
- Instruct the patient not to use bronchodilators or smoke for 6 hours before this test (if requested by physician).
- Withhold the use of small-dose meter inhalers and aerosol therapy before this study.
- Measure and record the patient's height and weight before this study to determine the predicted values.

- List on the laboratory slip any medications the patient is taking.

During

- Note the following procedural steps:

Spirometry and airflow rates

1. The unsedated patient is taken to the pulmonary function laboratory.
2. The patient breathes through a sterile mouthpiece and into a spirometer to measure and record the desired values.
3. The patient is asked to inhale as deeply as possible and then forcibly exhale as much air as possible. This is repeated several times (usually two to three times). The two best are used for calculations. This test may be repeated with bronchodilators if the patient's values are deficient.
4. From this, the machine computes FVC, FEV_1, FEV_1/FVC, PIFR, PEFR, and MMEF.
5. The patient is asked to breathe in and out as deeply and frequently as possible for 15 seconds. The total volume breathed is recorded and multiplied by 4 to obtain the MVV.
6. The patient is asked to breathe in and out normally into the spirometer and then exhale forcibly from the end tidal volume expiration point. This provides measurement of ERV.
7. The patient is asked to breathe in and out normally into the spirometer and then inhale forcibly from the end tidal volume expiration point. This provides measurement of IC.
8. The patient is asked to breathe in and out maximally (but not forced). This is a measure of VC and the calculated TLC.

Gas exchange/diffusing capacity of the lung (D_L)

1. The D_L of CO is usually measured by having the patient inhale a CO mixture.
2. D_LCO is calculated with an analysis of the amount of CO exhaled compared with the amount inhaled. Some procedures require arterial blood gases to be performed at the same time as the gas exchange maneuvers.

Inhalation tests (bronchial provocation studies)
1. These tests also may be performed during pulmonary function studies to establish a cause-and-effect relationship in some patients with inhalant allergies.
2. The *methacholine* or *histamine challenge* test is typically used to detect the presence of hyperactive airway diseases. This test would not be indicated for a patient known to have asthma. A positive methacholine challenge is a greater than 20% reduction in the patient's FEV_1.
3. Care is taken during this challenge test to reverse any severe bronchospasm with prompt administration of an inhalant bronchodilator (e.g., isoproterenol).

After
- Note that patients with severe respiratory problems are occasionally exhausted after the testing and will need rest.

Abnormal findings

Pulmonary fibrosis
Interstitial lung diseases
Tumor
Chest wall trauma
Emphysema
Chronic bronchitis
Asthma
Inhalant pneumonitis
Post pneumonectomy
Bronchiectasis
Airway infection
Pneumonia
Neuromuscular disease
Hypersensitivity bronchospasm

P

notes

rabies-neutralizing antibody test

Type of test Blood

Normal findings <1 : 16

Test explanation and related physiology

Identification and documentation of the presence of rabies-neutralizing antibody is important for veterinary health care workers and others who may be or may have been exposed to the rabies virus. This test is performed on patients who are at great risk for animal bites and have received the human diploid cell rabies vaccine (HDCV). A rabies titer of greater than 1:16 is considered to be protective.

The rabies antibody test is also used in making the diagnosis of rabies in a patient suspected to have been exposed to the virus. A fourfold rise in antibody titer over several weeks in a person not previously exposed to the HDCV indicates rabies exposure.

Procedure and patient care

Before

- Tell the patient that no fasting or special preparation is required.

During

- Collect 7 to 10 ml of venous blood in a red-top tube.

After

- Apply pressure to the venipuncture site.

Abnormal findings

Exposure to rabies vaccine
Recent bite exposure to rabies virus
Active rabies in patient or animal

notes

radioactive iodine uptake (RAIU, Iodine uptake test, ^{131}I uptake)

Type of test Nuclear scan

Normal findings
2 hours: 4% to 12% absorbed
6 hours: 6% to 15% absorbed
24 hours: 8% to 30% absorbed

Test explanation and related physiology

The RAIU is a useful guide to thyroid function. This test is based on the ability of the thyroid gland to trap and retain iodine. In this procedure a known quantity of radioactive iodine is given orally to the patient. A gamma ray detector placed over the thyroid gland determines the quantity or percentage of radioactive iodine taken up by the gland over a specific time.

Performing the measurement at different times after the iodine is given allows several aspects of thyroid function to be evaluated. Uptake determination at 30 minutes reflects the ability of the thyroid gland to trap iodine. When uptake is measured at 6 hours, the ability of the thyroid gland to bind iodine organically is evaluated. Maximal iodine uptake is observed within 24 hours. This measurement also is useful in determining the amount of radioactive iodine to be administered to patients requiring thyroid ablation therapy with radioactive iodine. Determinations of iodine uptake after 24 hours measure the ability of the gland to release iodine in the form of thyroid hormone.

Increased thyroid uptake of radioactive iodine is seen in patients with hyperthyroid states. Decreased uptake occurs in patients with hypothyroid conditions. The RAIU tends to be more accurate for diagnosing hyperthyroidism than hypothyroidism.

Contraindications
- Patients who are allergic to iodine or shellfish
- Patients who are pregnant

Potential complication
- Radioactive exposure to the thyroid gland
  This is minimized when ^{123}I or ^{125}I is used instead of ^{131}I.

R

Interfering factors

- In patients taking exogenous iodine preparations, the iodine increases the body's iodine pool and decreases uptake by the thyroid gland.
- Iodine-deficient patients trap increased amounts of iodine, resulting in increased uptake.
- Rebound thyroid stimulation after discontinuation of suppressive doses of thyroid medications results in falsely elevated RAIU levels.
- Recent x-ray studies using iodinated contrast material decrease uptake.
- Diarrhea caused by decreased absorption of tracer doses in the gastrointestinal tract results in decreased RAIU levels.
- Drugs that may cause *increased* levels include barbiturates, estrogen, lithium, phenothiazines, and thyroid-stimulating hormone.
- Drugs that may cause *decreased* levels include adrenocorticotropic hormone, antihistamines, corticosteroids, Lugol's solution, nitrates, saturated solution of potassium iodide, thyroid and antithyroid drugs, and tolbutamide.

Procedure and patient care

Before

- Explain the procedure to the patient.
- Assess the patient for allergies to iodine.
- Note that some laboratories prefer to keep the patient NPO after midnight on the day of the test.
- Restrict iodine and thyroid preparations 1 week before testing if indicated by the institution.
- Evaluate the patient's drug history for interfering factors.

During

- Note the following procedural steps:
  1. A tasteless dose of radioactive iodine, usually ^{123}I, is given by mouth to the patient. If RAIU is to be determined at 2 hours, the iodine is administered intravenously.
  2. The patient is given written instructions regarding the times to return to the radiology department for scanning.
  3. The patient is informed that he or she may usually eat 45 minutes to 1 hour after the dose of iodine has been given.

4. For the scanning, the patient is asked to lie in a supine position.
5. A gamma ray detector is placed over the patient's thyroid gland to determine RAIU.

- List on the laboratory slip the x-ray studies and drugs the patient has received that could affect test results.
- Note that this test is performed in approximately 30 minutes by a radiologic technologist.
- Inform the patient that this test is not uncomfortable.

After

- Inform the patient that the dose of radioactive iodine used in this test is minute and harmless. Tell him or her that no isolation or special urine precautions are necessary.

Abnormal findings

▲ **Increased levels**
  Hyperthyroidism

▼ **Decreased levels**
  Hypothyroidism

notes

R

red blood cell count (RBC count, Erythrocyte count)

Type of test Blood

Normal findings (million/mm³ or million/μl)

Adult/elderly
    Male: 4.7-6.1
    Female: 4.2-5.4
Children
    Newborn: 4.8-7.1
    2-8 wks: 4-6
    2-6 mos: 3.5-5.5
    6 mos-1 yr: 3.5-5.2
    1-6 yr: 4-5.5
    6-18 yr: 4-5.5

Test explanation and related physiology

This test is a count of the number of circulating red blood cells (RBCs) in 1 mm³ of peripheral venous blood. The RBC is routinely performed as part of a complete blood count. Within each RBC are molecules of hemoglobin that permit the transport and exchange of oxygen to the tissues and carbon dioxide from the tissues. The RBC is produced by the erythroid elements in the bone marrow. Under the stimulation of erythropoietin, RBC production is increased.

Normally RBCs survive in the peripheral blood for approximately 120 days. During that time, the RBC is transported through the bloodstream. In the smallest of capillaries, the RBC must fold and bend to conform to the size of these tiny vessels. Toward the end of the life of the RBC, the cell membrane becomes less pliable; the aged RBC is then lysed and extracted from the circulation by the spleen. Abnormal RBCs have a shorter life span and are extracted earlier (see RBC survival studies p. 715). Intravascular RBC trauma, such as that caused by artificial heart valves or peripheral vascular atherosclerotic plaques, also shorten the life of the RBC. An enlarged spleen, such as that caused by portal hypertension or leukemia, may inappropriately destroy and remove normal RBCs from the circulation.

Normal RBC values vary according to gender and age. Women tend to have lower values than do men, and RBC counts tend to decrease with age. When the value is decreased by more than 10% of the expected normal value, the patient is said to be anemic. Low RBC values are caused by many factors, including the following:

1. Hemorrhage, as in gastrointestinal bleeding or trauma
2. Hemolysis, as in glucose-6-phosphate dehydrogenase deficiency, spherocytosis, or secondary splenomegaly
3. Dietary deficiency, as of iron or vitamin B_{12}
4. Genetic aberrations, as in sickle cell anemia or thalassemia
5. Drug ingestion, as of chloramphenicol, hydantoins, or quinidine
6. Marrow failure, as in fibrosis, leukemia, or antineoplastic chemotherapy
7. Chronic illness, as in tumor or sepsis
8. Other organ failure, as in renal disease

RBC counts greater than normal can be physiologically induced as a result of the body's requirements for greater oxygen-carrying capacity (e.g., at high altitudes). Diseases that produce chronic hypoxia (e.g., congenital heart disease) also provoke this physiologic increase in RBCs. Polycythemia vera is a neoplastic condition involving uncontrolled production of RBCs.

Interfering factors

- Normal decreases are seen in the RBC during pregnancy because of normal body fluid increases and dilution of the RBCs.
- Persons living at high altitudes have increased RBCs.
- Hydration status: Dehydration factitiously increases the RBC count, and overhydration decreases the RBC count.
- Drugs that may cause *increased* RBC levels include gentamicin and methyldopa.
- Drugs that may cause *decreased* RBC levels include chloramphenicol, hydantoins, and quinidine.

Procedure and patient care

Before

- Explain the procedure to the patient.
- Tell the patient that no fasting is required.

During

- Collect approximately 5 to 7 ml of blood in a lavender-top tube.
- Thoroughly mix the blood with the anticoagulant by tilting the tube.

- Avoid hemolysis.
- List on the laboratory slip any drugs or other patient factors that may affect RBC levels.

After

- Apply pressure to the venipuncture site.

Abnormal findings

▲ **Increased levels**
  High altitude
  Congenital heart disease
  Polycythemia vera
  Dehydration/
    hemoconcentration
  Cor pulmonale
  Pulmonary fibrosis

▼ **Decreased levels**
  Hemorrhage
  Hemolysis
  Anemia
  Hemoglobinopathy
  Advanced cancer
  Bone marrow fibrosis
  Leukemia
  Antineoplastic chemo-
    therapy
  Chronic illness
  Renal failure
  Overhydration
  Multiple myeloma
  Pernicious anemia
  Rheumatoid disease
  Subacute endocarditis
  Pregnancy
  Dietary deficiency

notes

red blood cell indices (RBC indices, MCV, MCH, MCHC, Blood indices, Erythrocyte indices, Red cell distribution width [RDW])

Type of test Blood

Normal findings

Mean corpuscular volume (MCV)
Adult/elderly/child: 80-95 μm^3
Newborn: 96-108 μm^3

Mean corpuscular hemoglobin (MCH)
Adult/elderly/child: 27-31 pg
Newborn: 32-34 pg

Mean corpuscular hemoglobin concentration (MCHC)
Adult/elderly/child: 32-36 g/dl (or 32% to 36%)
Newborn: 32-33 g/dl (or 32% to 33%)

Red blood cell distribution width (RDW)
Adult: 11% to 14.5%

Test explanation and related physiology

The RBC indices provide information about the size (MCV and RDW), weight (MCH), and hemoglobin concentration (MCHC) of RBCs. This test is routinely performed as part of a complete blood count (CBC). The results of the RBC, hematocrit, and hemoglobin tests are necessary to calculate the RBC indices. When investigating anemia, it is helpful to categorize the anemia according to the RBC indices, as shown in Table 15. Cell size is indicated by the terms *normocytic*, *microcytic*, and *macrocytic*. Hemoglobin content is indicated by the terms *normochromic*, *hypochromic*, and *hyperchromic*. Additional information about the RBC size, shape, color, and intracellular structure is described in the blood smear study (see p. 151).

Mean corpuscular volume

The MCV is a measure of the average volume, or size, of a single RBC and is therefore used in classifying anemias. MCV is calculated as follows:

$$MCV = \frac{hematocrit\ (\%) \times 10}{RBC\ (million/mm^3)}$$

When the MCV value is increased, the RBC is said to be abnormally large, or *macrocytic*. This is most frequently seen in

TABLE 15 Categorization of anemia according to RBC indices

Normocytic,[1] normochromic[2] anemia
Iron deficiency (detected early)
Chronic illness (e.g., sepsis, tumor)
Acute blood loss
Aplastic anemia (e.g., chloramphenicol toxicosis)
Acquired hemolytic anemias (e.g., from a prosthetic cardiac valve)

Microcytic,[3] hypochromic[4] anemia
Iron deficiency (detected late)
Thalassemia
Lead poisoning

Microcytic, normochromic anemia
Renal disease (because of the loss of erythropoietin)

Macrocytic,[5] normochromic anemia
Vitamin B_{12} or folic acid deficiency
Hydantoin ingestion
Chemotherapy

---

[1]Normocytic—normal RBC size.
[2]Normochromic—normal color (normal hemoglobin content).
[3]Microcytic—smaller than normal RBC size.
[4]Hypochromic—less than normal color (decreased hemoglobin content).
[5]Macrocytic—larger than normal RBC size.

---

megaloblastic anemias (e.g., vitamin B_{12} or folic acid deficiency). When the MCV value is decreased, the RBC is said to be abnormally small, or *microcytic*. This is associated with iron deficiency anemia or thalassemia.

Mean corpuscular hemoglobin

The MCH is a measure of the average amount (weight) of hemoglobin within an RBC. MCH is calculated as follows:

$$MCH = \frac{\text{hemoglobin (g/dl)} \times 10}{\text{RBC (million/mm}^3)}$$

Because macrocytic cells generally have more hemoglobin and microcytic cells have less hemoglobin, the causes for these values closely resemble those for the MCV value.

Mean corpuscular hemoglobin concentration

The MCHC is a measure of the average concentration or percentage of hemoglobin within a single RBC. MCHC is calculated as follows:

$$MCHC = \frac{hemoglobin\ (g/dl) \times 100}{hematocrit\ (\%)}$$

When values are decreased, the cell has a deficiency of hemoglobin and is said to be *hypochromic* (frequently seen in iron deficiency anemia and thalassemia). When values are normal, the anemia is said be *normocytic* (e.g., hemolytic anemia). RBCs cannot be considered *hyperchromic*. Only 37 g/dl of hemoglobin can fit into the RBC.

Red blood cell distribution width

The RDW is an indication of the variation in RBC size. It is calculated by a machine using the MCV and RBC values. Variations in the width of the RBCs may be helpful when classifying certain types of anemia. The RDW is essentially an indicator of the degree of *anisocytosis*, a blood condition characterized by RBCs of variable and abnormal size.

Interfering factors

- Abnormal RBC size may affect indices.
- Extremely elevated white blood cell counts may affect RBC indices.
- Large red blood cell precursors, e.g., reticulocytes (see p. 732), cause an abnormally high MCV.
- The presence of cold agglutinins also falsely elevates MCHC, MCH and MCV.

R

Procedure and patient care

Before

- Tell the patient that no fasting is required.

During

- Collect approximately 5 to 7 ml of venous blood in a lavender-top tube.
- Avoid hemolysis.
- Transport the specimen to the hematology laboratory, where

the blood is passed through automated machines that calculate the RBC indices.

After

- Apply pressure to the venipuncture site.

Abnormal findings

▲ **Increased MCV**
Liver disease
Antimetabolite therapy
Alcoholism
Pernicious anemia
  (vitamin B_{12} deficiency)
Folic acid deficiency

▲ **Increased MCH**
Macrocytic anemia

▲ **Increased MCHC**
Spherocytosis
Intravascular hemolysis
Cold agglutinins

▲ **Increased RDW**
Iron deficiency anemia
B_{12} or folate deficiency anemia
Hemoglobinopathies (e.g., sickle cell disease)
Hemolytic anemias
Post hemorrhagic anemias

▼ **Decreased MCV**
Iron deficiency anemia
Thalassemia

▼ **Decreased MCH**
Microcytic anemia
Hypochromic anemia

▼ **Decreased MCHC**
Iron deficiency anemia
Thalassemia

notes

red blood cell survival study (RBC survival study, Splenic sequestration study)

Type of test Nuclear scan

Normal findings
Half-life of RBC: 26-30 days
Spleen/liver ratio: 1:1
Spleen/pericardium ratio: <2:1

Test explanation and related physiology

In patients with hemolytic anemia, the RBCs are destroyed and normally sequestered in the spleen. As a result of this ongoing RBC destruction, the RBC life span will be significantly reduced. This reduction in RBC survival indicates that active hemolysis is occurring and is the cause of the patient's anemia.

The nuclear medicine determination of the RBC life span can provide a semiquantitative measurement of the degree of hemolysis. This quantitation can be best performed by determining the half-life of the RBC within the circulation. This part of the test is performed by extracting some of the patient's RBCs, labeling them with chromium-51 (^{51}Cr), and reinjecting them into the patient. Subsequent blood levels of ^{51}Cr indicate the half-life of the labeled RBCs. As RBC survival decreases, more labeled RBCs are sequestered by the spleen. As a result, the amount of ^{51}Cr activity in the blood decreases.

The second part of the test is the imaging of the spleen, liver, and pericardium. In patients with hemolytic anemia associated with abnormal splenic sequestration, the spleen/liver ratio is in excess of 1:1. However, this abnormally high ratio can occur in patients who have splenomegaly caused by a disease other than hemolytic anemia. Therefore spleen/pericardium ratios are performed; those greater than 2:1 indicate abnormal splenic sequestration of hemolyzed RBCs. A normal spleen/pericardium ratio with an increased spleen/liver ratio indicates splenomegaly.

This splenic sequestration part of the study is also helpful in determining which patients with hemolytic anemia will benefit from splenectomy. Patients with increased splenic sequestration can be expected to improve greatly as a result of splenectomy.

R

Contraindications

- Patients who are pregnant because of the risk of fetal damage

Interfering factors

- Factors that can decrease RBC survival include recent RBC transfusion, increased RBC production, active bleeding, high white blood cell (WBC) counts in excess of 25,000, and high platelet counts greater than 500,000.
- Splenomegaly can increase spleen/pericardium ratios.
- Splenic infarctions can decrease spleen/pericardium ratios.

Procedure and patient care

Before

- Explain the procedure to the patient.
- Assure the patient that he or she will not be exposed to large amounts of radioactivity, because only tracer doses of the isotope are used.
- Tell the patient that no preparation or sedation is required.
- Notify the nuclear medicine technologist or physician if blood transfusion or hemorrhage has occurred shortly before or during the study.
- Note that usually a hematocrit, WBC count, platelet count, and reticulocyte count are performed before testing.

During

- Note the following procedural steps:
  1. Approximately 20 ml of blood is withdrawn from the patient, and the RBCs are labeled with ^{51}Cr.
  2. The RBCs are immediately reinjected into the patient.
  3. On the first day of testing, 10 ml of blood is withdrawn by a peripheral venipuncture into a red-top tube.
  4. The RBCs are quantitated for ^{51}Cr counts per minute.
  5. Nuclear imaging of the spleen, liver, and pericardium is carried out.
  6. This process is repeated three times a week for 3 weeks.
  7. The peripheral venous blood ^{51}Cr counts are plotted on a graph, and the half-life is determined.
  8. The spleen/liver and spleen/pericardium ratios and nuclear counts are determined.
- Note that this test takes place over 2 to 3 weeks. The results are available on the day after the study is completed. The study is performed by a nuclear medicine technologist or physician.

- Tell the patient that no pain or discomfort is associated with this procedure. The patient must lie still during the nuclear imaging part of the test.

After

- Inform the patient that, because only tracer doses of radioisotopes are used, no precautions need to be taken against radioactive exposure.

Abnormal findings

▲ **Increased splenic sequestration**
Hemolysis
Splenomegaly

▼ **Decreased RBC survival**
Hemolysis
Hemorrhage
Abnormally increased erythropoiesis
Recent transfusion

notes

R

renal biopsy (Kidney biopsy)

Type of test Microscopic examination of tissue

Normal findings No pathologic conditions

Test explanation and related physiology

Biopsy of the kidney affords microscopic examination of renal tissue. Renal biopsy is performed for the following purposes:

1. To diagnose the cause of renal disease (e.g., poststrep-tococcal glomerulonephritis, Goodpasture syndrome, lupus nephritis)
2. To detect primary and metastatic malignancy of the kidney in patients who may not be candidates for surgery
3. To evaluate the degree of rejection that occurs after kidney transplantation, which enables the physician to determine the appropriate dose of immunosuppressive agents

Renal biopsy is most often obtained percutaneously (Figure 29). During this procedure, a needle is inserted through the skin and into the kidney to obtain a sample of kidney tissue. The biopsy needle is more accurately placed when guided by ultrasonography or fluoroscopy. These techniques allow more precise localization of the desired kidney tissue.

Occasionally open renal biopsy is performed. This involves an incision through the flank and dissection to expose the kidney surgically.

Contraindications

- Patients with coagulation disorders because of the risk of excessive bleeding
- Patients with operable kidney tumors, because tumor cells may be disseminated during the procedure
- Patients with hydronephrosis, because the enlarged renal pelvis can be easily entered and cause a persistent urine leak requiring surgical repair
- Patients with urinary tract infections, because the needle insertion may disseminate the active infection throughout the retroperitoneum

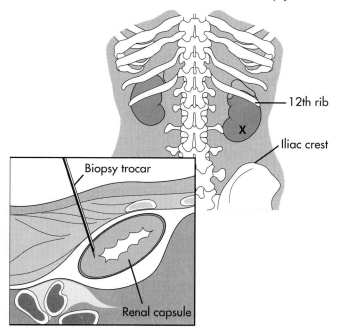

12th rib

Iliac crest

Biopsy trocar

Renal capsule

Figure 29 Renal biopsy. A biopsy needle is placed through the posterior lower chest wall and into the renal parenchyma from where tissue is extracted.

Potential complications

- Hemorrhage from the highly vascular renal tissue
- Inadvertent puncture of the liver, lung, bowel, aorta, and inferior vena cava
- Infection when an open biopsy is performed

Procedure and patient care

Before

- Explain the procedure to the patient.
- Ensure that written and informed consent for this procedure is obtained by the physician.
- Keep the patient NPO after midnight on the day of the test in the event that bleeding or inadvertent puncture of an abdominal organ may necessitate surgical intervention.

R

- Assess the patient's coagulation studies (prothrombin time, partial thromboplastin time).
- Check the patient's hemoglobin and hematocrit values.
- Note that the patient may need to be typed and crossmatched for blood in the event of severe hemorrhage requiring transfusions.
- Tell the patient that no sedative is required.
- Note that the needle stick may be done at the bedside.
- If fluoroscopic or ultrasound guidance is to be used, note that the needle stick is performed in the radiology or ultrasonography department.

During

- Note the following procedural steps:
  1. The patient is placed in a prone position with a sandbag or pillow under the abdomen to straighten the spine.
  2. Under sterile conditions the skin overlying the kidneys is infiltrated with a local anesthetic (lidocaine).
  3. While the patient holds his or her breath to stop kidney motion, the physician inserts the biopsy needle into the kidney and takes a specimen.
  4. After this procedure is completed, the needle is removed, and pressure is applied to the site for approximately 20 minutes.
- Note that this procedure is performed by a physician in approximately 10 minutes.
- Tell the patient that this procedure is uncomfortable, but only minimally if enough lidocaine is used.

After

- After the test, apply a pressure dressing.
- Turn the patient on his or her back and keep on bed rest for approximately 24 hours.
- Check the patient's vital signs, puncture site, and hematocrit values frequently during the 24-hour period.
- Instruct the patient to avoid any activity that increases abdominal venous pressure (e.g., coughing).
- Assess the patient for signs and symptoms of hemorrhage (e.g., decrease in blood pressure, increase in pulse, pallor, backache, flank pain, shoulder pain, lightheadedness).
- Evaluate the patient's abdomen for signs of bowel or liver penetration (e.g., abdominal pain and tenderness, abdominal muscle guarding and rigidity, decreased bowel sounds).

- Inspect all urine specimens for gross hematuria. Usually the patient's urine will contain blood initially, but this generally will not continue after the first 24 hours. Urine samples may be placed in consecutive chronologic order to facilitate comparison for evaluation of hematuria. This is referred to as *rack* or *serial* urine samples.
- Encourage the patient to drink large amounts of fluid to prevent clot formation and urine retention.
- Frequently obtain blood for hemoglobin and hematocrit determination after the biopsy specimen to assess for active bleeding. One purple-top tube of blood is needed.

🏠 Home care responsibilities

- Instruct the patient to avoid strenuous exercise (e.g., heavy lifting, contact sports, horseback riding) or any activity that could cause jolting of the kidney for at least 2 weeks.
- Teach the patient the signs and symptoms of renal hemorrhage, and instruct him or her to call the physician if any of these symptoms occur.
- Instruct the patient to report burning on urination or any temperature elevations. These could indicate a urinary tract infection.

Abnormal findings

Renal disease (e.g., poststreptococcal conditions, glomerulo-nephritis, lupus nephritis)
Primary and metastatic malignancy of the kidney
Rejection of kidney transplant

R

notes

renal scanning (Kidney scan, Radiorenography, Renography, Radionuclide renal imaging, Nuclear imaging of the kidney, DMSA renal scan, DTPA renal scan, Captopril renal scan)

Type of test Nuclear scan

Normal findings Normal size, shape, and function of the kidney

Test explanation and related physiology

Renal scans are to indicate the perfusion, function, and structure of the kidneys. They are also used to indicate the presence of ureteral obstruction or renovascular hypertension. Because this study uses no iodinated dyes (except when iodohippurate is used), it is safe to use on patients who have iodine allergies or compromised renal function. Renal scans are used to monitor renal function in patients with known renal disease. This scan also plays a large part of the diagnosis of renal transplant rejection.

This nuclear procedure provides visualization of the urinary tract after IV administration of a radioisotope. The radioactive material is detected by a scintillator camera, which can detect the gamma rays emitted by the radionuclide in the kidney. Scans do not interfere with the normal physiologic process of the kidney. The resultant image (scan) indicates distribution of the radionuclide within the kidney and ureters.

There are several different kinds of renal scans, depending on what information is needed to be obtained. Different isotopes may be more suitable for different scans, based on the manner in which the kidney handles the radioisotope.

Renal blood flow (perfusion) scan

This type of renal scan is used to evaluate the blood flow to each kidney. It is used to identify renal artery stenosis, renovascular hypertension, and rejection of renal transplant. Also, it is used to demonstrate hypervascular lesions (renal cell carcinoma) in the kidney.

Decreased gamma activity is noted in the kidney with arterial stenosis or renovascular hypertension. Decreased activity relative to the aorta is noted in a transplanted kidney that is experiencing rejection. Localized increased gamma activity is noted in the kidney that contains a hypervascular tumor (cancer).

Renal structural scan

This type of renal scan is performed to outline the structure of the kidney to identify pathology that may alter normal anatomic structure (e.g., tumor, cyst, abscess). Congenital disorders (e.g., hypoplasia or aplasia of the kidney, malposition of the kidney) can also be detected. A filling defect in the renal parenchyma may indicate a tumor, cyst, abscess, or infarction. Horseshoe-shaped kidney, pelvic kidney, or absence of a kidney may be evident. Also, information concerning postrenal transplants can be obtained with this scan. Anatomic alterations in the parenchymal distribution of tracer may indicate transplant rejection. Tc-DTPA or DSMA can be used for this scan.

Renal function scan (renogram)

Renal function can be determined by documenting the capability of the kidney to take up and excrete a particular radioisotope. A well-functioning kidney can be expected to rapidly assimilate the isotope and then excrete it. A poorly functioning kidney will not be able to take up the isotope rapidly nor excrete it in a timely manner. Renal function can be monitored by serially repeating this test and comparing results. Each radioactive tracer is handled by the kidney in a different manner. Different renal functions can be tested according to which isotope is used:

Technetium-99m diethylenetriamine pentaacetic acid (^{99m}Tc DTPA) measures glomerular filtration;

Tc disodium monomethanearsonate (DMSA) measures tubular cell secretion;

Iodine-131 (^{131}I) or ^{133}I hippurate measures both glomerular filtration and tubular cell secretion.

Renal hypertension scan

This scan is used to identify the presence and location of renovascular hypertension. It usually uses ACE inhibitors such as captopril. The *captopril scan* (captopril renography/scintigraphy) determines the functional significance of a renal artery or arteriole stenosis. These scans may predict the response of the blood pressure to medical treatment, angioplasty, or surgery.

Renal obstruction scan

This scan is performed to identify obstruction of the outflow tract of the kidney caused by obstruction of the renal pelvis, ureter, or bladder outlet.

Often several of these scans are combined to obtain the

maximum information about the renal system as possible. A *triple renal study* may use all of these techniques to evaluate renal blood perfusion, structure, and excretion. Radionuclear scans are also helpful in the evaluation of arterial trauma.

Contraindications

- Patients who are pregnant because of the risk of fetal damage

Procedure and patient care

Before

- Explain the procedure to the patient.
- Do not schedule a renal scan within 24 hours after an intravenous pyelogram.
- Assure the patient that he or she will not be exposed to large amounts of radioactivity because only tracer doses of isotopes are used.
- Note that Lugol's solution (10 drops) may be ordered if ^{131}I orthoiodohippurate is used. This minimizes thyroid uptake of the radioisotope.
- Remind the patient to void before the scan.
- Tell the patient that no sedation or fasting is required but that good hydration is essential.
- Instruct the patient to drink two to three glasses of water before the scan.

During

- Note the following procedural steps:
1. The unsedated, nonfasting patient is taken to the nuclear medicine department.
2. A peripheral IV injection of radionuclide is given. It takes only minutes for the radioisotopes to be concentrated in the kidneys.
3. While the patient assumes a prone or sitting position, a gamma ray scintography camera is passed over the kidney area and records the radioactive uptake on film.
4. Scans may be repeated at different intervals after the initial isotope injection.
5. Unique features of the various scans:
   a. For a *Lasix renal scan* or a *diuretic renal scan*, images are obtained for 10 to 20 minutes; then 40 mg of Lasix is administered IV, and another 20 minutes of images are obtained.

   b. For the *captopril renal scan*, the patient is scanned after the administration of captopril.

   c. For the *renal blood flow* and the *renal function scans*, scanning is started immediately after the injection

   d. For *structural renal scans*, the patient is asked to lie still for the entire time of the scan (30 minutes).

- Note that the duration of this test varies from 1 to 4 hours, depending on the specific information required. Perfusion scans are done in approximately 20 minutes, and functional scans in less than 1 hour. Static structure scans require 20 minutes to 4 hours for completion.
- Note that this study is performed by a nuclear medicine technologist or physician.
- Tell the patient that no pain or discomfort is associated with this procedure.
- Inform the patient that he or she must lie still during this study.

After

- Because only tracer doses of radioisotopes are used, inform the patient that no precautions need to be taken against radioactive exposure.
- Tell the patient that the radioactive substance is usually excreted from the body within 6 to 24 hours. Encourage the patient to drink fluids.

Abnormal findings

Urinary obstruction
Pyelonephritis
Renovascular hypertension
Absence of kidney function
Renal infarction
Renal arterial atherosclerosis
Glomerulonephritis
Renal tumor
Congenital abnormalities
Renal trauma
Transplant rejection
Acute tubular necrosis
Renal abscess
Renal cyst

R

renin assay, plasma (Plasma renin activity [PRA])

Type of test Blood

Normal findings

Adult/elderly

Upright position, *sodium-depleted* (sodium-restricted diet)
Ages 20-39 years: 2.9-24.0 ng/ml/hr
>40 years: 2.9-10.8 ng/ml/hr
Upright position, *sodium-repleted* (normal sodium diet)
Ages 20-39 years: 0.1-4.3 ng/ml/hr
>40 years: 0.1-3.0 ng/ml/hr

Child
0-3 years: <16.6 ng/ml/hr
3-6 years: <6.7 ng/ml/hr
6-9 years: <4.4 ng/ml/hr
9-12 years: <5.9 ng/ml/hr
12-15 years: <4.2 ng/ml/hr
15-18 years: <4.3 ng/ml/hr

Test explanation and related physiology

Renin is an enzyme released by the juxtaglomerular apparatus of the kidney into the renal veins in response to hyperkalemia, sodium depletion, decreased renal blood perfusion, or hypovolemia. Renin activates the renin-angiotensin system, which results in angiotensin II, a powerful vasoconstrictor that also stimulates aldosterone production from the adrenal cortex. Angiotensin and aldosterone increase the blood volume, blood pressure, and serum sodium (Figure 30).

Renin is not actually measured in this test. The PRA test actually measures the rate of generation of angiotensin. This is the most commonly used renin assay. The *plasma renin concentration (PRC)* is used to measure the maximum renin effect.

The PRA is a screening procedure for the detection of essential, renal, or renovascular hypertension. The PRA may be supplemented by other tests such as the renal vein renin assay (see p. 730). A determination of the PRA and a measurement of the plasma aldosterone level (see p. 31) are used in the differential diagnosis of primary versus secondary hyperaldosteronism. Patients with primary hyperaldosteronism (adrenal adenoma overproducing aldosterone-Conn's syndrome) have increased aldosterone production associated with decreased

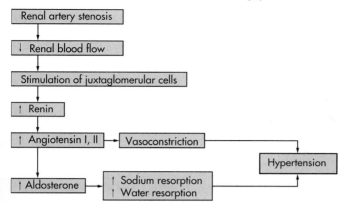

Figure 30 Physiology of renovascular hypertension.

renin activity. Patients with secondary hyperaldosteronism (caused by renovascular occlusive disease or primary renal disease) have increased levels of plasma renin.

The *renin stimulation test* can be performed to more clearly diagnosis and separate primary from secondary hyperaldosteronism. In this test PRA is obtained while the patient is in the recumbent and standing position. In primary hyperaldosteronism a change in position will not result in increased renin levels. In secondary hyperaldosteronism (or normals with essential hypertension), renin levels increase.

The PRA is assessed as part of the *captopril test*, a new screening test for renovascular hypertension (RVH). Patients with RVH have greater falls in blood pressure and increases in PRA after administration of angiotensin-converting enzyme (ACE) inhibitors than do those with essential hypertension.

Interfering factors

- Renin levels are affected by pregnancy, salt intake, and licorice ingestion.
- Values are higher in patients on low-salt diets, and when the patient is in an upright position.
- Posture affects renin levels. Renin is increased in the erect position and decreased in the recumbent position.
- Values are higher early in the day. There is a diurnal variation in renin production.

☙ Drugs that *increase* levels of renin include antihypertensives, ACE inhibitors, diuretics, estrogens, oral contraceptives, and vasodilators.

☙ Drugs that *decrease* renin levels include beta blockers, clonidine, potassium, licorice, and reserpine.

Procedure and patient care

Before

- Explain the procedure to the patient.
- Instruct the patient to maintain a normal diet with a restricted amount of sodium (approximately 3 g/day) for 3 days before the test. A high-sodium diet causes a decrease in renin.
- Instruct the patient to discontinue medications (e.g., diuretics, steroids, antihypertensives, vasodilators, oral contraceptives) and licorice for 2 to 4 weeks before the test.
- Usually draw a fasting blood sample because renin values are higher in the morning.
- For stimulation tests, instruct the patient to significantly reduce sodium intake (supplemented with potassium) for 3 days before testing.

During

- Usually perform the test with the patient in an upright position.
- For the stimulation tests, the blood is drawn in the recumbent and upright position.
- Ensure that the patient stands or sits upright for 2 hours before the blood is drawn.
- If a recumbent sample is ordered, have the patient remain in bed in the morning until the blood sample has been obtained.
- It is best to release the tourniquet immediately prior to obtaining the blood specimen because stasis can lower renin levels.
- Collect approximately 7 to 12 ml of venous blood and place it in a chilled lavender-top tube with ethylenediaminetetraacetic acid as an anticoagulant.
- Gently invert the blood tube to allow adequate mixing of the blood sample and the anticoagulant.
- Record the patient's position, dietary status, and time of day on the laboratory slip. Also note any medication that the patient is currently taking.

- Place the tube of blood on ice and immediately send it to the laboratory.

After

- Apply pressure to the venipuncture site.
- Tell the patient that usually a normal diet may be resumed.
- Note that medications that were withheld may be reordered.

Abnormal findings

▲ Increased levels
Essential hypertension
Malignant hypertension
Renovascular hypertension
Chronic renal failure
Salt-losing gastrointestinal disease (vomiting or diarrhea)
Addison's disease
Renin-producing renal tumor
Bartter syndrome
Cirrhosis
Hyperkalemia
Hemorrhage

▼ Decreased levels
Primary hyperaldosteronism
Steroid therapy
Congenital adrenal hyperplasia

notes

R

renin assay, renal vein

Type of test Blood

Normal findings Renin ratio of involved kidney to uninvolved kidney <1.4

Test explanation and related physiology

Renal vein assays for renin are used to diagnose renovascular hypertension, which is hypertension caused by inappropriately high renin levels in a diseased kidney or a hypoperfused kidney. See p. 726 for a full discussion of the physiology of renin. For this procedure a catheter is placed into each renal vein, and blood is withdrawn from each vein. If hypertension is caused by renal artery stenosis or renal pathology, the renal vein renin level of the affected kidney should be 1.4 or more times greater than that of the unaffected kidney. If the levels are the same, the hypertension is not caused by a renovascular source. Another cause for the patient's elevated blood pressure should be considered. This test is very helpful in determining whether a stenosis seen on a renal angiogram is significantly contributing to hypertension.

Contraindications

- Patients who are allergic to shellfish or iodinated dye

Potential complications

- Allergic reaction to iodinated dye.

Procedure and patient care

Before

- Explain the procedure to the patient.
- Ensure that written and informed consent for this procedure is obtained by the physician.
- Assess the patient for allergies to iodine.
- Place the patient on a "no added salt" diet and diuretics for 3 days before the examination.
- Keep the patient NPO after midnight on the day of the study.
- Instruct the patient to remain in the upright position for 2 hours before the test.
- Premedicate the fasting patient as ordered. Meperidine and atropine are typically used.

During

- Note the following procedural steps:
  1. The patient is taken to the radiology department and placed on the fluoroscopy table in a supine position.
  2. The patient's groin is prepared and draped in a sterile manner and then anesthetized.
  3. The femoral vein is punctured, and a catheter is placed into the vein and advanced into the inferior vena cava.
  4. Fluoroscopy is used to monitor the catheter placement.
  5. Dye is injected, and the renal veins are identified.
  6. The catheter is placed into one renal vein at a time, and separate blood specimens are withdrawn and labeled.
  7. The catheter is removed, and a pressure dressing is applied to the puncture site.
- Note that this procedure is usually performed by a radiologist in less than 1 hour.
- Inform the patient that the groin puncture needed for this study is uncomfortable.

After

- Usually place the patient on bed rest for several hours.
- Monitor the patient's vital signs.
- Usually send the blood to a commercial laboratory for analysis.
- Assess the patient for renal vein thrombosis, which may occur 1 to 7 days after the procedure. This will be manifested by costovertebral tenderness, hematuria, and elevated creatinine levels.
- Observe the venous puncture site frequently for hematoma or hemorrhage.
- Apply cold compresses to the puncture site if needed to reduce discomfort and swelling.
- See p. xviii for appropriate interventions concerning the care for patients with iodine allergy.

Abnormal findings

▲ **Increased levels**

Renal artery stenosis
Renal artery occlusion
Renin-producing renal tumor

reticulocyte count (Retic count)

Type of test Blood

Normal findings

Reticulocyte count:
  Adult/elderly/child: 0.5% to 2%
  Infant: 0.5% to 3.1%
  Newborn: 2.5% to 6.5%
Reticulocyte index: 1.0

Test explanation and related physiology

The reticulocyte count is a test for determining bone marrow function and evaluating erythropoietic activity. This test is also useful in classifying anemias. A reticulocyte is an immature red blood cell (RBC) that can be readily identified under a microscope. Normally there are a small number of reticulocytes in the bloodstream.

The reticulocyte count gives an indication of RBC production by the bone marrow. Increased reticulocyte counts indicate that the marrow is putting an increased number of RBCs into the bloodstream, usually in response to anemia. A normal or low reticulocyte count in a patient with anemia indicates that the marrow response to the anemia by way of production of RBCs is inadequate and perhaps contributing to or the cause of the anemia (as in aplastic anemia, iron deficiency, vitamin B_{12} deficiency, or depletion of iron stores). An elevated reticulocyte count found in patients with a normal hemogram indicates increased RBC production compensating for an ongoing loss of RBCs (hemolysis or hemorrhage).

Because the reticulocyte count is a percentage of the total number of RBCs, a normal to low number of reticulocytes can appear high in the anemic patient because the total number of mature RBCs is low. To determine if a reticulocyte count indicates an appropriate erythropoietic (RBC marrow) response in patients with anemia and a decreased hematocrit, one should calculate the *reticulocyte index*:

Reticulocyte index =

$$\text{Reticulocyte count (in \%)} \times \frac{\text{Patient's hematocrit}}{\text{Normal hematocrit}}$$

The reticulocyte index in a patient with a good marrow response to the anemia should be 1.0. If it is below 1.0, even though the reticulocyte count is elevated, the bone marrow response is inadequate in its ability to compensate.

Interfering factors

- Pregnancy may cause an increased reticulocyte count.
- RBCs containing Howell-Jolly bodies look like reticulocytes and are miscounted by the automated counter machines to be reticulocytes and give a falsely high number of reticulocytes.

Procedure and patient care

Before

- Tell the patient that no fasting is required.

During

- Collect approximately 5 to 7 ml of venous blood in a lavender-top tube.

After

- Apply pressure to the venipuncture site.

Abnormal findings

▲ **Increased levels**
  Hemolytic anemia
  Sickle cell anemia
  Hemorrhage (3 to 4 days later)
  Postsplenectomy
  Erythroblastosis fetalis
  Pregnancy
  Leukemias
  Recovery from nutritional anemias

▼ **Decreased levels**
  Pernicious anemia
  Folic acid deficiency
  Adrenocortical hypofunction
  Aplastic anemia
  Radiation therapy
  Marrow failure
  Anterior pituitary hypofunction
  Chronic infection
  Cirrhosis
  Malignancy

R

retrograde pyelography

Type of test X-ray with contrast dye

Normal findings Normal outline and size of the ureters and bladder

Test explanation and related physiology

Retrograde pyelography refers to radiographic visualization of the urinary tract through ureteral catheterization and the injection of contrast material. The ureters are catheterized during cystoscopy. A radiopaque material is injected into the ureters, and x-ray films are taken. This test can be performed even if the patient has an allergy to IV contrast dye, because none of the dye injected into the ureters is absorbed.

Retrograde pyelography is helpful in radiographically examining the ureters in patients when visualization with intravenous pyelography (IVP, see p. 497) is inadequate or contraindicated. When a ureter is obstructed, IVP will visualize only the ureter proximal to the obstruction, if at all. To visualize the distal part of the ureter, retrograde pyelography is necessary. Also, in patients with unilateral renal disease, the involved kidney and collecting system are not visualized because renal function is so poor. As a result, no dye will be filtered into the collecting system by the nonfunctioning kidney. To rule out ureteral obstruction as a cause of the unilateral kidney disease, retrograde pyelography must be done. Tumors, benign strictures, tortuous ureters, stones, scarring, and extrinsic compression may cause ureteral obstruction.

Potential complications

- Urinary tract infection
  Infections may be caused by the invasive nature of this procedure.
- Sepsis by seeding the bloodstream with bacteria from infected urine
- Perforation of the bladder or ureter
- Hematuria
- Temporary obstruction to ureteral urine flow
  Manipulation of the ureters may cause edema, which can result in temporary, partial obstruction to urine flow.
- Allergic reaction to iodinated dye
  This rarely occurs, because the dye is not administered intravenously.

Interfering factors

- Retained barium from previous x-ray studies could obscure visualization.

Procedure and patient care

Before

- Explain the procedure to the patient.
- Ensure that informed consent for this procedure is obtained.
- If enemas are ordered to clear the bowel, assist the patient as needed and record the results.
- If the procedure will be performed with the patient under general anesthesia, follow the routine general anesthesia precautions. Keep the patient NPO after midnight on the day of the test. Fluids may be given intravenously.
- Administer the preprocedural medications as ordered 1 hour before the study. Sedatives decrease the spasm of the bladder sphincter, thus decreasing the patient's discomfort.

During

- Note the following procedural steps:
  1. The ureteral catheters are passed into the ureters by means of cystoscopy (see p. 308).
  2. Radiopaque contrast material (Hypaque or Renografin) is injected into the ureteral catheters, and x-ray films are taken.
  3. The entire ureter and renal pelvis are demonstrated.
  4. As the catheters are withdrawn, more dye is injected, and more x-ray films are taken to visualize the complete outline of the ureters.
  5. A delayed film is often performed to assess the emptying capabilities of the ureter. This is usually done about 5 minutes after the last injection.
  6. If obstruction is noted, a stent may be left in the ureter so that the ureter can drain.
- Note that retrograde pyelography is performed by a urologist in approximately 1 hour in a cystoscopy room or operating room.
- Inform the patient that this study is uncomfortable. If awake, the patient will feel pressure and an urge to void.

R

After

- Check and record the patient's vital signs as ordered. Watch for a decrease in blood pressure and increase in pulse as an indication of bleeding.
- Observe the patient for signs and symptoms of sepsis (elevated temperature, flush, chills, decreased blood pressure, increased pulse).
- Assess the patient's ability to void for at least 24 hours. Urinary retention may be secondary to edema caused by instrumentation.
- Note the color of the urine; a pink tinge is typically present. Report bright-red blood or clots to the physician.
- Encourage the patient to increase intake of fluids. A dilute urine decreases dysuria. Fluids also maintain a constant flow of urine to prevent stasis and the accumulation of bacteria in the bladder.
- Monitor the patient for bladder spasms. Often, belladonna-and-opium suppositories are given to relieve bladder spasms.
- Administer analgesics as needed.

🏠 Home care responsibilities

- Observe the vital signs for indications of bleeding (decreased blood pressure, increased pulse) and sepsis (temperature, flush, chills).
- Monitor the urine output over the first 24 hours to detect urinary retention.
- Encourage the patient to drink lots of fluids to prevent stasis and to prevent the accumulation of bacteria in the bladder.

Abnormal findings

Tumor
Strictures
Stones
Ureteral obstruction
Intrinsic or extrinsic tumor affecting the ureters
Congenital anomaly

rheumatoid factor (RF)

Type of test Blood

Normal findings

Negative (<60 U/ml by nephelometric testing)
Elderly patients may have slightly increased values

Test explanation and related physiology

Rheumatoid arthritis (RA) is a chronic inflammatory disease that affects most joints, especially the metacarpal and phalangeal joints, the proximal interphalangeal joints, and the wrists; however, any synovial joint can be involved.

In this disease abnormal immunoglobulin G (IgG) antibodies produced by lymphocytes in the synovial membranes act as "antigens". Other IgG and IgM antibodies in the patient's serum react with the "fc" component of the abnormal synovial antigenic IgG to produce immune complexes. These immune complexes activate the complement system and other inflammatory systems to cause joint damage. The reactive IgM is called RF. Tissues other than the joints, including blood vessels, lungs, nerves, and heart, may also be involved in the autoimmune inflammation.

Tests for RF are directed toward identification of the IgM antibodies. The exact role, if any, that RF plays in the pathophysiology of the disease is not well known. Approximately 80% of patients with rheumatoid arthritis have positive RF titers. To be considered positive, RF must be found in a dilution of greater than 1:80; when RF is found in titers less than 1:80, diseases such as systemic lupus erythematosus, scleroderma, and other autoimmune conditions should be considered. Although the normal value is "no rheumatoid factor identifiable at low titers," a small number of normal patients will have RF present at a very low titer. Furthermore, a negative RF does not exclude the diagnosis of RA. RF is not a useful disease marker because its presence does not disappear in patients who are experiencing a remission from the disease symptoms.

Other autoimmune diseases (see Table 1, p. 80) such as systemic lupus erythematosus or Sjögren syndrome also may cause a positive RF test. RF is occasionally seen in patients with tuberculosis, chronic hepatitis, infectious mononucleosis, and subacute bacterial endocarditis as well.

Interfering factors

- Elderly patients often have false-positive results.

Procedure and patient care

Before

- Explain the procedure to the patient.
- Tell the patient that no fasting or preparation is required.

During

- Collect approximately 7 ml of venous blood in a red-top tube.

After

- Apply pressure to the venipuncture site.

Abnormal findings

▲ **Increased levels**

Rheumatoid arthritis
Other autoimmune diseases (e.g., systemic lupus erythematosus)
Chronic viral infection
Subacute bacterial endocarditis
Tuberculosis
Chronic hepatitis
Dermatomyositis
Scleroderma
Infectious mononucleosis
Leukemia
Cirrhosis
Syphilis
Renal disease

notes

rubella antibody test (German measles test, Hemagglutination inhibition [HAI])

Type of test Blood

Normal findings

Method	Result	Interpretation
HAI titer	<1:8	No immunity to rubella
HAI titer	>1:20	Immune to rubella
LA	negative	No immunity to rubella
ELISA — IgM	<0.9 IU/ml	No infection
ELISA — IgM	>1.1 IU/ml	Active infection
ELISA — IgG	<7 IU/ml	No immunity to rubella
ELISA — IgG	>10 IU/ml	Immune to rubella

LA, Latex agglutination; *ELISA,* enzyme-linked immunosorbent assay.

Possible critical values Evidence of susceptibility in pregnant women with recent exposure to rubella

Test explanation and related physiology

Screening for rubella antibodies is done to detect immunity to rubella. These tests detect the presence of IgG and/or IgM antibodies to rubella (the causative agent for German measles). They become elevated a few days to a few weeks after the onset of the rash, depending on what method of testing is used. IgM tends to disappear after about 6 weeks. IgG, however, persists at low but detectable levels for years. These antibodies become elevated in patients with active rubella infection or with past infections. It is vitally important to identify exposure to rubella infection and susceptibility status in pregnant women, because congenital rubella infection in the first trimester of pregnancy is associated with congenital abnormalities (heart defects, brain damage, deafness), abortion, or stillbirth. This test is sometimes used before pregnancy if a women is not sure if she has had rubella. If antibodies are not present, she can be immunized before pregnancy. The term TORCH (toxoplasmosis, other, rubella, cytomegalovirus, herpes) has been applied to infections with recognized detrimental effects on the fetus. The effects on the fetus may be direct or indirect (e.g., precipitating abortion or premature labor). All of these tests are discussed separately (see separate listings).

R

If the woman's titer is greater than $1:10$ to $1:20$, she is not susceptible to rubella. If the woman's titer is $1:8$ or less, she has little or no immunity to rubella. A fourfold increase in HAI rubella titer from the acute to the convalescent titer indicates that the rash was caused by an active rubella infection. Alternatively, an IgM antibody titer could be done. If the titer is positive, recent infection has occurred. IgM titers appear 1 to 2 days after onset of the rash and disappear 5 to 6 weeks after infection.

Anti-rubella antibody testing is also used to diagnose rubella in infants (congenital rubella). IgM anti-rubella antibodies cannot pass through the placenta. If an infant has IgM antibodies, acute congenital or newborn rubella is suspected. Antibody testing is often used in children with congenital abnormalities which may have come from congenital rubella infection.

Procedure and patient care

Before

- Explain the purpose of the test to the patient.

During

- Collect approximately 7 ml of venous blood in a red-top tube.

After

- Apply pressure to the venipuncture site.
- Inform the patient when to return for a follow-up HAI titer if indicated.

Abnormal findings

Active rubella infection
Previous rubella infection leading to immunity

notes

Schilling test (Vitamin B$_{12}$ absorption test)

Type of test Urine (24- to 48-hour); nuclear

Normal findings Excretion of 8% to 40% of radioactive vitamin B$_{12}$ within 24 hours

Test explanation and related physiology

The Schilling test is performed to evaluate vitamin B$_{12}$ absorption. Normally ingested vitamin B$_{12}$ combines with intrinsic factor (IF), which is produced by gastric mucosa, and is absorbed in the distal part of the ileum. Pernicious anemia results when absorption of vitamin B$_{12}$ is inadequate. This may be caused by a primary malabsorption problem of the intestinal tract or from lack of IF.

The two-stage Schilling test can detect a defect in vitamin B$_{12}$ absorption. With normal absorption the ileum absorbs more vitamin B$_{12}$ than the body needs and excretes the excess into the urine. With impaired absorption, however, little or no vitamin B$_{12}$ is excreted into the urine.

In the Schilling test urinary B$_{12}$ levels are measured after the ingestion of radioactive vitamin B$_{12}$. The test can be performed in one stage (without IF) or two stages (with IF). Patients with pernicious anemia from lack of IF will have an abnormal first-stage and a normal second-stage Schilling test. Patients with malabsorption from an intestinal source will have an abnormal first- and second-stage Schilling test. A combined one-stage and two-stage test is now commonly used.

All bone marrow and hematologic studies along with serum vitamin B$_{12}$ levels must be done before the Schilling's test. The vitamin B$_{12}$ that is administered during this test can significantly alter the test results.

Contraindications

- Patients who are pregnant
- Patients who are lactating

Interfering factors

- Radioactive nuclear material received 10 days before testing may affect results.
- Renal insufficiency may cause reduced excretion of radioactive vitamin B$_{12}$.

S

- Patients who are elderly or hypothyroid or who have diabetes may have reduced excretion of vitamin B_{12}.
- Drugs that may affect test results include laxatives, because they could *decrease* the rate of vitamin B_{12} absorption.

Procedure and patient care

Before

- Explain the procedure to the patient.
- Instruct the patient to remain NPO except for water 8 to 12 hours before the test. Food should not be given until after the patient receives the injections.
- Instruct the patient not to take laxatives during the test period.

During

- Note the following procedural steps:

First-stage Schilling test (without intrinsic factor)

1. Radioactive vitamin B_{12} is administered orally to the patient.
2. Shortly thereafter, nonradioactive vitamin B_{12} is administered to the patient intramuscularly to saturate tissue-binding sites and to permit some excretion of radioactive vitamin B_{12} in the urine if it is absorbed.
3. A 24- to 48-hour urine collection for vitamin B_{12} is obtained.
4. The patient is encouraged to drink fluids.

Second-stage Schilling test (with intrinsic factor)

1. If indicated, the second stage is performed approximately 1 week after the first stage.
2. The fasting patient is provided radioactive vitamin B_{12} combined with human intrinsic factor.
3. As before, an IM injection of nonradioactive vitamin B_{12} is administered.
4. Again, 24- to 48-hour urine collections are begun.

Combined one-stage and two-stage Schilling test

1. The fasting patient receives a capsule of cobalt-57-labeled vitamin B_{12} plus intrinsic factor.
2. A second capsule of cobalt-58-labeled vitamin B_{12} is also given.
3. One hour later an IM injection of nonradioactive vitamin B_{12} is administered.
4. Again the urine for vitamin B_{12} is collected for 24 to 48 hours.

5. Percentages of cobalt-57 and cobalt-58 are calculated. Cobalt-57-labeled vitamin B_{12} only will be present in patients with pernicious anemia secondary to lack of intrinsic factor. No vitamin B_{12} will be present in the urine of patients whose pernicious anemia is caused by primary bowel malabsorption.

After

- Ensure that the urine specimens are promptly transported to the laboratory.

Abnormal findings

▲ **Decreased levels**

Pernicious anemia
Intestinal malabsorption
Hypothyroidism
Liver disease

notes

scrotal nuclear imaging (Scrotal scan, Testicular imaging)

Type of test Nuclear medicine

Normal findings Symmetric and prompt blood flow to both testicles

Test explanation and related physiology

Scrotal imaging is helpful in the diagnosis of patients with a sudden onset of unilateral testicular swelling and pain. Scrotal imaging can differentiate unilateral testicular torsion from other causes of testicular pain (e.g., acute epididymitis, torsion of the testicular appendage, orchitis, strangulated hernia, testicular hemorrhage). Testicular torsion is a surgical emergency requiring prompt surgical exploration to salvage the involved testicle. It must be differentiated from other causes of testicular pain to provide immediate surgical care if the testicle is to be salvaged. The other causes of painful testicular swelling do not require surgery. Use of radionuclide scrotal imaging enables the surgeon to diagnose testicular torsion. This study is usually performed on an emergency basis and in the nuclear medicine department.

The patient is positioned under the gamma ray camera with the scrotum supported between the abducted thighs. Technetium-99m pertechnetate is administered, and a dynamic radionuclide angiogram is obtained. Static images are obtained immediately afterward. An area of decreased perfusion corresponding to the involved testes indicates a high probability of torsion of the testicle. If the clinically involved testes is normally perfused or hypervascular, a disease other than torsion of the testicle (as described earlier) exists. In 95% of all cases of testicular torsion, the scrotal image will make the diagnosis. This information can be obtained 10 to 15 minutes after injection of the nuclear material.

Procedure and patient care

Before

- Explain the procedure to the patient.
- Tell the patient that no fasting or premedication is required.
- Assure the patient that he will not be exposed to large amounts of radiation, because only tracer doses of isotope are used.

- If the patient is a child, encourage the parent(s) to be present.

During

- The patient is placed on a padded table in the supine position.
- The patient's legs are abducted, and the testicles are supported with tape or a lead shield. The penis is taped to the lower abdomen.
- A small IV injection of technetium-99m pertechnetate is administered.
- Radionuclide imaging is then immediately performed over both testicles. Both dynamic and static images are obtained.

After

- Because only tracer doses of radioisotopes are used, inform the patient that no precautions need to be taken by others against radiation exposure.
- If the patient is identified as having torsion of the testicle, prepare the patient for surgery.

Abnormal findings

▲ **Increased testicular blood flow**

Epididymitis
Torsion of the testicular appendage
Orchitis
Trauma

▼ **Decreased testicular blood flow**

Testicular torsion of the spermatic cord

notes

S

scrotal ultrasound (Ultrasound of testes)

Type of test Ultrasound

Normal findings Normal size, shape, and configuration of the testicles

Test explanation and related physiology

With the advent of scrotal ultrasound, a noninvasive, nonionizing, rapid method for scrotal examination was developed. Through the use of reflected sound waves, ultrasonography provides accurate visualization of the scrotum and its contents. Ultrasonography requires the emission of high-frequency sound waves from the transducer to penetrate the organ being studied. The sound waves are bounced back to the transducer and electronically converted into a pictorial image.

Present uses for scrotal ultrasound include:

1. Evaluation of scrotal masses
2. Measurement of testicular size
3. Evaluation of scrotal trauma
4. Evaluation of scrotal pain
5. Evaluation of occult testicular neoplasm
6. Surveillance of patients with prior primary or metastatic testicular neoplasms
7. Follow-up for testicular infections
8. Location of undescended testicles
9. Ultrasound guided needle biopsy of a suspected testicle tumor

With the real-time ultrasound transducer, the scrotum is examined. The testicle and extratesticular intrascrotal tissues are examined. The accuracy of scrotal ultrasound is 90% to 95%. Both benign and malignant tumors (primary and metastatic) can be identified with ultrasound. Benign abnormalities such as testicular abscess, orchitis, testicular infarction, and testicular torsion also can be identified. Extratesticular lesions such as hydrocele, hematocele (blood in the scrotum), and pyocele (pus in the scrotum) can be identified as well. Scrotal and groin ultrasound has been very helpful in locating cryptorchid (undescended) testicles.

There is very little discomfort associated with testicular ultrasound. It is usually performed by an ultrasound technologist and interpreted by an ultrasound physician.

Procedure and patient care

Before

- Explain the procedure to the patient.
- Tell the patient that no fasting is required.

During

- Note the following procedural steps:
  1. Careful examination of the scrotum is performed by the physician. Usually a short history is obtained.
  2. The scrotum is supported by a towel or cradled by the examiner's gloved hand.
  3. A greasy, conductive paste is applied to the scrotum before scanning. This paste enhances sound wave transmission and reception.
  4. Thorough scanning in the sagittal, transverse, and oblique projections is performed.
- The test takes approximately 20 to 30 minutes.

After

- Remove the coupling agent (grease) from the patient's scrotum.

Abnormal findings

Benign testicular tumor
Malignant testicular tumor
Occult testicular tumor
Testicular infection (orchitis)
Hydrocele
Hematocele
Pyocele
Varicocele
Epididymitis
Spermatocele
Scrotal hernia
Cryptorchidism
Hematoma
Testicular torsion

notes

S

secretin-pancreozymin (Pancreatic enzymes)

Type of test Fluid analysis

Normal findings
Volume: 2-4 ml/kg body weight
HCO_3^- (bicarbonate): 90-130 mEq/L
Amylase: 6.6-35.2 U/kg

Test explanation and related physiology

Cystic fibrosis is an inherited disease characterized by abnormal secretion by exocrine glands within the bronchi, small intestines, pancreatic ducts, bile ducts, and skin (sweat glands). Because of this abnormal exocrine secretion, children with cystic fibrosis develop mucous plugs that obstruct their pancreatic ducts. The pancreatic enzymes (e.g., amylase, lipase, trypsin, chymotrypsin) cannot be expelled into the duodenum and therefore are either completely absent or present only in diminished quantities within the duodenal aspirate. For the same reasons, bicarbonate and other neutralizing fluids cannot be secreted from the pancreas.

In this test, secretin and pancreozymin are used to stimulate pancreatic secretion of these enzymes and bicarbonate into the duodenum. The duodenal contents are then aspirated and examined for pH, bicarbonate, and enzyme levels; amylase is the most frequently measured enzyme. Diminished values are suggestive of cystic fibrosis. This test is indicated in children with recurrent respiratory tract infections, malabsorption syndromes, or failure to thrive.

Procedure and patient care

Before
- Explain the procedure to the patient and/or parents.
- Instruct the adult patient to fast for 12 hours before testing.
- Determine pediatric fasting times according to the patient's age.

During
- Note the following procedural steps:
  1. With the use of fluoroscopy, a Dreiling tube is passed through the patient's nose and into the stomach.

2. The distal lumen of the tube is placed within the duodenum.

3. The proximal lumen of the tube is placed within the stomach.

4. Both lumens are aspirated. The gastric lumen is continually aspirated to avoid contamination of the gastric contents in the duodenum aspirate.

5. A control specimen of the duodenal juices is collected for 20 minutes.

6. The patient is tested for sensitivity to secretin and pancreozymin by low-dose intradermal injection.

7. If no sensitivity is present, these hormones are administered intravenously. Secretin can be expected to stimulate pancreatic water and bicarbonate secretion. Pancreozymin can be expected to stimulate pancreatic enzyme (lipase, amylase, trypsin, chymotrypsin) secretion.

8. Four duodenal aspirates are collected at 20-minute intervals and placed in the specimen container.

9. Each specimen is analyzed for pH, volume, bicarbonate, and amylase levels.

- Note that a physician performs this test in approximately 2 hours in the laboratory or at the patient's bedside.
- Tell the patient that he or she may have discomfort and gagging during placement of the Dreiling tube.

After

- Place the aspirated specimens on ice. Send them to the chemistry laboratory as soon as the test is completed.
- Remove the Dreiling tube after completion of the test. Give appropriate nose and mouth care.
- Allow the patient to resume a normal diet.

Abnormal findings

Cystic fibrosis
Sprue

notes

semen analysis (Sperm count, Sperm examination, Seminal cytology, Semen examination)

Type of test Fluid analysis

Normal findings

Volume: 2-5 ml
Liquefaction time: 20 to 30 minutes after collection
pH: 7.12-8.00
Sperm count (density): 50-200 million/ml
Sperm motility: 60% to 80% actively motile
Sperm morphology: 70% to 90% normally shaped

Test explanation and related physiology

Semen analysis is one of the most important aspects of the fertility workup because the cause of a woman's inability to conceive often lies with the man. After 2 to 3 days of sexual abstinence, sperm is collected and examined for volume, sperm count, motility, and morphology.

The freshly collected semen is first measured for volume. After liquefaction of the white, gelatinous ejaculate, a sperm count is done. Men with very low or very high counts likely are infertile. The motility of the sperm is then evaluated; at least 60% should show progressive motility. Morphology is studied by staining a semen preparation and calculating the number of normal versus abnormal sperm forms. A single sperm analysis, especially if it indicates infertility, is inconclusive, because sperm count varies from day to day. A semen analysis should be done at least twice, and possibly a third time, 3 weeks apart.

Semen production depends on the function of the testicles. Semen analysis is a measure of testicular function. Inadequate sperm production can be the result of primary gonadal failure (Klinefelter syndrome, infection, radiation, or surgical orchidectomy) or secondary gonadal failure (caused by pituitary diseases). Men with *aspermia* (no sperm) or *oligospermia* (20 million/ml) should be evaluated endocrinologically for pituitary, thyroid, or testicular aberrations.

A normal semen analysis alone does not accurately assess the male factor unless the effect of the partner's cervical secretion on sperm survival is also determined (see Sims-Huhner test, p. 765). In addition to its value in infertility workups, semen analysis is also helpful in documenting adequate sterilization after a vasectomy. It is usually performed 6 weeks after the surgery. If any sperm are seen, the adequacy of the vasectomy must be questioned.

Interfering factors

☛ Drugs that may cause *decreased* semen levels include antineoplastic agents (e.g., nitrogen mustard, procarbazine, vincristine, methotrexate), cimetidine, estrogens, and methyltestosterone.

Procedure and patient care

Before

- Explain the procedure to the patient.
- Instruct the patient to abstain from sexual activity for 2 to 3 days before collecting the specimen. Prolonged abstinence before the collection should be discouraged because the quality of the sperm cells, and especially their motility, may diminish.
- Give the patient the proper container for the sperm collection.
- Instruct the patient to avoid alcoholic beverages for several days before the collection.
- For evaluation of the adequacy of vasectomy, the patient should ejaculate once or twice before the day of examination.

During

- Note that semen is best collected by ejaculation into a clean container. For best results, the specimen should be collected in the physician's office or laboratory by masturbation.
- Note that less satisfactory specimens can be obtained in the patient's home by coitus interruptus or masturbation. Note the following procedural steps:
  1. Instruct the patient to deliver these home specimens to the laboratory within 1 hour after collection.
  2. Tell the patient to avoid excessive heat and cold during transportation of the specimen.

After

- Record the date of the previous semen emission, along with the collection time and date of the fresh specimen.
- Tell the patient when and how to obtain the test results. Remember that abnormal results may have a devastating effect on the patient's sexuality.

S

Abnormal findings

Infertility
Vasectomy (obstruction of vas deferens)
Orchitis
Testicular atrophy
Testicular failure
Hyperpyrexia

notes

sexually transmitted disease cultures (STD cultures, culture of cervix, urethra, and anus)

Type of test Microscopic examination; blood

Normal findings No evidence of sexually transmitted disease

Test Explanation and related physiology

STDs can cause urethritis, vaginitis, endometritis, pelvic inflammatory disease, pharyngitis, proctitis, epididymitis, prostatitis, and salpingitis. Children born of infected mothers may develop conjunctivitis, pneumonia, neonatal blindness, neonatal neurologic injury, and even death.

Cultures for STD infections are performed on men and women with suggestive symptoms. If the culture is positive, sexual partners should be evaluated and treated. Cervical cultures are usually done for women; urethral cultures are done for men. Rectal and throat cultures are performed in persons who have engaged in anal and oral intercourse. Because rectal gonorrhea accompanies genital gonorrhea in a high percentage of women, rectal cultures are recommended in all women with suspected gonorrhea.

Other STDs are identified by culture or smear of a genital lesion, tissue biopsy, serologic testing, and observation of classic clinical lesion (see Table 16).

Interfering factors

- *N. gonorrhoeae* can be destroyed by the use of lubricants and disinfectants.
- Menses may alter test results.
- Female douching within 24 hours of a cervical culture makes fewer organisms available for culture.
- Male voiding within 1 hour of a urethral culture washes secretions out of the urethra.
- Fecal material may contaminate an anal culture.

Procedure and patient care

Before

- Explain the purpose and procedure to the patient. Use a matter-of-fact, nonjudgmental approach.
- Tell the patient that no fasting or sedation is required.

TABLE 16 Sexually transmitted diseases (STDs) and methods of diagnosis

Disease	Method of diagnosis
Gonorrhea	Cervical, urethral, anal, oropharyngeal cultures
Chlamydia Lymphogranuloma venereum *C. trachomatis*	Cervical, urethral culture, serology, DNA probe testing (see p. 227)
Herpes genitalis	Culture from lesion, serology (see p. 474)
Syphilis	Serology, fluid cultures (CNS), darkfield slide (see p. 797)
Hepatitis	Serology (see p. 470)
AIDS	Serology (see p. 23)
Trichomoniasis	Cervical, urethral, vaginal smear on a wet mount
Candida (Monilia)	Wet mount, Gram stain, fungal culture
Gardnerella vaginialis	Cervical, urethral, anal cultures

During

- Obtain cultures as follows:

Cervical culture

1. The female patient is told to refrain from douching and tub bathing before the cervical culture.
2. The patient is placed in the lithotomy position, and a moistened nonlubricated vaginal speculum is inserted to expose the cervix.
3. Cervical mucus is removed with a cotton ball held in a ring forceps.
4. A sterile cotton-tipped swab is inserted into the endocervical canal and moved from side to side to obtain the culture.
5. The swab is placed in sterile saline or a transporting fluid obtained from the laboratory. The specimen should be plated as soon as possible. The specimen should not be refrigerated.

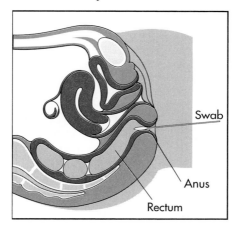

Figure 31 Rectal culture of the female. Method for obtaining an anorectal culture for sexually transmitted diseases on a female patient. (From Pagana KD, Pagana TJ: *Mosby's manual of diagnostic and laboratory tests,* St Louis, 1998, Mosby.)

Anal canal culture

1. An anal culture of the female or male patient is taken by inserting a sterile, cotton-tipped swab approximately 1 inch into the anal canal (see Figure 31).
2. If stool contaminates the swab, a repeat swab is taken.

Urethral culture

1. The urethral specimen should be obtained from the male patient before voiding. Voiding within 1 hour of collection washes secretions out of the urethra, making fewer organisms available for culture. The best time to obtain the specimen is before the first morning micturition.
2. A culture is taken by inserting a sterile swab gently into the anterior urethra (see Figure 32).
3. It is advisable to place the male patient in the supine position to prevent falling if vasovagal syncope occurs during introduction of the cotton swab or wire loop into the urethra.
4. The patient is observed for hypotension, bradycardia, pallor, sweating, nausea, and weakness.
5. Prostatic massage may increase the chances of obtaining positive cultures.

S

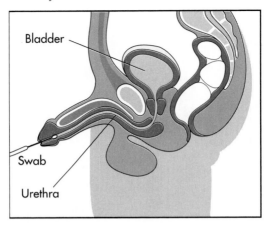

Figure 32 Urethral culture of the male. Method for obtaining an urethral culture for sexually transmitted diseases on a male patient. (From Pagana KD, Pagana TJ: *Mosby's manual of diagnostic and laboratory tests,* St Louis, 1998, Mosby.)

Oropharyngeal culture

1. This culture should be obtained in male and female patients who have engaged in oral intercourse.
2. A throat culture is best obtained by depressing the patient's tongue with a wooden tongue blade and touching the posterior wall of the throat with a sterile cotton-tipped swab.

After

- Place the swabs for gonorrhea in a Thayer-Martin medium and roll them from side to side.
- Label and send the culture bottle to the microbiology laboratory.
- Transport the specimen to the laboratory as soon as possible.
- Handle all specimens as though they were capable of transmitting disease.
- Do not refrigerate the specimen.
- Mark the laboratory slip with the collection time, date, source of specimen, patient's age, current antibiotic therapy, and clinical diagnosis.
- Advise the patient to avoid intercourse and all sexual contact until test results are available.

- If the culture results are positive, tell the patient to obtain treatment and to have sexual partners evaluated.
- Note that repeat cultures should be taken after completion of treatment to evaluate therapy.

Abnormal findings

STD

notes

S

sialography

Type of test X-ray

Normal findings No evidence of pathology in the salivary ducts and related structures

Test explanation and related physiology

Sialography is an x-ray procedure used to examine the salivary ducts (parotid, submaxillary, submandibular, sublingual) and related glandular structures after injection of a contrast medium into the desired duct. This procedure is used to detect calculi, strictures, tumors, or inflammatory disease in patients who complain of pain, tenderness, or swelling in these areas.

Contraindications

- Patients with mouth infections

Potential complication

- Allergic reaction to the iodinated dye
  This rarely occurs because the dye is not administered intravenously.

Procedure and patient care

Before

- Explain the procedure to the patient. The thought of a dye injection in the mouth is frightening to many patients. Provide emotional support.
- Obtain informed consent if required by the institution.
- Instruct the patient to remove jewelry, hairpins, and dentures, which could obscure x-ray visualization.
- Instruct the patient to rinse his or her mouth before the procedure with an antiseptic solution to reduce the possibility of introducing bacteria into the ductal structures.

During

- Note the following procedural steps:
  1. X-ray studies are taken before the dye injection to ensure that stones are not present, which could prevent the contrast material from entering the ducts.
  2. The patient is placed in a supine position on an x-ray table.
  3. The contrast medium is injected directly into the desired orifice via a cannula or a special catheter.

4. X-ray films are taken with the patient in various positions.
5. The patient is given a sour substance (e.g., lemon juice) orally to stimulate salivary excretion.
6. Another set of x-ray studies is taken to evaluate ductal drainage.

- Note that a radiologist performs this procedure in the radiology department in less than 30 minutes.
- Tell the patient that he or she may feel a little pressure as the contrast medium is injected into the ducts.

After

- Encourage the patient to drink fluids to eliminate the dye.

Abnormal findings

Calculi
Strictures
Tumor
Inflammatory disease

notes

S

sickle cell test (Sickle cell preparation, Sickledex, Hgb S test)

Type of test Blood

Normal findings No sickle cells present

Test explanation and related physiology

Both sickle cell disease (homozygous for hemoglobin [Hgb] S) and sickle cell trait (heterozygous for Hgb S) can be detected by this study. Sickle cell anemia results from a genetic homozygous defect and is caused by the presence of Hgb S instead of Hgb A. When Hgb S becomes deoxygenated, it tends to bend in a way that causes the red blood cell (RBC) to assume a sickle shape. These sickled RBCs cannot freely pass through the capillaries, and thus they cause plugging of the microvascular tree. This may compromise the blood supply to various organs. Hgb S is found in varying quantities in 8% to 10% of the black population.

The routine peripheral blood smear of patients with sickle cell disease does not contain sickled RBCs unless hypoxemia is present. In the sickle cell test a deoxygenating agent is added to the patient's blood. If 25% or more of the patient's hemoglobin is of the S variation, the cells will assume the crescent (sickle) shape, and the test is positive. If no sickling occurs, the test is negative. A negative test indicates that the patient has no or very little Hgb S. Other less common hemoglobin variants also may cause sickling.

This test is only a screening test, and its sensitivity varies according to the method used by the laboratory. The definitive diagnosis is made by hemoglobin electrophoresis (see p. 467), in which Hgb S can be identified and quantified.

Interfering factors

- Any blood transfusions within 3 to 4 months before the sickle cell test may cause false-negative results because the donor's normal hemoglobin may dilute the recipient's abnormal Hgb S.
- Polycythemia may cause false-negative results.
- Infants less than 3 months of age may have false-negative results.
- Drugs that may cause false-negative results include phenothiazines.

Procedure and patient care

Before
- Explain the procedure to the patient.
- Tell the patient that no fasting is required.

During
- Collect approximately 7 ml of venous blood in a lavender-top tube.

After
- Apply pressure to the venipuncture site.
- If the test is positive, offer the family genetic counseling. A patient with one recessive gene (heterozygous) is said to have sickle cell *trait*. A patient with two recessive genes (homozygous) has sickle cell *anemia*.
- Inform patients with sickle cell anemia that they should avoid situations in which hypoxia may occur (e.g., strenuous exercise, air travel in unpressurized aircraft, travel to high-altitude regions).

Abnormal findings

Sickle cell trait
Sickle cell anemia

notes

S

sigmoidoscopy (Proctoscopy, Anoscopy)

Type of test Endoscopy

Normal findings Normal anus, rectum, and sigmoid colon

Test explanation and related physiology

Endoscopy of the lower gastrointestinal (GI) tract allows one to visualize and perform biopsies of tumors, polyps, hemorrhoids, or ulcers of the anus, rectum, and sigmoid colon. *Anoscopy* refers to examination of the anus; *proctoscopy* to examination of the anus and rectum; and *sigmoidoscopy* (the most frequent procedure) to examination of the anus, rectum, and sigmoid colon. This test can be performed with a rigid or flexible sigmoidoscope. Because the lower GI tract is difficult to visualize radiographically, direct visualization by sigmoidoscopy is helpful.

Furthermore, sigmoidoscopy, as with colonoscopy, can be therapeutic. Reduction of sigmoid volvulus, removal of polyps, and obliteration of hemorrhoids can be performed through the sigmoidoscope.

Contraindications

- Patients who are uncooperative
- Patients with diverticulitis
- Patients with painful anorectal conditions (e.g., fissures, fistulas, hemorrhoids)
- Patients with severe bleeding
  Blood clots obstruct the view of the scope.
- Patients suspected of having perforated colon lesions

Potential complications

- Perforation of the colon
- Bleeding from biopsy sites

Interfering factors

- Poor bowel preparation may obscure visualization of the bowel mucosa.
- Rectal bleeding may obstruct the lens system and preclude adequate visualization.

Procedure and patient care

Before

- Explain the procedure to the patient.
- Obtain informed consent for this procedure.
- Assist the patient with bowel preparation. In most cases two Fleet enemas are sufficient.
- Instruct the patient to ingest only a light breakfast on the morning of the endoscopy.
- Assure patients that they will be properly draped to avoid unnecessary embarrassment.

During

- Note the following procedural steps:
  1. The patient is placed on the endoscopy table or bed in the left lateral decubitus position. Physicians often prefer the knee-chest position; many operating and examining tables are easily converted to make the knee-chest position more comfortable. This procedure also can be performed with the patient in the lithotomy position.
  2. Usually no sedation is required.
  3. The anus is mildly dilated with a well-lubricated finger.
  4. The rigid or flexible sigmoidoscope is placed into the rectum and advanced to its point of maximal penetration.
  5. Air is insufflated during the procedure to distend more fully the lower intestinal tract.
  6. The sigmoid, rectum, and anus are visualized.
  7. Biopsies can be obtained, and polypectomy performed at the time of sigmoidoscopy.
- Note that a physician trained in GI endoscopy usually performs this procedure in the GI laboratory, operating room, patient's bedside, or outpatient clinic setting in approximately 15 to 20 minutes.
- Tell the patient that he or she probably will feel discomfort and the urge to defecate as the sigmoidoscope is inserted.

After

- Inform the patient that because air has been insufflated into the bowel during the procedure, he or she may have flatulence or gas pains. Ambulation may help.
- Observe the patient for signs of abdominal distention, increased tenderness, or rectal bleeding.
- Tell the patient that slight rectal bleeding may occur if biopsies have been taken.

S

🏠 Home care responsibilities

- Observe for increasing abdominal pain, which may indicate bowel perforation.
- Note that fever and chills may indicate a bowel perforation.
- Inform the patient that frequent bloody bowel movements may indicate poor hemostasis if biopsy or polypectomy was performed.
- Observe for abdominal bloating and inability to pass flatus, which may indicate colon obstruction if a neoplasm was identified.

Abnormal findings

Tumor (benign or malignant)
Polyps
Ulcerative colitis
Pseudomembranous colitis
Crohn's disease (regional enteritis)
Intestinal ischemia
Irritable bowel syndrome

notes

Sims-Huhner test (Postcoital test, Postcoital cervical mucus test, Cervical mucus sperm penetration test)

Type of test Fluid analysis

Normal findings

Cervical mucus adequate for sperm transmission, survival, and
penetration
6 to 20 active sperm per high-power field

Test explanation and related physiology

The Sims-Huhner test consists of a postcoital examination of
the cervical mucus to measure the ability of the sperm to
penetrate the mucus and maintain motility. This test is used in
the evaluation of infertile couples. It evaluates interaction
between the sperm and the cervical mucus. It also measures the
quality of the cervical mucus. This test can determine the effect
of vaginal and cervical secretions on the activity of the sperm. It
is only performed after a previously performed semen analysis has
been determined to be normal.

This test is performed during the middle of the ovulatory
cycle, because at this time the secretions should be optimal
for sperm penetration and survival. During ovulation the
quantity of cervical mucus is maximal, whereas the viscosity is
minimal, thus facilitating sperm penetration. The *endocervical
mucus sample* is examined for color, viscosity, and tenacity
(*spinnbarkeit*) (Figure 33). The fresh specimen is then spread on
a clean glass slide and examined for the presence of sperm.
Estimates of the total number and of the number of motile
sperm per high-power field are reported. Normally, 6 to 20
active sperm cells should be seen in each microscopic high-power
field; if the sperm are present but not active, the cervical
environment is unsuitable (e.g., abnormal pH) for their survival.

After the specimen has dried on the glass slide, the mucus can
be examined for *ferning*. This pattern is correlated with estrogen
activity and is therefore present in all ovulatory women at
midcycle. When the cervical mucus is checked again immediately
before menstruation, no ferning is found because of progesterone activity. The Sims-Huhner study is invaluable in fertility
examinations; however, it is not a substitute for the semen
analysis. If the results of the Sims-Huhner test are less than

Figure 33 Cervical mucus test. Spinnbarkheit (elasticity) of the cervical mucus increases at ovulation.

optimal, the test is usually repeated during the same or next ovulatory cycle.

This analysis is also helpful in documenting cases of suspected rape by testing the vaginal and cervical secretions for sperm.

Procedure and patient care

Before

- Explain the procedure to the patient.
- Inform the patient that basal body temperature recordings should be used to indicate ovulation.
- Tell the patient that no vaginal lubrication, douching, or bathing is permitted until after the vaginal cervical examination, because these factors will alter the cervical mucus.
- Inform the patient that this study should be performed after 3 days of sexual abstinence.
- Instruct the patient to remain in bed for 10 to 15 minutes after coitus to ensure cervical exposure to the semen. After resting, the patient should report to her physician for examination of her cervical mucus within 2 hours after coitus.

During

- Note that, with the patient in the lithotomy position, the cervix is exposed by an unlubricated speculum. The specimen is aspirated from the endocervix and delivered to the laboratory for analysis.
- Note that this procedure is performed by a physician in approximately 5 minutes.
- Tell the patient that the only discomfort associated with this study is insertion of the speculum.

After

- Tell the patient how and when she may obtain the test results.

Abnormal findings

Infertility
Suspected rape

notes

S

skull x-ray

Type of test X-ray

Normal findings Normal skull and surrounding structures

Test explanation and related physiology

An x-ray film of the skull allows for visualization of the bones making up the skull, the nasal sinuses, and any cerebral calcification. This study is indicated for patients in whom a pathologic condition is suspected in any of these structures.

Skull fractures are easily seen as abnormal radiolucent lines in an otherwise radiopaque skull bone. Metastatic tumors of the skull can easily be seen as radiolucent spots in an otherwise normal skull. Opacification of the nasal sinuses may indicate sinusitis, hemorrhage, or tumor.

Located in the middle of the brain, the pineal gland is thought to regulate the biorhythms of mammals. This gland may become calcified after puberty. When calcified, the pineal gland is a very useful marker and allows the midline of the brain to be easily identified on the skull x-ray film. Conditions such as unilateral hematoma or tumor cause a shift of the midline structures (and the calcified pineal gland) to the side opposite the site of the pathologic condition. Simple skull x-ray films therefore allow for the easy detection of these unilateral, space-occupying lesions.

The *sella turcica* (an area of the bony cranium at the base of the skull) surrounds and protects the pituitary gland. Tumors of the pituitary gland may cause an increase in size or an erosion of the sella turcica. These changes can be detected by skull x-ray films.

Procedure and patient care

Before

- Explain the procedure to the patient.
- Instruct the patient to remove all objects above the neck because metal objects and dentures prevent x-ray visualization of the structures they cover.
- Avoid hyperextension and manipulation of the head if surgical injuries are suspected.
- Tell the patient that no sedation or fasting is required.

During

- Note that the patient is taken to the radiology department and placed on an x-ray table. Axial (submentovertical), half-axial (Towne), posteroanterior, and lateral views of the skull are usually taken.
- Note that a radiologic technologist takes skull films in a few minutes.
- Tell the patient that this test is painless.

After

- If a prosthetic eye is present, note this on the x-ray examination request, because it can present a confusing shadow on x-ray film.

Abnormal findings

Skull fracture
Metastatic tumor
Sinusitis
Hemorrhage
Tumor
Hematoma
Congenital anomaly

notes

sleep studies (Polysomnography [PSG])

Type of test electrodiagnostic; miscellaneous

Normal findings Respiratory disturbance index (RDI): <5-10 episodes per study

Test explanation and related physiology

Sleep studies are used to diagnose obstructive sleep apnea (OSA). OSA occurs as a result of complete upper airway obstruction associated with no ventilation for at least 10 seconds. These apneic spells may be associated with significant oxygen desaturation, cardiac rhythm disturbances, muscle spasms/seizures (restless leg syndrome), sleep interruption, and insomnia. As a result of the above symptoms, the patient's sleep is frequently interrupted. The preceding partial or near-complete upper airway obstruction causes excessive snoring. The daytime sequelae of sleep apnea is excessive daytime sleeping/narcolepsy.

Other nonairway obstructive forms of sleep apnea exist. Central sleep apnea is highlighted by simple cessation of breathing unrelated to obstructed airway. Primary cardiac events that lead to significant and transient reduction in cardiac output can also cause apnea.

Testing for OSA is performed in a sleep laboratory especially constructed for this type of testing. During the observation period (usually done during normal sleep hours), the patient is monitored by electrocardiogram (ECG), pulse oximetry, electroencephalogram (EEG), and electromyography (see pp. 335, 604, 340, and 343). Airflow in the mouth and nose is monitored. Chest and abdominal wall impedance as a measure of respiratory effort is also monitored.

Interfering factors

- Psychologic-induced insomnia associated with laboratory environmental changes compared to home may occur. Environmental noises, temperature changes, or others sensations may affect the sleep pattern.

Procedure and patient care

Before

- Explain the procedure to the patient.
- Caffeine should be avoided for several days before testing.

- Reassure the patient that monitoring equipment will not interrupt the patient's sleeping pattern.
- Allow the patient to express concerns about videotaping and other forms of monitoring.

During

- Electrodes for ECG, EEG, and electromyography are applied to the patient. Excess hair may need to be shaved on male patients.
- Airflow, oximetry, and impedance monitors are also applied.
- Once the patient is comfortable, the patient is allowed to sleep per normal routine.
- The lights are turned off, and monitoring begins before sleeping.

After

- On completion of the sleep cycle, the monitors and electrodes are removed.
- Test results take several days to collate and interpret.

Abnormal findings

Obstructive sleep apnea
Central sleep apnea
Cardiac sleep apnea

notes

S

small bowel follow-through (SBF, Small bowel enema)

Type of test X-ray with contrast dye

Normal findings

Normal positioning, motility, and patency of the small intestine
No evidence of intrinsic obstruction or extrinsic compression

Test explanation and related physiology

The SBF study is performed to identify abnormalities in the small bowel. Usually the patient is asked to drink barium; in patients who cannot drink, barium can be injected through a nasogastric tube. X-ray films are then taken at timed intervals (usually 30 minutes) to follow the progression of barium through the small intestine. Significant delays in transit time of the barium may occur with both benign and malignant forms of obstruction or diminished intestinal motility (ileus). On the other hand, the flow of barium is faster in patients who have hypermotility states of the small bowel (malabsorption syndromes). Failure of the progression through the small bowel can be seen in patients with partial mechanical small bowel obstruction or diminished intestinal motility, as seen in patients with diabetes. Furthermore, SBF series are helpful in identifying and defining the anatomy of small bowel fistulas (abnormal connections between the small bowel and other abdominal organs or skin).

A more accurate radiographic evaluation of the small intestine is provided by the *small bowel enema*. Unlike the SBF, in which the barium is swallowed by the patient, during the small bowel enema the barium is injected into a tube previously passed to the small bowel. This small bowel enema provides better visualization of the entire small bowel, because the barium is not diluted by gastric and duodenal juices, as occurs when the patient drinks barium. This test is especially useful in the evaluation of patients with partial small bowel obstruction of unknown etiology. Tumors, ulcers, and small bowel fistulas are more easily identified and defined with the enema.

Contraindications

- Patients with a complete small bowel obstruction
  The introduction of barium into an obstructed bowel may create a stonelike impaction; however, this is extremely rare.

- Patients suspected of having a perforated viscus
Barium should not be used in these patients because it may cause prolonged and recurrent abscesses if it leaks out of the bowel. Gastrografin, a water-soluble contrast medium, can be used if perforation is suspected. Unfortunately, Gastrografin becomes diluted very rapidly, minimizing the accuracy of the SBF with this contrast medium.
- Patients with unstable vital signs
These patients should be supervised during the time required for this study.

Potential complication

- Barium-induced small bowel obstruction

Interfering factors

- Barium within the intestinal tract from a previous barium x-ray film.
This may obstruct adequate visualization of the small bowel.
- Food or fluid within the gastrointestinal tract

Procedure and patient care

Before

- Explain the procedure to the patient.
- Instruct the patient not to eat anything for at least 8 hours before the test. Usually keep the patient NPO after midnight on the day of the test.
- Inform the patient that the SBF series may take several hours. Suggest that the patient bring reading material or some paperwork to occupy his or her time.
- Accompany the patient to the radiology department if his or her vital signs are not stable.
- Arrange for transportation of the hospitalized patient back to the nursing unit between serial films.

During

- Note the following procedural steps:
  1. A specially prepared drink containing barium sulfate is mixed as a milkshake, which the patient drinks through a straw.
  2. Usually, an upper GI series is performed concomitantly (see p. 854).
  3. The barium flow is followed through the upper GI tract fluoroscopically.

S

4. At frequent intervals (15 to 60 minutes), repeat x-ray films are taken to follow the flow of barium through the small intestine. These films are repeated until barium is seen flowing into the right colon. This usually takes 60 to 120 minutes, but in patients with delayed progression of the barium, the test may take as much as 24 hours to complete.

Small bowel enema

1. This is usually performed by placing a long, weighted tube transorally; however, a tube also can be placed into the upper small bowel endoscopically.
2. After the tube is in place, a thickened barium mixture is injected through the tube, and x-ray films are serially performed as described for the SBF.

- Note that this procedure is performed by a radiologist in the radiology department in approximately 30 minutes.
- Tell the patient that this test is not uncomfortable.

After

- Inform the patient of the need to evacuate adequately all the barium. Cathartics (e.g., magnesium citrate) are recommended. Initially stools will be white and should return to normal color with complete evacuation.

Abnormal findings

Small bowel tumor
Small bowel obstruction from intrinsic tumors
Small bowel obstruction from adhesions, extrinsic tumors, or hernia
Inflammatory small bowel disease (e.g., Crohn's disease)
Malabsorption syndromes (e.g., Whipple's disease, sprue)
Congenital anatomic anomaly (e.g., malrotation)
Congenital abnormalities (e.g., small bowel atresia, duplication, Meckel's diverticulum)
Small bowel intussusception
Small bowel perforation

notes

sodium (Na⁺), blood

Type of test Blood

Normal findings

Adult/elderly: 136-145 mEq/L or 136/145 mmol/L
  (SI units)
Child: 136-145 mEq/L
Infant: 134-150 mEq/L
Newborn: 134-144 mEq/L

Possible critical values <120 or >160 mEq/L

Test explanation and related physiology

Sodium is the major cation in the extracellular space, where serum levels of approximately 140 mEq/L exist. The concentration of sodium intracellularly is only 5 mEq/L. Therefore sodium salts are the major determinants of extracellular osmolality. The sodium content of the blood is a result of a balance between dietary sodium intake and renal excretion. Normally individual nonrenal (e.g., sweat) sodium losses are minimal.

Many factors regulate homeostatic sodium balance. Aldosterone causes conservation of sodium by decreasing renal losses. Natriuretic hormone, or third factor, increases renal losses of sodium. Antidiuretic hormone (ADH), which controls the resorption of water at the distal tubules of the kidney, also affects sodium serum levels.

Physiologically water and sodium are very closely interrelated. As free body water is increased, serum sodium is diluted, and the concentration may decrease. The kidney compensates by conserving sodium and excreting water. If free body water were to decrease, the serum sodium concentration would rise; the kidney would then respond by conserving free water. Aldosterone, adrenocorticotropic hormone (ADH), and natriuretic factor all assist in these compensatory actions of the kidney.

An average dietary intake of approximately 90 to 250 mEq/day is needed to maintain sodium balance in adults. Symptoms of hyponatremia may include weakness, confusion, lethargy, stupor, and coma. Symptoms of hypernatremia include dry mucous membranes, thirst, agitation, restlessness, hyperreflexia, mania, and convulsions.

S

Interfering factors

- Recent trauma, surgery, or shock may cause increased levels.
- Drugs that may cause *increased* levels include anabolic steroids, antibiotics, clonidine, corticosteroids, cough medicines, laxatives, methyldopa, carbenicillin, estrogens, and oral contraceptives.
- Drugs that may cause *decreased* levels include carbamazepine, diuretics, sodium-free IV fluids, sulfonylureas, triamterene, ACE inhibitors, captopril, haloperidol, heparin, nonsteroidal antiinflammatory drugs (NSAIDs), tricyclic antidepressants, and vasopressin.

Procedure and patient care

Before

- Explain the procedure to the patient.
- Tell the patient that no food or fluid is restricted.

During

- Collect 5 to 10 ml of venous blood in a red- or green-top tube.
- If the patient is receiving an IV infusion, obtain the blood from the opposite arm.
- List on the laboratory slip any drugs that may affect test results.

After

- Apply pressure to the venipuncture site.

Abnormal findings

▲ **Increased levels (hypernatremia)**

Increased sodium intake
Excessive dietary intake
Excessive sodium in IV fluids

Decreased sodium loss
Cushing's syndrome
Hyperaldosteronism

Excessive free body water loss
Excessive sweating
Extensive thermal burns
Diabetes insipidus
Osmotic diuresis

▼ **Decreased levels (hyponatremia)**

Decreased sodium intake
Deficient dietary intake
Deficient sodium in IV fluids

Increased sodium loss
Addison's disease
Diarrhea
Vomiting or nasogastric aspiration
Diuretic administration
Chronic renal insufficiency

Increased free body water
Excessive oral water intake
Excessive IV water intake
Congestive heart failure
Syndrome of inappropriate secretion of ADH (SIADH)
Osmotic dilution

Third-space losses of sodium
Ascites
Peripheral edema
Pleural effusion
Intraluminal bowel loss (ileus or mechanical obstruction)

S

notes

sodium (Na⁺), urine

Type of test Urine (24-hour)

Normal findings

40-220 mEq/L/day or 40-220 mmol/L (SI units)
Values vary greatly with dietary intake

Test explanation and related physiology

This test evaluates sodium balance in the body by determining the amount of sodium excreted in urine over 24 hours. Sodium is the major cation in the extracellular space. Measuring the amount of sodium in the urine is useful for evaluating patients with volume depletion, acute renal failure, adrenal disturbances, and acid-base imbalances. This test is important, especially when the serum sodium concentration is low. For example, in patients with hyponatremia caused by inadequate sodium intake, the urine sodium will be low. In patients with hyponatremia caused by chronic renal failure, however, the urine sodium concentration will be high.

The sodium content in urine is the result of the balance between the dietary sodium and the renal excretion of sodium. In the normal individual, nonrenal sodium losses are minimal. Many factors affect this delicate homeostatic sodium balance. For example, aldosterone tends to decrease urine sodium levels by stimulating conservation of sodium. Antidiuretic hormone, which increases the resorption of water in the distal tubules of the kidney, tends to increase urine sodium levels.

Interfering factors

- Dietary salt intake may increase sodium levels.
- Altered kidney function may affect levels.
- ⚕ Drugs that may cause *increased* levels include antibiotics, cough medicines, laxatives, and steroids.
- ⚕ Drugs that may cause *decreased* levels include diuretics (e.g., Lasix) and steroids.

Procedure and patient care

Before

- Explain the procedure to the patient.
- Tell the patient that no fasting is required.

During

- Instruct the patient to begin the 24-hour urine collection after urinating. Discard the initial specimen and start the 24-hour timing at that point.
- Collect all urine passed during the next 24 hours.
- Show the patient where to store the urine specimen.
- Keep the specimen on ice or refrigerated during the 24 hours.
- Indicate the starting time on the urine container and on the laboratory slip.
- Post the hours for urine collection in a noticeable place to prevent accidental discarding of the specimen.
- Instruct the patient to void before defecating so that urine is not contaminated by feces.
- Remind the patient not to put toilet paper in the collection container.
- Encourage the patient to drink fluids during the 24 hours.
- Instruct the patient to collect the last specimen as close as possible to the end of the 24-hour period. Add this urine to the container.

After

- Transport the urine specimen promptly to the laboratory.

Abnormal findings

▲ **Increased levels**
  Dehydration
  Starvation
  Adrenocortical insuffi-
    ciency
  Diuretic therapy
  Hypothyroidism
  Syndrome of inappropri-
    ate ADH secretion
    (SIADH)
  Diabetic ketoacidosis
  Toxemia of pregnancy

▼ **Decreased levels**
  Congestive heart failure
  Malabsorption
  Diarrhea
  Renal failure
  Cushing's syndrome
  Aldosteronism
  Diaphoresis
  Pulmonary emphysema
  Inadequate sodium intake

S

somatomedin C (Insulin-like growth factors I, IGF-1)

Type of test Blood

Normal findings

Adults: 42-110 ng/ml
Children:

Ages (yr)	Girls (ng/ml)	Boys (ng/ml)
0-8	7-110	4-87
9-10	39-186	26-98
11-13	66-215	44-207
14-16	96-256	48-255

Test explanation and related physiology

Growth hormone (GH) exerts its effects on many tissues through a group of peptides called somatomedins. The most commonly tested somatomedin is somatomedin-C (also called insulin-like growth factor [IGF-1]).

Great variation in GH secretion occurs during the day. A random GH assay result may significantly overlap between normal and abnormal values. To negate the common variations in GH secretion, screening for somatomedin C provides a more accurate reflection of the mean plasma concentration of growth hormone. Somatomedins are not affected by the time of day, food intake, or exercise as is GH because they circulate bound to proteins that are durable or long lasting. As a result, there is no overlap of results of somatomedin C among normal and abnormal values. Normally there is a large increase during the pubertal growth spurt.

Levels of somatomedin C depend on levels of GH. As a result, somatomedin levels are low when GH levels are deficient. See GH (p. 452) for a discussion of causes of and diseases associated with GH deficiency. Nonpituitary causes of reduced somatomedin C include malnutrition, severe chronic illnesses, severe liver disease, hypothyroidism and Larson's dwarfism. Abnormally low test results require an abnormally reduced or absent GH during a GH stimulation test to make the diagnosis of GH deficiency (see p. 452).

Interfering factors

- A radioactive scan performed within the week before the test may affect test results.
- Drugs that may cause decreased levels include high doses of estrogens.

Procedure and patient care

Before

- Explain the procedure to the patient.
- Tell the patient that an overnight fast is preferred.

During

- Collect one lavender- or red-top tube of venous blood.

After

- Apply pressure to the venipuncture site.

Abnormal findings

▲ **Increased levels**

Acromegaly
Gigantism
Hyperpituitarism
Obesity
Pregnancy
Precocious puberty

▼ **Decreased levels**

GH deficiency
Laron dwarfism
Inactive GH
Resistance to somato-
    medins
Nutritional deficiency
Delayed puberty
Pituitary tumor
Hypopituitarism
Cirrhosis of the liver

notes

S

spinal x-rays (Cervical, thoracic, lumbar, sacral, or coccygeal x-ray studies)

Type of test X-ray

Normal findings Normal spinal vertebrae

Test explanation and related physiology

Spinal x-ray studies may be performed to evaluate any area of the spine. They usually include anteroposterior, lateral, and oblique views of these structures. These x-ray films are often done to assess back or neck pain, degenerative arthritic changes, traumatic fractures, tumor metastasis, spondylosis (stress fracture of the vertebrae), and spondylolisthesis (slipping of one vertebral disk on the other). Cervical spine x-ray studies are routinely performed in cases of multiple trauma to ensure no fracture before the patient is moved or the neck is manipulated. Spinal x-rays are very helpful in evaluating children and adults for spinal alignment abnormalities (e.g., kyphosis, scoliosis).

Contraindications

- Patients who are pregnant

Procedure and patient care

Before

- Explain the procedure to the patient.
- Instruct the patient to remove any metal objects covering the area to be visualized.
- Immobilize the patient if a spinal fracture is suspected. Apply a neck brace if a cervical spine fracture is suspected.
- Tell the patient that no fasting or sedation is required; however, if a fracture is suspected, the patient may be kept NPO.

During

- Note that the patient is placed on an x-ray table. Anterior, posterior, lateral, and oblique x-ray films are taken of the desired area on the spinal cord.
- Note that a radiologic technologist takes spinal x-ray films in a few minutes.
- Tell the patient that no discomfort is associated with this study.

After
- Note that positioning and patient activity depend on test results.

Abnormal findings

Degenerative arthritis changes
Traumatic or pathologic fracture
Spondylosis
Spondylolisthesis
Metastatic tumor invasion

notes

sputum culture and sensitivity (C&S, Culture and Gram stain)

Type of test Sputum

Normal findings Normal upper respiratory tract

Test explanation and related physiology

Sputum cultures are obtained to determine the presence of pathogenic bacteria in patients with respiratory infections, such as pneumonia. A *Gram stain* is the first step in the microbiologic analysis of sputum. Staining of sputum provides an opportunity to classify bacteria as gram positive or gram negative. This may be used to guide drug therapy until the C&S report is complete. The sputum sample is then applied to a series of bacterial culture plates. The bacteria that grow on those plates 1 to 3 days later are then identified. Determinations of bacterial sensitivity to various antibiotics are done to identify the most appropriate antimicrobial drug therapy. This is done by observing a ring of growth inhibition around an antibiotic plug in the culture medium. Sputum for C&S should be collected before antimicrobial therapy is initiated, unless the test is being performed to evaluate the effectiveness of medications already being given. Preliminary reports are usually available in 24 hours. Cultures require at least 48 hours for completion. Sputum cultures for fungus and *Mycobacterium tuberculosis* may take 6 to 8 weeks.

Procedure and patient care

Before

- Explain the procedure for sputum collection to the patient.
- Remind the patient that sputum must be coughed up from the lungs and that saliva is not sputum.
- Hold antibiotics until after the sputum has been collected.
- If an elective specimen is to be obtained, give the patient a sterile sputum container on the night before the sputum is to be collected so that the morning specimen may be obtained on arising.
- Instruct the patient to rinse out his or her mouth with water before the sputum collection to decrease contamination of the sputum by particles in the oropharynx.

During

- Note that sputum specimens are best when the patient awakens in the morning before eating or drinking.
- Collect at least 1 teaspoon of sputum in a sterile sputum container.
- Usually obtain sputum by having the patient cough after taking several deep breaths.
- If the patient is unable to produce a sputum specimen, stimulate coughing by lowering the head of the patient's bed or giving the patient an aerosol administration of a warm, hypertonic solution.
- Note that other methods to collect sputum include endotracheal aspiration, fiberoptic bronchoscopy, and transtracheal aspiration.

After

- Inform the patient to notify the nurse as soon as the sputum is collected.
- Label the sputum and send it to the laboratory as soon as possible.
- Note any current antibiotic therapy on the laboratory slip.

Abnormal findings

Bacterial infection (e.g., pneumonia)
Viral infection
Atypical bacterial infection (e.g., tuberculosis)

notes

S

sputum cytology

Type of test Sputum

Normal findings Normal epithelial cells

Test explanation and related physiology

Tumors within the pulmonary system frequently slough cells into the sputum. When the sputum is gathered, the cells are examined. If the cytologic test is positive, malignant cells are seen, indicating a lung tumor. If only normal epithelial cells are seen, either no malignancy exists, or any existing tumor is not shedding cells. Therefore a positive test indicates malignancy; a negative test means nothing.

Bronchoscopy and percutaneous lung biopsy has supplanted the need for sputum cytology to a large degree. Now its greatest use is in patients who have an abnormal chest x-ray, productive cough, and nothing visible on bronchoscopy. It is also used to monitor smokers who have had some atypical changes on prior examination of the lower respiratory tract.

Procedure and patient care

Before

- Explain the procedure for sputum collection to the patient.
- Remind the patient that sputum must be coughed up from the lungs and that saliva is not sputum.
- Give the patient a sterile sputum container on the night before the sputum is to be collected so that the morning specimen may be obtained on arising.
- Instruct the patient to rinse out her or his mouth with water to decrease contamination of the sputum by particles in the oropharynx.

During

- Note that sputum specimens are best collected when the patient awakes in the morning.
- Collect at least 1 teaspoon of sputum in the sterile sputum container.
- Usually obtain sputum by having the patient cough after taking several deep breaths.
- If the patient is unable to produce a sputum specimen, stimulate coughing by lowering the head of the patient's bed or

giving the patient an aerosol administration of a warm, hypertonic solution.

- Note that other methods to collect sputum include endotracheal aspiration, fiberoptic bronchoscopy, and transtracheal aspiration.
- Usually collect sputum for cytology on three separate occasions.

After

- Instruct the patient to notify the nurse as soon as the sputum is collected.
- Label the specimen and send it to the laboratory as soon as possible.

Abnormal findings

Malignancies

notes

S

stool culture (Stool for culture and sensitivity [C&S], Stool for ova and parasites [O&P])

Type of test Stool

Normal findings Normal intestinal flora

Test explanation and related physiology

Normally stool contains many bacteria and fungi. The more common bacteria include *Enterococcus*, *Escherichia coli*, *Proteus*, *Pseudomonas*, *Staphylococcus aureus*, *Candida albicans*, *Bacteroides*, and *Clostridium*. Bacteria are indigenous to the bowel. Sometimes the normal stool flora can become pathogenic if overgrowth of the bacteria occurs as a result of antibiotics, immunosuppression, or overaggressive catharsis (e.g., *Clostridium difficile*). *Salmonella*, *Shigella*, *Campylobacter*, *Yersinia*, pathogenic *Escherichia coli*, *Clostridium*, and *Staphylococcus* are acquired bacteria that can infect the bowel. Parasites also may affect the stool. Common parasites are *Ascaris* (hookworm), *Strongyloides* (tapeworm), and *Giardia* (protozoans). Identification of any of these pathogens in the stool incriminates that "bug" as the etiology of the infectious enteritis.

Infections of the bowel from bacteria, virus, or parasites usually present as acute diarrhea, excessive flatus, and abdominal discomfort. Patients who have been drinking well water, have been on prolonged antibiotics, or have traveled out of the United States are especially susceptible.

Interfering factors

- Urine may inhibit the growth of bacteria. Therefore urine should not be mixed with the feces during collection of a stool sample.
- Recent barium studies may obscure the detection of parasites.
- ⚕ Drugs that may affect test results include antibiotics, bismuth, and mineral oil.

Procedure and patient care

Before

- Explain the method of stool collection to the patient. Be matter-of-fact to avoid any embarrassment to the patient.
- Instruct the patient not to mix urine or toilet paper with the stool specimen.

- Instruct the patient to use an appropriate collection container.

During

- Ask the patient to defecate into a clean bedpan.
- Place a small amount of stool in a sterile collection container.
- Send mucus and blood streaks with the specimen.
- If a rectal swab is to be used, wear gloves and insert the cotton-tipped swab at least 1 inch into the anal canal. Then rotate the swab for 30 seconds and place it into the clean container.

Tape test

- Use this test when pinworms (Enterobius) are suspected.
- Place a clear tape in the patient's perianal region. (This is especially helpful in children.)
- Because the female worm lays her eggs at night around the perianal area, apply the tape before bedtime and remove it in the morning before the patient gets out of the bed.
- Press the sticky surface of the tape directly to a glass slide and examine microscopically for pinworm ova.

After

- Handle the stool specimen carefully, as though it were capable of causing infection. Wear gloves when obtaining and handling the specimen.
- Indicate on the laboratory slip any antibiotics that the patient may be taking.
- Promptly send the stool specimen to the laboratory. Delays in transfer of the specimen may affect viability of the organism. If long delays are necessary, obtain a buffered glycerol-saline solution to be combined with the stool and use as a preservative.
- Note that some enteric pathogens occasionally take as long as 6 weeks to isolate.
- When pathogens are detected, maintain isolation of the patient's stool until therapy is completed.

Abnormal findings

Bacterial enterocolitis
Protozoan enterocolitis
Parasitic enterocolitis

stool for occult blood (Stool for OB)

Type of test Stool

Normal findings No occult blood within stool

Test explanation and related physiology

Normally only minimal quantities of blood are passed into the gastrointestinal (GI) tract. Usually, this bleeding is not significant enough to cause a positive result in stool for OB testing. Tumors of the intestine grow into the lumen and are subjected to repeated trauma by the fecal stream. Eventually the friable tumor ulcerates, and bleeding occurs. Most often, bleeding is so slight that gross blood is not seen in the stool. The blood can only be detected by chemical assay through the OB testing of the stool.

Benign and malignant GI tumors, ulcers, inflammatory bowel disease, arteriovenous malformations, diverticulosis, and hematobilia (hemobilia) can cause OB within the stool. Other more common abnormalities (e.g., hemorrhoids, swallowed blood from oral or nasal pharyngeal bleeding) may also cause OB within the stool. This test can detect occult blood when as little as 5 ml of blood is lost per day.

This test is a part of every routine physical examination. It is also a part of routine screening of asymptomatic individuals over the age of 50 years. It is important to note that many drugs and the ingestion of hemoglobin contained in red meats such as beef and pork may cause a false-positive OB stool test. The more sensitive the test method, the more false positives will be obtained.

A positive result obtained on multiple specimens performed on successive days warrants a thorough GI evaluation. Most would agree that four positives out of six specimens would constitute criteria for a more thorough evaluation.

Interfering factors

- Vigorous exercise
- Bleeding gums following a dental procedure
- Ingestion of red meat within the 3 days before testing
- Ingestion of fish, turnips, and horseradish
- Drugs that may cause GI bleeding include anticoagulants, aspirin, colchicine, iron preparations (large doses), nonsteroidal antiarthritics, and steroids.

✓ Drugs that may cause false-positive results include colchicine, iron, oxidizing drugs (e.g., iodine, bromides, boric acid), and rauwolfia derivatives.

✓ Drugs that may cause false-negative results include vitamin C.

Procedure and patient care

Before

- Explain the procedure to the patient.
- Instruct the patient to refrain from eating any red meat for at least 3 days before the test.
- Instruct the patient to refrain from drugs known to interfere with OB testing.
- Instruct the patient as to the method of obtaining appropriate stool specimens. Many procedures are available (e.g., specimen cards, tissue wipes, test paper). Tests may be done at home with specimen cards (Hemoccult) and mailed when collected.
- Instruct the patient not to mix urine with the stool specimen.
- Inform the patient as to the need for multiple specimens obtained on separate days to increase the test's accuracy.
- Note that in some centers a high-residue diet is recommended to increase the abrasive effect of the stool.
- Note on the laboratory slip any anticoagulant medications that the patient may be taking.
- Be gentle in obtaining stool by digital rectal examination. Traumatic digital examination can cause a false-positive stool, especially in patients with prior anorectal disease such as hemorrhoids.

During

Hemoccult slide test

- Place a stool sample on one side of guaiac paper.
- Place two drops of developer on the other side.
- Note that a bluish discoloration indicates OB in the stool.

Tablet test

- Place a stool sample on the developer paper.
- Place a tablet on top of the stool specimen.
- Put two or three drops of tap water on the tablet and allow to flow onto the paper.
- Note that a bluish discoloration indicates OB in the stool.

After

- Inform the patient as to the results.
- If the tests are positive, inquire whether the patient violated any of the preparation recommendations.

Abnormal findings

GI tumor
Polyps
Ulcer
Varices
Inflammatory bowel disease
Diverticulosis
Ischemic bowel disease
GI trauma
Recent GI surgery
Hemorrhoids
Esophagitis
Gastritis

notes

swallowing examination (Videofluoroscopy swallowing examination)

Type of test X-ray with contrast dye

Normal findings Normal swallowing function and complete clearing of radiographic material through the upper digestive tract

Test explanation and related physiology

This test is performed to identify the exact problems that exist in a patient who is unable to swallow. Problems in swallowing may result from local structural diseases such as tumors, upper esophageal diverticula, inflammation, extrinsic compression of the upper gastrointestinal (GI) tract, or surgery to the oropharyngeal tract. Motility disorders of the upper GI tract (such as Zenker's diverticulum) and neurologic disorders (such as stroke syndrome), Parkinson's disease, and neuropathies also may cause difficulty in swallowing. Videofluoroscopy of the swallowing function allows the speech pathologist to delineate more clearly the exact pathology in the swallowing mechanism. This videofluoroscopy then can be used to determine the most appropriate treatment and teach the patient proper swallowing technique.

This test is performed by asking the patient to swallow barium or a barium-containing meal. With the use of videofluoroscopy, the swallowing function is visualized and documented. Morphologic abnormalities and functional impairment can be identified easily using the slow-framed progression and reversal that is available with videofluoroscopy. Although this test is similar to the barium swallow (see p. 137), finer details of swallowing can be evaluated with the use of videofluoroscopy.

S

Contraindications

- Patients who obviously aspirate their saliva and are not candidates for swallowing, because they will require nonswallowing methods of alimentation

Procedure and patient care

Before

- Explain the procedure to the patient.
- Explain to the patient that no preparation is required.

During

- In the radiology department the patient is asked to swallow a barium-containing meal. The consistency of the meal will be determined by the speech therapist and radiologist. The meal consistency simulates foods to which the patient is to be initially reintroduced. The food may be in the form of a liquid, semisoft (e.g., applesauce), or solids (e.g., a tea biscuit). While the patient is swallowing, videofluoroscopy is recorded in both the lateral and the anterior positions.
- The video is then repeatedly examined and reexamined by the radiologist and speech pathologist.

After

- No catharsis is required.

Abnormal findings

Oral pharyngeal inflammation

Cancer

Extrinsic compression

Neuromuscular disorder

Achalasia

Upper GI motility disorder (e.g., stroke syndrome, Parkinson's disease, peripheral neuropathy)

Diffuse esophageal spasms

Zenker's diverticulum

notes

sweat electrolytes test (Iontophoretic sweat test)

Type of test Fluid analysis

Normal findings

Sodium values in children
Normal: <70 mEq/L
Abnormal: >90 mEq/L
Equivocal: 70-90 mEq/L

Chloride values in children
Normal: <50 mEq/L
Abnormal: >60 mEq/L
Equivocal: 50-60 mEq/L

Test explanation and related physiology

Patients with cystic fibrosis have increased sodium and chloride contents in their sweat. This forms the basis of this test, which is both sensitive and specific for cystic fibrosis. Cystic fibrosis is an inherited disease characterized by abnormal secretion by exocrine glands within the bronchi, small intestines, pancreatic ducts, bile ducts, and skin (sweat glands). Sweat induced by electrical current (*pilocarpine iontophoresis*) is collected, and its sodium and chloride contents are measured. The degree of abnormality is no indication of the severity of cystic fibrosis; it merely indicates that the patient has the disease.

In children with recurrent respiratory tract infections, malabsorption syndromes, or failure to thrive, this test is indicated to diagnose cystic fibrosis. This test is also used to screen children or siblings of cystic fibrosis patients for the disease. Almost all patients with cystic fibrosis have sweat sodium and chloride contents 2 to 5 times greater than normal values. In patients with suspicious clinical manifestations, these levels are diagnostic of cystic fibrosis.

Procedure and patient care

Before
- Explain the procedure to the patient and/or parents.
- Tell the patient and/or parents that no fasting is required.

During

- Note the following procedural steps:
  1. For iontophoresis, a low-level electrical current is applied to the test area (the thigh in infants, the forearm in older children).
  2. The positive electrode is covered by gauze and saturated with pilocarpine hydrochloride, a stimulating drug that induces sweating.
  3. The negative electrode is covered by gauze saturated with a bicarbonate solution.
  4. The electrical current is allowed to flow for 5 to 12 minutes.
  5. The electrodes are removed, and the arm is washed with distilled water.
  6. Paper disks are placed over the test site with the use of clean, dry forceps.
  7. These disks are covered with paraffin to obtain an air-tight seal, preventing evaporation of sweat.
  8. After 1 hour the paraffin is removed. The paper disks are transferred immediately by forceps to a weighing jar and sent for sodium and chloride analysis.
  9. A *screening* test may be done to detect sweat chloride levels. For screening, a test paper containing silver nitrate is pressed against the child's hand for several seconds. The test is positive when the excess chloride combines with the silver nitrate to form white-silver chloride on the paper (i.e, the child with cystic fibrosis will leave a "heavy" handprint on the paper).
  10. A positive screening test is usually validated by iontophoresis.
- Note that an experienced technologist performs the sweat test in approximately 90 minutes in the laboratory or at the patient's bedside.
- Inform the patient that the electrical current is small and no discomfort or pain is generally associated with this test.

After

- Initiate extensive education and counseling for the patient and/or parents if the results indicate cystic fibrosis.

Abnormal finding

Cystic fibrosis

syphilis detection test (Serologic test for syphilis [STS], Venereal Disease Research Laboratory [VDRL], Rapid plasma reagin [RPR], Fluorescent treponemal antibody test [FTA])

Type of test Blood

Normal findings Negative, or nonreactive

Test explanation and related physiology

These blood tests are used to diagnose and to document successful therapy of syphilis. Syphilis is caused by a spirochete *Treponema pallidum*. There are two groups of antibodies that form the basis for these tests. The first group of tests detects the presence of a nontreponemal antibody, called *reagin*, which reacts to phospholipids in the patient's body (which are probably similar to lipids in the membrane of *T. pallidum*). The nontreponemal antibody test are grouped as STS and are relatively nonspecific. These antibodies are most often detected by the *Wassermann test* or the *VDRL test*. A newer, more sensitive nontreponemal test is the RPR test. The VDRL and RPR tests, by virtue of their testing for a nonspecific antibody, have a high false-positive (or cross reactive) rate. The VDRL test becomes positive approximately 2 weeks after the patient's inoculation with *Treponema* and returns to normal after adequate treatment is administered. The test is positive in nearly all primary and secondary stages of syphilis and in two thirds of patients with tertiary syphilis.

If the VDRL or RPR test is positive, the diagnosis may be confirmed by the *Treponema* test, such as the *FTA absorption test* (FTA-ABS). This second group of tests detects antibodies directed against the *Treponema* organism itself. The FTA test, which tests for a more specific antibody, is more accurate than the VDRL and RPR tests.

False-positive and false-negative results are rare in all stages of the disease. The FTA test is required before the diagnosis of syphilis can be made with certainty.

Screening for syphilis is usually done during the first prenatal checkup for pregnant women. Syphilis, if untreated, may cause abortion, stillbirth, and premature labor. The effect on the fetus can be central nervous system damage, hearing loss, and possible death.

Interfering factors

- Excessive hemolysis and gross lipemia may affect test results.
- Excess chyle in the blood may interfere with the test results.
- Many conditions cause false-positive results when VDRL and RPR tests are used. Some of these conditions include *Mycoplasma* pneumonia, malaria, acute bacterial and viral infections, autoimmune diseases, and pregnancy.
- Recent ingestion of alcohol may alter the test results.

Procedure and patient care

Before

- Explain the procedure to the patient.
- Check with the laboratory regarding fasting requirements. Some prefer collecting the specimen before meals. Some laboratories request that the patient refrain from alcohol for 24 hours before the blood test.

During

- Collect approximately 7 ml of blood in a red-top tube.

After

- Apply pressure to the venipuncture site.
- If the test is positive, instruct the patient to inform recent sexual contacts so they can be evaluated.
- If the test is positive, be sure the patient receives the appropriate antibiotic therapy.

Abnormal finding

Syphilis

notes

testosterone (Total testosterone serum level)

Type of test Blood

Normal findings

Age	Male (ng/dl)	Female (ng/dl)
Newborn	75-400	20-64
1-5 mos	1-177	1-5
6-12 mos	2-7	2-5
1-5 yrs	2-25	2-10
6-9 yrs	3-30	2-20
puberty	5-800	2-40
adult	280-1100	15-70

Test explanation and related physiology

Testosterone is made in the male by the Leydig cells in the testicle; this accounts for 95% of the circulating testosterone in men. In women the ovary and adrenal gland secrete small amounts of testosterone; the majority of the testosterone in the female is made as a derivative of metabolism of androstenedione (see p. 53). Approximately 60% of circulating testosterone binds strongly to sex hormone-binding globulin. Most of the remaining testosterone is bound loosely to albumin, and approximately 2% is unbound.

Testosterone levels are used to evaluate ambiguous sex characteristics, precocious puberty, virilizing syndromes in the female, and infertility in the male. This test can also be used as a tumor marker for rare tumors of the ovary and testicle.

Physiologically testosterone stimulates spermatogenesis and influences the development of male secondary sexual characteristics. Overproduction of this hormone in the young male may cause precocious puberty. This can be caused by testicular, adrenal, or pituitary tumors or adrenal hyperplasia. Overproduction of this hormone in females causes masculinization, which is demonstrated by amenorrhea and excessive growth of body hair (hirsutism). Ovarian and adrenal tumors/hyperplasia and medications (e.g., danazol) are all potential causes of masculinization in the female. Reduced levels of testosterone in the male suggest hypogonadism or Klinefelter syndrome.

Several *testosterone stimulation tests* can be performed to more accurately evaluate hypogonadism. Human chorionic gonado-

T

tropin, clomiphene, and GnRH can be used to stimulate testosterone secretion.

Interfering factors

- Drugs that may cause *increased* testosterone levels include anticonvulsants, barbiturates, estrogens, and oral contraceptives.
- Drugs that may cause *decreased* testosterone levels include androgens, dexamethasone, diethylstilbestrol, digoxin, alcohol, steroids, ketoconazole, phenothiazine, and spironolactone.

Procedure and patient care

Before

- Explain the procedure to the patient.
- Tell the patient that no fasting is required.
- Because testosterone levels are highest in the early morning hours, blood should be drawn in the morning.

During

- Collect 7 ml of peripheral venous blood in a red-top tube.

After

- Apply pressure to the venipuncture site.

Abnormal findings

▲ **Increased levels (male)**
  Idiopathic sexual precocity
  Pinealoma
  Encephalitis
  Congenital adrenal hyperplasia
  Adrenocortical tumor
  Testicular or extragonadal tumor
  Hyperthyroidism
  Testosterone resistance syndromes

▼ **Decreased levels (male)**
  Klinefelter syndrome
  Cryptorchidism
  Primary and secondary hypogonadism
  Down syndrome
  Orchidectomy
  Hepatic cirrhosis

▲ **Increased levels (female)**
Ovarian tumor
Adrenal tumor
Congenital adrenocortical hyperplasia
Trophoblastic tumor
Polycystic ovaries
Idiopathic hirsutism

notes

T

therapeutic drug monitoring

Type of test Blood

Normal findings See Table 17.

Test explanation and related physiology

Therapeutic drug monitoring (TDM) entails taking measurements of blood drug levels to determine effective drug dosages and to prevent toxicity. It is also used to identify noncompliant patients. Patient age and size, extent and rate of drug absorption or excretion, and metabolic rate can all affect drug levels. Measurement of drug levels is very important in patients who are beyond the normal range in regard to variables that affect drug metabolism. TDM is helpful in patients who take other medicines that may affect drug levels or act in a synergistic or antagonistic manner with the drug to be tested. TDM is helpful in prescribing medicines (e.g., antiarrhythmics, bronchodilators, antibiotics, anticonvulsants, cardiotonics) that have a very narrow therapeutic margin (i.e., the difference between therapeutic and toxic drug levels is small).

Table 17 lists the therapeutic and toxic ranges for most patients. These ranges may not apply to all patients because clinical response is influenced by many factors (e.g., noncompliance, concurrent drug use, other clinical conditions, patient's age and size, extent and rate of drug absorption, metabolism). Also, note that different laboratories use different units for reporting test results and normal ranges. It is important that sufficient time pass between the administration of the medication and the collection of the blood sample to allow for therapeutic levels to occur.

Blood samples can be taken at the drug's *peak* level (the highest concentration) or at the trough level (the lowest concentration). Peak levels are useful when testing for toxicity, and trough levels are useful for demonstrating a satisfactory therapeutic level. Trough levels are often referred to as *residual* levels. The time when the sample should be drawn after the last dose of the medication varies according to whether a peak or trough level is requested and according to the half-life of the drug.

TABLE 17 Therapeutic drug monitoring data

Drug	Use	Therapeutic level*	Toxic level*
Acetaminophen	Analgesic, antipyretic	Depends on use	<250 µg/ml
Amikacin	Antibiotic	15-25 µg/ml	>25 µg/ml
Aminophylline	Bronchodilator	10-20 µg/ml	>20 µg/ml
Amitriptyline	Antidepressant	120-150 ng/ml	>500 ng/ml
Carbamazepine	Anticonvulsant	5-12 µg/ml	>12 µg/ml
Chloramphenicol	Antiinfective	10-20 µg/ml	>25 µg/ml
Desipramine	Antidepressant	150-300 ng/ml	>500 ng/ml
Digitoxin	Cardiac glycoside	15-25 ng/ml	>25 ng/ml
Digoxin	Cardiac glycoside	0.8-2.0 ng/ml	>2.4 ng/ml
Disopyramide	Antiarrhythmic	2-5 µg/ml	>5 µg/ml
Ethosuximide	Anticonvulsant	40-100 µg/ml	>100 µg/ml
Gentamicin	Antibiotic	5-10 µg/ml	>12 µg/ml
Imipramine	Antidepressant	150-300 ng/ml	>500 ng/ml
Kanamycin	Antibiotic	20-25 µg/ml	>35 µg/ml
Lidocaine	Antiarrhythmic	1.5-5.0 µg/ml	>5 µg/ml
Lithium	Manic episodes of manic-depression psychosis	0.8-1.2 mEq/L	>2.0 mEq/L

Continued

T

TABLE 17 Therapeutic drug monitoring data—cont'd

Drug	Use	Therapeutic level*	Toxic level*
Methotrexate	Antitumor agent	>0.01 µmol	>10 µmol/24 hr
Nortriptyline	Antidepressant	50-150 ng/ml	>500 ng/ml
Phenobarbital	Anticonvulsant	10-30 µg/ml	>40 µg/ml
Phenytoin	Anticonvulsant	10-20 µg/ml	>30 µg/ml
Primidone	Anticonvulsant	5-12 µg/ml	>15 µg/ml
Procainamide	Antiarrhythmic	4-10 µg/ml	>16 µg/ml
Propranolol	Antiarrhythmic	50-100 ng/ml	>150 ng/ml
Quinidine	Antiarrhythmic	2-5 µg/ml	>10 µg/ml
Salicylate	Antipyretic, antiinflammatory, analgesic	100-250 µg/ml	>300 µg/ml
Theophylline	Bronchodilator	10-20 µg/ml	>20 µg/ml
Tobramycin	Antibiotic	5-10 µg/ml	>12 µg/ml
Valproic acid	Anticonvulsant	50-100 µg/ml	>100 µg/ml

*Levels vary according to the institution performing the test.

Procedure and patient care

Before

- Explain the procedure to the patient.
- Tell the patient that no food or fluid restrictions are needed.

During

- Collect approximately 7 to 10 ml of venous blood in a tube designated by the laboratory. *Peak* levels are usually obtained 1 to 2 hours after oral intake, approximately 1 hour after IM administration, and approximately 30 minutes after IV administration. *Residual* (trough) levels are usually obtained shortly before (0 to 15 minutes) the next scheduled dose. Consult with the pharmacy for specific times.

After

- Apply pressure to the venipuncture site.
- Clearly mark all blood samples with the following information: patient's name, diagnosis, name of drug, time of last drug ingestion, time of sample, and any other medications the patient is currently taking.
- Promptly send the specimen to the laboratory.

Abnormal findings

Nontherapeutic levels of drugs
Toxic levels of drugs

notes

thoracentesis and pleural fluid analysis (Pleural tap)

Type of test   Fluid analysis

Normal findings

Gross appearance: Clear, serous, light yellow, 50 ml
Red blood cells (RBCs): None
White blood cells (WBCs): 300/ml
Protein: <4.1 g/dl
Glucose: 70-100 mg/dl
Amylase: 138-404 U/L
Alkaline phosphatase
    Adult male: 90-240 U/L
    Female: <45 years: 76-196 U/L
    Female: >45 years: 87-250 U/L
Lactate dehydrogenase (LDH): Similar to serum lactate dehydrogenase
Cytology: No malignant cells
Bacteria: None
Fungi: None
Carcinoembryonic antigen (CEA): <5 ng/ml

Test explanation and related physiology

Thoracentesis is an invasive procedure that entails insertion of a needle into the pleural space for removal of fluid (or rarely air) (Figure 34). Pleural fluid is removed for diagnostic and therapeutic purposes. *Therapeutically* it is done to relieve pain, dyspnea, and other symptoms of pleural pressure. Removal of this fluid also permits better radiographic visualization of the lung.

Diagnostically thoracentesis is performed to obtain and analyze fluid to determine the etiology of the pleural effusion. Pleural fluid is classified according to transudate or exudate. This is an important differentiation and is very helpful in determining the etiology of the effusion. *Transudates* are most frequently caused by congestive heart failure, cirrhosis, nephrotic syndrome, and hypoproteinemia. *Exudates* are most often found in inflammatory, infectious, or neoplastic conditions. However, collagen vascular disease, pulmonary infarction, trauma, and drug hypersensitivity also may cause an exudative effusion.

Pleural fluid is usually evaluated for the following features.

Figure 34 Thoracentesis. A needle is placed through the chest wall and into the fluid contained within the pleural cavity. A special one-way valve system is placed between the needle and the syringe to allow aspiration of fluid when the plunger of the syringe is pulled back and diversion of the fluid to a container when the plunger is pushed in. (From Beare PG, Myers JM: *Principles and practice of adult health nursing,* ed 2, St Louis, 1994, Mosby.)

Gross appearance

The color, optical density, and viscosity are noted as the pleural fluid appears in the aspirating syringe. Empyema is characterized by the presence of a foul odor and thick, puslike fluid. An opalescent, pearly fluid is characteristic of chylothorax (chyle in the pleural cavity).

Cell counts

The white blood cell (WBC) and differential counts are determined. A WBC count exceeding 1000/ml is suggestive of an exudate. The predominance of polymorphonuclear leukocytes usually is an indication of an acute inflammatory condition (e.g., pneumonia, pulmonary infarction, early tuberculosis effusion). When over 50% of the WBCs are small lymphocytes, the effusion is usually caused by tuberculosis or tumor. Normally no RBCs should be present. The presence of RBCs may indicate neoplasms, tuberculosis, or intrathoracic bleeding.

Protein content

Total protein levels greater than 3 g/dl are characteristic of exudates, whereas transudates usually have a protein content of less than 3 g/dl. The *albumin gradient* between serum and pleural fluid can differentiate better between the transudate and exudate nature of pleural fluid than can the total protein content. This gradient is obtained by subtracting the pleural albumin value from the serum albumin value. Values of 1.1 g/dl or more suggest a transudate. Values less than 1.1 g/dl suggest an exudate but will not differentiate the potential cause of the exudate (malignancy from infection or inflammation). The total protein ratio (fluid/serum) has been considered to be another accurate criterion differentiating transudate from exudate. A total protein ratio of fluid to serum of greater than 0.5 is considered to be an exudate.

Lactic dehydrogenase

A pleural fluid/serum LDH ratio greater than 0.6 is typical of an exudate. An exudate is identified with a high degree of accuracy if the pleural fluid/serum protein ratio is greater than 0.5 and the pleural fluid/serum LDH ratio is greater than 0.6.

Glucose

Usually pleural glucose levels approximate serum levels. Low values appear to be a combination of glycolysis by the extra cells and impairment of glucose diffusion because of damage to the pleural membrane. Values less than 60 mg/dl are occasionally seen in tuberculosis or malignancy and typically occur in rheumatoid arthritis and empyema.

Amylase

In a malignant effusion the amylase concentration is slightly elevated. Amylase levels above the normal range for serum or two times the serum level are seen when the effusion is caused by pancreatitis or rupture of the esophagus associated with leakage of salivary amylase.

Triglyceride

Measurement of triglyceride levels is an important part of identifying chylous effusions. These effusions are usually produced by obstruction or transection of the lymphatic system caused by lymphoma, neoplasm, trauma, or recent surgery. The triglyceride value in a chylous effusion exceeds 110 mg/dl.

Gram stain and bacteriologic culture

These tests are routinely performed when bacterial pneumonia or empyema is a possible cause of the effusion. If possible, these should be done before initiation of antibiotic therapy.

Cultures for *Mycobacterium tuberculosis* and fungus

Tuberculosis is less often a cause for pleural effusion in the United States today than it was in the past. Fungus may be a cause of pulmonary effusion in patients with compromised immunologic defenses.

Cytology

A cytologic study is performed to detect tumor cells in approximately 50% to 60% of patients with malignant effusions. Breast and lung are the two most frequent tumors; lymphoma is the third.

Carcinoembryonic antigen

Pleural fluid CEA levels are elevated in various malignant (gastrointestinal, breast) conditions. See p. 201.

Special tests

The pH of pleural fluid is usually 7.4 or greater. The pH is typically less than 7.2 when empyema is present. The pH may be 7.2 to 7.4 in tuberculosis or malignancy.

In some instances, the rheumatoid factor (see p. 737) and the complement levels (see p. 260) are also measured in pleural fluid.

Pleural fluid antinuclear antibody (ANA) levels and pleural fluid/serum ANA ratios are often used to evaluate pleural effusion secondary to systemic lupus erythematosus.

Contraindications

- Patients with significant thrombocytopenia

Potential complications

- Pneumothorax because of puncture of the visceral pleura or entry of air into the pleural space
- Interpleural bleeding because of puncture of tissue or a blood vessel
- Hemoptysis caused by needle puncture of a pulmonary vessel or by inflammation
- Reflex bradycardia and hypotension
- Pulmonary edema
- Seeding of the needle tract with tumor when malignant pleural effusion exists

Procedure and patient care

Before

- Explain the procedure to the patient.
- Obtain informed consent for this procedure.
- Tell the patient that no fasting or sedation is necessary.
- Inform the patient that movement or coughing should be minimized to avoid inadvertent needle damage to the lung or pleura during the procedure.
- Administer a cough suppressant before the procedure if the patient has a troublesome cough.
- Note that an x-ray film or ultrasound scan is often used to assist in location of the fluid. Fluoroscopy also may be used.

During

- Note the following procedural steps:
  1. The patient is usually placed in an upright position, with the arms and shoulders raised and supported on a padded overhead table. This position spreads the ribs and enlarges the intercostal space for insertion of the needle.
  2. Patients who cannot sit upright are placed in a side-lying position on the unaffected side with the side to be tapped uppermost.
  3. The thoracentesis is performed under strict sterile technique.
  4. The needle insertion site, which is determined by percussion, auscultation, and examination of a chest x-ray film, ultrasound scan, or fluoroscopy, is aseptically cleansed and anesthetized locally.
  5. The needle is positioned in the pleural space, and the fluid is withdrawn with a syringe and a three-way stopcock.
  6. Various mechanisms to stabilize the pleural needle are available to secure the needle depth during the fluid collection.
  7. A short polyethylene catheter may be inserted into the pleural space for fluid aspiration; this decreases the risk of puncturing the visceral pleura and inducing a pneumothorax.
  8. Also, large volumes of fluid may be collected by connecting the catheter to a gravity-drainage system.
- Note that this procedure is performed by a physician at the patient's bedside, in a procedure room, or in the physician's office in less than 30 minutes.
- Monitor the patient's pulse for reflex bradycardia and evaluate the patient for diaphoresis and the feeling of faintness during the procedure.

- Although local anesthetics eliminate pain at the insertion site, tell the patient that he or she may feel a pressurelike pain when the pleura is entered and the fluid is removed.

After

- Place a small bandage over the needle site. Usually turn the patient on the unaffected side for 1 hour to allow the pleural puncture site to heal.
- Label the specimen with the patient's name, date, source of fluid, and diagnosis. Send the specimen promptly to the laboratory.
- Obtain a chest x-ray study as indicated to check for pneumothorax.
- Monitor the patient's vital signs.
- Observe the patient for coughing or expectoration of blood (hemoptysis), which may indicate trauma to the lung.
- Evaluate the patient for signs and symptoms of pneumothorax, tension pneumothorax, subcutaneous emphysema, and pyogenic infection (e.g., tachypnea, dyspnea, diminished breath sounds, anxiety, restlessness, fever).
- Assess the patient's lung sounds for diminished breath sounds, which could be a sign of pneumothorax.
- If the patient has no complaints of dyspnea, normal activity usually can be resumed 1 hour after the procedure.

Abnormal findings

Exudate
Empyema
Pneumonia
Tuberculosis effusion
Pancreatitis
Ruptured esophagus
Tumors
Lymphoma
Pulmonary infarction
Collagen vascular disease
Drug hypersensitivity

Transudate
Cirrhosis
Congestive heart failure
Nephrotic syndrome
Hypoproteinemia
Trauma

T

thoracoscopy

Type of test Endoscopy

Normal findings Normal pleura and lung

Test explanation and related physiology

This procedure is used to directly visualize the pleura, lung, and mediastinum. Tissue can be obtained for testing. It is also helpful in assisting in the staging and dissection of lung cancers.

With this technique the parietal pleura, visceral pleura, and mediastinum can be directly visualized. Tumor involving the chest cavity can be staged by direct visualization. Any abnormality can be biopsied. Collections of fluid can be drained and aspirated for testing. Dissection for lung resection can be carried out with the thoracoscope (*video-assisted thoracotomy*), thereby minimizing the extent of a thoracotomy incision.

Contraindications

- Patients with previous lung surgery, because it is difficult to obtain access to the free pleural space.

Potential complications

- Bleeding
- Infection or empyema
- Prolonged pneumothorax

Procedure and patient care

Before

- Explain the procedure to the patient.
- Ensure that an informed consent for this procedure is obtained.
- An open thoracotomy may be required because of the possibility of intrathoracic injury. Be sure the patient is aware of this.
- Because the procedure is usually performed with the patient under general anesthesia, follow the routine general anesthesia precautions.
- Shave and prepare the patient's chest as ordered.
- Keep the patient NPO after midnight on the day of the test. IV fluids may be given.

During

- Note the following procedural steps:
  1. Thoracoscopy is performed in the operating room. The patient is initially placed in the lateral decubitus position.
  2. After the thorax is cleansed, a blunt-tipped (Verres) needle is inserted through a small incision, and the lung is collapsed.
  3. A thoracoscope is inserted through a trocar to examine the chest cavity. Other trocars can be placed as conduits for other instrumentation.
  4. After the desired procedure is completed, the scope and trocars are removed.
  5. Usually a small chest tube is placed to ensure full reexpansion of the lung.
  6. The incision(s) is closed with a few skin stitches and covered with an adhesive bandage.

After

- Assess the patient frequently for signs of bleeding (increased pulse rate, decreased blood pressure). Report any significant findings to the physician.
- Provide analgesics to relieve the minor to moderate pain that may be experienced.
- If a surgical procedure has been performed thoracoscopically, provide appropriate specific postsurgical care.
- A chest x-ray is performed after the procedure to ensure complete reexpansion of the lung.

Abnormal findings

Primary lung cancer
Metastatic cancer to the lung or pleura
Empyema
Pleural tumor
Pleural infection
Pleural inflammation
Pulmonary infection

T

throat culture and sensitivity (C&S)

Type of test Microscopic examination

Normal findings Negative

Test explanation and related physiology

Because the throat is normally colonized by many organisms, culture of this area serves only to isolate and identify a few particular pathogens (e.g., streptococci, meningococci, gonococci, *Bordetella pertussis, Corynebacterium diphtheriae*). Recognition of these organisms requires treatment. Streptococci are most often sought, because a beta-hemolytic streptococcal pharyngitis may be followed by rheumatic heart disease or glomerulonephritis. This type of streptococcal infection most frequently affects children between the ages of 3 and 15 years. Therefore all children with a sore throat and fever should have a throat culture done to attempt to identify streptococcal infections. In adults, however, fewer than 5% of patients with pharyngitis have a streptococcal infection. Therefore throat cultures in adults are only indicated when the patient has severe or recurrent sore throat, often associated with fever and palpable lymphadenopathy. These adults often have a history of streptococcal infections.

Rapid immunologic tests (*strept screen*) with antiserum against group A streptococcus antigen are now available and are very accurate. With these newer kits, the streptococcus organism can be identified directly from the swab specimen without culture. These tests can be performed in about 15 minutes. If the test is negative, no streptococcus infection exists.

All cultures should be performed before antibiotic therapy is initiated. Otherwise, the antibiotic may interrupt the growth of the organism in the laboratory. Most organisms take approximately 24 hours to grow in the laboratory, and a preliminary report can be given at that time. Occasionally a period of 48 to 72 hours is required for growth and identification of the organism. Cultures may be repeated on completion of appropriate antibiotic therapy to identify resolution of the infection.

Interfering factors

✶ Drugs that may affect test results include antibiotics and antiseptic mouthwashes.

Procedure and patient care

Before

- Explain the procedure to the patient.

During

- Obtain a throat culture by depressing the tongue with a wooden tongue blade and touching the posterior wall of the throat and areas of inflammation, exudation, or ulceration with a sterile cotton swab. Two swabs are preferred. Growth of streptococcus from both swabs is more accurate, and the second swab can also be used in the strept screen.
- Avoid touching any other part of the mouth.
- Wear gloves and handle the specimen as if it were capable of transmitting disease.
- Place the swab in a sterile container and send it to the microbiology laboratory within 30 minutes.
- Indicate on the laboratory slip any medications that the patient may be taking that could affect test results.

After

- Notify the physician of any positive results so that appropriate antibiotic therapy can be initiated.

Abnormal findings

Bacterial pathogens (e.g., streptococci)

notes

T

thyroid scanning (Thyroid scintiscan)

Type of test Nuclear scan

Normal findings

Normal size, shape, position, and function of the thyroid gland
No areas of decreased or increased uptake

Test explanation and related physiology

Thyroid scanning allows the size, shape, position, and physiologic function of the thyroid gland to be determined with the use of radionuclear scanning. A radioactive substance such as technetium-99m is given to the patient to visualize the thyroid gland. A scanner is passed over the neck area, and an image is recorded.

Thyroid nodules are easily detected by this technique. Nodules are classified as functioning (warm/hot) or nonfunctioning (cold), depending on the amount of radionuclide taken up by the nodule. A functioning nodule could represent a benign adenoma or a localized toxic goiter. A nonfunctioning nodule may represent a cyst, carcinoma, nonfunctioning adenoma or goiter, lymphoma, or localized area of thyroiditis.

Scanning is useful in:
1. Patients with a neck or substernal mass
2. Patients with a thyroid nodule. Thyroid cancers are usually nonfunctioning (cold) nodules.
3. Patients with hyperthyroidism. Scanning assists in differentiating Graves' disease (diffusely enlarged hyperfunctioning thyroid gland) from Plummer's disease (nodular hyperfunctioning gland).
4. Patients with metastatic tumors without a known primary site. A normal scan excludes the thyroid gland as a possible primary site.
5. Patients with a well-differentiated form of thyroid cancer. Areas of metastasis may show up on subsequent whole-body nuclear scans.

Another form of thyroid scan is called the *whole body thyroid scan*. This scan is performed on patients who have previously had a thyroid cancer treated. Iodine-125 is injected intravenously, and the entire body is scanned to look for metastatic thyroid tissue. A hot spot indicates recurrent tumor. This test is routinely (every 1 to 2 years) performed on patients who have had a thyroid cancer larger than 1 cm.

Contraindications

- Patients who are allergic to iodine or shellfish
- Patients who are pregnant

Potential complication

- Radiation-induced oncogenesis
  This complication is eliminated if technetium or low-radioactive iodine isomers are used instead of iodine-131.

Interfering factors

- Iodine-containing foods
- Recent administration of x-ray contrast agents
- Drugs that may affect test results include cough medicines, multiple vitamins, oral contraceptives (some), and thyroid drugs.

Procedure and patient care

Before

- Explain the procedure to the patient.
- Check the patient for allergies to iodine.
- Instruct the patient about medications that need to be restricted for weeks before the test (e.g., thyroid drugs, medications containing iodine).
- Obtain a history concerning previous contrast x-ray studies, nuclear scanning, or intake of any thyroid-suppressive or antithyroid drugs.
- Tell the patient that fasting is usually not required. Check with the laboratory.

During

- Note the following procedural steps:
  1. A standard dose of radioactive technetium is usually given to the patient by mouth. The capsule is tasteless.
  2. Scanning is usually performed 24 hours later. If technetium is used, scanning may be performed 2 hours later.
  3. At the designated time, the patient is placed in a supine position and a detector is passed over the thyroid area.
  4. The radioactive counts are recorded and displayed.
- Note that this study is performed by a radiologic technologist in less than 30 minutes.
- Tell the patient that no discomfort is associated with this study.

T

After

- Assure the patient that the dose of radioactive technetium used in this test is minute and therefore harmless. No isolation and no special urine precautions are needed.

Abnormal findings

Adenoma
Toxic and nontoxic goiter
Cyst
Carcinoma
Lymphoma
Thyroiditis
Graves' disease
Plummer's disease
Metastasis
Hyperthyroidism
Hypothyroidism
Hashimoto's disease

notes

thyroid-stimulating hormone (TSH, Thyrotropin)

Type of test Blood

Normal findings

Adult: 2-10 µU/ml or 2-10 mU/L (SI units)
Newborn: 3-18 µU/L or 3-18 mU/L
Cord: 3-12 µU/L or 3-12 mU/L
Values vary between laboratories

Test explanation and related physiology

The TSH concentration aids in differentiating primary from secondary hypothyroidism. Pituitary TSH secretion is stimulated by hypothalamic thyroid-releasing hormone (TRH). Low levels of triiodothyronine and thyroxine (T_3, T_4) are the underlying stimuli for TRH and TSH. Therefore a compensatory elevation of TRH and TSH occurs in patients with primary hypothyroid states such as surgical or radioactive thyroid ablation; patients with burned-out thyroiditis, thyroid agenesis, idiopathic hypothyroidism, or congenital cretinism; or patients taking antithyroid medications.

In secondary hypothyroidism the function of the hypothalamus or pituitary gland is faulty because of tumor, trauma, or infarction. Therefore TRH and TSH cannot be secreted, and plasma levels of these hormones are near 0 despite low T_3 and T_4 levels.

The TSH test is used as well to monitor exogenous thyroid replacement. The goal of thyroid replacement therapy is to provide an adequate amount of thyroid medication so that TSH secretion is minimal, indicating a euthyroid state. Therefore doses of medication are given to keep the TSH level less than 2. Even lower TSH levels are preferred if thyroid suppression is the clinical goal. This test is also done to detect primary hypothyroidism in newborns with low screening T_4 levels. TSH and T_4 levels are frequently measured to differentiate pituitary from thyroid dysfunction. A decreased T_4 and normal or elevated TSH level can indicate a thyroid disorder. A decreased T_4 with a decreased TSH level can indicate a pituitary disorder.

Interfering factors

- Recent radioisotope administration may affect test results.
- Severe illness may cause decreased TSH levels.

✶ Drugs that may cause *increased* levels include antithyroid medications, lithium, potassium iodide, and TSH injection.

✶ Drugs that may cause *decreased* levels include aspirin, dopamine, heparin, steroids, and T_3.

Procedure and patient care

Before

- Explain the procedure to the patient.
- Tell the patient that no food or drink restrictions are necessary.

During

- Collect approximately 5 ml of venous blood in a red-top tube.
- Use a heel stick to obtain blood from newborns.

After

- Apply pressure to the venipuncture site.

Abnormal findings

▲ **Increased levels**

Primary hypothyroidism (thyroid dysfunction)
Thyroiditis
Thyroid agenesis
Congenital cretinism

▼ **Decreased levels**

Secondary hypothyroidism (pituitary dysfunction)
Hyperthyroidism
Pituitary hypofunction

notes

thyroid-stimulating hormone stimulation test (TSH stimulation test)

Type of test Blood

Normal findings Increased thyroid function with administration of exogenous TSH

Test explanation and related physiology

The TSH stimulation test is used to differentiate *primary* (or thyroidal) hypothyroidism from *secondary* (or hypothalamic-pituitary) hypothyroidism. Normal people and patients with hypothalamic-pituitary hypothyroidism can increase thyroid function when exogenous TSH is given. However, patients with primary thyroidal hypothyroidism are not; their thyroid gland is inadequate and cannot function, no matter how much stimulation it receives. Patients with less than a 10% increase in radioactive iodine uptake (RAIU) or less than a 1.5 μg/dl rise in thyroxine (T_4) are considered to have a primary cause for their hypothyroid state. If the initially low uptake is caused by inadequate pituitary stimulation of an intrinsically normal thyroid gland, the RAIU should increase at least 10%, and the T_4 level should rise 1.5 μg/dl or more. This is characteristic of secondary hypothyroidism.

Procedure and patient care

Before
- Explain the procedure to the patient.
- Obtain baseline levels of RAIU (see p. 705) or T_4 (see p. 830) as indicated.
- Tell the patient that no fasting is required.

During
- Administer 5 to 10 U of TSH intramuscularly for 3 days.
- Repeat the levels of RAIU or T_4 as indicated.

After
- Apply pressure to the venipuncture site.

Abnormal findings

Primary (thyroidal) hypothyroidism
Secondary (hypothalamic-pituitary) hypothyroidism

thyroid ultrasound (Thyroid echogram, Thyroid sonogram)

Type of test Ultrasound

Normal findings Normal size, shape, and position of the thyroid gland

Test explanation and related physiology

Ultrasound examination of the thyroid gland is valuable for distinguishing cystic from solid thyroid nodules. If the nodule is found to be purely cystic (fluid filled), the fluid can simply be aspirated (cysts are not cancerous), and surgery is avoided. If the nodule has a mixed or solid appearance, however, a tumor may be present, and surgery may be required for diagnosis and treatment.

This study may be repeated at intervals to determine the response of a thyroid mass to medical therapy. This test is also the procedure of choice for studying the thyroid gland of pregnant patients because no radioactive material is used.

Procedure and patient care

Before
- Explain the procedure to the patient.
- Tell the patient that breathing or swallowing will not be affected by the placement of a transducer on the neck.
- Inform the patient that a liberal amount of lubricant will be applied to the neck to ensure effective transmission and reception of sound waves.
- Tell the patient that no fasting or sedation is required.

During
- Note the following procedural steps:
  1. The patient is taken to the ultrasonography department (usually in the radiology department) and placed in the supine position with the neck hyperextended.
  2. Gel is applied to the patient's neck.
  3. A sound transducer is passed over the nodule.
  4. Photographs are taken of the image displayed.
- Note that an ultrasound technologist usually performs this study in approximately 15 minutes and that a radiologist evaluates the results.

- Tell the patient that no discomfort is associated with this study.

After

- Assist the patient in removing the lubricant from his or her neck.

Abnormal findings

Cyst
Tumor
Thyroid adenoma
Thyroid carcinoma
Goiter

notes

thyrotropin-releasing hormone test (TRH test, Thyrotropin-releasing factor test [TRF test])

Type of test Blood

Normal findings

Baseline TSH: <10 (μU/ml)
Stimulated TSH: more than double baseline

Test explanation and related physiology

The TRH test assesses the responsiveness of the anterior pituitary gland via its secretion of thyroid-stimulating hormone (TSH) to an IV injection of TRH. After the TRH injection the normally functioning pituitary gland should secrete TSH. In hyperthyroidism either slight or no increase in the TSH level is seen because pituitary TSH production is suppressed by the direct effect of excess circulating thyroxine and triiodothyronine (T_4, T_3) on the pituitary gland. A normal result is considered reliable evidence for excluding the diagnosis of thyrotoxicosis. The TRH test is one of the most reliable confirmatory procedures for hyperthyroidism; other tests are often compared with it to determine their accuracy.

In addition to assessing the responsiveness of the anterior pituitary gland, this test aids in the detection of primary, secondary, and tertiary hypothyroidism. In primary hypothyroidism (thyroid gland failure) the increase in the TSH level is two or more times the normal result. With secondary hypothyroidism (anterior pituitary failure), no TSH response occurs. Tertiary hypothyroidism (hypothalamic failure) may be diagnosed by a delayed rise in the TSH level. Multiple injections of TRH may be needed to induce the appropriate TSH response in this case.

The TRH test also may be useful in differentiating primary depression from manic-depressive psychiatric illness and from secondary types of depression. In primary depression the TSH response is blunted in most patients, whereas patients with other types of depression have a normal TRH-induced TSH response.

Interfering factors

- Pregnancy may increase the TSH response to TRH.
- Drugs that may modify the TSH response include antithyroid drugs, aspirin, corticosteroids, estrogens, levodopa, and T_4.

Procedure and patient care

Before

- Explain the procedure to the patient.
- Instruct the patient to discontinue thyroid preparations for 3 to 4 weeks before the TRH test.
- Assess the patient for medications currently being taken.
- Tell the patient that no fasting or sedation is required.

During

- Administer a 500-mg IV bolus of TRH.
- Obtain venous blood samples at intervals and measure for TSH levels.

After

- Apply pressure to the venipuncture site.
- Indicate on the laboratory slip if the patient is pregnant.
- List any medications that the patient is taking.

Abnormal findings

Hyperthyroidism
Hypothyroidism
Psychiatric primary depression
Acute starvation
Old age (especially in men)
Pregnancy

notes

T

thyroxine-binding globulin (TBG, thyroid-binding globulin)

Type of test Blood

Normal findings

Age	Male (mg/dl)	Female (mg/dl)
1-5 days	2.2-4.2	2.2-4.2
1-11 mos	1.6-3.6	1.7-3.7
1-9 yrs	1.2-2.8	1.5-2.7
10-19 yrs	1.4-2.6	1.4-3.0
>20 yrs	1.7-3.6	1.7-3.6
Oral contraceptives	—	1.5-5.5
Pregnancy (third trimester)	—	4.7-5.9

Test explanation and related physiology

TBG is the major thyroid hormone protein carrier. When it is elevated, T_3 and T_4 are also elevated. This may give the false sense that the patient has hyperthyroidism when, in fact, the patient just has elevated TBGs. When total T_4 is elevated, one must ascertain whether that elevation is caused by an elevation in TBG or a real elevation in T_4 alone, which is associated with hyperthyroidism.

The most common causes of elevated TBGs are pregnancy, hormone replacement therapy, or use of oral contraceptives. Elevated TBGs are also present in some cases of porphyria and in infectious hepatitis. Decreased TBGs are commonly associated with other causes of hypoproteinemia (e.g., nephrotic syndrome, gastrointestinal malabsorption, and malnutrition).

Interfering factors

- Previous administration of diagnostic radioisotopes may confound test results because TBG is measured by radioimmunoassay.
- Drugs that *increase* TBG include estrogens, methadone, tamoxifen, and oral contraceptives.
- Drugs that *decrease* TBG include steroids, androgens, danazol, phenytoin, and propanolol.

Procedure and patient care

Before
- Explain the procedure to the patient.
- Tell the patient that no fasting is required.

During

- Collect approximately 5 to 7 ml of venous blood in a red-top tube.
- List on the laboratory slip any drugs that may affect test results.

After

- Apply pressure to the venipuncture site.

Abnormal findings

▲ **Increased levels**

Pregnancy
Estrogen replacement
 therapy
Estrogen-producing
 tumors
Infectious hepatitis
Genetic increased TBG
Acute intermittent
 porphyria

▼ **Decreased levels**

Protein-losing enter-
 opathy
Protein-losing ne-
 phropathy
Malnutrition
Testosterone-producing
 tumors
Ovarian failure
Major stress

notes

T

thyroxine, free (FT₄)

Type of test Blood

Normal findings
0-4 days: 2-6 ng/dl
2 weeks-20 years: 0.8-2 ng/dl
Adult: 0.8-2.7 ng/dl

Test explanation and related physiology

This test is used to determine thyroid function, especially when the patient has concurrent clinical situations that may alter protein blood levels. Greater-than-normal levels indicate hyperthyroid states, and subnormal values are seen in hypothyroid states.

Thyroid hormone is made up of thyroxine (T_4) and triiodothyronine (T_3). Over 90% of thyroid hormone is made up of T_4. Ninety-nine percent of T_4 is bound to proteins (thyroid-binding globulin [TBG] and albumin). Only 1% to 5% of total T_4 is unbound or "free." The free T_4 is the metabolically active thyroid hormone. When measuring total T_4 (see p. 830), the bound and the unbound are measured. Abnormalities in protein levels can have significant effect on the results of the total T_4. Pregnancy and hormone replacement therapy increase TBG and cause T_4 to be falsely elevated, suggesting that hyperthyroidism exists when, in fact, the patient is euthyroid. If the free T_4 is measured in these patients, it would be normal, indicating that free T_4 is a more accurate indicator of thyroid function than total T_4. Likewise, in cases in which TBG is reduced (e.g., hypoproteinemia), the total T_4 is likewise reduced, suggesting hypothyroidism. Measurement of free T_4 would indicate normal levels and thereby discount the abnormal total T_4 as merely a result of the reduced TBG and not as a result of hypothyroidism.

Interfering factors

- Neonates have higher levels than do older children and adults.
- Prior use of radioisotopes can alter test results as the method used to determine free T_4 levels is radioimmunoassay.
- Drugs that *increase* free T_4 levels include heparin, aspirin, danazol, and propanolol.
- Drugs that *decrease* free T_4 levels include furosemide, phenytoins, methadone, and rifampicin.

☙ Exogenously administered thyroxine causes elevated free T_4 results.

Procedure and patient care

Before

- Evaluate the patient's medication history.
- If indicated, instruct the patient to stop exogenous T_4 medication one month before testing.
- Tell the patient that no fasting is required.

During

- Collect a venous blood specimen in a red-top tube.
- List on the laboratory slip any drugs that may affect test results.

After

- Apply pressure to the venipuncture site.

Abnormal findings

▲ **Increased levels**
    Graves' disease
    Plummer's disease
    Toxic thyroid adenoma
    Acute thyroiditis
    Factitious hyperthyroidism
    Struma ovarii

▼ **Decreased levels**
    Cretinism
    Surgical ablation
    Myxedema
    Pituitary insufficiency
    Hypothalamic failure
    Iodine insufficiency
    Renal failure
    Cushing's disease
    Cirrhosis
    Advanced cancer

notes

T

thyroxine, total (T₄, Thyroxine screen)

Type of test Blood

Normal findings

1-3 days: 11-22 μg/dl
1-2 weeks: 10-16 μg/dl
1-4 mos: 8-16 μg/dl
1-5 yrs: 7-15 μg/dl
5-10 yrs: 6-13 μg/dl
10-15 yrs: 5-12 μg/dl
Adult male: 4-12 μg/dl
Adult female: 5-12 μg/dl
Adult >60 yrs: 5-11 μg/dl

Possible critical values

Newborn: <7 μg/dl
Adult: <2 μg/dl if myxedema coma possible; >20 μg/dl if
thyroid storm possible

Test explanation and related physiology

The serum thyroxine (T_4) study is a direct measurement of the total amount of T_4 present in the patient's blood. T_4 makes up nearly all of what we call thyroid hormone. Greater-than-normal levels indicate hyperthyroid states, and subnormal values are seen in hypothyroid states. Newborns are screened by T_4 tests to detect hypothyroidism. Mental retardation can be prevented by early diagnosis.

This is a very reliable test of thyroid function; however, results are affected by thyroid-binding globulin (TBG). Because T_4 is bound by serum proteins such as TBG, any increase in these proteins (as in pregnant women and patients taking oral contraceptives) will cause factitiously elevated levels of T_4 and, to some extent, triiodothyronine (T_3). T_4 testing is also used to monitor replacement and suppressive therapy.

Interfering factors

- T_4 levels may be increased after x-ray iodinated contrast studies.
- Pregnancy causes increased levels.
- Drugs that may cause *increased* levels include clofibrate, estrogens, heroin, methadone, and oral contraceptives.

☛ Drugs that may cause *decreased* levels include anabolic steroids, androgens, antithyroid drugs (e.g., propylthiouracil), lithium, phenytoin (Dilantin), and propranolol (Inderal).

Procedure and patient care

Before

- If indicated, instruct the patient to stop exogenous T_4 medication 1 month before testing.
- Tell the patient that no fasting is required.

During

Adult
- Collect a venous blood specimen in a red-top tube.

Newborn
- Perform a heel stick to obtain blood.
- Thoroughly saturate the circles on the filter paper with blood.
- Note that prompt collection and processing are crucial to the early detection of hypothyroidism.
- Note that the optimal collection time is 2 to 4 days after birth.
- All newborns should be screened before discharge (regardless of age), however, because of the consequences of delayed diagnosis.

After

- Apply pressure to the venipuncture site.

Abnormal findings

▲ **Increased levels**

Graves' disease
Plummer's disease
Toxic thyroid adenoma
Acute thyroiditis
Familial dysalbuminemic hyperthyroxinemia
Factitious hyperthyroidism
Struma ovarii
Pregnancy
Hepatitis
Congenital hyperproteinemia

▼ **Decreased levels**

Cretinism
Surgical ablation
Myxedema
Pituitary insufficiency
Hypothalamic failure
Protein depleted disease states
Iodine insufficiency
Renal failure
Cushing's syndrome
Cirrhosis

T

thyroxine index, free (FTI, FT₄ index)

Type of test Blood

Normal findings 0.8-2.4 ng/dl or 10-31 pmol/L (SI units)

Test explanation and related physiology

The FT_4I study measures the amount of free thyroxine (T_4), which is only 1% of the total T_4. Free T_4 is the unbound T_4 that enters the cell and is metabolically active. The diagnostic value of measuring the FT_4I is that it is not affected by thyroid-binding globulin (TBG) abnormalities; therefore it correlates more closely with the true hormonal status than do total T_4 or tri-iodothyronine (T_3) determinations. To determine the FT_4I, T_3 uptake is measured and multiplied by the measured T_4 (see p. 830). The following mathematic computation

$$FT_4I = \frac{T_4 \text{ (total)} \times T_3 \text{ uptake (\%)}}{100}$$

corrects the estimated total T_4 assay for the effects of TBG protein alterations. If TBG is increased, the T_3 uptake decreases and corrects for the increased T_4 associated with the increased TBG. However when the TBG is normal and the T_4 is elevated, the FT_4 will be increased, indicating true hyperthyroidism. Therefore the FT_4I indicates the same information as the free T_4 radioimmunoassay (p. 828).

This index is useful in diagnosing hyperthyroidism and hypothyroidism, especially in patients with abnormalities in TBG levels. High FTI calculations suggest hyperthyroidism; low FTI values suggest hypothyroidism. The FTI study also aids in the evaluation of the thyroid status of pregnant women and patients who have abnormal TBG levels as a result of being treated with certain drugs (e.g., estrogen, phenytoin, salicylates).

Interfering factor

- Recent radionuclear scan

Procedure and patient care

Before

- Explain the procedure to the patient.
- Obtain the T_4 value and T_3 uptake ratio.

During

- Multiply the T_3 uptake value by the T_4 value to obtain the FTI (see p. 832).

After

- Apply pressure to the venipuncture site.

Abnormal findings

▲ **Increased levels**

Graves' disease
Plummer's disease
Toxic thyroid adenoma
Acute thyroiditis
Factitious hyperthyroidism
Struma ovarii

▼ **Decreased levels**

Hypothyroid states
Cretinism
Surgical ablation
Myxedema
Pituitary insufficiency
Hypothalamic failure
Iodine insufficiency

notes

T

TORCH test

The term TORCH (*T*oxoplasmosis, *O*ther, *R*ubella, *C*yto-megalovirus, *H*erpes) has been applied to infections with recognized detrimental effects on the fetus. The effects on the fetus may be direct or indirect (e.g., precipitating abortion or premature labor). Included in the category of *other* are infections such as syphilis. All of these tests are discussed separately:

Toxoplasmosis, p. 839
Rubella, p. 739
Cytomegalovirus, p. 314
Herpes virus, p. 474

notes

toxicology screening

Type of test Blood; urine

Normal findings See Tables 18 and 19 for blood toxicology and urine toxicology, respectively.

Test explanation and related physiology

This section includes a discussion of the detection of the most commonly abused nonprescription mood altering drugs. These are the drugs most commonly used in suicide attempts and chemical poisons.

Testing for drug overdose and poisoning is best performed on blood. Results indicate the immediate drug levels that can indicate or alter therapy. Screening for use or abuse of nonprescription drugs is usually done on urine. Urine specimens are easily obtained without any invasive procedure. Often the specimen is obtained several hours or days after the drug administration. Blood levels are low, but urine levels are high. Further, drug metabolic products exist in the urine for even longer periods of time, thereby allowing detection of any drug use in the past few hours or days. Urine temperature, specific gravity, and creatinine are often done on the urine specimen to ensure that the specimen has not been altered. It is important to define the appropriate chain of transfer of the specimen from the moment it is obtained to the point of testing to avoid any potential tampering.

Toxicology studies are used to incriminate drugs as a cause or factor in the death of a person. They are also used to assess patients when drug abuse or poisoning is contributing to an illness.

A list of commonly abused drugs and toxins follows.

Marijuana (cannabis)
Cocaine
Crack
Phencyclidine (PCP)
Amphetamines (especially methamphetamine)
Morphine (or other narcotic alkaloids)
Barbiturates
Lead
Other heavy metals

T

TABLE 18 Blood toxicology screening

Drug	Type	Therapeutic level*	Toxic level*
Acetaminophen	Analgesic, antipyretic	Depends on the use	>250 µg/ml
Alcohol	—	None	80-200 mg/dl (mild to moderate intoxication)
			250-400 mg/dl (marked intoxication)
			>400 mg/dl (severe intoxication)
Amobarbital	Sedative, hypnotic	0.5-3.0 µg/ml	>10 µg/ml
Butabarbital	Sedative, hypnotic	0.5-3.0 µg/ml	>10 µg/ml

Carboxyhemoglobin (COHb, carbon monoxide)	Gas	>30% COHb (beginning of coma)
Glutethimide	Sedative	>10 μg/ml
Lead	—	>40 μg/dl
Lithium	Manic episodes of manic-depression psychosis	>2.0 mEq/l
Meprobamate	Antianxiety agent	>10 μg/ml
Methyprylon	Hypnotic	>10 μg/ml
Phenobarbital	Anticonvulsant	>40 μg/ml
Phenytoin (Dilantin)	Anticonvulsant	>20 μg/ml
Salicylate	Antipyretic, anti-inflammatory, analgesic	>300 μg/ml

None	
0.5-3.0 μg/ml	
None	
0.8-1.2 mEq/l	
0.5-3.0 μg/ml	
0.5-3.0 μg/ml	
15-30 μg/ml	
10-20 μg/ml	
100-250 μg/ml	

*Levels vary according to the institution performing the test.

T

TABLE 19 Urine toxicology screening for amphetamines

Drug	Therapeutic level*	Toxic level*
Amphetamine	2-3 µg/ml	>3 µg/ml
Dextroamphetamine	0.1-1.5 µg/ml	>15 µg/ml
Methamphetamine	3-5 µg/ml	>40 µg/ml
Phenmetrazine	5-30 µg/ml	>50 µg/ml

*Levels vary according to the institution performing the test.

Procedure and patient care

Before

- Explain the procedure to the patient or significant others.
- If the specimen is obtained for medicolegal testing, ensure that the patient or family member has signed a consent form.
- Obtain as much information as possible about the drug type, amount, and ingestion time.
- Carefully assess the patient for respiratory distress (a common adverse reaction of drug overdosage).

During

- Collect blood as designated by the laboratory or urine specimens as indicated. Urine specimens are usually collected in the presence of the nurse.
- Collect gastric contents for analysis if indicated.
- Note that hair and nail samples may be used to detect or document exposure to arsenic and mercury.

After

- Apply pressure to the venipuncture site.
- Assess the patient for respiratory distress (a common adverse reaction of drug overdosage).
- Refer the patient for appropriate drug and psychiatric counseling.

Abnormal findings

Abuse or use of nonprescription drugs
Heavy metal and lead poisoning
Toxic levels of drugs in suicide attempts

toxoplasmosis antibody titer

Type of test Blood

Normal findings

Titers <1:16 indicate no previous infection
Titers 1:16-1:256 are usually prevalent in general population
Titers >1:256 suggest recent infection
Rising titers are of great significance

Test explanation and related physiology

Toxoplasmosis is a protozoan disease caused by *Toxoplasma gondii*, which is found in poorly cooked or raw meat and in the feces of cats. Most often, humans are asymptomatic from the infection. When symptoms occur, this disease is characterized by central nervous system lesions, which may lead to blindness, brain damage, and death. The condition may occur congenitally or postnatally. Because approximately 25% to 50% of the adult population are asymptomatically affected with toxoplasmosis, the Centers for Disease Control and Prevention (CDC) recommends that patients who are pregnant be serologically tested for this disease.

The presence of antibodies before pregnancy indicates prior exposure and chronic asymptomatic infection. The presence of these antibodies probably ensures protection against congenital toxoplasmosis in the child. Fetal infection occurs if the mother acquires toxoplasmosis after conception and passes it to the fetus through the placenta. Repeat testing of pregnant patients with low or negative titers may be done before the twentieth week and before delivery to identify antibody converters and determine appropriate therapy (e.g., therapeutic abortion at 20 weeks, treatment during the remainder of the pregnancy, or treatment of the newborn).

Hydrocephaly, microcephaly, chronic retinitis, and convulsions are complications of congenital toxoplasmosis. Congenital toxoplasmosis is diagnosed when the antibody levels are persistently elevated or a rising titer is found in the infant 2 to 3 months after birth. Toxoplasmosis is an infection included in the acronym TORCH (*t*oxoplasmosis, *o*ther, *r*ubella, *c*ytomegalovirus, *h*erpes) which is associated with recognized detrimental effects on the fetus.

T

Procedure and patient care

Before

- Explain the procedure to the patient.

During

- Collect approximately 5 ml of blood in a red-top tube.
- Indicate on the laboratory slip if the patient is pregnant or has been exposed to cats.

After

- Apply pressure to the venipuncture site.

Abnormal finding

Toxoplasmosis infection

notes

transesophageal echocardiography (TEE)

Type of test   Endoscopy/ultrasound

Normal findings   Normal position, size, and movement of the heart muscle, valves, and heart chambers

Test explanation and related physiology

TEE provides ultrasonic imaging of the heart from a retrocardiac vantage point, avoiding interference with the ultrasound by the interposed subcutaneous tissue, bony thorax, and lungs. In this procedure a high-frequency ultrasound transducer placed in the esophagus by endoscopy provides better resolution than that of images obtained with routine transthoracic echocardiography (see p. 332). For TEE, the distal end of the endoscope is advanced into the esophagus. The transducer is positioned behind the heart (Figure 35). Controls on the handle of the endoscope permit the transducer to be rotated and flexed in both the anteroposterior and right-left lateral planes. TEE images have better resolution than those obtained by routine transthoracic echocardiography because of the higher-frequency sound waves and closer proximity of the transducer to the cardiac structures.

TEE is helpful in the evaluation of structures that are inaccessible or poorly visualized by the transthoracic probe approach. It is especially helpful in patients who are obese or have large lung-air spaces.

This test is performed for the following reasons:

1. To better visualize the mitral valve
2. To differentiate intracardiac from extracardiac masses and tumors
3. To better visualize the atrial septum (for atrial septal defects)
4. To diagnose thoracic aortic dissection
5. To better detect valvular vegetation indicative of endocarditis
6. To determine cardiac sources of arterial embolism
7. To detect coronary artery disease

TEE can also be used intraoperatively to monitor high-risk patients for ischemia. Ischemic muscle movement is much different from normal muscle movement; therefore TEE is a very sensitive indicator of myocardial ischemia. TEE can be used to

T

Figure 35 Transesophageal echocardiography. Diagram illustrates location of the transesophageal endoscope within the esophagus.

monitor patients undergoing major abdominal, peripheral vascular, and carotid artery procedures who are at high risk for intraoperative ischemia because of coronary artery disease.

TEE is more sensitive than electrocardiography (ECG) for detecting ischemia. It is also used intraoperatively to evaluate surgical results of valvular or congenital heart diseases. Furthermore, TEE is also the most sensitive technique for detecting air emboli, a serious complication of neurosurgery performed with the patient in the upright position (cervical laminectomy).

Contraindications

- Patients with known upper esophageal pathology
- Patients with known esophageal varices

- Patients with Zenker's diverticulum
- Patients with esophageal abnormalities (e.g., stricture diverticula, scleroderma, esophagitis)
- Patients with bleeding disorders
- Patients who have had prior esophageal surgery
- Patients who cannot cooperate with the procedure

Potential complications

- Esophageal perforation or bleeding
- Cardiac arrhythmias

Procedure and patient care

Before

- Explain the procedure to the patient.
- Instruct the patient to fast for 4 to 6 hours before the test.
- Removal all oral prostheses.
- Obtain IV access.

During

- Intravenous sedation is commonly provided with a short-acting benzodiazepine. Other sedation may be provided.
- Apply ECG leads and continually monitor heart rhythm.
- Apply a blood pressure cuff and monitor blood pressure periodically.
- Pulse oximetry is monitored to determine oxygen saturation in sedated patients.
- Note the following procedural steps:
  1. The pharynx is anesthetized with a local topical agent to depress the gag reflex.
  2. The patient is placed in the left lateral decubitus position.
  3. Intubation is carried out through the mouth and into the upper esophagus.
  4. The patient is asked to swallow, and the transducer is advanced into position behind the heart.
  5. The room is darkened, and the ultrasound images are displayed on a monitor. Views can be obtained of the ultrasound image after desired images are visualized.
- The procedure is performed by a cardiologist and/or a gastrointestinal endoscopist in approximately 20 minutes in the endoscopy suite. It also can be performed at the bedside.
- Very little discomfort is associated with this test.

T

After

- Naloxone or mazicon may be administered to reverse the sedative effects of the narcotics.
- Observe the patient closely for approximately 1 hour after the procedure, until the effects of sedation have worn off.

Abnormal findings

Myocardial ischemia
Myocardial infarction
Valvular heart disease
Intracardiac thrombi
Cardiac valvular vegetation
Ventricular and atrial septal defects
Cardiomyopathy
Marked cardiac chamber dilation
Cardiac tumors

notes

triglycerides (TGs)

Type of test Blood

Normal findings

Adult/elderly
  Male: 40-160 mg/dl or 0.45-1.81 mmol (SI units)
  Female: 35-135 mg/dl or 0.40-1.52 mmol/L (SI units)

Child	Male	Female
0-5 years:	30-86 mg/dl	32-99 mg/dl
6-11 years:	31-108 mg/dl	35-114 mg/dl
12-15 years:	36-138 mg/dl	41-138 mg/dl
16-19 years:	40-163 mg/dl	40-128 mg/dl

Critical values >400 mg/dl.

Test explanation and related physiology

TGs are a form of fat that exists within the bloodstream. They are transported by very low-density lipoproteins (VLDLs) and low-density lipoproteins (LDLs). TGs are produced in the liver by using glycerol and other fatty acids as building blocks. A TG acts as a storage source for energy. When TG levels in the blood are in excess, TGs are deposited into the fatty tissues. TGs are a part of a lipid profile that also evaluates cholesterol (see p. 232) and lipoproteins (see p. 528). A lipid profile is performed to assess the risk of coronary and vascular disease.

Interfering factors

- Ingestion of fatty meals may cause elevated TG levels.
- Ingestion of alcohol may cause elevated levels.
- Pregnancy may cause increased levels.
- ✶ Drugs that may cause *increased* TG levels include cholestyramine, estrogens, and oral contraceptives.
- ✶ Drugs that may cause *decreased* levels include ascorbic acid, asparaginase, clofibrate, and colestipol.

Procedure and patient care

Before

- Explain the procedure to the patient.
- Instruct the patient to fast for 12 to 14 hours before the test. Only water is permitted.
- Tell the patient not to drink alcohol for 24 hours before the test.

T

- Inform the patient that dietary indiscretion for as much as 2 weeks before this test will influence results.

During

- Collect 5 to 10 ml of venous blood in a red-top tube.

After

- Apply pressure to the venipuncture site.
- Mark the patient's age and gender on the laboratory slip.
- Instruct the patient with increased TG levels regarding diet, exercise, and appropriate weight.

Abnormal findings

▲ **Increased levels**
Glycogen storage disease
Hyperlipidemias
Hypothyroidism
High-carbohydrate diet
Poorly controlled diabetes
Risk of arteriosclerotic occlusive coronary disease and peripheral vascular disease
Nephrotic syndrome
Hypertension
Alcoholic cirrhosis
Pregnancy
Myocardial infarction

▼ **Decreased levels**
Malabsorption syndrome
Malnutrition
Hyperthyroidism

notes

triiodothyronine (T_3 radioimmunoassay [T_3 by RIA])

Type of test Blood

Normal findings

1-3 days: 100-740 ng/dl
1-11 mos: 105-245 ng/dl
1-5 yrs: 105-270 ng/dl
6-10 yrs: 95-240 ng/dl
11-15 yrs: 80-215 ng/dl
16-20 yrs: 80-210 ng/dl
20-50 yrs: 70-205 ng/dl
>50 yrs: 40-180 ng/dl

Test explanation and related physiology

As with the thyroxine (T_4) test, the serum T_3 test is an accurate measure of thyroid function. T_3 is less stable than T_4 and occurs in minute quantities in the active form. Only about 7% to 10% of thyroid hormone is composed of T_3. Seventy percent of that T_3 is bound to proteins (thyroid-binding globulin [TBG] and albumen). This test is a measurement of total T_3, (i.e., the free and the bound T_3). Generally, when the T_3 level is below normal, the patient is in a hypothyroid state.

Other severe nonthyroidal diseases can decrease T_3 levels by diminishing the conversion of T_4 to T_3 in the liver. This makes T_3 levels less useful in indicating hypothyroid states. Further, there is considerable overlap between hypothyroid states and normal thyroid function. Because of this, T_3 levels are mostly just used to assist in the diagnosis of hyperthyroid states. An elevated T_3 indicates hyperthyroidism, especially when the T_4 is also elevated. There is a rare form of hyperthyroidism called *T_3 toxicosis,* in which the T_4 is normal and the T_3 is elevated.

T

Interfering factors

- Radioisotope administration before the test may alter the results.
- T_3 values are increased in pregnancy.
- ⚕ Drugs that may cause *increased* levels include estrogen, methadone, and oral contraceptives.
- ⚕ Drugs that may cause *decreased* levels include anabolic steroids, androgens, phenytoin (Dilantin), propranolol (Inderal), reserpine, and salicylates (high dose).

Procedure and patient care

Before
- Explain the procedure to the patient.
- Determine whether the patient is taking any exogenous T_3 medication, because this will affect test results.
- Withhold drugs that may affect results (with physician's approval).
- Tell the patient that no fasting is required.

During
- Collect approximately 5 to 10 ml of venous blood in a red-top tube.
- List on the laboratory slip any medications the patient is currently taking.

After
- Apply pressure to the venipuncture site.

Abnormal findings

▲ **Increased levels**

Graves' disease
Plummer's disease
Toxic thyroid adenoma
Acute thyroiditis
Factitious hyper-
    thyroidism
Struma ovarii
Pregnancy
Hepatitis
Congenital hyper-
    proteinemia

▼ **Decreased levels**

Hypothyroidism
Cretinism
Thyroid surgical ablation
Myxedema
Pituitary insufficiency
Hypothalamic failure
Protein malnutrition and
    other protein depleted
    states (e.g., nephrotic
    syndrome)
Iodine insufficiency
Renal failure
Cushing's syndrome
Cirrhosis
Liver diseases

notes

tuberculin test (PPD skin test)

Type of test Skin

Normal findings Negative; reaction <5 mm

Test explanation and related physiology

Although this test is used to detect tuberculosis (TB) infection, it is unable to indicate whether the infection is active or dormant. For this test, a *purified protein derivative* (PPD) of the tubercle bacillus is injected intradermally. If the patient is infected with TB (whether active or dormant), lymphocytes will recognize the PPD antigen and cause a local reaction; if the patient is not infected, no reaction will occur. If the test is negative and the physician strongly suspects TB, a "second-strength" PPD can be used. If this test is then negative, the patient does not have TB. (See p. 851 for tuberculosis culture.) The PPD skin test usually becomes positive 6 weeks after infection. Once positive, the reaction usually persists for life.

The PPD test also can be used as part of a series of skin tests done to assess the immune system. If the immune system is nonfunctioning because of poor nutrition or chronic illness (e.g., neoplasia, infection), the PPD test will be negative despite the patient having had an active or a dormant TB infection. Other skin tests used to test immune function include *Candida*, mumps virus, and *Trichophyton*, organisms to which most people in the United States have been exposed.

Testing for TB is usually performed as part of the routine prenatal evaluation in pregnant women. Often this may be the mother's first contact with the health care system in several years.

When a patient known to have active TB receives a PPD test, the local reaction may be so severe as to cause a complete skin slough requiring surgical care. When these patients are eliminated from PPD testing, the test has no complications. The PPD test will not cause active TB, because no live organisms exist in the test solution.

Contraindications

- Patients with known active TB
- Patients who have received *bacille Calmette-Guérin* (BCG) immunization against PPD, because these patients will

T

demonstrate a positive reaction to the PPD vaccination even
though they have never had TB infection

Procedure and patient care

Before

- Explain the procedure to the patient.
- Assure the patient that she or he will not develop TB from
  this test.
- Assess the patient for previous history of TB. Report a posi-
  tive history to the physician.
- Evaluate the patient's history for previous PPD results and
  BCG immunization.

During

- Prepare the patient's forearm with alcohol and allow it to dry.
- Intradermally inject the PPD. A skin wheal will occur.
- Circle the area with indelible ink.
- Record the time at which the PPD was injected.

After

- Read the results in 48 to 72 hours.
- Examine the test site for induration (hardening). Measure the
  area of induration (not redness) in millimeters.
- If the test is positive, ensure that the physician is notified and
  the patient treated appropriately.
- If the test is positive, check the patient's arm 4 to 5 days after
  the test to be certain that a severe skin reaction has not
  occurred.

Abnormal findings

Positive results
TB infection
Nontuberculous mycobacteria infections

Negative result
Possible immunoincompetence

notes

tuberculosis culture (TB culture, BACTEC method, Polymerase chain reaction)

Type of test Microbiology culture

Normal findings Negative for tuberculosis

Test explanation and related physiology

Diagnosis of TB can be made only by identification and culture of *Mycobacterium tuberculosis* in the specimen. Conventional culture techniques for growth, identification, and susceptibility of acid-fast mycobacterium take 4 to 6 weeks. Because the patient suspected of having TB cannot be isolated for that duration, the disease may spread to many other people while he or she waits for the diagnosis. With the resurgence and increasing incidence of TB in the U.S. population (especially among immunocompromised patients with acquired immunodeficiency syndrome), newer, more rapid culture techniques have been identified and are now being performed.

The *BACTEC* method is a culture technique in which the growth medium for culturing mycobacteria is supplanted with a substrate labeled with radioactive carbon (^{14}C). This substrate is used by mycobacteria; during metabolism radioactive carbon dioxide ($^{14}CO_2$) is produced from the substrate. The $^{14}CO_2$ is detected and quantitated. This permits quick identification of mycobacterial growth.

Polymerase chain reaction culture methods also have recently been developed. With the addition of a deoxyribonucleic acid (DNA) polymerase, genetic chromosomal parts can be multiplied. This allows amplification of genomes, which then can be detected by genetic DNA probes. With the newer techniques already described, *M. tuberculosis* can be identified in as few as 36 to 48 hours. With this reduction in diagnostic time, treatment can be started earlier. Thus it is anticipated that the spread of tuberculosis will be greatly reduced. The average detection time, however, is longer for extrapulmonary specimens than for sputum specimens. The time for identification is greatly reduced when numerous mycobacteria are present. Generally organisms in specimens from patients already receiving antituberculosis treatment take longer to grow.

After identification and growth of mycobacteria, antibiotic susceptibility testing is performed to identify the most effective

T

antimycobacterial drugs. The culture specimen can be performed on sputum, body fluids, cerebrospinal fluid, and even biopsy tissue specimens.

When tuberculosis is suspected, a *sputum smear for acid-fast bacillus (AFB)* can be obtained. After taking up a dye such as fuchsin, *M. tuberculosis* is not decolorized by acid alcohol (i.e., it is acid-fast). It is seen under the microscope as a red, rod-shaped organism. If this bacillus is seen, the patient may have active TB. At least 5000 organisms must be present in each milliliter of specimen to be seen on a microscope smear. Other specimens such as cerebrospinal fluid, tissue, and synovial fluid may be used. Smears may be negative as much as 50% of the time, even with positive cultures. AFB is also used to monitor treatment for TB. If after adequate therapy (2 months), the sputum still contains AFB (even though the culture may be negative due to anti-TB drugs), treatment failure should be considered.

Interfering factors

☒ Antituberculosis drugs

Procedure and patient care

Before

- Explain the procedure to the patient.
- Tell the patient that no fasting is required.

During

- For *sputum*, obtain an early morning specimen. It is best to induce sputum production with an ultrasonic or nebulizing device.
- Collect three to five early morning specimens. All specimens must contain mycobacteria to make the diagnosis of TB.
- For *urine* collection obtain three to five single, clean-voided specimens early in the morning.
- *Swabs*, *intestinal washings*, and *biopsy* specimens should be transported to the laboratory immediately for preparation.
- Follow the institution's policy for universal specimen handling.
- Once the specimen is received by the laboratory, a decontamination process is applied to it to kill all nonmycobacteria. The specimen is then cultured in the appropriate medium.
- With the rapid growth techniques, the specimen is evaluated every 24 hours.

- When cultural growth is considered adequate, the organisms are stained for acid-fast bacillus and identified.
- With genetic probes, the *Mycobacterium* species is identified.
- At this point, if *M. tuberculosis* is present, the report will read "culture more positive for mycobacteria." If the species has been identified, this also will be reported.
- Drug-susceptibility testing then will be carried out and subsequently reported.

After

- Instruct the patient as to appropriate isolation of sputum and other body fluids to avoid potential spread of suspected TB.

Abnormal findings

TB
Atypical mycobacterial nontuberculosis disease

notes

T

upper gastrointestinal x-ray study (Upper GI series, UGI)

Type of test X-ray with contrast dye

Normal findings Normal size, contour, patency, filling, positioning, and transit of barium through the lower esophagus, stomach, and upper duodenum

Test explanation and related physiology

The upper GI study consists of a series of x-ray films of the lower esophagus, stomach, and duodenum, usually using barium sulfate as the contrast medium. When there is concern for leakage of x-ray contrast through a perforation of the GI tract, however, Gastrografin (a water-soluble contrast) is used. This test can be performed in conjunction with a barium swallow or a small bowel series (see pp. 137 and 772), which can precede or succeed the upper GI study, respectively.

The purpose of this examination is to detect ulcerations, tumors, inflammations, or anatomic malpositions (e.g., hiatal hernia) within these organs. Obstruction of the upper GI tract is also easily detected.

In this test the patient is asked to drink barium. As the contrast descends, the lower esophagus is examined for position, patency, and filling defects (e.g., tumors, scarring, varices). As the contrast enters the stomach, the gastric wall is examined for benign or malignant ulcerations, filling defects (most often in cancer), and anatomic abnormalities (e.g., hiatal hernia). The patient is placed in a flat or head-down position, and the gastroesophageal area is examined for evidence of gastroesophageal reflux of barium.

As the contrast leaves the stomach, patency of the pyloric channel and the duodenum is evaluated. Benign peptic ulceration is the most common pathologic condition affecting these areas. Extrinsic compression caused by tumors, cysts, or enlarged pathologic organs (e.g., liver) near the stomach also can be identified by anatomic distortion of the outline of the upper GI tract. The small intestine can then be studied (see discussion of small bowel follow-through, p. 772).

Contraindications

- Patients with complete bowel obstructions
- Patients suspected of upper GI perforation

Water-soluble Gastrografin should be used instead of barium.
- Patients with unstable vital signs
  These patients should be supervised during the time required for this test.
- Patients who are uncooperative because of the necessity of frequent position changes

Potential complications
- Aspiration of barium
- Constipation or partial bowel obstruction caused by inspissated barium in the small bowel or colon

Interfering factors
- Previously administered barium
  This may block visualization of the upper GI tract.
- Poor performance status of the patient
  Incapacitated patients cannot assume the multiple positions required for the study.
- Food and fluid in the stomach
  This gives the false impression of filling defects within the stomach, precluding adequate evaluation of the gastric mucosa.

Procedure and patient care

Before
- Explain the procedure to the patient. Allow the patient to verbalize concerns.
- Instruct the patient to abstain from eating for at least 8 hours before the test. Usually keep the patient NPO after midnight on the day of the test.
- Assure the patient that the test will not cause any discomfort.

During
- Note the following procedural steps:
  1. The patient is asked to drink approximately 16 ounces of barium sulfate. This is a chalky substance usually suspended in milkshake form and drunk through a straw. Usually the drink is flavored to increase palatability.
  2. After drinking the barium, the patient is moved through several position changes (e.g., prone, supine, lateral) to promote filling of the entire upper GI tract.
  3. Films are taken at the discretion of the radiologist observing the flow of barium fluoroscopically.
  4. The flow of barium is followed through the lower esophagus, stomach, and duodenum.

U

5. Several films are taken throughout the course of the test.
6. In an *air-contrast upper GI study*, the patient is asked to swallow rapidly carbonated powder. This creates carbon dioxide in the stomach, providing air contrast to the barium within the stomach and increased visualization of the gastric mucosa.

- Note that a radiologist performs this procedure in approximately 30 minutes.
- Tell the patient that he or she may be uncomfortable lying on the hard x-ray table and occasionally may experience the sensation of bloating or nausea during the test.

After

- Inform the patient that, if Gastrografin was used, he or she may have significant diarrhea. Gastrografin is an osmotic cathartic.
- Instruct the patient to use a cathartic (e.g., milk of magnesia) if barium sulfate was used as the contrast medium. Water absorption may cause the barium to harden and create a fecal impaction if catharsis is not carried out.
- Instruct the patient to watch his or her stools to ensure that all of the barium has been removed. The stools should return to normal color after completely expelling the barium, which may take as much as a day and a half.

Abnormal findings

Esophageal cancer
Esophageal varices
Hiatal hernia
Esophageal diverticula
Gastric cancer
Gastric inflammatory disease (e.g., Ménétrier's disease)
Benign gastric tumor (e.g., leiomyoma)
Extrinsic compression by pancreatic pseudocysts, cysts, pancreatic tumors, or hepatomegaly
Perforation of the esophagus, stomach, or duodenum
Congenital abnormalities (e.g., duodenal web, pancreatic rest, malrotation syndrome)
Gastric ulcer (benign and malignant)
Gastritis
Duodenal ulcer
Duodenal cancer
Duodenal diverticulum

urea nitrogen blood test (Blood urea nitrogen [BUN], Serum urea nitrogen)

Type of test Blood

Normal findings

Adult: 10-20 mg/dl or 3.6-7.1 mmol/L (SI units)
Elderly: may be slightly higher than those of adults
Child: 5-18 mg/dl
Infant: 5-18 mg/dl
Newborn: 3-12 mg/dl
Cord: 21-40 mg/dl

Possible critical values >100 mg/dl (indicates serious impairment of renal function)

Test explanation and related physiology

The BUN measures the amount of urea nitrogen in the blood. Urea is formed in the liver as the end product of protein metabolism. During ingestion protein is broken down into amino acids. In the liver these amino acids are catabolized, and free ammonia is formed. The ammonia is combined to form urea, which is then deposited into the blood and transported to the kidneys for excretion. Therefore the BUN is directly related to the metabolic function of the liver and the excretory function of the kidney. It serves as an index of the function of these organs. Patients who have elevated BUN levels are said to have azotemia.

Nearly all renal diseases cause an inadequate excretion of urea, which causes the blood concentration to rise above normal. If the disease is unilateral, however, the unaffected kidney can compensate for the diseased kidney, and the BUN may not become elevated. The BUN also increases in conditions other than primary renal disease. For example, when excess amounts of protein are available for hepatic catabolism (from a high-protein diet or gastrointestinal [GI] bleeding), large quantities of urea are made. BUN levels also may vary according to the state of hydration, with increased levels seen in dehydration and decreased levels seen in overhydration. Finally, one must be aware that the synthesis of urea depends on the liver. Patients with severe primary liver disease will have a decreased BUN. With combined liver and renal disease (as in hepatorenal syndrome),

U

the BUN can be normal not because renal excretory function is good but because poor hepatic functioning has resulted in decreased formation of urea.

The BUN is interpreted in conjunction with the creatinine test (see p. 294). These tests are referred to as *renal function studies.*

Interfering factors

- Changes in protein intake may affect BUN levels.
- Advanced pregnancy may cause increased levels.
- Overhydration and underhydration will affect levels.
- ✹ Drugs that may cause *increased* BUN levels include allopurinol, aminoglycosides, cephalosporins, chloral hydrate, cisplatin, furosemide, guanethidine, indomethacin, methotrexate, methyldopa, nephrotoxic drugs (e.g., aspirin, amphotericin B, bacitracin, carbamazepine, colistin, gentamicin, methicillin, neomycin, penicillamine, polymyxin B, probenecid, vancomycin), propranolol, rifampin, spironolactone, tetracyclines, thiazide diuretics, and triamterene.
- ✹ Drugs that may cause *decreased* levels include chloramphenicol and streptomycin.

Procedure and patient care

Before

- Explain the procedure to the patient.
- Tell the patient that no fasting is required.

During

- Collect approximately 5 ml of blood in a red-top tube.
- Avoid hemolysis.

After

- Apply pressure or a pressure dressing to the venipuncture site.

Abnormal findings

▲ **Increased levels**

Prerenal causes
Hypovolemia
Shock
Burns
Dehydration
Congestive heart failure
Myocardial infarction
GI bleeding
Excessive protein ingestion
Alimentary tube feeding
Excessive protein catabolism
Starvation
Sepsis

Renal causes
Renal disease (e.g., glomerulonephritis, pyelonephritis, acute tubular necrosis)
Renal failure
Nephrotoxic drugs

Postrenal azotemia
Ureteral obstruction
Bladder outlet obstruction

▼ **Decreased levels**

Liver failure
Overhydration caused by fluid overload or SIADH syndrome
Negative nitrogen balance (e.g., malnutrition or malabsorption)
Pregnancy
Nephrotic syndrome

notes

U

uric acid, blood and urine

Type of test Blood/urine

Normal findings

Blood

Adult

Male: 2.1-8.5 mg/dl or 0.15-0.48 mmol/L

Female: 2-6.6 mg/dl or 0.09-0.36 mmol/L

Elderly: values may be slightly increased

Child: 2.5-5.5 mg/dl or 0.12-0.32 mmol/L

Newborn: 2-6.2 mg/dl

Urine: 250-750 ml/24 hr or 1.48-4.43 mmol/day (SI units)

Possible critical values Blood: >12 mg/dl

Test explanation and related physiology

Uric acid is a nitrogenous compound that is a product of purine (a deoxyribonucleic acid [DNA] building block) catabolism. Uric acid is excreted to a large degree by the kidney and to a smaller degree by the intestinal tract. When uric acid levels are elevated (hyperuricemia), the patient may have gout. Causes of hyperuricemia can be overproduction or decreased excretion of uric acid (e.g., kidney failure). Overproduction of uric acid may occur in patients with a catabolic enzyme deficiency that stimulates purine metabolism or in patients with cancer in whom purine and DNA turnover is great. Other causes of hyperuricemia may include alcoholism, leukemias, metastatic cancer, multiple myeloma, hyperlipoproteinemia, diabetes mellitus, renal failure, stress, lead poisoning, and dehydration caused by diuretic therapy. Ketoacids (as occur in diabetic or alcoholic ketoacidosis) may compete with uric acid for tubular excretion and may cause decreased uric acid excretion. Many causes of hyperuricemia are undefined and therefore labeled as *idiopathic*.

Elevated uric acid in the urine is called uricosuria. Uric acid can become supersaturated in the urine and crystallize to form kidney stones that can block the renal system. Urinary excretion of uric acid depends on uric acid levels in the blood, along with glomerular filtration and tubular secretion of uric acid into the urine. Uric acid is less well saturated in an acidic urine. As the urine pH rises, more uric acid can exist without crystallization and stone formation. Therefore, when a person is known to have high uric acid in the urine, the urine can be alkalinized by ingestion of a strong base to prevent stone formation.

Interfering factors

- Stress may cause increased uric acid levels.
- Recent use of x-ray contrast agents may cause decreased serum levels.
- Recent use of x-ray contrast agents may increase uric acid levels in the urine.
- Drugs that may cause *increased* serum levels include alcohol, ascorbic acid, aspirin (low dose), caffeine, cisplatin, diazoxide, diuretics, epinephrine, ethambutol, levodopa, methyldopa (Aldomet), nicotinic acid, phenothiazines, and theophylline.
- Drugs that may cause *decreased* serum levels include allopurinol, aspirin (high dose), azathioprine (Imuran), clofibrate, corticosteroids, estrogens, glucose infusions, guaifenesin, mannitol, probenecid, and warfarin.
- Drugs that may cause *increased* urine levels include ascorbic acid, calcitonin, citrate, dicumarol, estrogens, steroids, iodinated dyes, glyceryl guaiacolate, phenolsulfonphthalein, probenecid, salicylates, and outdated tetracycline.

Procedure and patient care

Before
- Explain the procedure to the patient.
- Follow the institution's requirements regarding fasting. (Some recommend that the patient fast.)

During

Blood
- Collect approximately 5 to 7 ml of venous blood in a red-top tube.
- List on the laboratory slip any drugs that may affect test results.

Urine
- Instruct the patient to begin the 24-hour urine collection after voiding. Discard the initial specimen and start the 24-hour timing at that point.
- Collect all the urine passed during the next 24 hours. A preservative may be used.
- Show the patient where to store the urine container.
- Keep the specimen on ice or refrigerated during the entire 24 hours. (Note that some laboratories do not require refrigeration.)
- Indicate the starting time on the urine container and laboratory slip.

U

- Post the hours for the urine collection in a noticeable place to prevent accidental discarding of the specimen.
- Instruct the patient to void before defecating so the urine is not contaminated by feces.
- Remind the patient not to put toilet paper in the collection container.
- Encourage the patient to drink fluids during the 24 hours.
- Instruct the patient to collect the last specimen as close as possible to the end of the 24-hour period. Add this urine to the container.

After

Blood

- Apply pressure to the venipuncture site.

Urine

- Transport the urine specimen promptly to the laboratory.

Abnormal findings

▲ **Increased blood levels (hyperuricemia)**

Gout
Increased ingestion of purines
Genetic inborn error in purine metabolism
Metastatic cancer
Multiple myeloma
Leukemias
Cancer chemotherapy
Hemolysis
Rhabdomyolysis (e.g., heavy exercise, burns, crush injury, epileptic seizure, or myocardial infarction)
Chronic renal disease
Acidosis (ketotic or lactic)
Hypothyroidism
Toxemia of pregnancy
Hyperlipoproteinemia
Alcoholism
Shock or chronic blood volume depletion states
Idiopathic

▼ **Decreased blood levels**

Wilson's disease
Fanconi syndrome
Lead poisoning
Yellow atrophy of the liver

▲ **Increased urine levels (uricosuria)**
Gout
Metastatic cancer
Multiple myeloma
Leukemias
Cancer chemotherapy
High purine diet
Lead toxicity

▼ **Decreased urine levels**
Kidney disease
Eclampsia
Chronic alcohol ingestion
Acidosis (ketotic or lactic)

notes

U

urinalysis (UA)

Type of test Urine

Normal findings

Appearance: clear
Color: amber yellow
Odor: aromatic
pH: 4.6-8.0 (average 6.0)
Protein
   None or up to 8 mg/dl
   50-80 mg/dl (at rest)
   <250 mg/dl (exercise)
Specific gravity
   Adult: 1.005-1.030 (usually 1.010-1.025)
   Elderly: values decrease with age
   Newborn: 1.001-1.020
Leukocyte esterase: negative
Nitrites: negative
Ketones: negative
Crystals: negative
Casts: none present
Glucose (see urine glucose discussion, p. 439)
   Brand new specimen: negative
   24-hour specimen: <0.5 g/dl or <70 mmol/day (SI units)
White blood cells (WBCs): 0-4 per low-power field
WBC casts: negative
Red blood cells (RBCs): up to 2
RBC casts: none

Test explanation and related physiology

A total urinalysis involves multiple routine tests on a urine specimen. This specimen is not necessarily a clean-catch specimen. However, if urinary tract infection is suspected, often a midstream, clean-catch specimen is obtained. This urine is then split into two parts. One is sent for urinalysis, and the other is held in the laboratory refrigerator and cultured (see p. 878) if the urinalysis indicates infection. Routinely a urinalysis includes remarks about the color, appearance, and odor of the urine. The pH is determined. The urine is tested for the presence of proteins, glucose, ketones, blood, and leukocyte esterase. The urine is examined microscopically for RBCs, WBCs, casts, crystals, and bacteria.

Examination of the urine sediment provides a significant amount of information about the urinary system. The test is done on a centrifuged urinary sediment. There are many different methods to prepare the sediment for microscopic review. As a result, normal values may vary significantly among laboratories. Reference ranges have been provided to recognize marked abnormalities.

Appearance and color

Urine appearance and color are noted as part of routine urinalysis. The appearance of a normal urine specimen should be clear. Cloudy urine may be caused by the presence of pus, RBCs, or bacteria; however, normal urine also may be cloudy because of ingestion of certain foods (e.g., large amounts of fat, ureates, or phosphates). The color of urine ranges from pale yellow to amber because of the pigment urochrome. The color indicates the concentration of the urine and varies with specific gravity. Dilute urine is straw colored, and concentrated urine is deep amber.

Abnormally colored urine may result from a pathologic condition or the ingestion of certain foods or medicines. For example, bleeding from the kidney produces dark-red urine, whereas bleeding from the lower urinary tract produces bright-red urine. Dark-yellow urine may indicate the presence of urobilinogen or bilirubin. *Pseudomonas* organisms may produce green urine. Beets may cause red urine, and rhubarb can color the urine brown. Many frequently used drugs also may affect urine color (see Table 20).

Odor

Determination of urine odor is a part of routine urinalysis. The aromatic odor of fresh, normal urine is caused by the presence of volatile acids. Urine of patients with diabetic ketoacidosis has the strong, sweet smell of acetone. In patients with a urinary tract infection, the urine may have a very foul odor. Patients with a fecal odor to their urine may have an enterobladder fistula.

pH

The analysis of the pH of a freshly voided urine specimen indicates the acid-base balance of the patient. An alkaline pH is obtained in a patient with alkalemia. Also, bacteria, urinary tract infection, or a diet high in citrus fruits or vegetables may cause

U

TABLE 20 Frequently used drugs that may affect urine color

Generic and brand names	Drug classification	Urine color
Anisindione (Miradon)	Oral anticoagulant	Red-orange in alkaline urine
Cascara sagrada	Stimulant laxative	Red in alkaline urine; yellow-brown in acid urine
Chloroquine (Aralen)	Antimalarial	Rusty yellow or brown
Chlorzoxazone (Paraflex)	Skeletal muscle relaxant	Orange or purple-red
Docusate calcium (Doxidan, Surfak)	Laxative	Pink to red to red-brown
Furazolidone (Furoxone)	Antiinfective, antiprotozoal	Brown
Iron preparations (Ferotran, Imferon)	Hematinic	Dark brown or black on standing
Levodopa	Antiparkinsonian	Dark brown on standing

Drug	Use	Urine color
Methylene blue (Urolene Blue)	Antimethemoglobinemic	Blue-green
Nitrofurantoin (Macrodantin, Nitrodan)	Antibacterial	Brown
Phenazopyridine (Pyridium)	Urinary tract analgesic	Orange to red
Phenindione (Eridione)	Anticoagulant	Red-orange in alkaline urine
Phenolphthalein (Ex-Lax)	Contact laxative	Red or purplish pink in alkaline urine
Phenothiazines (e.g., prochlorperazine [Compazine])	Antipsychotic, neuroleptic, antiemetic	Red-brown
Phenytoin (Dilantin)	Anticonvulsant	Pink, red, red-brown
Riboflavin (vitamin B)	Vitamin	Intense yellow
Rifampin	Antibiotic	Red-orange
Sulfasalazine (Azulfidine)	Antibacterial	Orange-yellow in alkaline urine
Triamterene (Dyrenium)	Diuretic	Pale blue fluorescence

U

an increased urine pH. Certain medications (e.g., streptomycin, neomycin, kanamycin) are effective in treating urinary tract infections when the urine is alkaline. Acidic urine is generally obtained in patients with acidemia, which can result from metabolic or respiratory acidosis, starvation, dehydration, or a diet high in meat products or cranberries.

The urine pH is useful in identifying crystals in the urine and determining the predisposition to form a given type of stone. Acidic urine is associated with xanthine, cystine, uric acid, and calcium oxalate stones. To treat or prevent these urinary calculi, urine should be kept alkaline. Alkaline urine is associated with calcium carbonate, calcium phosphate, and magnesium phosphate stones; for these stones urine should be kept acidic.

Protein

Evaluation of protein is a sensitive indicator of kidney function. Normally protein is not present in the urine because the spaces in the normal glomerular filtrate membrane are too small to allow its passage. If the glomerular membrane is injured, as in glomerulonephritis, the spaces become much larger, and protein seeps out into the filtrate and then into the urine. If this persists at a significant rate, the patient can become hypoproteinemic because of the severe protein loss through the kidneys. This decreases the normal capillary oncotic pressure that holds fluid within the vasculature and causes severe interstitial edema. The combination of proteinuria and edema is known as the nephrotic syndrome.

Proteinuria is probably the most important indicator of renal disease. The urine of all pregnant women is routinely checked for proteinuria, which can be an indicator of preeclampsia. In addition to screening for nephrotic syndrome, urinary protein also screens for complications of diabetes mellitus, glomerulonephritis, amyloidosis, and multiple melanoma (see test for Bence Jones protein, p. 140).

Glucose

See discussion on pp. 439 to 441.

Specific gravity

The specific gravity is a measure of the concentration of particles, including wastes and electrolytes, in the urine. A high specific gravity indicates a concentrated urine; a low specific gravity indicates dilute urine. Specific gravity refers to the weight of the urine compared to that of distilled water (which has a specific gravity of 1.000). It is the particles in the urine that give the urine it weight or specific gravity.

The specific gravity is used to evaluate the concentrating and excretory power of the kidney. Renal disease tends to diminish the concentrating capability of the kidney. As a result, chronic renal diseases are associated with a low specific gravity. The specific gravity must be interpreted in light of the presence or absence of glycosuria and proteinuria. The specific gravity is also a measurement of the hydration status of the patient. An overhydrated patient will have a more dilute urine with a lower specific gravity. The specific gravity of the urine in a dehydrated patient can be expected to be abnormally high. The measurement of urine specific gravity is easier and more convenient than the measurement of osmolality (see p. 600). The specific gravity correlates roughly with osmolality. Knowledge of the specific gravity is needed for interpreting the results of most parts of the urinalysis. Specific gravity is usually evaluated by the use of a refractometer or a dipstick.

Leukocyte esterase (WBC esterase)

Leukocyte (WBC) esterase is a screening test used to detect leukocytes in the urine. When positive, this test indicates a urinary tract infection. This examination uses chemical testing with a leukocyte esterase dipstick; a shade of purple is considered positive. Some laboratories have established screening protocols in which a microscopic examination (see p. 878) is only performed if a leukocyte esterase test is positive.

Nitrites

Like the leukocyte esterase, the nitrite test is a screening test for the identification of urinary tract infections. This test is based on the principle that many bacteria produce an enzyme called *reductase,* which can reduce urinary nitrates to nitrites. Chemical testing is done with a dipstick containing a reagent that reacts with nitrites to produce a pink color, thus indirectly suggesting the presence of bacteria. A positive test result would indicate the need for a urine culture. Nitrite screening enhances the sensitivity of the leukocyte esterase test to detect urinary tract infections.

Ketones

Normally no ketones are present in the urine; however, a patient with poorly controlled diabetes who is hyperglycemic may have massive fatty acid catabolism. The purpose of this catabolism is to provide an energy source when glucose cannot be transferred into the cell because of an insufficiency of insulin. Ketones (beta-hydroxybutyric acid, acetoacetic acid, and acetone) are the end products of this fatty acid breakdown. As with glucose, ketones spill over into the urine when the blood levels of patients with diabetes are elevated. The excess production of ketones in the urine is usually associated with poorly controlled diabetes. This test for ketonuria is also important in evaluating ketoacidosis associated with alcoholism, fasting, starvation, high-protein diets, and isopropanol ingestion. Ketonuria may occur with acute febrile illnesses, especially in infants and children.

Crystals

Crystals found in the urinary sediment on microscopic examination indicate that renal stone formulation is imminent, if not already present. Urea crystals occur in patients with high serum uric acid levels (gout). Phosphate and calcium oxalate crystals occur in the urine of patients with parathyroid abnormalities or malabsorption states. The type of crystal found varies with the disease and the pH of the urine (see above discussion on urinary pH).

Casts

Casts are clumps of materials or cells. They are formed in the renal distal and collecting tubules where the material is maximally concentrated. These amorphous clumps of material and cells have the shape of the tubule, thus the term cast. Casts are most usually associated with some degree of proteinuria and stasis within the renal tubules. There are two kinds of casts: hyaline and cellular.

Hyaline casts are conglomerations of protein and indicate proteinuria. A few hyaline casts are normally found, especially after strenuous exercise.

Cellular casts, conglomerations of degenerated cells, are described in the following paragraphs.

Granular casts result from the disintegration of cellular material into granular particles within a WBC or epithelial cell cast. Granular casts are found after exercise and in patients with various renal diseases. The basic etiology is the same as their cellular component.

In some diseases the epithelial cells desquamate into the renal tubule. As the cell degenerates, fatty deposits within the cell coalesce and become incorporated with protein into *fatty casts.*

These casts are all associated with the nephrotic syndrome/nephrosis. Free oval fat bodies may also be associated with fatty emboli that occur in patients with bone fractures.

Waxy casts may be cell casts, hyaline casts, or renal failure casts. Waxy casts probably represent further degeneration of granular casts. They occur when urine flow through the renal tubule is diminished, giving time for granular casts to degenerate. Waxy casts are found especially in patients with chronic renal diseases and are associated with chronic renal failure. They also occur in patients with diabetic nephropathy, malignant hypertension, and glomerulonephritis.

Epithelial cells can enter the urine anywhere along the process of urinary excretion. The presence of occasional epithelial cells is not remarkable. Large numbers, however, are abnormal and can conglomerate into *tubular (epithelial) casts*. These are most suggestive of glomerulonephritis.

Normally few WBCs are found in the urine sediment on microscopic examination. The presence of five or more WBCs in the urine indicates a urinary tract infection involving the bladder, kidney, or both. A clean-catch urine culture should be done for further evaluation. *WBC casts* are most frequently found in patients with infections within the kidney, such as acute pyelonephritis.

Any disruption in the blood-urine barrier whether at the glomerular, tubular, or bladder level will cause RBCs to enter the urine. The bleeding can be microscopic or gross hematuria. *RBC casts* suggest glomerulonephritis. RBC casts are also seen in patients with acute necrosis, pyelonephritis, renal trauma, or renal tumor.

Interfering factors

- Certain foods affect urine color. Carrots may cause a dark-yellow color. Beets may cause a red-colored urine. Rhubarb may cause a red or brown discoloration.
- Urine color darkens with prolonged standing.
- Some foods (e.g., asparagus) produce characteristic urine odors.
- When urine stands for a long time and begins to decompose, it has an ammonia-like smell.
- The urine pH becomes alkaline on standing because of the action of urea-splitting bacteria, producing ammonia.
- The urine pH of an uncovered specimen will become alkaline because carbon dioxide will vaporize from the urine and into the air.

U

- Dietary factors affect urine pH
  An alkaline urine is observed in people who eat large quantities of citrus fruits, dairy products, and vegetables. Acidic urine is observed with a diet high in meat and certain foods (e.g., cranberries).
- A transient proteinuria may be associated with severe emotional stress, excess exercise, and cold baths.
- Radiopaque contrast media received within the last 3 days may cause false-positive results for protein in the urine.
- Urine contaminated with vaginal secretions may cause proteinuria.
- Recent use of radiographic dyes in the urine increases specific gravity.
- False-positive leukocyte esterase results may occur in specimens contaminated with vaginal secretions (e.g., heavy menstrual discharge, *Trichomonas* infection, and parasites).
- False-negative leukocyte esterase results may occur in specimens containing high levels of protein or ascorbic acid.
- Special diets (carbohydrate-free, high-protein, high-fat) may cause ketonuria.
- Radiographic dyes may cause precipitation of urinary crystals.
- Vaginal discharge may contaminate the urine specimen and factitiously cause WBCs in the urine.
- Strenuous physical exercise may cause RBC casts.
  Traumatic urethral catheterization may cause RBCs in the urine.
- Many drugs affect urine color and appearance (see Table 20).
- Drugs that may affect urine color include antibiotics and vitamins.
- Drugs that may cause acidic urine include ammonium chloride, chlorothiazide diuretics, and methenamine mandelate.
- Drugs that may cause alkaline urine include acetazolamide, potassium citrate, and sodium bicarbonate.
- Drugs that may cause *increased* protein levels include acetazolamide, aminoglycosides, amphotericin B, cephalosporins, colistin, griseofulvin, lithium, methicillin, nafcillin, nephrotoxic drugs (e.g., arsenicals, gold salts), oxacillin, penicillamine, penicillin G, phenazopyridine, polymixin B, salicylates, sulfonamides, tolbutamide, and vancomycin.
- Drugs that may cause *increased* specific gravity include dextran and sucrose.
- Drugs that may cause false-positive results for ketones include Bromsulphalein (BSP), isoniazid, isopropanol, levodopa, paraldehyde, phenazopyridine, and PSP dye.

Procedure and patient care

Before
- Explain the procedure to the patient.

During
- Collect a fresh urine specimen in a urine container.
- If the urine specimen contains vaginal discharge or bleeding, a clean-catch or midstream specimen will be needed. This requires meticulous cleaning of the urinary meatus with an iodine preparation to reduce contamination of the specimen by external organisms. The cleansing agent then must be completely removed or it will contaminate the specimen. The *midstream collection* is obtained by:
  1. Having the patient begin to urinate in a bedpan, urinal, or toilet and then stop urinating (this washes the urine out of the distal urethra)
  2. Correctly positioning a sterile urine container into which the patient voids 3 to 4 ounces of urine
  3. Capping the container
  4. Allowing the patient to finish voiding
- For ketones this test can be performed immediately after collection by placing a drop of urine on an Acetest tablet. If acetone is present, shades of lavender will appear at the designated time.
- With a Ketostix, dip the reagent into the urine specimen and remove it. Read the strip in 15 seconds by comparing it with the color chart.
- For urine specific gravity, a first-voided specimen is best obtained.
- For protein, again the first-voided specimen is best; however, occasionally a 24-hour urine collection (see p. 381) is preferred.

After
- Transport the urine specimen to the laboratory promptly.
- If the specimen cannot be processed immediately, refrigerate it.
- If a 24-hour urine collection is requested, the specimen should be refrigerated or preserved with formalin during the collection time.
- Casts will break up as urine is allowed to sit. Urine examinations for casts should be performed on fresh specimens.

U

Abnormal findings

Appearance and color

Bacteria
Pus
Red blood cells
Certain foods (e.g., beets,
  carrots)
Drug therapy (see Table 20)
Pathologic conditions (e.g.,
  bleeding from the kidney)

Dehydration
Overhydration
Diabetes insipidus
Fever
Excessive sweating
Jaundice

Odor

Infection
Ketonuria
Urinary tract infection
Rectal fistula

Maple sugar urine
  disease
Phenylketonuria
Hepatic failure

pH

▲ **Increased levels**

Respiratory alkalosis
Metabolic alkalosis
Urea-splitting bacteria
Vegetarian diet
Renal failure with inability
  to form ammonia
Gastric suction
Vomiting
Diuretic therapy
Renal tubular acidosis
Urinary tract infection

▼ **Decreased levels**

Metabolic acidosis
Diabetes mellitus
Diarrhea
Starvation
Respiratory acidosis
Emphysema
Sleep
Pyrexia

Protein

▲ **Increased levels**
Nephrotic syndrome
Diabetes mellitus
Multiple myeloma
Preeclampsia
Glomerulonephritis
Congestive heart failure
Malignant hypertension
Polycystic disease
Diabetic glomerulo-
   sclerosis

▼ **Decreased levels**
Amyloidosis
Lupus erythematosus
Goodpasture syndrome
Renal vein thrombosis
Heavy-metal poisoning
Galactosemia
Bacterial pyelonephritis
Nephrotoxic drug therapy
Bladder tumor

Specific gravity

▲ **Increased levels**
Dehydration
Pituitary tumor or trauma
   that causes syndrome of
   inappropriate release of
   excessive antidiuretic
   hormone (SIADH)
Decrease in renal blood
   flow (as in heart failure,
   renal artery stenosis, or
   hypotension)
Glycosuria and proteinuria
Water restriction
Fever
Excessive sweating
Vomiting
Diarrhea
X-ray contrast dye

▼ **Decreased levels**
Overhydration
Diabetes insipidus
Renal failure
Diuresis
Hypothermia
Glomerulonephritis
Pyelonephritis

Leukocyte esterase
Possible urinary tract infection

Nitrites
Possible urinary tract infection

U

Ketones

Uncontrolled diabetes mellitus

Starvation

Excessive aspirin ingestion

Ketoacidosis of alcoholism

Febrile illnesses in infants and
  children

Weight reduction diets

Following anesthesia

Prolonged vomiting

Anorexia

Fasting

High-protein diets

Isopropanol ingestion

Dehydration

Crystals

Renal stone formation

Drug therapy

Urinary tract infection

Granular casts

Acute tubular necrosis

Urinary tract infection

Glomerulonephritis

Pyelonephritis

Nephrosclerosis

Chronic lead poisoning

Reaction after exercise

Stress

Renal transplant rejection

Fatty casts

Nephrotic syndrome

Diabetic nephropathy

Glomerulonephritis

Chronic renal disease

Epithelial casts

Glomerulonephritis

Eclampsia

Heavy-metal poisoning

Ethylene glycol intoxication

Acute renal allograft rejection

Waxy casts

Chronic renal disease

Chronic renal failure

Diabetic nephropathy

Malignant hypertension

Glomerulonephritis

Renal transplant rejection

Nephrotic syndrome

Hyaline casts

Proteinuria

Fever

Strenuous exercise

Stress

Glomerulonephritis

Pyelonephritis

Congestive heart failure

Chronic renal failure

Red blood cells and casts

▲ **Increased RBC levels**

Glomerulonephritis
Interstitial nephritis
Acute tubular necrosis
Pyelonephritis
Renal trauma
Renal tumor
Renal stones
Cystitis
Prostatitis
Traumatic bladder
catheterization

White blood cells and casts

▲ **Increased WBC levels**

Bacterial infection in the
urinary tract

▲ **Increased RBC cast levels**

Glomerulonephritis
Subacute bacterial
endocarditis
Renal infarct
Goodpasture syndrome
Vasculitis
Sickle cell anemia
Malignant hypertension
Systemic lupus ery-
thematosus

▲ **Increased WBC cast levels**

Acute pyelonephritis
Glomerulonephritis
Lupus nephritis

notes

U

urine culture and sensitivity (C&S)

Type of test   Urine; microscopic

Normal findings

Negative: fewer than 10,000 bacteria per milliliter of urine
Positive: greater than 100,000 bacteria per milliliter of urine

Test explanation and related physiology

Urine cultures and sensitivities are obtained to determine the presence of pathogenic bacteria in patients with suspected urinary tract infections. Most often, urinary tract infections are limited to the bladder. However, the kidneys, ureters, bladder, or urethra can be the source of infection. All cultures should be performed before antibiotic therapy is initiated; otherwise the antibiotic may interrupt the growth of the organism in the laboratory. Most organisms require approximately 24 hours to grow in the laboratory, and a preliminary report can be given at that time. Occasionally 48 to 72 hours are required for growth and identification of the organism. Cultures may be repeated after appropriate antibiotic therapy to assess for complete resolution of the infection (especially in urinary tract infections).

To save money in some institutions, urine cultures are only done if the urinalysis suggests a possible infection (e.g., increased number of white blood cells [WBCs], bacteria, high pH, positive leukocyte esterase). In these institutions urine is collected and "split." One half is sent for urinalysis, and the other is held in the laboratory refrigerator and evaluated only if the urinalysis indicates a possible infection.

An important part of any routine culture is to assess the sensitivity of any bacteria that is growing within the urine to various antibiotics. The physician can then more appropriately recommend the correct antibiotic therapy. Antibiotics that are safest, least expensive, and most effective for the treatment of that specific bacteria are prescribed.

Interfering factors

- Contamination of the urine with stool, vaginal secretions, hands, or clothing will cause false positives.
- ✔ Drugs that may affect test results include antibiotics.

Procedure and patient care

Before

- Explain to the patient the procedure for collecting a clean-catch (midstream) urine collection.
- Hold antibiotics until after the urine specimen has been collected.
- Provide the patient with the necessary supplies for the collection.

During

- Note that a *clean-catch* or *midstream urine* collection is required for C&S testing. This requires meticulous cleansing of the urinary meatus with an iodine preparation to reduce contamination of the specimen by external organisms. Then the cleansing agent must be completely removed or it will contaminate the urine specimen. The midstream collection is obtained by:
  1. Having the patient begin to urinate in a bedpan, urinal, or toilet and then stop urinating (this washes the urine out of the distal urethra.)
  2. Correctly positioning a sterile urine container, into which the patient voids 3 to 4 ounces of urine
  3. Capping the container
  4. Allowing the patient to finish voiding
- Note that *urinary catheterization* may be needed for patients unable to void. This procedure is not usually performed, however, because of the risk of inducing organisms and because of patient discomfort.
- For inpatients with an *indwelling urinary catheter*, obtain a specimen by attaching a small-gauge (e.g., No. 25) needle to a syringe and aseptically inserting the needle into the catheter at a point distal to the sleeve leading to the balloon. Urine is aspirated and then placed in a sterile urine container. (Usually the catheter tubing distal to the puncture site needs to be clamped for 15 to 30 minutes before the aspiration of urine to allow urine to fill the tubing. After the specimen is withdrawn, the clamp is removed.)
- Note that *suprapubic aspiration* of urine is a safe method of obtaining urine in neonates and infants. The abdomen is prepared with an antiseptic, and a 25-gauge needle is inserted into the suprapubic area 1 inch above the symphysis pubis.

U

Urine is aspirated into the syringe and then transferred to a sterile urine container.

- Collect specimens from infants and young children in a disposable pouch called a *U bag*. This bag has an adhesive backing around the opening to attach to the child.
- Note that, for patients with a *urinary diversion* (e.g., an ileal conduit), catheterization should be done through the stoma.
- Urine should *not* be collected from the ostomy pouch.
- Indicate on the laboratory slip any medications that may affect test results.

After

- Transport the specimen to the laboratory immediately (at least within 30 minutes). If this is not possible, the specimen may be refrigerated up to 2 hours.
- Notify the physician of any positive results so that appropriate antibiotic therapy can be initiated.

Abnormal finding

Urinary tract infection

notes

urine flow studies (Uroflowmetry, Urodynamic studies)

Type of test Urodynamic

Normal findings Depend on the patient's age, gender, and volume voided

Test explanation and related physiology

Uroflowmetry is the simplest of the urodynamic techniques, being noninvasive and requiring uncomplicated and relatively inexpensive equipment. This study measures the volume of urine expelled from the bladder per second. This test is indicated to investigate dysfunctional voiding or suspicious outflow tract obstruction. It is also done before and after any procedure designed to modify the function of the urologic outflow tract.

The urine flow depends greatly on the volume of urine voided. The flow rates are highest and most predictable in the urine volume range of 200 to 400 ml. When the bladder contains more than 400 ml of urine, the efficiency of the bladder muscle is greatly decreased. Nomograms of maximal flow versus voided volume may be used for accurate test result interpretation, taking into account the patient's gender and age. If the flow rates are abnormally low, the test should be repeated to check for accuracy.

Modern urine flowmeters provide a permanent graphic recording. If flowmeters are not available, the patient can time the urinary stream with a stopwatch and record the voided volume; from this, the average flow is calculated.

In some cases it is more valuable to analyze several voided volumes and flow rates rather than a single flow rate. If this is to be done, the patient is taught to use a flowmeter. A graph of flow versus volume can be plotted. Together with clinical observation, this provides very valuable information on the severity of outflow obstruction, the likelihood of urinary retention, and the state of compensation or decompensation of the detrusor muscle.

Procedure and patient care

Before

- Explain the procedure to the patient.
- Instruct the patient how to void into the urine flowmeter.
- Determine the number of flow rates that will be needed.

During

- Note that this test should be performed when the patient has a normal desire to void and in conditions suitable for privacy. The bladder should be adequately full. Essentially, all the patient must do is urinate into the flowmeter. Several different types of flowmeters are available.
- Tell the patient that no discomfort is associated with this test.
- Note that the duration of this test is several seconds.

After

- Record the position of the patient, the method of filling the bladder (it should be natural), and whether this study was part of another evaluation.

Abnormal findings

Dysfunctional voiding
Urethral stricture
Prostate cancer
Prostatic hypertrophy

notes

uroporphyrinogen-I-synthase

Type of test Blood

Normal findings 1.27-2 mU/g of hemoglobin or
81.9-129.6 U/mol Hgb (SI units)

Test explanation and related physiology

Porphyria is a group of genetic disorders characterized by an accumulation of porphyrin products, usually in the liver. This group of disorders results from enzymatic deficiencies in synthesis of heme (a part of hemoglobin). Acute intermittent porphyria (AIP) is the most common form of the liver porphyrias; it is caused by a deficiency in uroporphyrinogen-I-synthase (also called porphobilinogen deaminase). This enzyme is necessary for erythroid cells to make heme.

Most patients with AIP have no symptoms (latent phase) until the acute phase is precipitated by medication or some other factor. The acute phase is highlighted by symptoms of abdominal and muscular pain, nausea, vomiting, hypertension, mental confusion, sensory loss, and hemolysis.

This enzyme is significantly reduced during the acute and latent phases of this disorder. It is important to identify this deficiency to prevent acute bouts of porphyria. The acute phase can be prevented by avoiding factors that can precipitate the acute symptoms.

Procedure and patient care

Before

- Tell the patient that no fasting is required.

During

- Collect 7 ml of peripheral venous blood in a purple-top tube.
- Because this test is based on the hemoglobin measurement, concurrently obtain a hemoglobin level on the patient.

After

- Indicate on the laboratory slip if the patient is having symptoms of acute porphyria.
- Apply pressure to the venipuncture site.

Abbreviated finding

▼   **Decreased levels**
   Acute intermittent porphyria

U

vanillylmandelic acid and catecholamines (VMA and epinephrine, norepinephrine, metanephrine, normetanephrine, dopamine)

Type of test Urine (24-hour)

Normal findings

VMA

Adult/elderly: 2-7 mg/24 hr or 10-35 μmol/24 hr (SI units)
Adolescent: 1-5 mg/24 hr
Child: 1-3 mg/24 hr
Infant: <2 mg/24 hr
Newborn: <1 mg/24 hr

Catecholamines

Epinephrine
Adult/elderly: 0.5-20 μg/24 hr or <275 nmol/24 hr (SI units)
Child
   0-1 years: 0-2.5 μg/24 hr
   1-2 years: 0-3.5 μg/24 hr
   2-4 years: 0-6 μg/24 hr
   4-7 years: 0.2-10 μg/24 hr
   7-10 years: 0.5-14 μg/24 hr

Norepinephrine
Adult/elderly: 15-80 μg/24 hr
Child
   0-1 years: 0-10 μg/24 hr
   1-2 years: 0-17 μg/24 hr
   2-4 years: 4-29 μg/24 hr
   4-7 years: 8-45 μg/24 hr
   7-10 years: 13-65 μg/24 hr

Dopamine
Adult/elderly: 65-400 μg/24 hr
Child
   0-1 years: 0-85 μg/24 hr
   1-2 years: 10-140 μg/24 hr
   2-4 years: 40-260 μg/24 hr
   >4 years: 65-400 μg/24 hr

Metanephrine
24-96 μg/24 hr

Normetanephrine
75-375 μg/24 hr

Test explanation and related physiology

This 24-hour urine test for VMA and catecholamines is primarily performed to diagnose hypertension secondary to pheochromocytoma. This test is also used to detect the presence of neuroblastomas and rare adrenal tumors.

A *pheochromocytoma* is an adrenal tumor that frequently secretes abnormally high levels of epinephrine and norepinephrine. These hormones cause episodic or persistent hypertension by causing peripheral arterial vasoconstriction. Dopamine is the precursor of epinephrine and norepinephrine. Metanephrine and normetanephrine are catabolic products of epinephrine and norepinephrine, respectively. VMA is the product of catabolism of both metanephrine and normetanephrine. In patients with pheochromocytoma, one or all of these substances will be present in excessive quantities in a 24-hour collection of urine.

A 24-hour urine test is preferable to a blood test because catecholamine secretion from the tumor may be episodic and could potentially be missed at any one time during the day. The urine provides the laboratory with a specimen that reflects catecholamine production over 1 whole day. It is best to perform testing when the symptoms (hypertension) of the potential adrenal tumor are significant. At that time, catecholamine production is greatest and will be more assuredly identified.

Interfering factors

- Increased levels of VMA may be caused by certain foods (e.g., tea, coffee, cocoa, vanilla, chocolate).
- Vigorous exercise, stress, and starvation may cause increased VMA levels.
- Falsely decreased levels of VMA may be caused by uremia, alkaline urine, and radiographic iodine contrast agents.
- ✗ Drugs that may cause *increased* VMA levels include caffeine, epinephrine, levodopa, lithium, and nitroglycerin.
- ✗ Drugs that may cause *decreased* VMA levels include clonidine, disulfiram (Antabuse), guanethidine, imipramine, monoamine oxidase inhibitors, phenothiazines, and reserpine.
- ✗ Drugs that may cause *increased* catecholamine levels include alcohol (ethyl), aminophylline, caffeine, chloral hydrate, clonidine (chronic therapy), contrast media (iodine containing), disulfiram, epinephrine, erythromycin, insulin, methenamine, methyldopa, nicotinic acid (large doses), nitroglycerin, quinidine, riboflavin, and tetracyclines.

V

☛ Drugs that may cause *decreased* catecholamine levels include guanethidine, reserpine, and salicylates.

Procedure and patient care

Before

- Explain the dietary restrictions and the 24-hour urine collection procedure to the patient.
- For 2 or 3 days before the 24-hour collection for VMA and throughout the collection, place the patient on a VMA-restricted diet. Generally, instruct the patient to avoid coffee, tea, bananas, chocolate, cocoa, licorice, citrus fruit, all foods and fluids containing vanilla, and also aspirin. Obtain specific restrictions from the laboratory.
- Restrict the patient from taking antihypertensive medications and sometimes all medications during this period and possibly even longer.

During

- Collect the 24-hour urine specimen using a preservative.
- Instruct the patient to begin the 24-hour urine collection after voiding. Discard the initial specimen and note the time; this is the starting time.
- Collect all urine passed during the next 24 hours. Refrigerate or keep on ice during the collection period.
- Post the hours for the urine collection in a prominent place to avoid accidental discarding of the specimen.
- Remind the patient to void before defecating so that the urine is not contaminated by feces.
- Instruct the patient not to put toilet paper in the collection container.
- Encourage the patient to drink fluids during the 24 hours unless contraindicated for medical purposes.
- Collect the last specimen as close as possible to the end of the 24-hour period. Add this urine to the container.
- Indicate the time of the last specimen collected on the laboratory slip or urine container.
- Identify and minimize factors contributing to patient stress and anxiety. Excessive physical exercise and emotion may alter catecholamine test results by causing an increased secretion of epinephrine and norepinephrine.

After

- Send the specimen to the laboratory as soon as the test is completed.

- Allow the patient to have foods and drugs that have been restricted in preparation for the test.

Abnormal findings

▲ **Increased levels**
   Pheochromocytomas
   Neuroblastomas
   Ganglioneuromas
   Ganglioblastomas
   Severe stress
   Strenuous exercise
   Acute anxiety

notes

V

venography of lower extremities (Phlebography, Venogram)

Type of test X-ray with contrast dye

Normal findings No evidence of venous thrombosis or obstruction

Test explanation and related physiology

Venography is an x-ray study designed to identify and locate thrombi within the venous system of the lower extremities. During this study dye is injected into the venous system of the affected extremity. X-ray films are then taken at timed intervals to visualize the venous system. Obstruction to the flow of dye or a filling defect within the dye-filled vein indicates that thrombosis exists. A positive study accurately confirms the diagnosis of venous thrombosis; however, a normal study, although not as accurate, does make the diagnosis of venous thrombosis very unlikely. Often both extremities are studied, even though only one leg is suspected to contain deep-vein thrombosis. The normal extremity is used for comparison with the involved extremity. Unlike venous plethysmography (see p. 652), venography is accurate for thrombi in veins below the knee.

Contraindications

- Patients with severe edema of the legs, making venous access impossible
- Patients who are uncooperative
- Patients who are allergic to iodinated dye or shellfish
- Patients with renal failure, because the iodinated dye is nephrotoxic

Potential complications

- Allergic reaction to iodinated dyes
- Renal failure, especially in elderly people who are chronically dehydrated or may have a mild degree of renal failure
- Subcutaneous infiltration of the dye, causing cellulitis and pain
- Venous thrombophlebitis caused by the dye
- Bacteremia caused by a break in sterile technique
- Venous embolism caused by dislodgment of a deep-vein clot induced by the dye injection

- Hypoglycemia or acidosis may occur in patients who are taking Glucophage and receive iodine dye.

Procedure and patient care

Before

- Explain the procedure to the patient.
- Obtain informed consent for this procedure.
- Assess the patient for allergies to iodinated dyes and shellfish.
- If needed, provide appropriate pain medication so the patient is able to lie still during the procedure.
- Ensure that the patient is appropriately hydrated before testing. Injection of the iodinated contrast may cause renal failure, especially in the elderly.

During

- Note the following procedural steps:
  1. The patient is taken to the radiology department and placed in a supine position on the x-ray table.
  2. Catheterization of a superficial vein on the foot is performed. This may require a surgical cutdown.
  3. An iodinated, radiopaque dye is injected into the vein.
  4. X-ray films are taken to follow the course of the dye up the leg.
  5. Frequently a tourniquet is placed on the leg to prevent filling of the superficial saphenous vein. Therefore all of the dye goes to filling the deep venous system, which contains the most clinically significant thrombosis that can embolize.
- Note that a radiologist performs this study in approximately 30 to 90 minutes.
- Tell the patient that the venous catheterization is only as uncomfortable as a cutaneous heel stick or a small incision in the foot.
- The dye may cause the patient to feel a warm flush. (This is not as severe as that noted with arteriography.) Inform the patient that occasionally mild degrees of nausea, vomiting, or skin itching also may occur.

After

- Continue appropriate hydration of the patient to prevent dehydration caused by the diuretic action of the dye.
- Observe the puncture site for infection, cellulitis, or bleeding.
- Assess the patient's vital signs for signs of bacteremia (e.g., high temperature, tachycardia, chills, fever).

V

- See p. xviii for appropriate interventions concerning the care for patients with iodine allergy.

Abnormal findings

Obstructed venous systems
Acute deep-vein thrombosis

notes

vitamin B$_{12}$ (cyanocobalamin)

Normal findings 100-700 pg/ml or 74-517 pmol/L

Test explanation and related physiology

Vitamin B$_{12}$ is necessary for conversion of the inactive form of folate to the active form. This function is most notable in the formation and function of red blood cells (RBCs). Vitamin B$_{12}$ deficiency, like folic acid deficiency, causes anemia. The RBCs formed in light of these deficiencies result in large megaloblastic RBCs. These RBCs cannot conform to the size of small capillaries. Instead they fracture and hemolyze. The shortened life span ultimately leads to anemia.

In the stomach gastric acid detaches vitamin B$_{12}$ from its binding proteins. Intrinsic factor (IF), necessary for Vitamin B$_{12}$ absorption in the small intestine, is made in the stomach mucosa. Without IF, vitamin B$_{12}$ cannot be absorbed. Deficiency of IF is the most common cause of vitamin B$_{12}$ deficiency (pernicious anemia [PA]). The next most common cause of vitamin B$_{12}$ deficiency is lack of gastric acid to separate the ingested vitamin B$_{12}$ from its binding proteins. A third cause of vitamin B$_{12}$ deficiency is malabsorption caused by diseases of the small terminal ileum.

Interfering factors

- ✔ Chloral hydrate is known to *increase* vitamin B$_{12}$ levels.
- ✔ Drugs known to *decrease* vitamin B$_{12}$ levels include alcohol, aminoglycosides, ASA, anticonvulsants, colchicine, and oral contraceptives.

Procedure and patient care

Before

- Explain the procedure to the patient.
- Tell the patient that no fasting is usually required. (However, some laboratories prefer an 8-hour fast.)
- Instruct the patient not to consume alcoholic beverages before the test.
- Draw the specimen before starting vitamin B$_{12}$ therapy.

During

- Collect approximately 5 to 10 ml of venous blood in a red-top tube.

V

- Indicate on the laboratory slip any medications that may affect test results.

After
- Apply pressure to the venipuncture site.
- Transport the blood immediately to the laboratory after collection.

Abnormal findings

▲ **Increased levels**
Leukemia
Polycythemia vera
Severe liver dysfunction
Myeloproliferative disease

▼ **Decreased levels**
Pernicious anemia
Malabsorption syndromes
Inflammatory bowel disease
Intestinal worm infestation
Atrophic gastritis
Zollinger-Ellison syndrome
Large proximal gastrectomy
Resection of terminal ileum
Achlorhydria
Pregnancy
Vitamin C deficiency
Folic acid deficiency

notes

white blood cell count and differential count
(WBC and differential, Leukocyte count, Neutrophil count, Lymphocyte count, Monocyte count, Eosinophil count, Basophil count)

Type of test Blood

Normal findings

Total WBCs

Adult/child >2 years: 5000-10,000/mm^3 or 5-10 × 10^9/L
(SI units)
Child ≤2 years: 6200-17,000/mm^3
Newborn: 9000-30,000/mm^3

Differential count

	(%)	Absolute (per mm^3)
Neutrophils	55 to 70	2500-8000
Lymphocytes	20 to 40	1000-4000
Monocytes	2 to 8	100-700
Eosinophils	1 to 4	50-500
Basophils	0.5 to 1	25-100

Possible critical values WBCs <2500 or >30,000/mm^3

Test explanation and related physiology

   The WBC count has two components. The first is a count of the total number of WBCs (leukocytes) in 1 mm^3 of peripheral venous blood. The other component, the differential count, measures the percentage of each type of leukocyte present in the same specimen. An increase in the percentage of one type of leukocyte means a decrease in the percentage of another. Neutrophils and lymphocytes make up 75% to 90% of the total leukocytes. These leukocyte types may be identified easily by their morphology on a venous blood smear. The total leukocyte count has a wide range of normal values, but many diseases may induce abnormal values. An increased total WBC count (leukocytosis: WBC >10,000) usually indicates infection, inflammation, tissue necrosis, or leukemic neoplasia. Trauma or stress, either emotional or physical, may increase the WBC count. A decreased total WBC count (leukopenia: WBC <4,000) occurs in many forms of bone marrow failure (e.g., following antineoplastic chemotherapy or radiation therapy, marrow infiltrative diseases,

W

overwhelming infections, dietary deficiencies, and autoimmune diseases).

The major function of the WBCs is to fight infection and react against foreign bodies or tissues. Five types of WBCs may easily be identified on a routine blood smear. These cells, in order of frequency, include neutrophils, lymphocytes, monocytes, eosinophils, and basophils. All of these WBCs arise from the same "pluripotent" stem cell within the bone marrow, as does the red blood cell (RBC). Beyond this origin, however, each cell line differentiates separately. Most mature WBCs are then deposited into the circulating blood.

White blood cells are divided into granulocytes and nongranulocytes. Granulocytes include neutrophils, basophils, and eosinophils. Granulocytes have multilobed nuclei and are sometimes referred to as polymorphonuclear leukocytes (PMNs or "polys").

Neutrophils are the most common PMN and are produced in 7 to 14 days and exist in the circulation for only 6 hours. The primary function of the neutrophil is phagocytosis (killing and digestion of bacterial microorganisms). Acute bacterial infections and trauma stimulate neutrophil production, resulting in an increased WBC count. Often, when neutrophil production is significantly stimulated, early immature forms of neutrophils enter the circulation. These immature forms are called *band* or *stab* cells. This occurrence, referred to as a "shift to the left" in WBC production, is indicative of an ongoing acute bacterial infection.

Basophils (also called mast cells), and especially *eosinophils*, are involved in the allergic reaction. Parasitic infestations also are capable of stimulating the production of these cells. These cells are capable of phagocytosis of antigen-antibody complexes. As the allergic response diminishes, the eosinophil count decreases. Eosinophils and basophils do not respond to bacterial or viral infections.

Nongranulocytes (agranulocytes) include lymphocytes and monocytes (the count also includes histiocytes). They have no cytoplasmic granules and have a small single rounded nuclei. *Lymphocytes* are divided into two types: T cells and B cells. T cells are primarily involved with cellular-type immune reactions, whereas B cells participate in humoral immunity (antibody production). The primary function of the lymphocytes is fighting chronic bacterial infection and acute viral infections. The differential count does not separate the T and B cells but rather counts the combination of the two.

Monocytes are phagocytic cells capable of fighting bacteria in a way very similar to that of neutrophils. However monocytes can be produced more rapidly and can spend a longer time in the circulation than neutrophils.

The WBC and differential count are routinely measured as part of the complete blood count (see p. 262). Serial WBC counts and differential counts have both diagnostic and prognostic value. For example, a persistent increase in the WBC count may indicate a worsening of an infectious process (e.g., appendicitis). A dramatic decrease in the WBC count below the normal range may indicate marrow failure. In patients receiving chemotherapy, a reduced WBC count may delay further chemotherapy.

Interfering factors

- Eating, physical activity, and stress may cause an increase in WBC and differential values.
- Pregnancy (final month) and labor may cause increased WBC levels.
- Patients who have had a splenectomy have a persistent, mild elevation of WBC counts.
- ▮ Drugs that may cause *increased* WBC levels include adrenalin, allopurinol, aspirin, chloroform, epinephrine, heparin, quinine, steroids, and triamterene (Dyrenium).
- ▮ Drugs that may cause *decreased* WBC levels include antibiotics, anticonvulsants, antihistamines, antimetabolites, antithyroid drugs, arsenicals, barbiturates, chemotherapeutic agents, diuretics, and sulfonamides.

Procedure and patient care

Before
- Explain the procedure to the patient.
- Tell the patient that no fasting is required.

During
- Collect approximately 5 to 7 ml of venous blood in a lavender-top tube.

After
- Apply pressure to the venipuncture site.

W

Abnormal findings

▲ **Increased WBC count (leukocytosis)**

Infection
Leukemic neoplasia
Trauma
Stress
Tissue necrosis
Inflammation

▼ **Decreased WBC count (leukopenia)**

Drug toxicity (e.g., chloramphenicol)
Bone marrow failure
Overwhelming infections
Dietary deficiency
Autoimmune disease
Bone marrow infiltration (e.g., myelofibrosis)
Congenital marrow aplasia

▲▼ **Increased/decreased differential count**
See Table 21.

notes

TABLE 21 Causes for abnormalities in the WBC differential count

Type of WBC	Elevated	Decreased
Neutrophils	*Neutrophilia* Physical or emotional stress Acute suppurative infection Myelocytic leukemia Trauma Cushing's syndrome Inflammatory disorders (e.g., rheumatic fever, thyroiditis, rheumatoid arthritis) Metabolic disorders (e.g., ketoacidosis, gout, eclampsia)	*Neutropenia* Aplastic anemia Dietary deficiency Overwhelming bacterial infection (especially in the elderly) Viral infections (e.g., hepatitis, influenza, measles) Radiation therapy Addison's disease Drug therapy: myelotoxic drugs (as in chemotherapy)
Lymphocytes	*Lymphocytosis* Chronic bacterial infection Viral infection (e.g., mumps, rubella) Lymphocytic leukemia Multiple myeloma Infectious mononucleosis Radiation Infectious hepatitis	*Lymphocytopenia* Leukemia Sepsis Immunodeficiency diseases Lupus erythematosus Later stages of human immunodeficiency virus infection Drug therapy: adrenocorticosteroids, antineoplastics Radiation therapy

W

TABLE 21 Causes for abnormalities in the WBC differential count—cont'd

Type of WBC	Elevated	Decreased
Monocytes	*Monocytosis* Chronic inflammatory disorders Viral infections (e.g., infectious mononucleosis) Tuberculosis Chronic ulcerative colitis Parasites (e.g., malaria)	*Monocytopenia* Drug therapy: prednisone
Eosinophils	*Eosinophilia* Parasitic infections Allergic reactions Eczema Leukemia Autoimmune diseases	*Eosinopenia* Increased adrenosteroid production
Basophils	*Basophilia* Myeloproliferative disease (e.g., myelofibrosis, polycythemia rubra vera) Leukemia	*Basopenia* Acute allergic reactions Hyperthyroidism Stress reactions

white blood cell scan (WBC scan, inflammatory scan)

Type of test Nuclear scan

Normal findings No signs of WBC localization outside the liver or spleen.

Test explanation and related physiology

This test is based on the fact that WBCs are attracted to an area of infection or inflammation. When the patient is suspected of having had infection or inflammation, yet the site cannot be localized, the injection of radiolabeled WBCs may identify and localize that area of inflammation or infection. This is especially helpful in patients who have a fever of unknown origin, suspected occult intraabdominal infection, or suspected (yet radiographically inapparent) osteomyelitis. The scan can differentiate infectious from noninfectious processes. For example, it is used to indicate whether or not an abnormal mass (e.g., a pancreatic pseudocyst) is infected or not.

Areas of non-infectious inflammation (e.g., inflammatory bowel disease) also take up the radiolabeled WBCs.

This scan requires drawing blood from the patient, separating out the WBCs, labeling the WBCs with technetium or indium, and reinjecting them back into the patient. Four to 24 hours later, imaging of the whole body may show an area of increased radioactivity suggestive of accumulation of the radiolabeled WBCs in an area of infection or inflammation.

The liver, spleen, and bone marrow normally tend to accumulate radiolabeled WBCs, thereby obscuring vision behind these organs.

Procedure and patient care

Before

- Explain the procedure to the patient.
- Assure the patient that he or she will not be exposed to large amounts of radioactivity, because only tracer doses of the isotope are used.
- Tell the patient that no preparation or sedation is required.

During

- Note the following procedural steps:
  1. Approximately 40 to 50 ml of blood is withdrawn from the patient, and the WBCs are extracted from the rest of the blood cells. This is usually done by centrifugation.

W

With leukopenia, the WBC count is so low that separating WBCs out from the other blood cellular components would be very difficult. In these instances donor WBCs are used instead of autologous WBCs. Donor WBCs are also used for human immunodeficiency virus-positive patients to minimize the risk to laboratory workers.

2. The WBCs are suspended in saline and tagged with ^{99m}Technetium (^{99m}Tc) or ^{111}Indium (^{111}In) lipid-soluble product. ^{99m}Tc is preferable to ^{111}In because its half-life is longer. Therefore it is cheaper and more readily available for the infrequent times this scan is requested.

3. The tagged WBCs are reinjected into the patient.

4. In 4, 24, and 48 hours after injection, a gamma ray detector/camera is placed over the body.

5. The patient is placed in supine, lateral, and prone positions so that all surfaces of the body scan be visualized.

6. The radionuclide image is recorded on film.

After

- Inform the patient that, because only tracer doses of radioisotopes are used, no precautions need to be taken against radioactive exposure.

Abnormal findings

Infection (e.g., abscess or osteomyelitis)
Inflammation (e.g., inflammatory bowel disease, arthritis)

notes

wound culture and sensitivity (C&S)

Type of test Microscopic examination

Normal findings Negative

Test explanation and related physiology

Wound cultures are obtained to determine the presence of pathogens in patients with suspected wound infections. Wound infections are most often caused by pus-forming organisms.

All cultures should be performed before antibiotic therapy is initiated. Otherwise, the antibiotic may interrupt the growth of the organism in the laboratory. More often than not, however, the physician will want to institute antibiotic therapy before the culture results are reported. In these instances a *Gram stain* of the specimen smeared on a slide is most helpful and can be reported in less than 10 minutes. All forms of bacteria are grossly classified as gram positive (blue staining) or gram negative (red staining). Knowledge of the shape of the organism (e.g., spheric, rod shaped) also may be very helpful in the tentative identification of the infecting organism. With knowledge of the Gram stain results, the physician can institute a reasonable antibiotic regimen based on past experience as to the organism's possible identity. Most organisms require approximately 24 hours to grow in the laboratory, and a preliminary report can be given at that time. Occasionally 48 to 72 hours are required for growth and identification of the organism. Cultures may be repeated after appropriate antibiotic therapy to assess for complete resolution of the infection.

Interfering factors

⚑ Drugs that may alter test results include antibiotics.

Procedure and patient care

Before

- Explain the procedure to the patient.

During

- Aseptically place a sterile cotton swab into the pus of the patient's wound, and then place the swab into a sterile, covered test tube. (Culturing specimens from the skin edge is much less accurate than culturing the suppurative material.)

W

- If an anaerobic organism is suspected, obtain an anaerobic culture tube from the microbiology laboratory.
- If wound cultures are to be obtained on a patient requiring wound irrigation, obtain the culture before the wound is irrigated.
- If any antibiotic ointment or solution has been previously applied, remove it with sterile water or saline before obtaining the culture.
- Handle all specimens as though they were capable of transmitting disease.
- Indicate on the laboratory slip any medications the patient may be taking that could affect test results.

After

- Transport the specimen to the laboratory immediately after testing (at least within 30 minutes).
- Notify the physician of any positive results so that appropriate antibiotic therapy can be initiated.

Abnormal finding

Wound infection

notes

D-xylose absorption test (Xylose tolerance test)

Type of test Blood; urine

Normal findings

Age	60 min-plasma (mg/dl)	120 min-plasma (mg/dl)	Urine (g/5 hr) [%]
Child	>15-20	>20	>4, [16-32]
Adult	20-57	30-58	>3.5-4, [>14]

Test explanation and related physiology

D-Xylose is a monosaccharide that is easily absorbed by the normal intestine. In patients with malabsorption, intestinal D-xylose absorption is diminished, and as a result, blood levels and urine excretion are reduced. D-xylose is the monosaccharide chosen for the test because it is not metabolized by the body. Its serum levels directly reflect intestinal absorption.

This particular monosaccharide is used because absorption does not require pancreatic or biliary exocrine function. Its absorption is directly determined by the small intestine. This test is used to separate patients with diarrhea caused by maldigestion (pancreatic/biliary dysfunction) from those with diarrhea caused by malabsorption (sprue, Whipple's disease, Crohn's disease).

In this test the patient is asked to drink a fluid containing a prescribed amount of D-xylose. Blood and urine levels are subsequently evaluated. Excellent gastrointestinal absorption is documented by high blood levels and a good urine secretion of D-xylose. Poor intestinal absorption is marked by decreased blood levels and urine excretion.

Contraindications

- Patients with abnormal kidney function
- Patients who are dehydrated

Interfering factors

☛ Drugs that may affect test results include aspirin, atropine, and indomethacin.

Procedure and patient care

Before

- Explain the procedure to the patient.
- Instruct the adult patient to fast for 8 hours before testing.

X

- Tell the pediatric patient or the parents that the patient should fast for at least 4 hours before testing.

During

- Collect approximately 7 ml of venous blood in a red-top tube before the patient ingests the D-xylose.
- Collect a first-voided morning urine specimen and send it to the laboratory.
- Ask the patient to drink 25 g of D-xylose dissolved in 8 ounces of water. Record the time of ingestion.
- Calibrate pediatric doses according to the patient's body weight.
- Repeat venipunctures to obtain blood in exactly 2 hours for an adult and 1 hour for a child.
- Collect urine for a designated time, usually 5 hours. Refrigerate the urine during the collection period.
- Observe the patient for nausea, vomiting, and diarrhea, which may occur as side effects of D-xylose.
- Instruct the patient to remain in a restful position. Intense physical activity may alter the digestive process and affect the test results.

After

- Apply pressure to the venipuncture site.
- Provide the patient with food or drink and inform the patient that normal activity may be resumed after completion of the study.

Abnormal findings

▼ **Decreased levels**

Sprue
Lymphatic obstruction
Enteropathy (e.g., radiation)
Crohn's disease
Whipple's disease
Small intestine bacterial overgrowth
Hookworm
Viral gastroenteritis
Giardia lamblia infestation
Short-bowel syndrome

Appendix A: List of tests by body system

Tests in this list are grouped by the following body systems: cancer, cardiovascular, endocrine, gastrointestinal, hematologic, hepatobiliary, immunologic, miscellaneous studies, nervous, pulmonary, reproductive, skeletal, and urologic.

CANCER STUDIES

Acid phosphatase, 7
Bence Jones protein, 140
Bone scan, 166
CA 27.29 and CA 15-3 tumor markers, 182
CA 19-9 tumor marker, 184
CA-125 tumor marker, 186
Carcinoembryonic antigen, 201

Estrogen-receptor assay, 383
Gallium scan, 420
Lymphangiography, 559
Mammography, 572
Octreotide scan, 593
Papanicolaou smear, 606
Progesterone receptor assay, 678
Prostate-specific antigen, 684
Sputum cytology, 786

CARDIOVASCULAR SYSTEM

Adenosine stress test, 211
Aldosterone assay, blood, 31
Antimyocardial antibodies, 77
Antistreptolysin O titer, 91
Apolipoproteins, 99
Arteriography, 113
Aspartate aminotransferase, 130
Cardiac catheterization, 203
Cardiac exercise stress testing, 211
Cardiac nuclear scanning, 216
Carotid duplex scanning, 221
Catecholamines, 885
Chest x-ray, 224
Cholesterol, 232
Computed tomography of chest, 271

Creatine phosphokinase, 290
Cryoglobulin, 299
Digital subtraction angiography, 113
Dipyridamole-thallium scan, 211
Dobutamine stress test, 211
Doppler studies, 329
Echocardiography, 332
Electrocardiography, 335
Electrophysiologic study, 354
Holter monitoring, 477
Isonitrile scan, 216
Lactate dehydrogenase, 511
Lipoproteins, 528
MUGA scan, 216
Myoglobin, 586
Pericardiocentesis, 631
Plethysmography
   Arterial, 650

ENDOCRINE SYSTEM

GASTROINTESTINAL SYSTEM

HEMATOLOGIC SYSTEM

HEPATOBILIARY SYSTEM

IMMUNOLOGIC SYSTEM

MISCELLANEOUS TESTS

NERVOUS SYSTEM

PULMONARY SYSTEM

RENAL/UROLOGIC SYSTEM

Urine pH, 864
Urine specific gravity, 864
Vanillylmandelic acid, 884

Waxy casts, 864
White blood cells and casts, 864

REPRODUCTIVE SYSTEM

Alpha-fetoprotein, 39
Amniocentesis, 43
Antispermatozoal antibody, 87
Breast cancer genetic screening, 171
Breast scintography, 173
Breast sonogram, 175
CA 27.29 and CA 15-3 tumor markers, 182
CA-125 tumor marker, 186
Chlamydia, 227
Chorionic villus sampling, 238
Colposcopy, 258
Cytomegalovirus, 314
Endometrial biopsy, 358
Estriol excretion, 379
Fetal biophysical profile, 398
Fetal contraction stress test, 401
Fetal nonstress test, 405
Fetal scalp blood pH, 407
Fetoscopy, 409
Follicle-stimulating hormone, 554

Gonorrhea culture, 753
Herpes genitalis, 474
Hysterosalpingography, 487
Hysteroscopy, 489
IUD localization, 277
Lamellar body count, 43
Laparoscopy, 518
Luteinizing hormone assay, 554
Mammography, 572
Obstetric ultrasonography, 623
Papanicolaou smear, 606
Phenylketonuria test, 635
Pregnancy tests, 670
Pregnanediol, 673
Progesterone assay, 676
Rubella antibody test, 739
Semen analysis, 750
Sexually transmitted disease cultures, 755
Sims-Huhner test, 765
Syphilis detection test, 797
TORCH test, 834
Toxoplasmosis antibody titer, 839

SKELETAL SYSTEM

Aldolase, 29
Alkaline phosphatase, 35
Arthrocentesis with synovial fluid analysis, 120
Arthrography, 124
Arthroscopy, 126
Bone densitometry, 156
Bone scan, 166
Bones x-ray, 169

Electromyography, 343
HLA-B27 antigen, 479
Lactate dehydrogenase, 511
Magnetic resonance imaging, 568
Myoglobin, 586
Rheumatoid factor, 737
Spinal x-rays, 782
Uric acid, 860

Appendix B: List of tests by type

Tests in this list are grouped by the following types: blood, electrodiagnostic, endoscopy, fluid analysis, manometric, microscopic examination, nuclear scan, other studies, sputum, stool, ultrasound, urine, and x-ray.

BLOOD TESTS

Acetylcholine receptor antibody, 5
Acid phosphatase, 7
Adrenocorticotropic hormone, 12
  Stimulation test, 15
Agglutinins, febrile/cold, 21
AIDS serology, 23
Alanine aminotransferase, 27
Aldolase, 29
Aldosterone assay, 31
Alkaline phosphatase, 35
Alpha$_1$-antitrypsin, 37
Alpha-fetoprotein, 39
Ammonia level, 41
Amylase, 49
Androstenedione, 53
Angiotensin-converting enzyme, 55
Anion gap, 57
Anticardiolipin antibodies, 62
Anticentromere antibody test, 64
Antideoxyribonuclease-B titer, 65
Antidiuretic hormone, 66
Anti-DNA antibody, 69
Anti-extractable nuclear antigens antibody, 71
Antiglomerular basement membrane antibody, 73

Antimitochondrial antibody, 75
Antimyocardial antibodies, 77
Antineutrophil cytoplasmic antibody, 78
Antinuclear antibody test, 80
Antiscleroderma antibody, 83
Anti-smooth muscle antibody, 85
Antispermatozoal antibody, 87
Anti-SS-A and anti-SS-B antibody, 89
Antistreptolysin O titer, 91
Antithrombin III, 93
Antithyroglobulin antibody, 95
Antithyroid microsomal antibody, 97
Apolipoproteins, 99
Aspartate aminotransferase, 130
Bilirubin, 142
Bleeding time, 146
Blood culture and sensitivity, 149
Blood gases, 104
Blood smear, 151
Blood typing, 154
Breast cancer genetic screening, 171

MICROSCOPIC EXAMINATIONS

NUCLEAR SCANS

OTHER STUDIES

list of tests by type

SPUTUM TESTS

Acid-fast bacilli, 852
Culture and sensitivity, 784

Cytology, 786

STOOL TESTS

Clostridial toxin assay, 244
Culture, 788
Fecal fat, 393

Occult blood testing, 790
Ova and parasites, 788

ULTRASOUND TESTS

Abdominal ultrasound, 1
Breast sonogram, 175
Carotid duplex scanning, 221
Doppler studies, 329
Echocardiography, 332
Fetal biophysical profile, 398
IUD localization, 277
Kidney sonogram, 1
Liver and pancreaticobiliary
    system ultrasonography, 1
Obstetric ultrasonography,
    623

Prostate/rectal sonogram,
    682
Scrotal ultrasound, 746
Testicular ultrasound, 746
Thyroid ultrasound, 822
Transesophageal echocardi-
    ography, 841
Transrectal ultrasonography,
    682

URINE TESTS

Aldosterone, 31
Amylase, 49
Appearance and color, 864
Bence Jones protein, 140
Cortisol, 283
Creatinine clearance, 296
Crystals, 864
Culture and sensitivity, 860
Delta-aminolevulinic acid,
    318
Dexamethasone suppression
    test, 321
Epithelial casts, 864
Estriol excretion, 379
Ethanol, 385
Fatty casts, 864

Flow studies, 881
Glucose, 434
Glucose tolerance test, 444
Granular casts, 864
Hyaline casts, 864
17-Hydroxycorticosteroids,
    482
5-Hydroxyindoleacetic acid,
    485
Ketones, 864
17-Ketosteroids, 506
Leucine aminopeptidase, 524
Leukocyte esterase, 864
Metyrapone, 18
Nitrites, 864
Odor, 864

X-RAY EXAMINATIONS

Appendix C: Typical abbreviations and units of measurement

<	Less than
≤	Less than or equal to
>	Greater than
≥	Greater than or equal to
C	Celsius
cc	Cubic centimeter
cg	Centigram
cm	Centimeter
cm H_2O	Centimeter of water
cu	Cubic
dl	Deciliter (100 ml)
fmol	Femtomole
g	Gram
hr	Hour
IU	International unit
ImU	International milliunit
IμU	International microunit
K	Kilo
kg	Kilogram
L	Liter
m	Meter
m^2	Square meter
m^3	Cubic meter
mEq	Milliequivalent
mEq/L	Milliequivalent per liter
mg	Milligram
min	Minute
ml	Milliliter
mm	Millimeter
mm^3	Cubic millimeter
mM	Millimole
mm Hg	Millimeter of mercury
mm H_2O	Millimeter of water
mol	Mole
mmol	Millimole
mOsm	Milliosmole
mμ	Millimicron

mU	Milliunit
mV	Millivolt
ng	Nanogram
nm	Nanometer
nmol	Nanomole
Pa	Pascal
pg	Picomole (or micromicrogram)
pl	Picoliter
pm	Picometer
pmol	Picomole
sec	Second
SI units	International System of Units
μ	Micron
μ^3	Cubic micron
μg	Microgram
IμU	Microinternational unit
μl	Microliter
μm	Micrometer
μm^3	Cubic micrometer
μmol	Micromole
μU	Microunit
U	Unit
yr	Year

bibliography

Aspelin P: Ultrasound examination of soft tissue injury of the lower limb in athletes, *Am J Sports Med* 20(5):601-603, 1992.

Ball EM et al: Diagnosis and treatment of sleep apnea within the community: the Walla Walla project, *Arch Intern Med* 157(4):419-424, 1997.

Barrick B, Vogel S: Application of laboratory diagnostics in HIV testing, *Nursing Clin North Am* 31(1):41-45, 1996.

Bates SE: Clinical applications of serum tumor markers, *Ann Intern Med* 115(8):623-634, 1991.

Braunwald E, editor: *Heart disease: a textbook of cardiovascular medicine,* ed 4, Philadelphia, 1992, WB Saunders.

Brooks MJ et al: The infectious etiology of peptic ulcer disease: diagnosis and implications for therapy, *Primary Care* 23(3):443-454, 1996.

Brunzel NA: *Fundamentals of urine and body fluid analysis,* Philadelphia, 1994, WB Saunders.

Bubien RS et al: What you need to know about radiofrequency ablation, *Am J Nurs* 93(7):30-36, 1993.

Byers T et al: American Cancer Society guidelines for screening and surveillance for early detection of colorectal polyps and cancer: update 1997, *Cancer* 47(3):154-160, 1997.

Carnaille B et al: Scintiscans and carcinoid tumors, *Surgery* 116(6): 1118-1122, 1994.

Casperson DS: Focus on oncology: prostatic specific antigen testing, *Urol Nurs* 11(1):31-34, 1992.

Cheney AM, Maquindang ML: Patient teaching for x-ray and other diagnostics, *RN* 56(4):54-56, 1993.

Clifford EJ et al: Scintimammography in the diagnosis of breast cancer, *Am J Surg* 172:483-486, 1996.

Couch FJ et al: BRCA 1 mutations in women attending clinics that evaluate the risk of breast cancer, *N Engl J Med* 336(20):1409-1415, 1997.

Coulter JS: Red blood cell distribution width and mean corpuscular volume: clinical applications, *Adv Clin Care* 6(6):13, 1991.

Creasy RK, Resnik R: *Maternal-fetal medicine: principles and practice,* ed 3, Philadelphia, 1994, WB Saunders.

Cupp MR, Oesterling JE: Prostate-specific antigen, digital rectal examination, and transrectal ultrasonography: their role in diagnosing early prostate cancer, *Mayo Clin Proc* 68:297-306, 1993.

Dalence CR et al: Amniotic fluid lamellar body count: a rapid and reliable fetal lung maturity test, *Obstet Gynecol* 86(2):235-239, 1995.

De Veciana M et al: Postprandial versus preprandial blood glucose monitoring in women with gestational diabetes mellitus requiring insulin therapy, *N Engl J Med* 333(19):1237-1241, 1995.

Frank AP et al: Anonymous HIV testing using home collection and telemedicine counseling, *Arch intern Med* 157(3):309-313, 1997.

Gawlikowski J: White cells at war, *Am J Nurs* 92(3):44-51, 1992.

Gregor CL: Antepartum fetal assessment techniques: an update for today's perinatal nurse, *J Perinatal Neonatal Nurs* 5(4):1-15, 1992.

Greenberg LR, Moore TR, Murphy H: Gestational diabetes mellitus: antenatal variables as predictors of postpartum glucose intolerance, *Gest Diabetes* 86(1):97-101, 1995.

Halfman-Francy M: Recognition and management of bleeding following cardiac surgery, *Crit Care Nurs Clin North Am* 3(4):675-689, 1991.

Hancock RD: Venipuncture vs. arterial catheter-activated partial thromboplastin times in heparinized patients, *DCCN* 12(5):238-245, 1993.

Henry JB: *Clinical diagnosis and laboratory management by laboratory methods,* ed 18, Philadelphia, 1991, WB Saunders.

Isselbacher KJ et al, editors: *Harrison's principles of internal medicine,* ed 13, New York, 1994, McGraw-Hill.

Kee JL, Hayes ER: Assessment of patient laboratory data in the acutely ill, *Nurs Clin North Am* 25(4):751-759, 1990.

Kikuchi S et al: Serum anti-*Helicobacter pylori* antibody and gastric carcinoma among young adults, *Cancer* 75(12):2789-2792, 1995.

Koepke JA, editor: *Practical laboratory hematology,* New York, 1991, Churchill Livingstone.

Kuhlman JE: Oral and IV contrast-enhanced abdominal CT, *Appl Radiol* 21(10):20-21, 1992.

Kvols LK et al: Evaluation of a radiolabeled somatostatin analog (1-123 octreotide) in the detection and localization of carcinoid and islet cell tumors, *Radiology* 187 (1), 129-133, 1993.

Lancaster LE: Immunogenetic basis of tissue and organ transplantation and rejection, *Crit Care Nurs Clin North Am* 4(1):1-24, 1992.

Lavin J: Anergy testing—a vital weapon, *RN* 56(9):31-33, 1993.

Lee GR et al, editors: *Wintrobe's clinical hematology,* ed 9, Philadelphia, 1993, Lea & Febiger.

Leitch AM et al: American Cancer Society guidelines for the early detection of breast cancer: update 1997, *Cancer* 47(3):150-153, 1997.

Lensing AW et al: A comparison of compression ultrasound with color Doppler ultrasound for diagnosis of symptomless postoperative deep vein thrombosis, *Arch Intern Med* 157(7):758-762, 1997.

Littrup PJ, Goodman AC, Mettlin CJ: The benefit and cost of prostate cancer early detection, *CA Cancer J Clin* 43(3):134-149, 1993.

Lowry WS: Tumor suppressor genes and risk of metastasis in ovarian cancer, *Br Med J* 307(6903):542, 1993.

McClatchey KD, editor: *Clinical laboratory medicine,* Baltimore, 1994, Williams & Wilkins.

Melillo KD: Interpretation of laboratory values in older adults, *Nurse Pract* 18(7):59-67, 1993.

Merva J: A closer look at the heart SAECG, *RN* 56(5):50-53, 1993.

Mettler FA et al: Benefits versus risks from mammography, *Cancer* 77(5):903-908, 1996.

Miller KE: Sexually transmitted diseases, *Primary Care* 24(1):179-193, 1997.

Moore S: Screening for prostate cancer: PSA blood test, rectal examination, and ultrasounds, *Urol Nurs* 12(3):106-107, 1992.

Norris MKG: Assessing fibrin-split products, *Nursing* 22(6):29, 1992.

Pagana KD, Pagana TJ: Mosby's manual of diagnostic and laboratory tests, St Louis, 1998, Mosby.

Rao JK et al: The role of antineutrophil cytoplasmic antibody (c-ANCA) testing in the diagnosis of Wegener granulomatosis, *Ann Intern Med* 123(12):925-932, 1995.

Resnick ML, Rifkin MD, editors: *Ultrasonography of the urinary tract,* ed 3, Baltimore, 1991, Williams & Wilkins.

Robie BH: Cardiovascular technology: noninvasive diagnosis of cardiovascular disease using ultrasound imaging, *J Cardiovasc Nurs* 6(2): 36-42, 1992.

Schwartz SL et al, editors: *Principles of surgery,* ed 6, New York, 1994, McGraw-Hill.

Sistrom C: Liver CT for cancer staging, *Appl Radiol* 21(6):19-24, 1992.

Spiro HM: *Clinical gastroenterology,* ed 4, New York, 1993, McGraw-Hill.

Taillefer R et al: Technetium-99m Sestamibi prone scintimammography to detect primary breast cancer and axillary lymph node involvement, *J Nuclear Med* 36(10):1758-1765, 1995.

Tanagho EA, McAninch JW, editors: *Smith's general urology,* ed 13, Norwalk, Conn, 1992, Appleton & Lange.

Taylor A, Datz FL, editors: *Clinical application of nuclear medicine,* New York, 1991, Churchill Livingstone.

Thompson EJ: Transesophageal echocardiography: a new window on the heart and great vessels, *Crit Care Nurse* 13(10):55-56, 1993.

Thompson S: Ultrasonography: intraoperative diagnosis of choledocholithiasis, *AORN J* 51(4):983-985, 1990.

Tonin P et al: Frequency of recurrent BRCA 1 and BRCA 2 mutations in Ashkenazi Jewish breast cancer families, *Nature Med* 2(11):1179-1183, 1996.

Wozniak-Petrofsky J: Prostate-specific antigen in prostate cancer, *J Urol Nurs* 12(3):104-105, 1992.

Wozniak-Petrofsky J: Basics of urodynamics, *J Urol Nurs* 12(2):434-463, 1993.

Young DS: *Effects of drugs on clinical laboratory tests,* ed 3, Washington, DC, 1990, AACS Press.

Zoloth SR: Anergy compromise screening for tuberculosis in high-risk populations, *Am J Public Health* 83(5):749-751, 1993.

Index

Page numbers designated *i* refer
to illustrations; those designated
t refer to tables.

Beta Hydroxybutylate < .4

Beta Hydroxybutarate. less than .4

	HSV-2	Herpes simplex virus, type 2
	HTLV	Human T-cell lymphotrophic virus
I	Ig	Immunoglobulin
	INR	International normalization ratio
	IV-GTT	Intravenous glucose tolerance test
	IVP	Intravenous pyelography
	IVU, IUG	Intravenous urography
K	K	Potassium
	KS	Ketosteroid
	KUB	Kidney, ureter, and bladder x-ray study
L	LAP	Leucine aminopeptidase
	LATS	Long-acting thyroid stimulator
	LDH	Lactic dehydrogenase
	LDL	Low-density lipoprotein
	LE	Lupus erythematosus
	LFTs	Liver function tests
	LH	Luteinizing hormone
	LP	Lumbar puncture
	L/S ratio	Lecithin/sphingomyelin ratio
	LS spine	Lumbosacral spine
M	MCH	Mean corpuscular hemoglobin
	MCHC	Mean corpuscular hemoglobin concentration
	MCV	Mean corpuscular volume
	Mg	Magnesium
	MRI	Magnetic resonance imaging
	MUGA	Multigated acquisition cardiac scan
N	Na	Sodium
	NMR	Nuclear magnetic resonance
	NST	Nonstress test
O	O&P	Ova and parasites
	OB	Occult blood
	OCT	Oxytocin challenge test
	OGTT	Oral glucose tolerance test
	17-OHCS	17-Hydroxycorticosteroids
	OPG	Oculoplethysmography
P	P	Phosphorus
	PAP	Prostatic acid phosphatase
	Pb	Lead
	P_{CO_2}	Partial pressure of carbon dioxide
	PET	Positron emission tomography
	PFTs	Pulmonary function tests
	pH	Hydrogen ion concentration
	PKU	Phenylketonuria
	PMN	Polymorphonuclear
	PNH	Paroxysmal nocturnal hemoglobinuria
	P_{O_2}	Partial pressure of oxygen
	P_{O_4}	Phosphate
	PPBS	Postprandial blood sugar